Eyelid Surgery

Principles and Techniques

Eyelid Surgery

Principles and Techniques

Clinton D. McCord, Jr., M.D.
Director, Southeastern Oculoplastic Center,
Atlanta, Georgia

Associate Author
Mark A. Codner, M.D.
Paces Plastic Surgery and Recovery Center,
Atlanta, Georgia

With Special Contributions by
T. Roderick Hester, Jr., M.D.
Director, Paces Plastic Surgery and Recovery Center,
Atlanta, Georgia

Lippincott - Raven
PUBLISHERS
Philadelphia • New York

Lippincott-Raven Publishers, 227 East Washington Square, Philadelphia, PA 19106-3780

Made in the United States of America

Library of Congress Cataloging in Publication Data

McCord, Clinton D.
Eyelid surgery : principles and techniques / Clinton D. McCord, Jr., Mark A. Codner, T. Roderick Hester, Jr.
p. cm.
Includes bibliographical references and index.
ISBN 0-7817-0293-3 (alk. paper)
1. Eyelids—Surgery. I. Codner, Mark A. II. Hester, T. Roderick. III. Title.
[DNLM: 1. Eyelids—surgery. WW 205 M478e 1995]
RE121.M37 1995
617.7′71059—dc20
DNLM/DLC
for Library of Congress 95-12660
CIP

The material contained in this volume was submitted as previously unpublished material, except in the instances in which some of the illustrative material was derived.

Great care has been taken to maintain the accuracy of the information contained in the volume. However, neither Lippincott-Raven nor the editors can be held responsible for errors or for any consequences arising from the use of the information contained herein.

9 8 7 6 5 4 3 2 1

To my lovely wife and daughters,
Cissy, Hollis, and Marty

Contents

Preface

This book contains detailed descriptions and illustrations of the eyelid surgical procedures that are used most frequently by the authors. Many of the procedures described are "time honored" but have been modified. Some techniques described in the text are new and, although routinely used for a period of time, have not been previously published. Discussions of surgical techniques are supplemented with discussions of the evaluation and management of the problem for which the surgery is intended. Management of problems arising from surgery is also discussed.

The book has been written primarily from the oculoplastic surgeon's (C.D.McC.) point of view. The contributing authors (M.A.C. and T.R.H.) have introduced the viewpoint of the plastic surgeon.

Because of the inclusion of introductory chapters on anatomy and basic surgical techniques, detailed discussions of problem evaluation and management, and the presentation of a broad scope of surgical procedures, the text addresses the interests of both the entry-level and the experienced surgeon.

Eyelid Surgery

Principles and Techniques

CHAPTER 1

Eyelid Anatomy

EYELIDS

Eyelids are the protective covering of the eye, consisting of an anterior lamella of skin and orbicularis muscle and a posterior lamella of tarsus and conjunctiva. Eyelid surgery requires a thorough knowledge of the structural anatomy, innervation, vascularity, and function of the eylids, all of which will be covered in this chapter.

Superficial Eyelid Anatomy

The topographic anatomy of the eyelids and facial area is shown in Fig. 1. The *palpebral fissure* is the opening between the eyelid margins; the standard opening is 28–30 mm horizontally and 9–10 mm vertically when the lids are open. The upper eyelid rests at the upper limbus in the young and about 1.5–2 mm below in the adult. The lower eyelid is generally found positioned at the lower limbus. The highest point of the curved upper eyelid is slightly nasal to the pupil. The lowest point of the lower eyelid is slightly temporal. The *commissures* are the junction points where the upper and lower eyelids meet medially and laterally, whereas the *medial* and *lateral canthi* are the angles formed by the eyelids at these commissures. The lateral commissure rests on the globe, whereas the medial commissure is separated from the globe by the caruncle and plica semilumaris (1).

The *upper eyelid crease* is formed by the insertion of levator fibers in the pretarasal skin. In patients undergoing blepharoplasty or levator surgery, the lid crease must be reformed by attachment of the eyelid skin and pretarsal orbicularis muscle to the levator aponeurosis or superior tarsal margin. The eyelid crease in Asians is only several millimeters from the eyelid margin because the superior orbital septum inserts on the levator aponeurosis at this low level, thus preventing the higher cutaneous insertion seen in Occidentals in whom the crease forms at 9–10 mm above the lashes in adults and 5–7 mm in children. The *pretarsal space* is the area of skin above the eyelashes in which the skin and muscle is firmly attached to the underlying tarsal plate and is normally not folded or wrinkled. It is visible in varying degrees depending on the amount of overhanging *upper lid fold,* which is the loose skin above the upper lid crease. Restoration of the pretarsal space visibility is the goal of upper lid blepharoplasty and maintaining the integrity of the pretarsal space is important in ptosis surgery (see Chapter 26). Another excessive skin fold in the upper lid is an epicanthal fold, which is present if the inner canthus is obscured by an extension of an upper lid fold.

The *orbital sulcus* is the usually concave area between the upper eyelid crease and the superior orbital margin. A sulcus may not be present with relaxation of the upper septum and outward folding of skin. Focal bulgings or convexities into the superior sulcus, especially medially, denote herniating orbital fat. With orbital volume loss seen in aging or after enucleation, the superior sulcus skin and muscle can become more concave because of lack of support of orbital tissue.

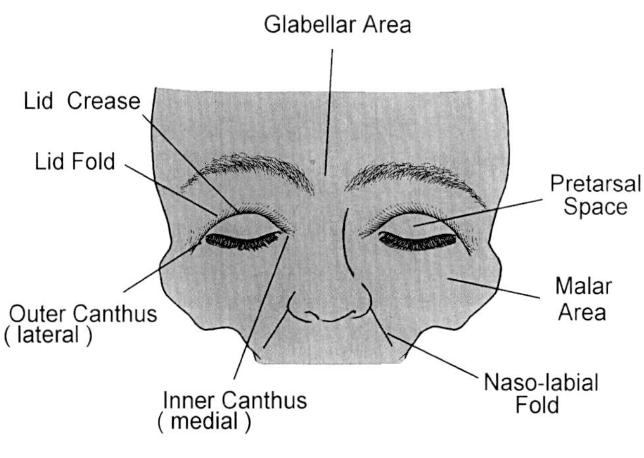

The *lower eyelid crease* is less well defined as can be seen in where the retractors superficially insert. The lower eyelid crease begins medially 4–5 mm from the eyelid margin and slopes slightly as it moves temporally. In the *malar area,* a less well-defined *malar crease* can be seen representing the junction between the orbicularis muscle and the malar fat, and the thin skin of the eyelid and the thicker skin of the cheek. The *nasolabial fold* marks the inferior border of the malar fat pad. A dense fibrous layer, the *submuscular aponeurotic system* (SMAS), anchors the nasolabial fold to the maxilla.

Skin wrinkles result from the interaction of contracting facial muscles and the overlying skin. The horizontal forehead furrows reflect attempts of the frontalis muscle to compensate for eyelid ptosis, dermatochalasis, and eyebrow ptosis. A horizontal fold across the *glabella area* indicates procerus contraction causing depression of the medial eyebrows. The vertical fold through the medial eyebrow represents corrugator action. The clinical importance of using these lines for planning surgical incisions is discussed in Chapter 2.

SKIN–MUSCLE–CONNECTIVE TISSUE

Skin

The skin of the eyelids is quite thin, and that of the medial upper eyelid is the thinnest in the body. Transition to the thick skin of the eyebrow above and to the malar region below is rather abrupt. Edema fluid and hemoglobin pigment from bruising will rapidly engorge the loose subcutaneous eyelid tissues with a specific border identifiable at junctures with the surrounding cheek area, which has thicker skin and denser subcutaneous fibroadipose tissue.

Tarsal Plates

The *tarsal plates* are dense, fibrous tissues that form the skeleton of the eyelids. They are about 25 mm in length, 1 mm in thickness, and 10 and 4 mm in height vertically in the upper and lower eyelids, respectively. A maximal height of about 10 mm is measured centrally in the upper eyelid. Most accounts cite a vertical height of 5 mm for the lower tarsus (1). However, one study measured the vertical height of the lower eyelid tarsus of 20 patients submitting to lower eyelid resections and the lower tarsus of 17 cadavers and the tarsal height was found to be 3.7 and 3.9 mm, respectively (2). The lower tarsus should be clearly identified in procedures involving eyelid repair or eyelid reconstruction so that tension bearing sutures can be placed through the tarsus. Medially and laterally the tarsal plates have fibrous connections to the orbital rims, traditionally termed "canthal ligaments." The principal attachments of the eyelids are formed by insertions of orbicularis muscles, which form a large portion of the "canthal tendons." Orbicularis muscle is densely fixed to the entire anterior surface of the tarsal plate of the upper and lower lid. Posteriorly, the tarsal plates are lined by a tightly adherent conjunctiva that continues on the eyelid margin to the mucocutaneous junction. In youth, the tarsal plates and canthal tendons hold the eyelids firmly against the eye. With aging the tendons and the tarsus itself may stretch, allowing the eyelids to mechanically be distracted from the globe by several millimeters.

Orbicularis Muscle

The *orbicularis oculi muscle* is subcutaneous and serves as the closure muscle (protractor) of the eyelids. It extends over the eylids and into the forehead, temple, and cheeks. The muscle is divided into an orbital and preseptal and pretarsal parts (Fig. 2) (3).

Medial Canthus

Medially the pretarsal orbicularis forms two heads that pass superficial and deep to the canaliculi (Fig. 3). The anterior (superficial) pretarsal orbicularis muscle forms the anterior crus of the medial canthal tendon that inserts into the frontal process of the maxillary bone. The posterior (deep) pretarsal orbicularis inserts into the posterior lacrimal crest (Horner's muscle). The muscle fibers arising closest to the palpebral margin send fibers the most deeply. The deep pretarsal heads insert on the posterior lacrimal crest and the lacrimal fascia, whereas the deep preseptal fibers insert chiefly

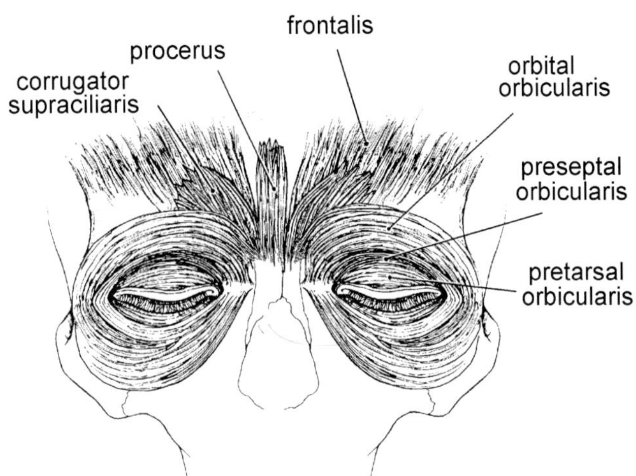

FIG. 2. Eyelid and facial muscles including orbicularis eyelid protractors, corrugator supraciliaris, and procerus brow depressors and frontalis muscle, brow elevator.

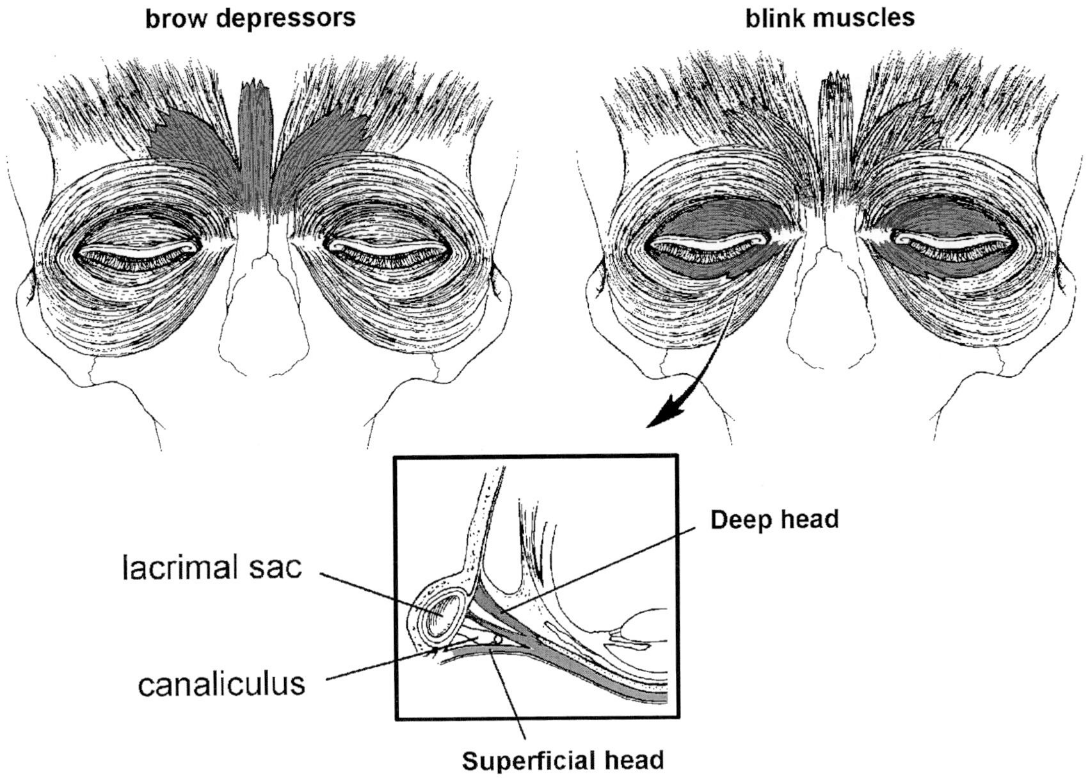

FIG. 3. Shaded muscles show the muscles most commonly used in certain eyebrow and eyelid actions. The interdigitation of the orbital orbicularis and corrugator muscles act in unison for brow depression. The canthal pretarsal orbicularis muscle fibers appear to have the greatest activity with simple blinking. The bulk of orbicularis fibers are recruited only in the act of forcible eyelid contracture. The posterior extensions of the preseptal and pretarsal fibers are shown in inset.

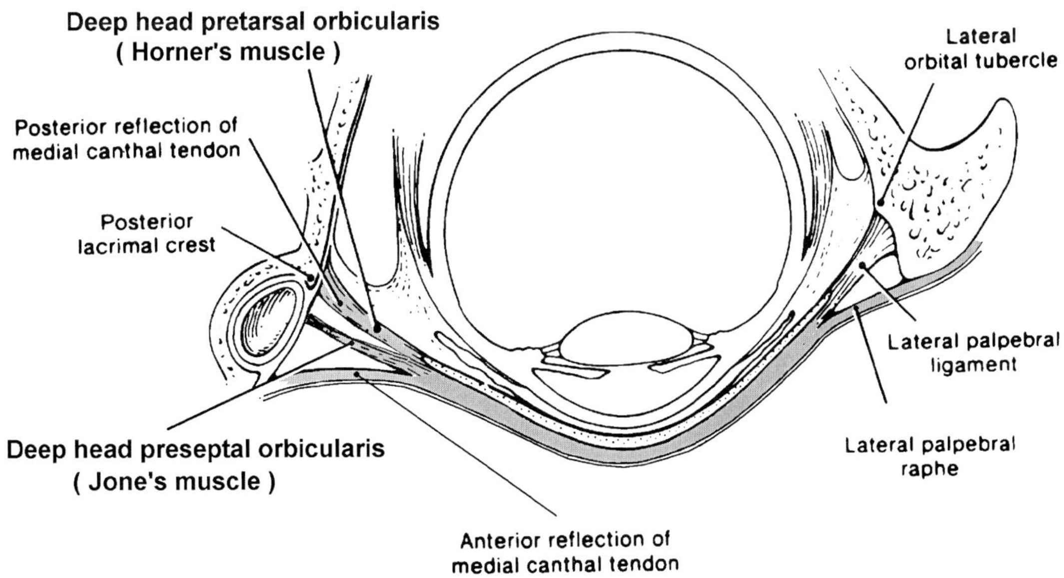

FIG. 4. Axial view of the medial and lateral canthal eyelid attachments. The preseptal and pretarsal orbicularis fibers send deep heads to insert on the lacrimal diaphragm and the posterior reflection of the medial canthal tendon. Laterally, there is also a deep and superficial insertion of fibers.

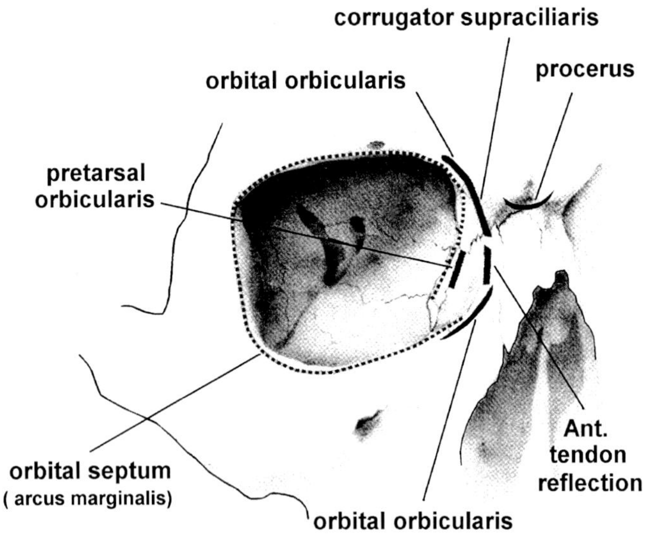

FIG. 5. Site of bony attachment of facial and eyelid muscles and orbital septum. Note that the orbital septum attachment is not continuous around the orbit and there is a separation in the lacrimal sac area. The superior septum inserts posterior to the lacrimal sac and posterior reflection of the canthal muscles (tendon).

on the lacrimal fascia (Jones' muscle). The preseptal muscle forms the horizontal raphe laterally and also medially inserts into the anterior crus of the medial canthal tendon (Fig. 4). The posterior placement of the medial deep pretarsal muscles (Horner's muscle) at the insertion along the lacrimal fascia and posterior lacrimal crest provides a posterior anchor allowing the eyelids to follow and cover the convex globe. The orbital orbicularis, in addition to attaching to the medial canthal tendon, attaches to the nasal part of the frontal bone and along the inferiomedial orbital margin (Figs. 5 and 6) (4,5). Laterally, the orbital portion of the orbicularis completes an ellipse around the orbit without interruption at the lateral canthus. The space between the superficial and deep, lateral heads of the preseptal and pretarsal orbicularis may be filled with fat. Anderson described a superior supporting branch of the anterior medial canthal tendon that inserts into the periosteum of the frontal bone, which may be found with some consistancy (6). Contraction of the muscle draws the eyelids (especially the lower) medially and posteriorly. The resulting lateral pull on the lacrimal diaphragm creates a negative pressure in the lacrimal sac that draws the tears from the canaliculi. The lacrimal ampullae are encased in pretarsal muscle at the medial edge of the tarsal plates and are compressed with muscle shortening; the fluid contained within the ampulla is pushed toward the sac. The pretarsal and preseptal muscles and their contractions that create this effect are called the "lacrimal pump" by Jones (Fig. 7) (7,8). Weakening of the eyelid muscles can cause epiphora through loss of an effective lacrimal pump, despite a normally positioned punctum and eyelid.

A small strip of pretarsal orbicularis at the lid margin is referred to as Riolan's muscle and forms the "gray line" of the lid margin. The pretarsal orbicularis is tightly adherent to the tarsus and can be separated only by sharp dissection. The preseptal and orbital components are less adherent except where attached to bone (the lateral palpebral raphe, the supraorbital ridge, the nasoorbital groove) and the malar crease. Mild, unforced orbicularis contraction (blinking) results in eyelid closure primarily through pretarsal orbicularis contracture (Fig. 3) (8). Increasingly greater forced eyelid closure recruits more orbicularis fibers and, with increasing contracture, overriding of preseptal and or-

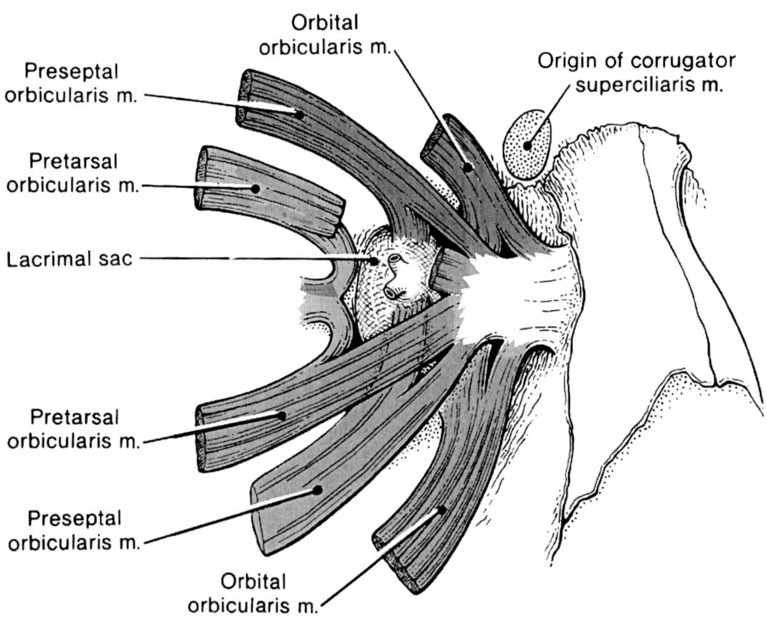

FIG. 6. Diagrammatic representation of the insertion of the preseptal and pretarsal orbicularis. The preseptal orbicularis sends a reflection to the lacrimal sac diaphragm that contracts during a blink and adds to the pumping mechanism of the eyelid (Jones' muscle). Extensions of the pretarsal orbicularis posterior to the sac compose the posterior reflection (Horner's muscle) and accompany the posterior medial canthal tendon.

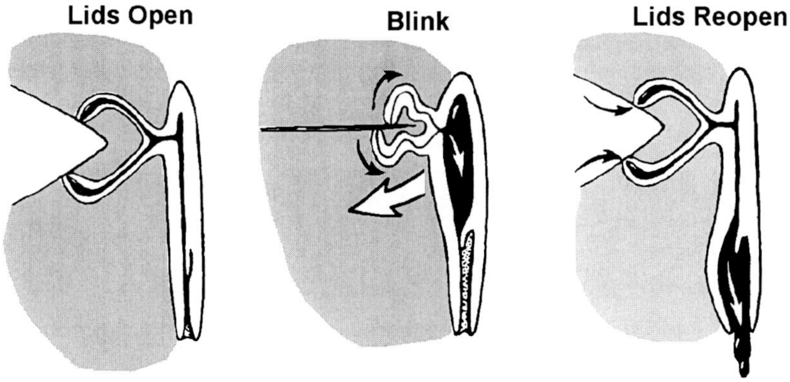

FIG. 7. Diagrammatic representation of the action of the canaliculi and tear sac during a blink. With closure, a negative pressure is created in the tear sac from contracture of the preseptal fibers of orbicularis and the fluid that had been present in the canaliculus squirts into the lacrimal sac. On opening the lid the lacrimal sac negative pressure subsides and is transferred to the ampulla so that tears are drained into the ampulla for the next cycle.

bital orbicularis components. The deep insertions of the pretarsal orbicularis muscle within the orbital rim allow a posterior pull on the eyelids to maintain their apposition to the globe (9–11).

The *medial retinaculum* is located in the periorbita just behind the posterior lacrimal crest. It is formed by the deep head of pretarsal orbicularis, the orbital septum, the medial end of Lockwood's ligament, the medial horn of the levator aponeurosis, check ligaments of the medial rectus muscle, and Whitnall's ligament.

Lateral Canthus

The pretarsal muscle is attached laterally to the lateral orbital tubercle by the *lateral canthal tendon* and lateral palpebral ligament, which is a band of connective tissue attached to the tarsi. At the lateral canthus, the preseptal and orbital orbicularis fibers pass uninterrupted along the orbital rim where the superficial muscle attaches to the zygoma along a horizontal lateral palpebral raphe. Fibrous strands continuous with the tarsus attach to the lateral orbital tubercle behind the deep pretarsal orbicularis fibers. The fibrous (ligament) component of the lateral attachment was in the past generally not felt to be substantial as compared to the pretarsal muscular component. There has been controversy in this area (Fig. 4).

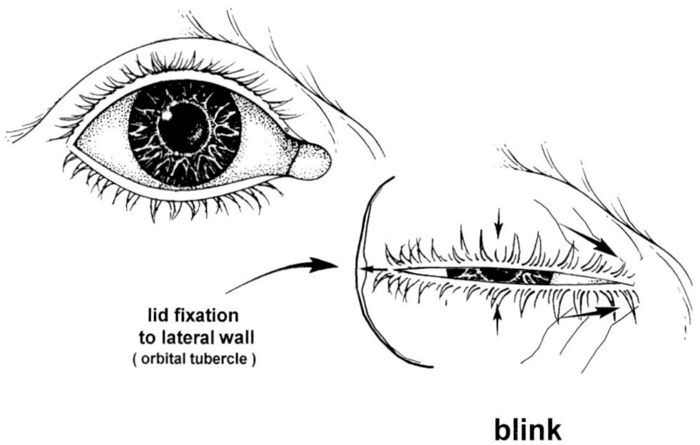

FIG. 8. Diagrammatic representation of lid movement during a blink. The diagram emphasizes that the eyelid movement occurs in the manner of a bow string contracture of the inner canthal muscles against the relatively fixed lateral canthal rim, pulling the upper lid downward and, to a lesser degree, the lower lid upward. Impairment of either lateral fixation or weakness of the canthal muscles will impair lid closure.

The *lateral retinaculum* is formed by the lateral horn of the levator aponeurosis, lateral canthal tendon, inferior suspensory (Lockwood's) ligament, Whitnall's ligament (via the intralacrimal gland fibrous septae), and check ligaments of the lateral rectus muscle. The lateral retinaculum inserts into the lateral orbital tubercle.

A lax lower eyelid can result in epiphora because of tear pump failure; with advanced laxity, frank ectropion occurs. The laxity rarely reflects elongation of the tarsus. It is more commonly laxity of either the lateral or medial canthal tendons, or a combination of the two structures. The lateral canthal tendon is most commonly implicated in cases of lower eyelid laxity.

Gioia et al. further clarified the anatomy of the fibrous component of lateral canthal ligament (LCT) and the findings are worth describing (12). In their dissections, the LCT arose as a fibrous attachment from the lateral ends of the tarsal plates and was identifiable as a broad band of connective tissue that ran from the lateral end of the tarsal plate to the lateral orbital tubercle. Laterally, the LCT was seen to pass deep to the septum and inserted 1.5 mm posterior to the orbital rim. Superiorly, the LCT was contiguous with the lateral horn of the levator aponeurosis. The inferior edge of the LCT curved downward near its insertion on the rim. The posterior aspect of the LCT was contiguous with the check ligament of the lateral rectus muscle (Fig. 9). Pretarsal orbicularis fibers were seen to pass posterior to the orbital septum and intermingle with the connective tissue of the LCT. Immediately anterior to the LCT was found a pocket of adipose tissue (Eisler's pocket, previously described). The check ligament of the lateral rectus muscle was seen posterior to the LCT at its insertion to the orbital tubercle and

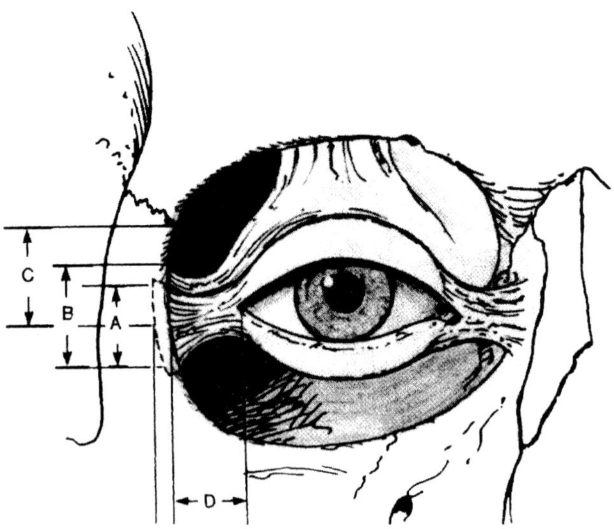

FIG. 9. Lateral canthal tendon (after Gioia et al., 12). This diagram shows the measurements made in cadaver dissections of the dimensions of the lateral canthal tendon. **A:** Vertical width of tendon approximately 6.6 mm. **B:** Vertical width of tendon and contiguous lateral horn of the levator aponeurosis approximately 10.2 mm. **C:** Distance from the frontozygomatic suture to the midpoint of the tendon, approximately 9.7 mm. **D:** Length of the lateral canthal tendon measured from the canthal angle to its insertion 10.6 mm.

some fibers of the LCT were seen to run posteriorly in the direction of the check ligament. These findings suggest that the attachment of the lateral canthal angle to the orbital rim is a combined tendon–ligament that connects the pretarsal orbicularis and the tarsal plates to the lateral orbital tubercle (Fig. 10).

The observation of fibrous connections between the LCT and the check ligament of the lateral rectus muscle also suggested a functional relationship between the two. In the study (12), a consistent lateral displacement of the canthal angle during lateral gaze was observed with an average of 2 mm displacement with extreme abduction of the globe. These findings suggest that the LCT not only provides structural fixation of the lids to the lateral canthus but imparts mobility to the canthal angle by its posterior fibrous attachments to the check ligament of the lateral rectus muscle.

Reconstructive surgery of the lateral canthus is frequently required for trauma, tumor resection, and correction of eyelid malpositions. Surgical techniques that provide fixation of the lateral canthus to the inner aspect of the orbital rim will reproduce normal positioning and pull of the lids against the globe. Attachment of the lid to the edge or anterior surface of the orbital rim should be avoided because it will pull the lids away from the globe.

Orbital Septum

Immediately beneath the orbicularis muscle is the orbital septum (septum orbitale), which is a fibrous sheath. It attaches to the edge of the orbital rim at the *arcus marginalis* and at that point is a thickening of the periosteum (Figs. 5 and 11). The orbital septum forms the anterior barrier of the orbital contents, confining the orbital fat. Medially, it inserts at the posterior lacrimal crest and is posterior to Horner's muscle. It then crosses the midlacrimal fossa and adheres to the lacrimal fascia as far as the anterior lacrimal crest. At the lateral canthus the orbital septum is also bilayered; the septum posterior to the superficial orbicularis joins at the lateral canthal tendon and a sheath of septum posterior to the deep orbicularis muscle inserts at the lateral orbital tubercle behind the muscle. In the eyelid proper, the septum inserts on the inferior tarsus after joining with the lower eyelid retractors 4–5 mm below this structure. The superior orbital septum usually in-

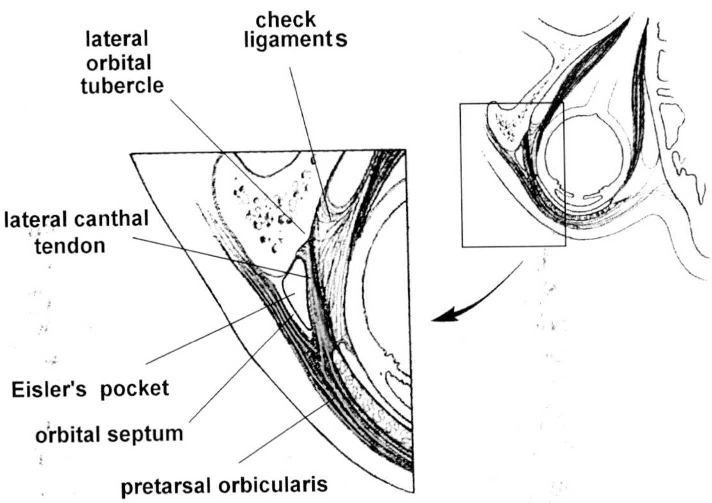

FIG. 10. Axial view of the lateral orbit (after Gioia et al., 12). Shows the insertion of the lateral canthal tendon and the fatty tissue in the space in front of the tendon known as Eisler's pocket. Insertions of check ligaments of the lateral rectus muscle and horns of the levator aponeurosis at the lateral retinaculum are shown.

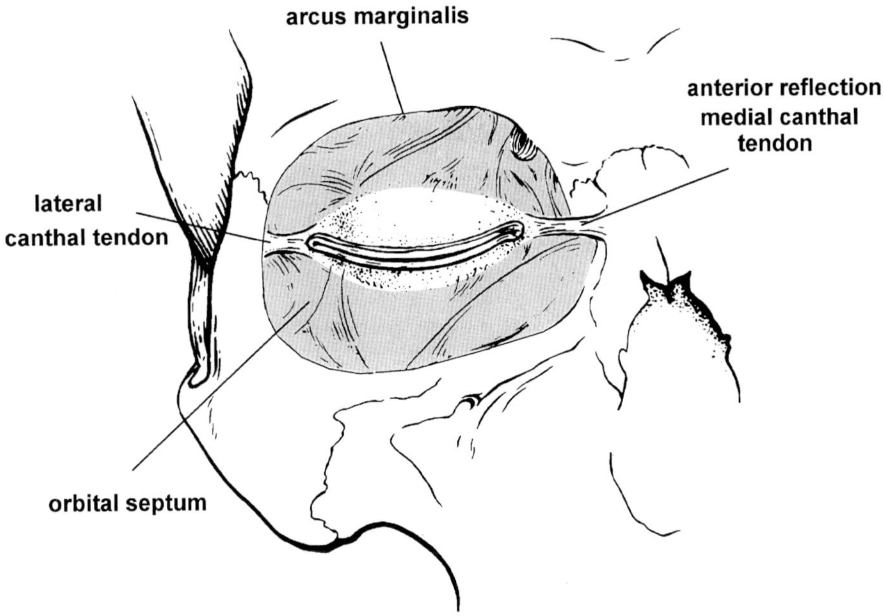

FIG. 11. Diagrammatic representation of the orbital septum following removal of orbicularis fibers showing its position and attachments.

serts on the levator aponeurosis about 10 mm above the superior eyelid margin superior to the tarsal plate (13–15). Immediately posterior to the septum is orbital fat. Nasally, the orbital septum is thinnest. Septum strength may attenuate with age, allowing orbital fat to herniate forward.

There are ethnic differences in septal anatomy. In Caucasians the orbital septum, as previously described, inserts above the superior border of the tarsus into the levator aponeurosis. In Asians the orbital septum inserts more inferiorly on the levator aponeurosis over the tarsus, allowing the anterior orbital fat to extend to the anterior tarsal space. In Asians the inferior extension of the orbital fat prevents the levator aponeurosis fibers from fanning out to the subcutaneous tissue to form the eyelid crease (16,17).

Preseptal (Retro-orbicularis) Eyelid Fat

A submuscular fatty layer is present in the eyebrow area and commonly extends downward onto the eyelid in the preseptal or retroorbicularis space (Figs. 12–14).

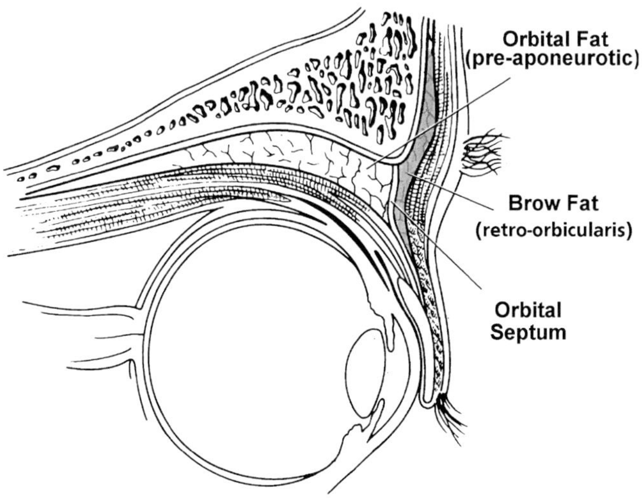

FIG. 12. The brow fat, originating in the submuscular plane, is shown in its location in the brow area and its extension into the preseptal area on the eyelid (Weiss, 18).

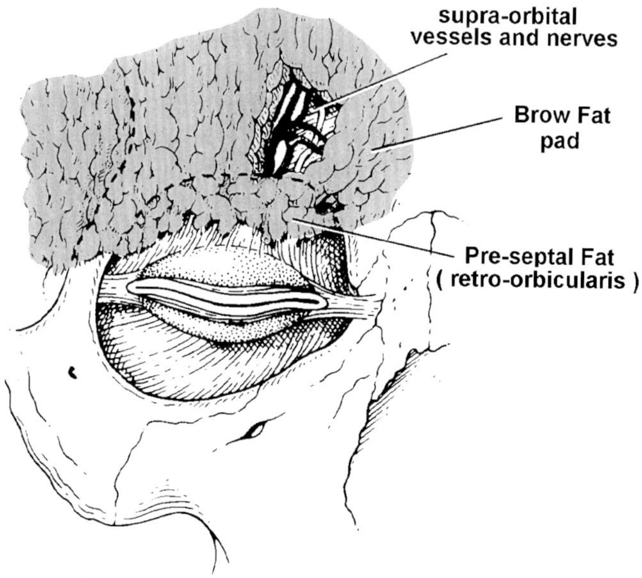

FIG. 13. Frontal view of the brow fat pad (after Weiss, 18). It extends varying degrees from the brow area down into the eyelid in the preseptal or retro-orbicularis plane.

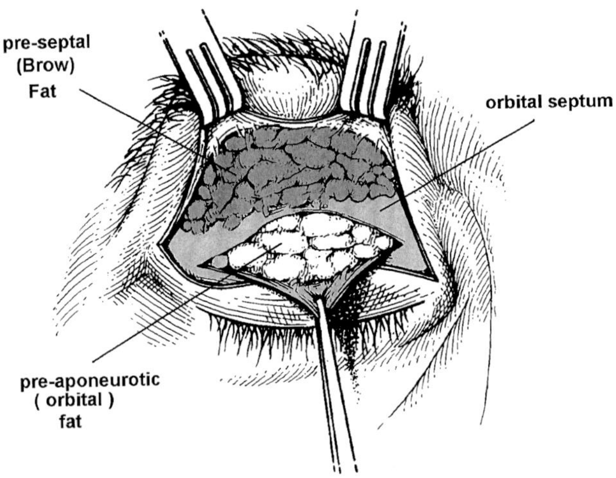

FIG. 14. View showing the brow fat (preseptal or retro-orbicularis fat) extending on the surface of the orbital septum (after Weiss, 18). The orbital septum has been opened and the preaponeurotic fat (orbital fat) can be seen. These two layers of fat in the upper lid are commonly seen in patients undergoing blepharoplasty or ptosis surgery.

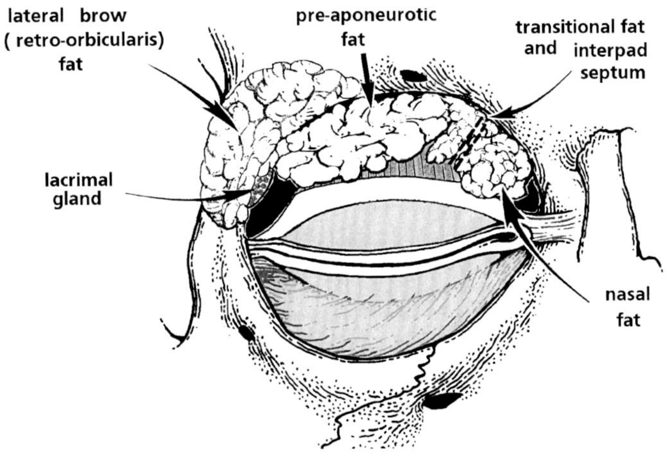

FIG. 16. Fat compartments (or location of fat) in the upper lid and brow area. In the past two fat pads in the upper lid have been described in the postseptal area: the nasal fat pad and the preaponeurotic fat pad. Commonly there is a grouping of fat in the zone between the preaproneurotic fat and nasal fat around a vertically oriented fibrous structure (interpad septum) that trails back to the area of the superior oblique tendon. The superior ophthalmic vein is also commonly seen in this area. The lateral brow fat occurs on the surface of the bony brow and extends in the preseptal plain onto the lid in many cases.

Its removal may be considered an integral part of blepharoplasty and is further discussed in Chapter 14 (18–20).

Postseptal Eyelid Fat Compartments

The anterior extension of the extraconal orbital fat lies immediately posterior to the orbital septum (Figs. 14 and 15). In the upper lid there are generally considered to be two fat pockets. The preaponeurotic fat pad is more yellow and is bordered posteriorly by the levator aponeurosis, medially by the trochlea, and temporally by the orbital lobe of the lacrimal gland. The nasal fat pad, lying beneath the trochlea, is whitish in color as is the nasal fat pad in the lower eyelid. Between the nasal fat pad and the preaponeurotic pad is a distinct accumulation of fat that seems to be separate from the nasal and loosely associated with the preaponeurotic pad—the transitional fat. The trochlear and supraorbital branch of the superior ophthalmic vein lie beneath it (Fig. 13). A strand of fibrous tissue extending vertically from Whitnall's tendon is commonly found—the interpad septum (Fig. 16).

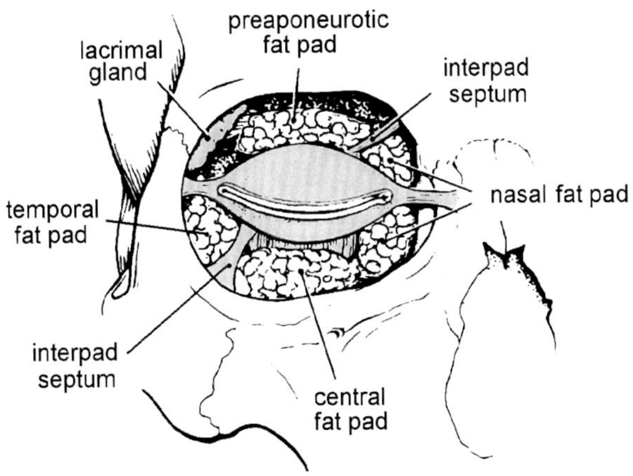

FIG. 15. General location of the fatty pads in the upper and lower lid.

In the lower eyelid there are three fat pads. The nasal fat pad is separated posteriorly from the central fat pad by the inferior oblique muscle. The central and lateral pads are connected in deeper layers but anteriorly are divided into two pads by a dense septal partition (Fig. 17) (1,16).

Eyelid Retractor Muscles

The levator palpebrae superioris and superior tarsal muscle (Müller's muscle) provide elevating movement to the upper eyelid combined with blinking and forced closure. The lower eyelid does not move appreciably in the vertical direction when the eye is looking straight ahead but does move in vertical gaze; the lower lid's movement is primarily horizontal with blinking (10,11). There are extensions to the lower eyelid from the inferior rectus that serve to depress the eyelid several millimeters in downgaze. Despite a difference in size and function, the upper and lower lids exhibit similarities in structure and function (Figs. 18 and 20).

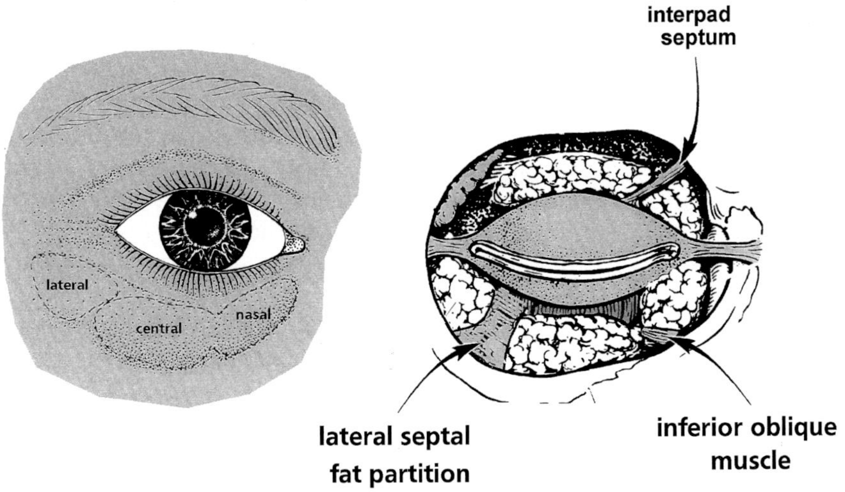

FIG. 17. Lower lid fat compartments. The fatty pads in the lower lid have been arbitrarily designated as lateral, central, and nasal depending on their visible protuberances. Anatomic dissections show that much of the fat is connected and its clinical presentation as discrete pads is influenced by the positioning of fibrous septal fat partitions. This is particularly true with the lateral and the central fat pocket with a discrete lateral septal fat petition being present that is usually retained during surgery. The inferior oblique muscle generally separates the nasal and central fat pocket.

The lifting muscle of the eyelid, *levator palpebrae superioris,* originates from the lesser sphenoid wing above the annulus of Zinn in the orbita apex periorbita. The origin of the levator is lateral to the superior oblique muscle origin and above the superior rectus muscle origin. It is innervated in its inner posterior one third by the superior division of the third nerve after the nerve passes through the superior rectus muscle.

The levator extends anteriorly in the superior orbit with a thin layer of fat, the supraorbital artery, the frontal nerve, and the trochlear nerve separating it from the orbital roof. The levator lies above and rests on the superior rectus. The levator and superior rectus are easily separated, except along their medial borders, where they are attached by a fascial sheath. Both muscles are innervated by the superior division of the oculomotor nerve, which enters the muscles on their undersides, about 12–13 mm from the orbital apex. The nerve to the levator usually passes around the lateral side of the superior rectus but may pass directly through it. The muscle sheath of the levator is thin, similar to the sheaths of the other extraocular muscles except on its medial edge where it joins with the superior rectus. The levator muscle extends anteriorly for 40 mm and becomes tendinous in front of Whitnall's ligament.

Immediately behind the superior orbital rim is a transverse band of fibrous condensation that attaches superiorly to the widening levator, the *superior transverse (Whitnall's) ligament,* which fans out medially and laterally to the orbital retinaculae. Whitnall's ligament is the condensed fascial sheath of the levator muscle approximately 18–20 mm above the superior border of the tarsus. It extends from the fascia of the trochlea and reflected superior oblique tendon to the capsule of the lacrimal gland (Fig. 19). It functions to

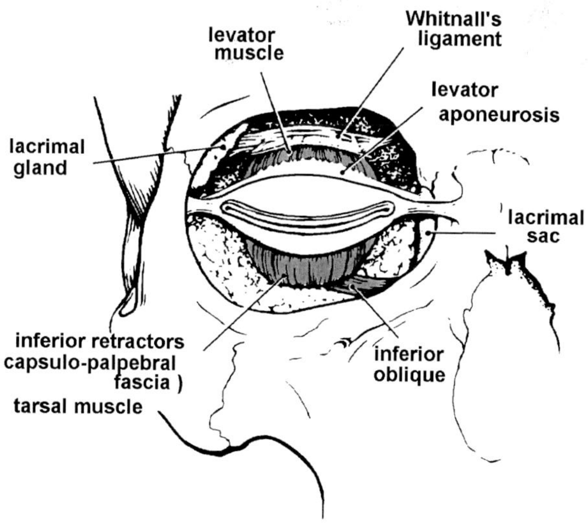

FIG. 18. General view of the retractor muscles and supporting elements in the upper and lower lid.

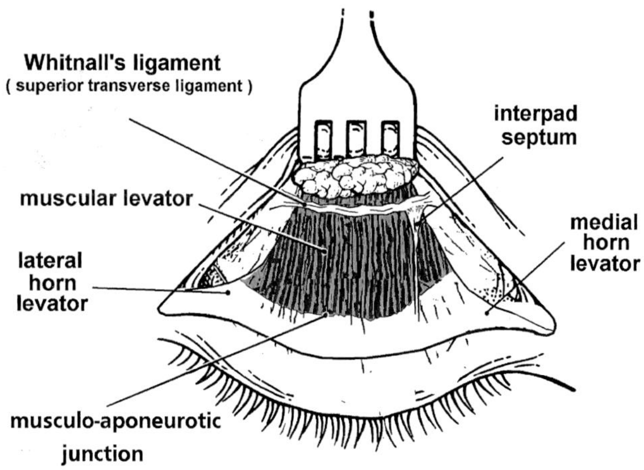

FIG. 19. Upper lid retractor. View showing the levator muscle as seen on a downward stretch. The lateral and medial horns extend to the lateral and medial retinaculum and are conjoined with the check ligaments of the medial and lateral canthal tendon. It is common to see a specific strand extend vertically from the area of Whitnall's ligament to the aponeurosis below nasally.

convert the anterior posterior pulling force of the levator muscle to a superior–inferior direction, which raises and lowers the eyelid (21,22). Whitnall's ligament medially terminates in fascia about the trochlea, in fibrous strands to bone beneath the superior oblique muscle more posteriorly. Laterally, the ligament joins with the capsule of the lacrimal gland and the frontal bone. Whitnall described the function of this structure as a check ligament of the levator because it limited the posterior pull of the muscle in the cadaver and because its location is analogous to the check ligaments of the other extraocular muscles. The importance of the ligament is support for the upper eyelid (23). Larger levator resections are necessary for elevations of the eyelid during ptosis surgery if the ligament is cut. Commonly a vertical strand of fibrous tissue, presumably an extension of Whitnall's ligament, is seen to extend to the aponeurosis in the nasal part of the lid. Severing this strand during ptosis surgery will reduce lagophthalmos in the lid postoperatively. Codere suggested that a sheet-like extension of Whitnall's ligament occurs beneath Müller's muscle and may commonly be seen during levator recession or resection (24).

About 8–10 mm below the point where the superior transverse ligament crosses the levator muscle, a transition in the levator occurs from a fleshy extraocular muscle to a fibrous aponeurotic sheath. Whitnall gives a length of 7 mm of the shealth from the musculoaponeurotic junction to the orbicularis and cutaneous insertions (21). Anteriorly, the levator aponeurosis fuses with the orbital septum above the superior border of the tarsus and sends fibrous strands between the orbisularis oculi muscle septa to the skin forming a supratarsal eyelid crease, 8–10 mm above the margin. The levator aponeurosis inserts an additional 7–8 mm onto the anterior surface of the tarsus (Fig. 20).

In addition to the palpebral insertions, the levator aponeurosis expands into a broad, fibrous sheet to insert into medial and lateral retinaculae behind the medial and lateral canthal tendons. These insertions, termed medial and lateral *"horns" of the levator,* may be severed during levator resection surgery to allow adequate stretchability of the levator muscle during ptosis procedures. The lateral horn is a strong, fibrous band incompletely dividing the lacrimal gland into two lobes and continuing inferiorly to insert on the lateral orbital tubercle behind the lateral canthal tendon. In contrast, the medial horn becomes thin as it passes over the reflected superior oblique tendon to reach its insertion behind the posterior lacrimal crest (25,26).

Müller's Muscle

The sympathetic smooth muscle of the eyelid *(Müller's)* forms at terminal striated muscle fibers of

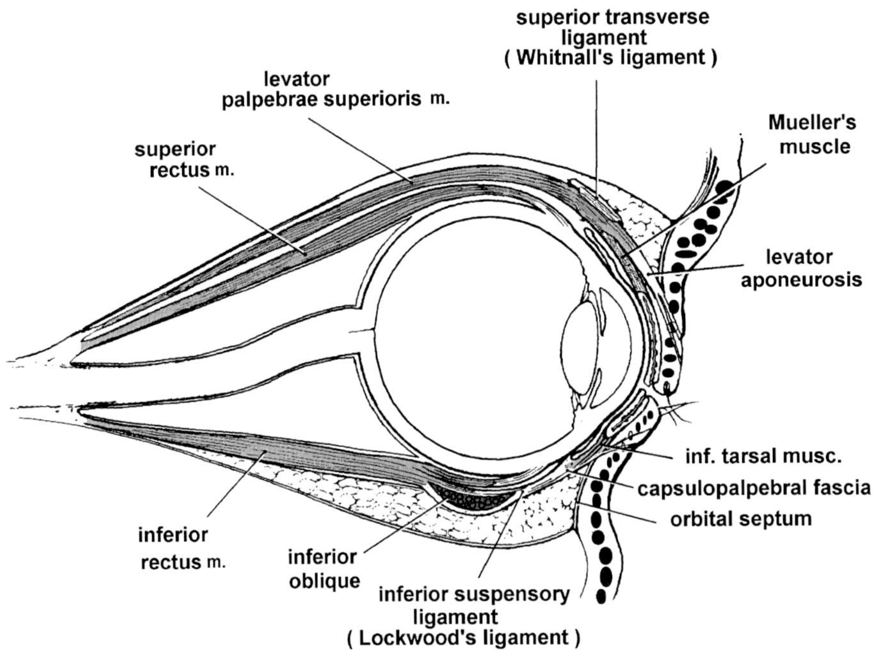

FIG. 20. Sagittal view of the retractor elements in the upper and lower lids with support structures. The lower lid is similar to the upper lid in that there are muscular retractor components attached to the tarsal plate covered by an aponeurotic system that inserts in the skin beneath the lashes. A condensation of connective tissue occurs in the superior orbit that supports the levator aponeurosis, Whitnall's ligament. Correspondingly, in the lower lid there is a condensation of tissue supporting the globe and inferior elements that is the strongest in the area just in front of the inferior oblique and its sheaths, called Lockwood's ligament.

the levator palpebrae superioris. It lies posterior to the aponeurosis, is firmly adherent to the conjunctiva, and is attached to the superior edge of the tarsus. It arises from the underside of the striated levator muscle about 8–10 mm above the superior tarsal border (Fig. 20). It is firmly attached to the levator only at its origin and may easily be separated from the latter below to form the postaponeurotic space. It functions as an additional insertion of the levator protractor muscle. Interruption of sympathetic innervation from the superior cervical ganglion results in 2 mm of blepharoptosis (Horner's syndrome). The exact course of sympathetic nerves to this smooth muscle is unknown. Infiltration and scarring occurs in Müller's muscle with thyroid disease and often it is selectively excised or detached in this condition in association with levator aponeurosis recession (27).

Lower Lid Retractors

The structures of the lower eyelid are analogous to those of the upper eyelid (28). The *capsulopalpebral fascia* (CPF) is analogous to the levator. It is formed by the capsulopalpebral head of the inferior rectus muscle. Shortly past this origin, the first fibers of the inferior tarsal muscle begin. The *capsulopalpebral head* splits around and fuses with the sheath of the inferior oblique muscle. Anterior to the inferior oblique muscle, the two heads fuse to form *Lockwood's ligament* (analogous to Whitnall's in the upper lid). The CPF is anterior to Lockwood's ligament. The superior portion of the CPF sends strands to the inferior fornix and becomes Tenon's fascia, extending onto the globe. The inferior portion of the CPF fuses anteriorly with the orbital septum 5 mm below the inferior tarsal border. Inferior tarsal muscle fibers extend to about 2.5 mm below the inferior tarsal border (Fig. 20). The inferior tarsal muscle, CPF, and orbital septum insert at a fusion point into the anterior and inferior surface and base of the tarsus. Some of the CPF extend through the orbicularis to the eyelid skin and form a lower eyelid crease. This is more evident in the young and is 2–3 mm below the lid margin and 5–6 mm laterally.

BLOOD SUPPLY

Arteries

Both the internal and external carotid arteries supply blood to the eyelids and a vascular network of the eyelid is formed by anastomoses from the internal carotid via branches of the ophthalmic artery with terminal branches of vessels derived from the external carotid system (29).

Internal Carotid Supply

The *dorsal nasal artery, supratrochlear artery, supraorbital artery,* and *lacrimal artery* are the contribution of the internal carotid artery to the eyelid vascular system and are terminal branches of the *ophthalmic artery*. The *lacrimal artery* arises from the ophthalmic artery laterally, close to the optic foramen, gives off a branch that passes through the superior orbital fissure and anastomoses with the middle meningeal artery through the meningeal foramen near the front of the frontosphenoid suture. The lacrimal artery then proceeds anteriorly along the superior border of the lateral rectus to the lacrimal gland (Figs. 21 and 22).

External Carotid Supply

The branches of the external carotid artery supplying the eyelid are the *facial*, the *internal maxillary,* and the *superficial temporal arteries* (Fig. 22). The *facial artery* crosses the mandible anterior to the masseter muscle, courses diagonally to the nasolabial fold, and rises beneath the levators of the lip, becoming more superficial to lie between the levator labii superioris and levator alae nasi muscles. It becomes the *angular artery,* which is superficial at the medial canthus, lying beneath the orbicularis muscle 6–8 mm medial to the canthus and 5 mm arterior to the lacrimal sac. The

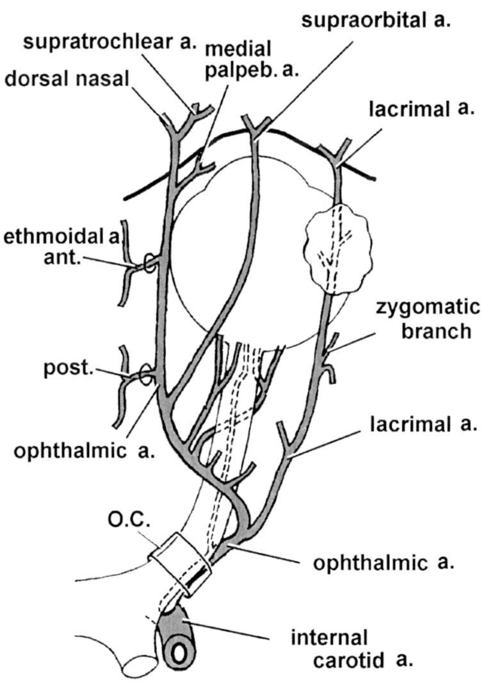

FIG. 21. Arterial supply of the orbit and eyelid. Axial view shows the ophthalmic artery arising from the internal carotid artery. The various branches of the ophthalmic artery are shown as they extend anteriorly into the eyelid area.

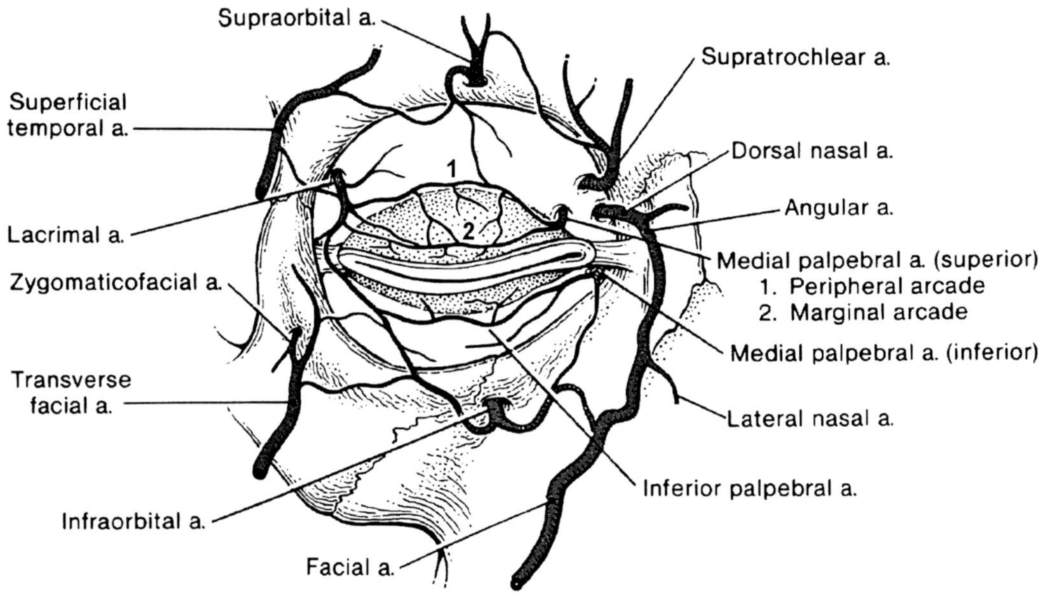

FIG. 22. Arterial supply of the eyelid (frontal view). This shows the vascular supply of the eyelid as derived from the ophthalmic artery. It also shows anastomotic branches with vessels from the external carotid: facial artery, transverse facial artery, superficial temporal artery, and infraorbital artery.

angular artery then perforates the orbital septum above the medial canthal tendon to anastomose with branches of the ophthalmic artery.

The *superficial temporal artery* is a terminal branch of the external carotid and freely anastomoses with the arteries of the scalp. After surfacing in front of the ear, it lies superficially in the superficial muscle plane above the muscles, separated from the skin by a varying amount of subcutaneous tissue. Three named branches arise from the superficial temporal artery lateral to the orbit and forehead and serve the eyelids; the *frontal,* the *zygomaticofacial,* and the *transverse facial,* which run nasally to anastomose with the lacrimal and supratrochlear arteries.

The *internal maxillary artery* continues as the *infraorbital artery* and traverses the inferior orbital fissure, pterygopalatine fossa, infraorbital groove and canal, and exits through the infraorbital foramen, to supply blood to the lower eyelid. It then anastomases with terminal branches of the dorsal nasal artery.

Eyelid Vascular Arcades

Anastomoses of the ophthalmic artery through the lacrimal and medial palpebral artery traverse the upper eyelid as the tarsal arcades. The *medial palpebral artery* arises from the ophthalmic artery temporal to the trochlea and divides into an inferior and superior branch just before traversing the orbital septum. The upper and lower eyelid arcades connect medially with the superior and inferior medial palpebral arteries and laterally with the terminal branches of the lacrimal artery, two lateral palpebral arteries.

The upper lid arcade consists of a *peripheral arcade,* which is located between Müller's muscle and the levator aponeurosis at the upper border of the tarsus, and a *marginal arcade,* just above the lash follicles in the pretarsal space. The marginal arcade lies on the anterior tarsal surface 2–3 mm from the eyelid margin and is encountered during reconstructive eyelid sharing techniques. The peripheral arcade lies above the tarsus in the pretarsal space (the most inferior portion of the postaponeurotic Jones space). This peripheral arcade system supplies the superior conjunctival fornix and communicates with the anterior ciliary arteries near the corneoscleral limbus (Fig. 23).

A lesser developed arcade system arises in the lower eyelid medially from the inferior palpebral artery and laterally anastomoses with the lacrimal and zygomaticofacial branch of the superficial temporal artery. The *inferior palpebral artery* travels along the inferior border of the tarsus in the pretarsal space.

Recent dissections by Tucker and Linberg further defined the configuration of the blood supply in the eyelid and, with quantitative casting, implied relative blood flow (30). Their dissections showed an *inferior palpebral vessel,* a branch from the superior palpebral vessel that descends vertically downward 10 mm, coursing deep to the canaliculi and medial canthal tendon and continuing as the inferior arcade. In their dissections, the largest contribution to the inferior arcade is from a branch of the facial artery (angular artery), which joins the inferior arcade at its most medial as-

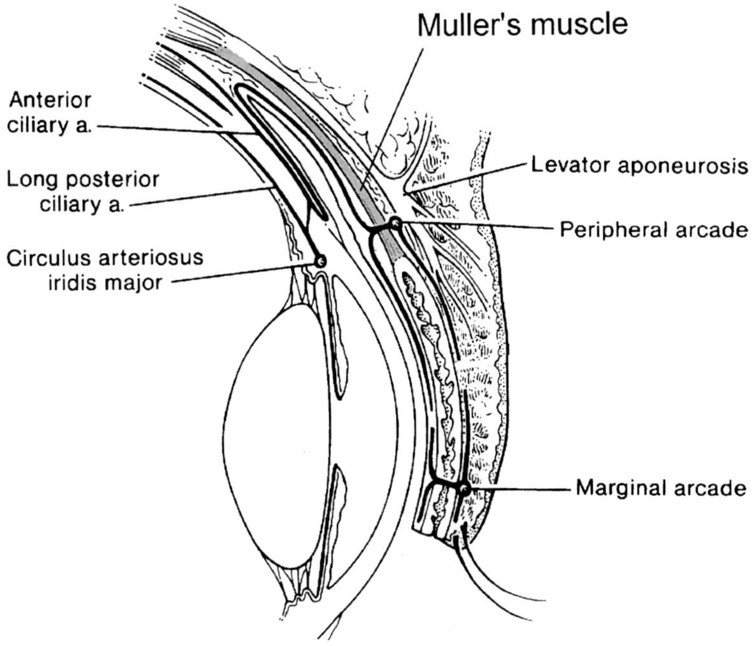

FIG. 23. Sagittal view of the arterial supply of the upper eyelid showing the vascular arcades and their supply of the upper fornix and anastamosis with the eye.

pect. The medial aspect of the lower eyelid also is supplied by branches from the infraorbital artery. Additional anastomoses of the external carotid supply with the inferior marginal arcade are with branches of the infraorbital artery and anterior deep temporal artery.

Tucker and Linberg (30) also found that the zygomaticofacial artery was a branch of the anterior deep temporal artery and not a branch of the superficial temporal artery as previously described (Fig. 24). In their study, examination of the size and shape of vessel casts allowed better understanding of the configuration and quantitation of blood flow in the eyelids. Medially, the upper marginal arcade was redundant and thrown into loops and then straightened out and narrowed in caliber laterally. The inferior marginal arcade was not as tortuous as compared with the superior eyelid but was also diminished in diameter laterally. The eyelid vessels were larger in caliber at their medial aspect, and the medial third of the upper and lower marginal arcades contained prominent vascular loops. This may be the result of the increased metabolic requirement of the orbicularis in that area, which is constantly active from blinking. Most of the excessive bleeding in blepharoplasty comes from this area and most surgeons note more bleeding medially than laterally in the eyelid during surgery.

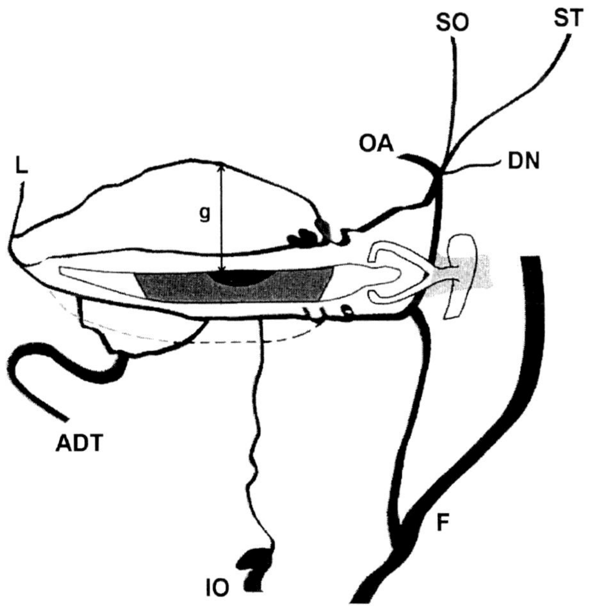

FIG. 24. Schematic diagram of eyelid arterial vascularity (after Tucker and Linberg, 30). IO, infraorbital; L, lacrimal; OA, ophthalmic; ADT, anterior deep temporal; F, facial; DN, dorsal nasal; SO, supraorbital; ST, supratrochlear. *G* = distance from the eyelid margin to the upper peripheral arcade (averages 9.2 mm).

A better understanding of the eyelid vascularity should allow modification of surgical techniques and reduce postoperative complications after eyelid surgery.

Veins

Anastomosis between the superficial facial and deep orbital venous systems also characterizes the veins of the eyelids. The *anterior facial vein* is the main superficial venous structure. The facial vein follows roughly the same course as the facial artery but is superficial to it and more lateral. The facial vein is called the *angular vein* near the medial canthus; it then becomes the *supratrochlear vein* and forms a deep anastomosis

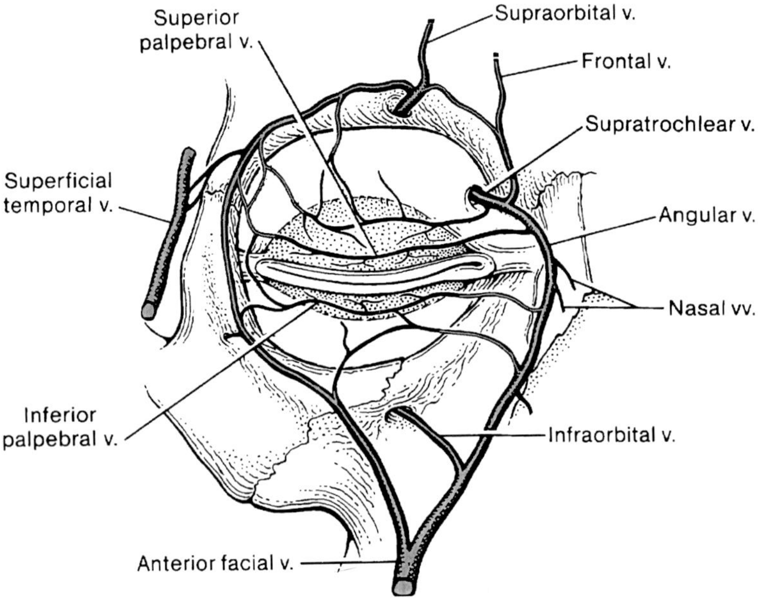

FIG. 25. Frontal view of venous drainage of the eyelid and periorbital area. There can be dual drainage of the area into the internal jugular via the deep orbital drainage and cavernous sinus or to the external jugular through the anterior facial and superior temporal veins.

superomedially in the orbit with the superior ophthalmic vein via the supraorbital vein. The angular vein lies temporal to the angular artery over the insertion of the medial canthal tendon, 8 mm from the medial commissure, and is often visible through the thin skin of this region. Laterally the *supraorbital vein* runs below the orbicularis oculi muscle on the frontalis muscle to communicate with frontal branches of the superficial temporal vein. Medially the supraorbital vein runs horizontally beneath the orbicularis and does not surface to join the *frontal vein* until it communicates with the superior ophthalmic vein of the orbit (Fig. 25). A confluence of angular, supraorbital, and supratrochlear veins forms the *superior ophthalmic vein*. The superior ophthalmic vein can be encountered with overaggressive removal of fat from the nasal or transitional area during upper lid blepharoplasty (see Chapter 14). The superior ophthalmic vein then passes posterolaterally, piercing the muscle cone in the midorbit. It then receives the venous drainage from the globe and, traveling along the lateral border of the superior rectus, enters the superior orbital fissure above the annulus of Zinn on its way to the cavernous sinus (Fig. 26) (1,16,31).

The orbital veins have no valves and in the facial area infection is dangerous because a superficial sepsis can spread to the cavernous sinus via the angular, supraorbital, and superior ophthalmic veins. The supraorbital vein also forms a deep preauricular plexus lateral to the lateral canthus underneath the orbicularis and passes posteriorly to the ear via the superficial temporal vein.

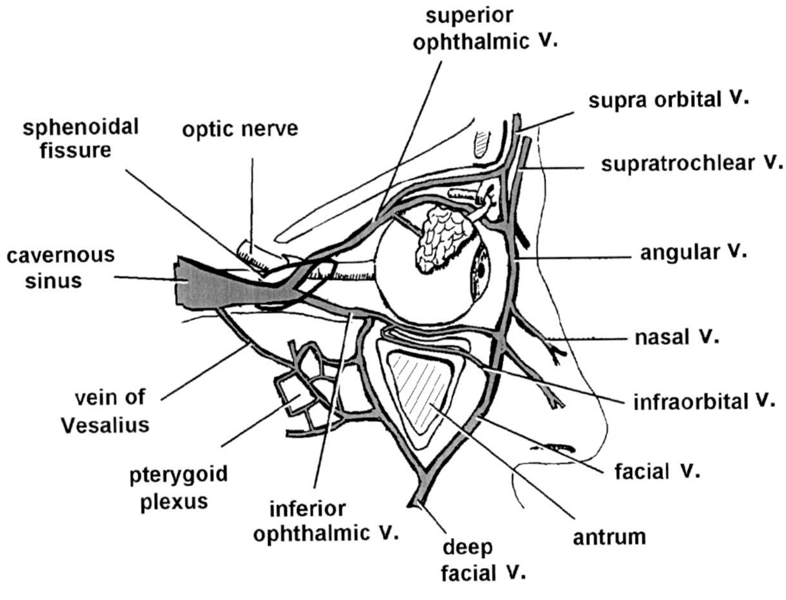

FIG. 26. Eyelid, orbital, and facial venous drainage. The superior ophthalmic vein originates from the angular and is attributable to the angular and supraorbital vein and enters the orbit in its nasal superior aspect in relationship to the trochlear and superior oblique tendon. It travels in the superior orbit in a transverse manner toward the lateral apex where it drains into the sphenoidal fissure and is joined by the inferior ophthalmic vein.

A second superficial to deep communication occurs between the facial vein and the pterygoid plexus via the deep facial vein. The pterygoid plexus communicates with the cavernous sinus directly and has drainage from the inferior ophthalmic vein through the inferior orbital fissure.

LYMPHATICS

Lymphatic drainage from the eyelids exists through a medial pathway draining to the submaxillary lymph nodes and larger lateral channels draining to the parotid lymph nodes. Medial lymphatics of the eyelids and conjunctiva follow the anterior facial vein to the submandibular lymph nodes. The lateral group drains the remainder of the lids to the superficial parotid lymph nodes anterior to the ear (Fig. 27). Sebaceous, squamous cell, and mucoepidermoid carcinomas commonly spread to the parotid nodes and all patients should be evaluated for this spread (see Chapter 25) (1,16,31).

NERVES

Sensory

The ophthalmic (V1), maxillary (V2), and mandibular (V3) nerves are the three divisions of the trigeminal (fifth cranial) nerve which provide sensory innervation to the eyelids (Fig. 28). The *ophthalmic division* traverses the cavernous sinus in its lateral wall and enters the orbit through the superior orbital fissure. Here it divides into the *frontal, nasociliary,* and *lacrimal nerves*. Frontal and lacrimal nerves lie in the superior orbital fissure above the annulus of Zinn. The nasociliary nerve provides sensory branches to ciliary ganglion lateral to the optic nerve. It gives off the two long posterior ciliary nerves and then runs forward superionasally with the ophthalmic artery, giving off the anterior and posterior ethmoidal nerves. The *infratrochlear nerve,* the terminal branch of the nasociliary nerve, supplies the side and tip of the nose, medial conjunctiva, caruncle, and lacrimal sac. The lacrimal nerve courses along the superior border of the lateral rectus muscle to the lacrimal sac. The lacrimal nerve courses along the superior border of the lateral rectus muscle to the lacrimal gland. It pierces the orbital septum and innervates the skin and conjunctiva of the lateral part of the upper eyelid. The frontal nerve, the largest of the three divisions of the ophthalmic nerve, runs directly forward between the periorbita and levator palpebrae superioris. Centrally in the orbit, it divides into the *supraorbital* and *supratrochlear nerves* (Fig. 29). Proceeding anteriorly above the trochlea, the supratrochlear nerve innervates the skin of the glabella, forehead, medial upper eyelid, and medial conjunctiva. The supraorbital nerve exits the orbit through a supraorbital notch or foramen and provides sensory innervation to the skin and conjunctiva of the upper eyelid and scalp. The *maxillary division* passes forward in the lower lateral wall of the cavernous sinus and exits the middle fossa via the foramen rotundum. It crosses the pterygopalatine fossa and enters the orbit in the inferior orbital fissure. In the posterior orbit, it becomes the *infraorbital nerve* and lies in the infraorbital groove. Continuing in the infraorbital canal, the anterior superior alveolar nerve is given off. The infraorbital nerve then emerges through the infraorbital canal. The nasal, labial, and palpebral branches carry sensation to the skin of the nose, upper and lower eyelids, and face. The *zygomatic nerve* branches from the maxillary nerve in the pterygopalatine fossa. It enters the orbit in the inferior orbital fissure and divides into the *zygomaticofacial* and *zygomaticotemporal* nerves. The zygomaticotemporal nerve runs along the lateral orbital wall and traverses the zygomaticotemporal foramen posterior to the anterior lateral orbital rim to supply sensation to the anterior temporal region. In the inferior lateral orbit, posterior to the orbital rim, the zygomaticofacial nerve exits its foramen to innervate the malar eminence (Figs. 30 and 31) (1,16,31).

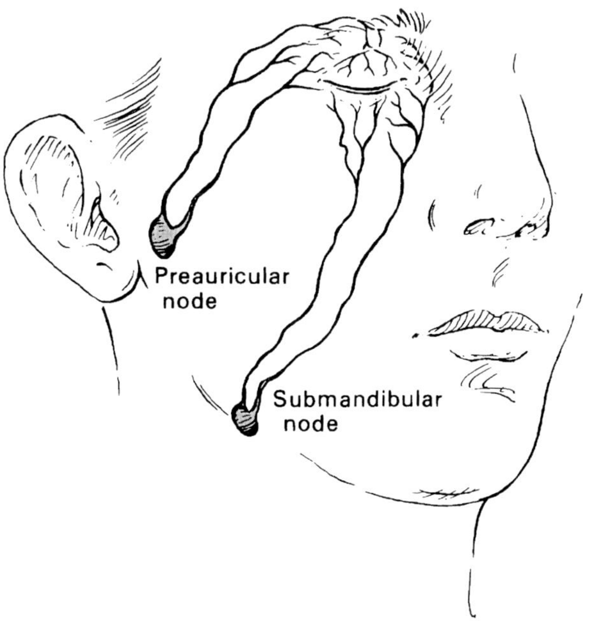

FIG. 27. Lymphatic drainage of the eyelid periorbital area.

Motor

The facial (seventh cranial) nerve, originating in the pons, emerges from the stylomastoid foramen and runs in the substance of the parotid gland. Posterior to the ramus of the mandible, it divides into *superior temporofacial* and *inferior cervicofacial branches* (Fig. 32).

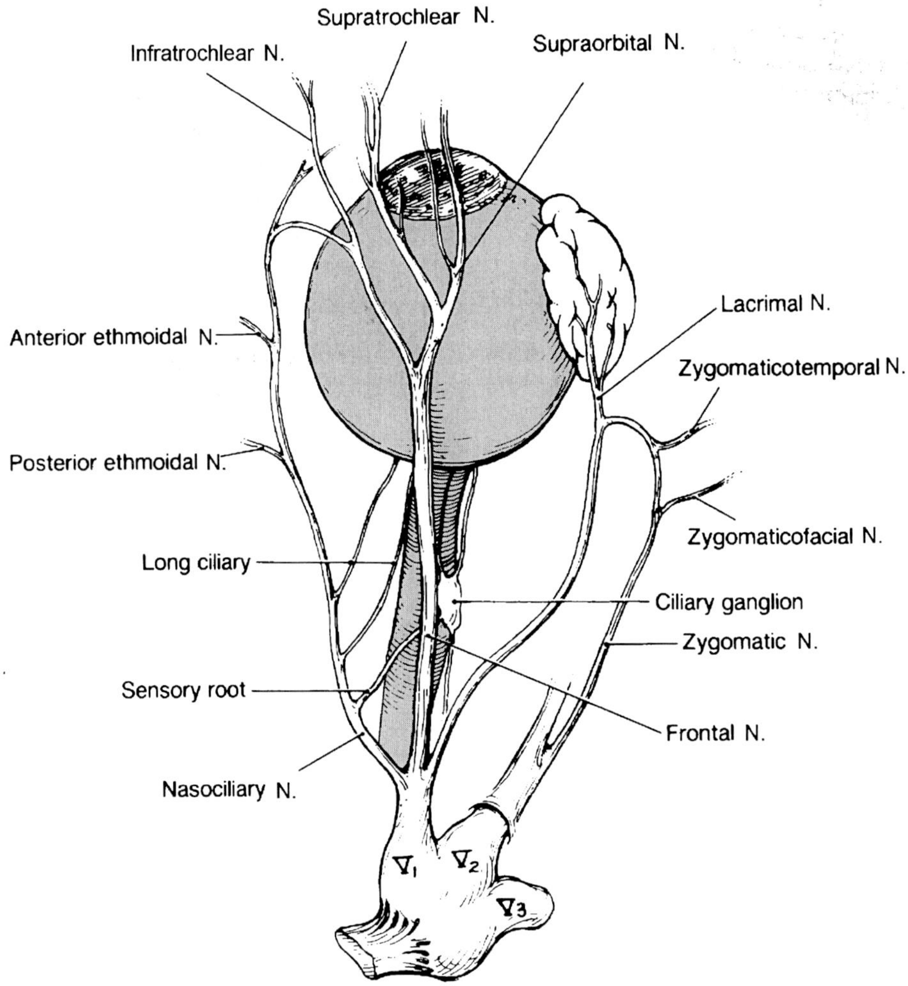

FIG. 28. Sensory nerves to the orbit and eyelid from branches of the fifth, or trigeminal, nerve.

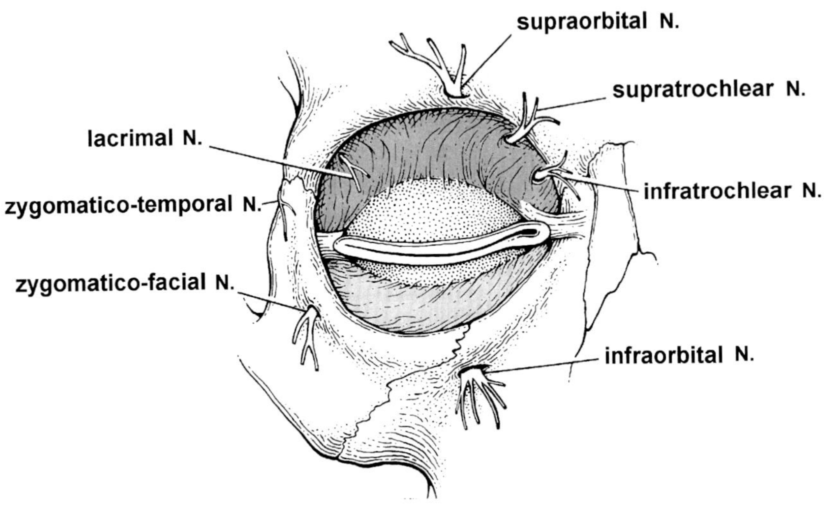

FIG. 29. Frontal view of terminal sensory branches of the fifth (trigeminal nerve).

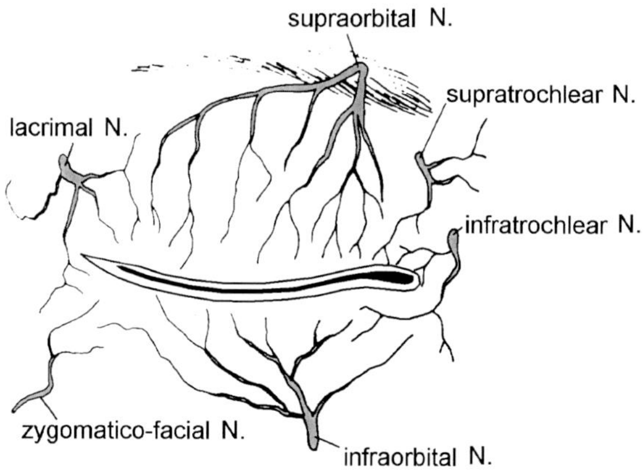

FIG. 30. Frontal view showing more detail of regional sensory innervation of the eyelid and periorbital area from the fifth nerve.

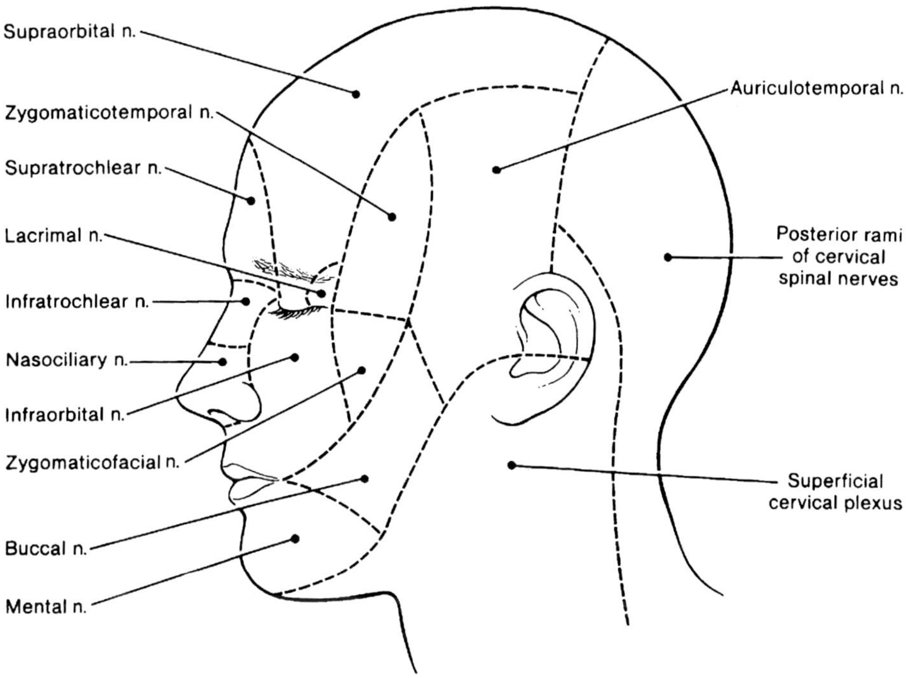

FIG. 31. Fields of cutaneous sensibility from innervation from the fifth cranial nerve.

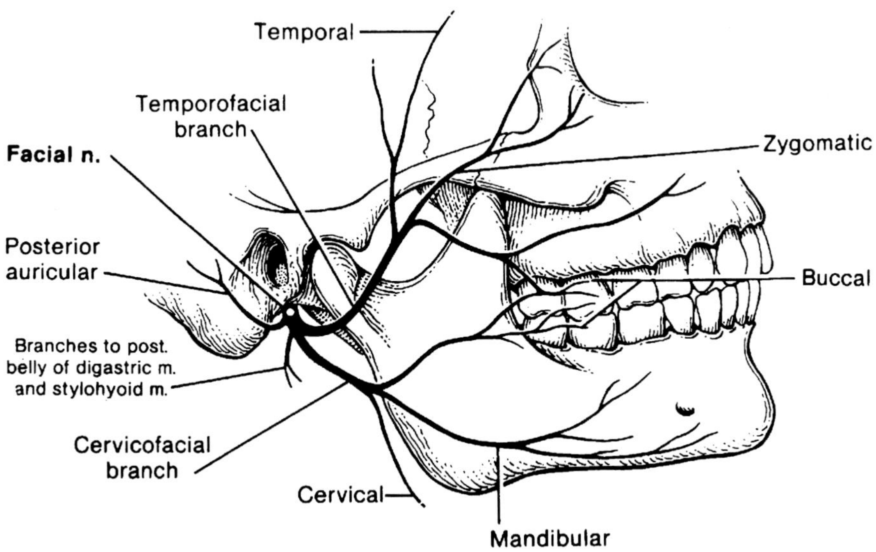

FIG. 32. Standard branching pattern of the seventh nerve or motor innervation to the eyelid facial area.

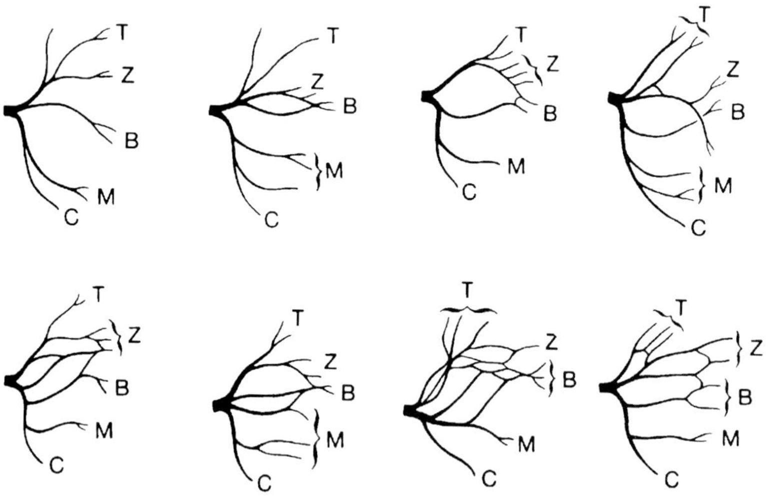

FIG. 33. Variation in branching patterns of the seventh facial nerve to the eyelid facial area. T, temporal; Z, zygomatic; B, buccal; M, mandibular; C, cervical.

The temporofacial nerve divides into the *temporal, zygomatic,* and *buccal* nerves. The temporal branch of the facial nerve lies on the periosteum of the zygomatic bone about 3 cm anterior to the external auditory meatus. This nerve innervates the frontalis, corrugator, and procerus muscles on their undersurface. The frontal nerve branches from the temporal and always travels along the undersurface of the superficial temporal fascia. The cervicofacial nerve divides into the *buccal, mandibular,* and *cervical nerves*. However, there are major variations in the branching and anastomosis pattern of the facial nerve (Fig. 33). The eyelid muscles and muscles of the facial expression are innervated on their deep surfaces by the facial nerve. Further discussion of the facial nerve can be found in Chapter 27 (1,32).

BROW, FOREHEAD, AND TEMPORAL REGION

The eyebrows extend over the superior orbital rim and consist of four layers: skin, muscle, fat, and galea. The skin of the brow is much thicker than eyelid skin. There are four muscles of the brow: frontalis, procerus, corrugator superciliaris, and orbicularis oculi. The *frontalis muscle* is a paired subcutaneous muscle that inserts into the skin of the brow. The *procerus muscle* is continuous with the frontalis and inserts into the nasal bones, pulls inferiorly, and is responsible for horizontal wrinkles of the *glabella area*. The *corrugator superciliaris* is obliquely oriented and after its insertion in the frontal bone medially extends 3 cm superolaterally and blends with the orbicularis oculi and frontalis muscles. It is responsible for vertical glabellar furrows (Figs. 2 and 3). The galea separates to envelope these muscles. Underneath the frontalis and orbicularis muscle sheaths lie the *eyebrow fat pad* that continues inferiorly into the space in the eyelid between the orbicularis muscle and the orbital septum. The eyebrow fat pad is firmly attached to the frontal bone at the superior orbital rim. This fat pad extends over the medial two thirds of the brow, corresponding to the supraorbital ridge (this structure is further discussed in Chapter 13) (Figs. 12–14). Laterally, vertically oriented orbicularis fibers are firmly attached on their undersurfaces to zygomatic bone at the horizontal raphe. This attachment results in "laugh lines." The supraorbital nerve and artery lie in the deep fat pad and pierce the frontalis muscle 2–3 cm above the supraorbital ridge. The supratrochlear nerve and artery pierce the corrugator to rise on the glabella. The supratrochlear vein is subcutaneous and connects to the angular vein anteriorly.

Posterolateral to the frontalis muscle, the *galea* is continous with the *superficial temporal fascia*. The superficial temporal artery and vein lie in this subcutaneous plane. Below this superficial fascia lies the *deep temporal fascia,* which is continuous with the *periosteum of the cranial bones*. The deep temporal fascia splits inferiorly to envelop a fat pad above the zygomatic bone and then fuses with zygomatic bone periosteum. The *temporalis muscle* fills the temporal fossa, originating at the *superior temporal line* and inserting on the coronoid process and anterior surface of the ramus. The motor branch of the mandibular division of the fifth cranial nerve innervates the temporalis muscle on its inner inferior surface. The temporalis muscle closes the jaws (Fig. 34) (1,34).

Eyelid Margin

The eyelid margin is divided into a medial lacrimal portion and a lateral palpebral portion by the lacrimal punctum. Medial to the punctum, the edge is rounded, without lashes, and carries the lacrimal canaliculus a variable depth beneath its surface. The lacrimal papilla is a fibrous ring within the medial end of the tarsus; the canaliculus travels posteriorly to the tarsus from

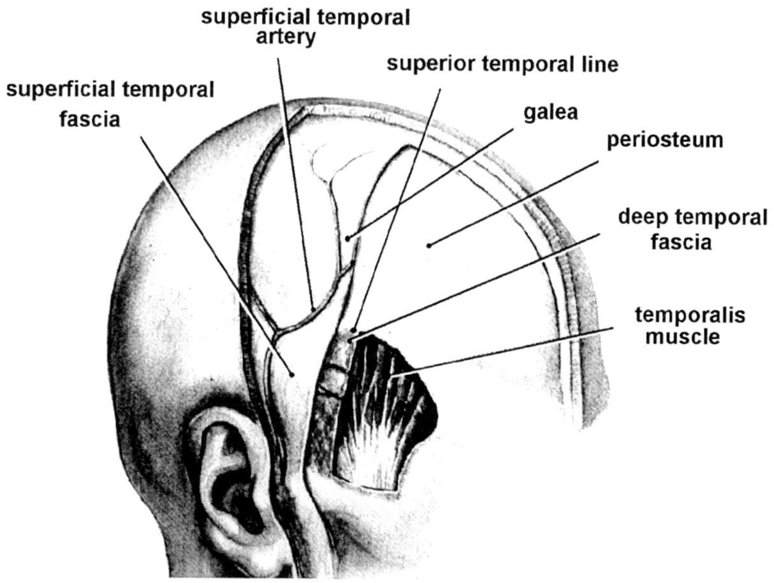

FIG. 34. Connective tissue layers in the forehad scalp temporal area. The periosteum is continuous to the deep temporal fascia and the galea is continuous to the superior temporal fascia. The superior portion of the temporalis muscle originates at the superior temporal line.

the ampulla. The palpebral portion of the eyelid margin has squared-off architecture with a mucous membrane–lined surface on the posterior edge and a keratinized surface on the anterior edge meeting in the middle. At the mucocutaneous junction, the margin of the eyelid exhibits a central fine line, the "*gray line,*" serving as a dissection guide to split the eyelid into an anterior lamella of skin muscle and lashes and a posterior tarsoconjunctival layer. This gray line is formed by Riolan's muscle (Fig. 35). Such a division is only approxi-

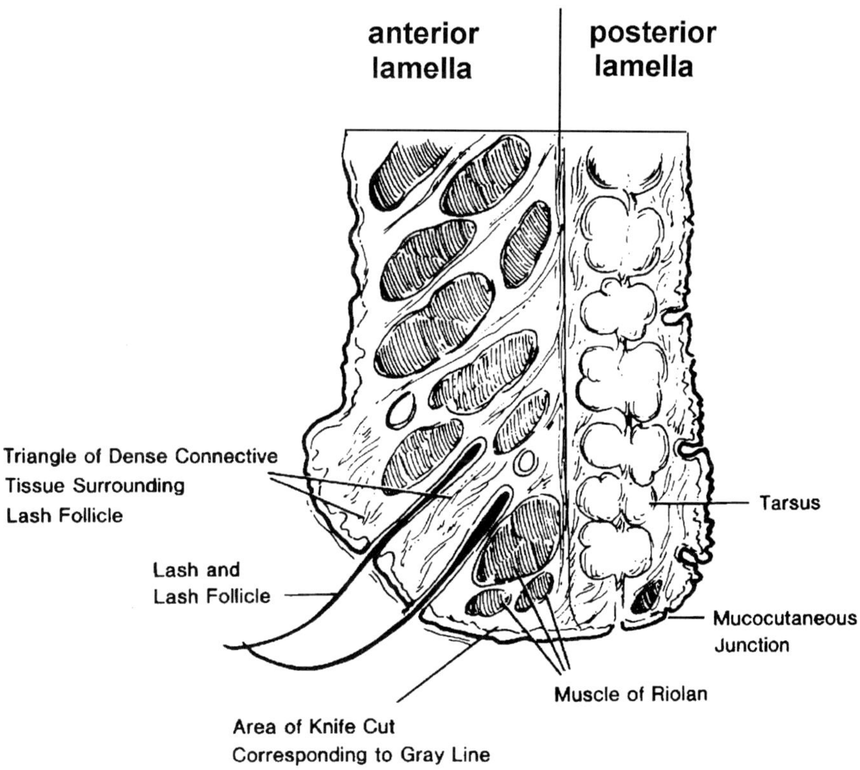

FIG. 35. Schematic vertical section through an eyelid (after Wulc and Dryden et al., 35). This demonstrates the separation in the lid into two components: the anterior lamella composed of skin and muscle, and the posterior lamella composed of tarsoconjunctiva. The gray line of the eyelid is seen on the eyelid margin and is a surgical landmark commonly used to make an incision to split the eyelid margin. The gray-appearing tissue corresponds to the muscle of Riolan, which lies in the anterior lamella.

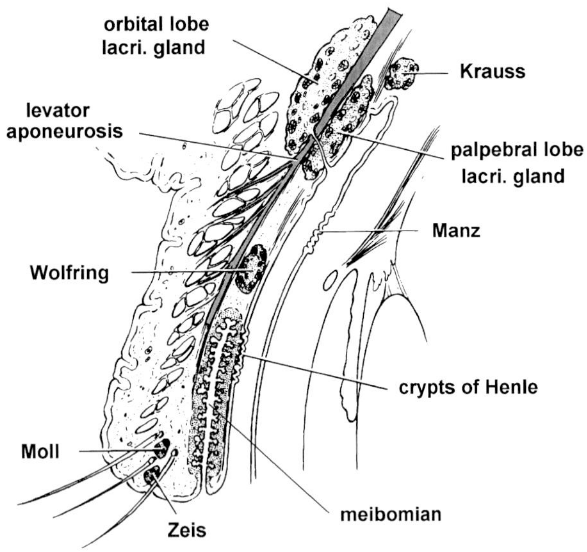

FIG. 36. Cross-section of the upper lid in the temporal section of the eyelid showing the relationship of the palpebral and orbital lobes of the lacrimal gland to the levator aponeurosis. The lacrimal ductules from the orbital lobe of the lacrimal gland pass through the aponeurosis and tissue lateral to the aponeurosis into the palpebral lobe of the lacrimal gland, which lies on the undersurface of the levator. Other accessory lacrimal glands are shown. Aqueous tear production can occur from the glands of Krause and Wolfring. Sebaceous elements of tears are derived from the glands of Zeis and Moll and the tarsal meibomian glands. Mucin glands are present in the conjunctiva with concentrations in the crypts of Henle and area of Manz.

mate since fibrous tissue from the tarsus splays anteriorly (35). Follicles may extend posteriorly to imbed in the tarsus, and orbicularis elements are seen posterior to the cilia and meibomian glands. The cilia number more than 100 in the upper eyelid and 50 in the lower lid. Pilosebaceous glands of Zeis empty into each follicle. Between each follicle is a spiral apocrine (sweat) gland of Moll ending on the eyelid margin (Fig. 36).

LUBRICATING SYSTEM OF THE EYELIDS

The tear layer is a three-layered structure consisting of oils secreted by the meibomian and Zeis glands, an aqueous component that is produced by the main lacrimal gland and the accessory lacrimal glands of Krause and Wolfring, and a basal mucinous layer secreted by conjunctival goblet cells. The *superficial oily layer* is the outer layer of the tear film and serves to slow the evaporation of tears by a factor of 15. The *aqueous component* is the middle layer and is uniformly about 6.5 μm thick across the cornea. It is actually a salt solution that contains the bactericidal lysozyme and lysin proteins. Because of considerable surface tension factors, there is little downflow of the aqueous film providing the surface corneal epithelium is intact. The *mucous layer* is the inner layer and is important for proper wetting of the corneal surface; corneal drying can occur despite an adequate aqueous film production in conditions that destroy the conjunctival goblet cells (36).

Jones proposed that the secretory system be divided into *basic secretors* and *reflex secretors* (5). The basic secretors are the mucin and oil glands, as well as the *accessory lacrimal glands of Krause* and *Wolfring*, and are thought to produce the tear film under ordinary conditions. The main lacrimal gland (orbital and palpebral lobes), which has a parasympathetic nerve supply, is thought to participate primarily in reflex lacrimation (i.e., stimulus from foreign body sensation or emotions). Removal of the main lacrimal gland, however, can produce keratitis sicca despite normally functioning accessory lacrimal glands. Clinical testing of lacrimal production is done by variations of the Schirmer test using filter paper strips in the inferior lateral conjunctival fornix (and by tear breakup time).

The *main lacrimal gland* resides superotemporally in the orbit in a shallow fossa in the frontal bone. The gland is divided on its medial and anterior surfaces by the lateral horn of the levator, dividing it into a larger orbital lobe above and a lesser palpebral lobe below. Division is not complete because a posterior wall of parenchyma persists between the lobes. The *upper (orbital) lobe* conforms to the space between the orbital wall and the globe, extending from the lateral border of the levator aponeurosis on which it rests, down to the frontozygomatic suture; it is bound in front by the orbital septum and the preaponeurotic fat pad, behind by orbital fat, medially by the intermuscular membrane between the superior and lateral recti, and laterally by bone. The *lower (palpebral) lobe* lies underneath the levator aponeurosis in the subaponeurotic space; it is separated from conjunctiva only medially where Müller's muscle intervenes (Fig. 36). Secretory ducts from the palpebral lobe drain into the superotemporal conjunctival fornix as do those from the orbital lobe. The upper lobe secretory ducts pass through the palpebral lobe parenchyma or remain tightly bound to its capsule so removal of the palpebral lobe will interrupt drainage from the orbital portion left behind (1).

Arterial blood to the lacrimal gland is supplied by the lacrimal branch of the ophthalmic artery, often by a contribution from the recurrent meningeal artery, which may join the lacrimal artery or enter the gland independently, and by a branch of the infraorbital artery.

The lacrimal gland receives innervation from the fifth and seventh cranial nerves as well as from sympathetics of the superior cervical ganglion. Sympathetic nerves arrive with the lacrimal artery with parasympathetics in the zygomatic nerve. The lacrimal nerve is sensory (although it may carry some sympathetic fibers gained while traversing the cavenous sinus). The seventh nerve supply to the lacrimal gland (via the zygomatic) provides the main secretomotor function, whereas the sympathetics are thought to stimulate basal secretion. Blocking the sphenopalatine ganglion will greatly diminish tear production but not eliminate it entirely.

The *accessory lacrimal glands of Krause and Wolfring* structurally resemble the lacrimal gland, may develop identical types of metaplasia, but differ in that they lack parasympathetic innervation. About 30 glands are located in the superior conjunctival fornix and perhaps half that number are in the inferior fornix. Several can be found along the upper border of the superior tarsus, in the caruncle, and in the plica semilunaris.

Oil Glands

The tarsus is in many places replaced by branched acinal glands with a long central duct extending nearly the vertical height of the plate. The *tarsal,* or *meibomian, glands* (about 30 in the upper tarsus and perhaps 15 more in the lower) are sebaceous, secreting an oil along the eyelid margin contributing to the outer, oily layer of the tear film. The meibomian gland orifice is located just anterior to the mucocutaneous junction, and the ductal epithelium is lined by keratinized epithelium. Following chronic inflammation the meibomian gland orifices may develop abnormal distichiatic hair follicles. This is explained by the fact that the glands represent a primitive sebaceous gland for a secondary row of eyelashes that has disappeared in humans. In the very young eyelid the meibomian gland orifices are seen very closely spaced, which suggests that growth produces horizontal lengthening. The glands themselves also increase in diameter and length with tarsal growth. The *pilosebaceous glands of Zeis* attached to the hair follicles and the *apocrine glands of Moll* also contribute to the oily layer (Fig. 36).

Aqueous Glands

As stated previously, the aqueous component of the tear layer is produced by the main lacrimal gland and the accessory lacrimal glands of Krause and Wolfring.

Mucous-Secreting Glands

Mucous-secreting goblet cells are located throughout the conjunctiva but are most concentrated at the lid margins, the conjunctival fornices, and near the corneoscleral limbus. They produce the thin, inner lining of the tear film contributing to the wettability of the corneal epithelium (Fig. 36).

CONJUNCTIVA

The *tarsoconjunctiva* covers the tarsal plates at the posterior eyelid margins and posterior tarsal surfaces. In the upper lid, the *palpebral portion* of the conjunctiva continues to the superior fornix and is attached to Müller's muscle immediately above the tarsus. The conjunctiva and Müller's muscle are tightly adherent. The superior fornix reflection of conjunctiva is about 13 mm from the margin with the eyes open and 20–25 mm with the eyes closed. The *suspensory ligament of the superior fornix* consists of smooth muscle and fibrous tissue arising from the conjoining of the levator and superior rectus muscles, which causes elevation of the fornix in upgaze. The upper forniceal attachments may become dehisced with overzealous dissection in levator resections for ptosis and a conjunctival prolaspe may occur (1).

In the lower eyelid, the conjunctiva can be elevated from the lower eyelid retractors without difficulty. The inferior fornix reflection remains 9–10 mm from the lower eyelid margin because the lower eyelid does not significantly elevate with closure. The *inferior suspensory ligament* arises from the inferior rectus extension that ensheaths the inferior oblique muscle.

Bulbar conjunctiva on the globe surface is less vascular and loosely adherent to the underlying Tenon's fascia until it reaches the cornea, where it is tightly bound to the episclera.

REFERENCES

1. Bergin D. Anatomy. In: McCord CD, Jr, Tanenbaum M, Nunery WR, eds. *Oculoplastic surgey.* 3rd ed. New York: Raven Press; 1995;51–83.
2. Wesley RE, McCord CD, Jones NA. Height of the tarsus in the lower lid. *Am J Ophthalmol* 1980;90:102–105.
3. Bergin D, McCord CD. Anatomy relevant to blepharospasm. In: Bosniak S, ed. *Advances in ophthalmic plastic and reconstructive surgery: Blepharospam.* Philadelphia: Harper and Row; 1985.
4. Tanenbaum M, McCord CD. The lacrimal drainage system. In: Tasman W, Jager EA, eds. *Duane's clinical ophthalmology.* Philadelphia: JB Lippincott; 1991.
5. Jones LT, Reeh M, Wirtschafter JD. *Ophthalmic anatomy.* Rochester, MN: American Academy of Ophthalmology and Otolaryngology; 1970.
6. Anderson RL. Medial canthal tendon branches out. *Arch Ophthalmol* 1977;95:2051–2052.
7. Doane MG. Blinking and the machanics of lacrinal drainage system. *Ophthalmology* 1981;88:844–851.
8. Gordon G. Observations upon movements of the eylids. *Br J Ophthalmal* 1951;35:339–351.
9. Blork A, Kugelberg E. The electrical activity of the eye and eyelids in various positions and during movement. *EEG Clin Neurophysiology* 1953;5:595–602.
10. Kennard DW, Glaser GH. An analysis of eyelid movements. *J Nerv Ment Dis* 1969;139:31–48.

11. McCord CD. Surgery of the eyelids. In: Duane TD, Jager EA, eds. *Clinical ophthalmology*. vol 51. New York: Harper and Row; 1983.
12. Gioia VM, Linberg JV, McCormick SA. The anatomy of the lateral canthal tendon. *Arch Ophthalmol* 1987;105:429–532.
13. Beard C, Quickert M. *Anatomy of the orbit*. Birmingham, AL: Aesculapius; 1977.
14. Putterman AM, Urist MJ. Surgical anatomy of the orbital septum. *Ann Ophthalmol* 1974;6:290–294.
15. Koorneef L. Orbital septa: anatomy and function. *Ophthalmology* 1979;86:876–880.
16. Doxanas MT, Anderson RL. *Clinical orbital anatomy*. Baltimore: Williams and Wilkins; 1984.
17. Doxanas MT, Anderson RL. Oriental eyelids: an anatomic study. *Arch Ophthalmol* 1984;102:1232–1235.
18. Weiss RA. Thesis for Am Soc Ophthal Plast Reconst Surg, 1988 (personal communication).
19. Lemke BN, Stasior OG. The anatomy of eyebrow ptosis. *Arch Ophthalmol* 1982;100:981.
20. McCord CD, Doxanas MT. Brow plasty and browpexy; an adjunct to blepharoplasty. *Plast Reconst Surg* 1990;86:248.
21. Whitnall SE. *Anatomy of the human orbit and accessory organs of vision*. Cambridge: Oxford University Press; 1932.
22. Anderson RL, Dixon RS. The role of Whitnall's ligament in ptosis surgery. *Arch Ophthalmol* 1979;97:705–707.
23. Goldberg RA, Wu JC, Jesmanowicz A, Hyde JS. Eyelid anatomy revisited: dynamic high-resolution magnetic resonance images of Whitnall's ligament and upper eyelid structures with the use of a surface coil. *Arch Ophthalmol* 1992;100:1598–1600.
24. Codere F. Presentation Am Soc Ophthal Plast Reconst Surg, San Francisco, 1994.
25. Anderson RL, Beard C. The levator aponeurosis: attachments and their clinical signficance. *Arch Ophthalmol* 1977;95:1437–1441.
26. Beard C. *Ptosis*. 3rd ed. St. Louis: CV Mosby; 1981.
27. Beard C. Mueller's superior tarsal muscle: anatomy, physiology, and clinical significance. *Ann Plast Surg* 1985;14:324–333.
28. Hawes MJ, Dortzbach RK. The microscopic anatomy of the lower eyelid retractors. *Arch Ophthalmol* 1982;100:1313–1318.
29. Hayreh SS. The ophthalmic artery. 111: Branches. *Br J Ophthalmol* 1962;46:212.
30. Tucker SM, Linberg JV. Vascular anatomy of the eyelids. *Ophthalmology* 1994;101:1118–1121.
31. Warwick R. Eugene Wolff's *Anatomy of the eye and orbit*. 7th ed. Philadelphia; WB Saunders; 1976.
32. McCormack LJ, Gluldwell EW, Anson BJ. The surgical anatomy of the facial nerve with specific reference to the parotid gland. *Surg Gynecol Obstet* 1945;80:620.
34. Hollinshead WH. *Anatomy for surgeons*. vol 1. *The head and neck*. 3rd ed. New York: Harper and Row; 1982.
35. Wulc A, Dryden RM, Khatchaturian T. Where is the grayline? *Arch Ophthalmol* 1987;105:1092–1098.
36. Maurice DM. The dynamics and drainage of tears. In: Holly FJ, Lemp MA, eds. The preocular tear film and dry eye syndromes. *Int Ophthalmol Clin* 1973;13:103–116.

CHAPTER 2

Basic Principles of Wound Closure

BASIC PRINCIPLES

The techniques involved in the management of skin and soft tissues provide the fundamental principles that should be applied to a wide variety of surgical procedures to ensure optimal results. The final surgical result depends directly on the basic principles of incision placement, suturing techniques, gentle handling of tissue, wound healing, and postoperative care. These concepts apply to all aspects of surgical procedures ranging from closure of a simple laceration to more complex procedures.

LOCATION OF SKIN INCISIONS

Although all skin incisions will inevitably result in a scar, the final appearance of the scar is dependent on several factors. Scar visibility can be minimized by the avoidance of beveled edges and by placement of the incision within or parallel to adjacent skin lines. A skin incision perpendicular to the surface results in the most rapid healing of the epithelium and a narrower scar width (1). An oblique incision will result in dermal overlap, which causes elevation of the epidermis and scar visibility. The incision should always be made with the skin held taut in a single, continuous motion. In order to avoid having blood obscure the incision markings, one should always proceed in an uphill direction with respect to skin contour.

Planning the location of the incision will influence the surgical outcome. The basic principles of incision placement suggest that scar results are improved when the incision is placed within an exiting skin line or crease. An upper eyelid incision placed within the lid crease is an example of this principle. When a distinct crease is not apparent, the incision should be placed parallel to the relaxed skin tension lines (Fig. 1). The relaxed tension lines of the skin are caused by underlying muscle contraction and are perpendicular to the axis of the musculature. These lines of minimal tension generally parallel the wrinkle lines and lines of facial expression (Fig. 2).

Scars are less conspicuous if placed within or parallel to the relaxed skin tension lines. The preferred incision placement is horizontal in the forehead and upper and lower eyelid regions, and vertical in the glabellar region. An incision near the eyebrow can be concealed by placement in the superior or inferior brow margin. Incisions in the cheek and lateral canthal areas should be more oblique, parallel to the nasojugal fold. Wound closure is facilitated by maximal extensibility of adjacent tissue. The lines of maximal extensibility are perpendicular to the lines of relaxed skin tension. Primary closure and flap advancement techniques are facilitated by movement of tissue along the lines of maximal extensibility.

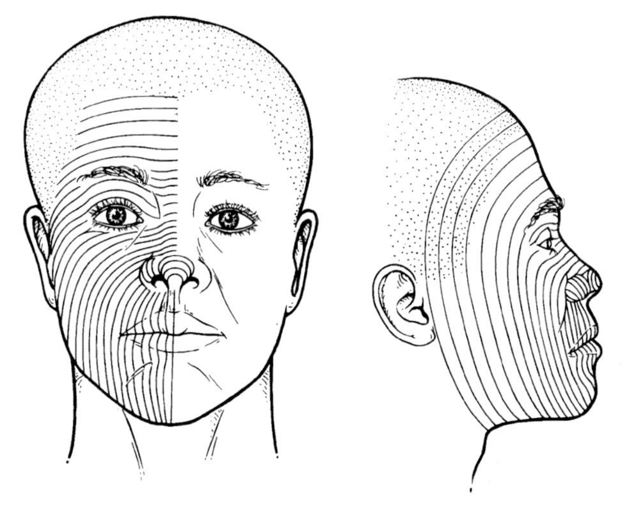

FIG. 1. Orientation of incisions parallel to the relaxed skin tension lines will minimize scar formation.

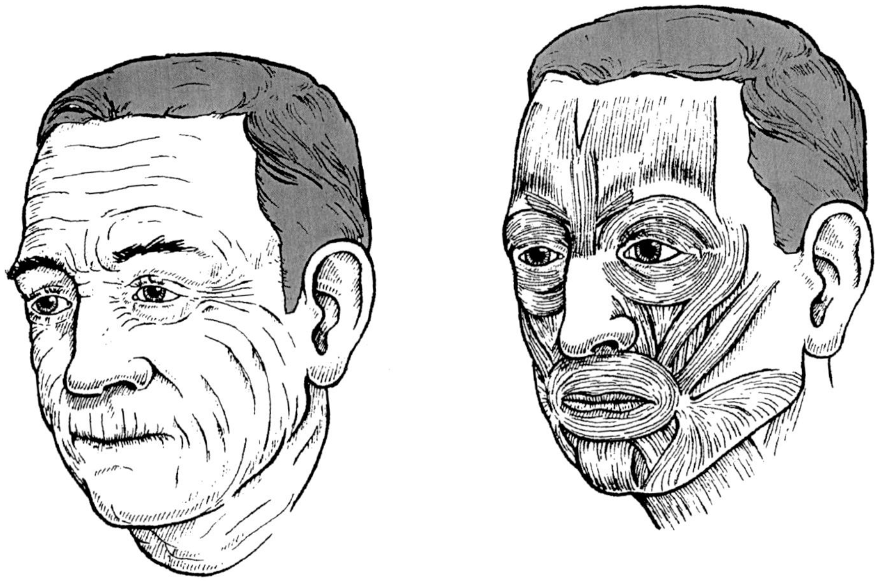

FIG. 2. Wrinkle lines are generally parallel to the relaxed skin tension lines and are perpendicular to the axes of the underlying musculature.

LOCAL ANESTHESIA

In order to safely administer local anesthesia, the basic pharmacology should be understood including dosage, metabolism, and toxicity. The most commonly used local anesthetic agents are lidocaine (Xylocaine) and marcaine with epinephrine and hyaluronidase (Wydase). Excellent hemostasis can be maintained with the use of epinephrine, which reduces bleeding by causing vasoconstriction of the subdermal plexus. Allow 7–8 min for this effect after injection (3). In order to minimize the pain associated with the injection of the local anesthetic, slow infiltration with a 27-gauge needle should be performed. The addition of 1 cm^3 8.4% sodium bicarbonate per 10 cm^3 of anesthesia will change the pH of lidocaine with epinephrine from 4.0 to a more neutral pH, thereby reducing the pain associated with local acidity.

The maximal dosage of lidocaine with epinephrine is 7 mg/kg and 4.5 mg/kg when used without epinephrine. Maximal dosages should be calculated prior to surgery. Since the half-life is 130 min, supplemental dosage can be safely administered after 60 min if necessary. Signs of toxicity include restlessness, which can progress to convulsions and respiratory arrest. Treatment includes immediate recognition with respiratory support and intravenous valium for seizure control. Strict adherence to maximal dosage, particularly in children, and avoidance of intravenous injection should prevent toxic complications.

Although lidocaine with epinephrine is generally used for hemostasis, special clinical situations, such as retrobulbar block, temporal artery biopsy, and upper eyelid ptosis adjustments, may require the avoidance of epinephrine. The use of hyaluronidase promotes widespread penetration of the local anesthesia, which eliminates tissue distortion. The use of regional nerve blocks should include frontal block in the upper eyelid and infraorbital and zygomaticofacial block in the lower eyelid. The amount of local anesthetic agent injected in the eyelids is reduced when combined with regional blocks and a reduction in eyelid tremor.

SUTURE AND SURGICAL INSTRUMENTS

Prior to closure, correct suture material and needle size as well as the appropriate instruments are selected depending on the wound depth and width. Sutures are classified as absorbable and nonabsorbable types. Absorbable sutures include catgut, chromic, and plain, as well as polyglycolic acid derivates such as vicryl, dexon, maxon, PDS, and monocryl. Nonabsorbable sutures cause less tissue reaction and include synthetic monofilament material such as nylon and prolene. Silk is a braided nonabsorbable suture that has the best tying properties and is most pliable. In general, 4-0 and 5-0 are used for deep layers and 6-0 and 7-0 for skin closure.

Absorbable sutures are frequently used with a buried knot to close deep layers or repair mucous membranes. Catgut is made from the submucosal layer of sheep intestine. Plain catgut is fast absorbing and retains tensile strength for 4–7 days. Chromic catgut is created by treatment with a chromic salt solution, which coagulates the proteins extending strength to 30 days with complete absorption by 90 days. Catgut is absorbed by proteolytic enzyme degradation followed by phagocytosis. Dexon and vicryl are stronger than catgut and lose tensile strength at 30 days with absorption by 90 days. PDS and monocryl retain tensile strength for 60 days with complete absorption at 180 days. Since the suture is a monofilament and undergoes degradation with hydrolysis, less inflammatory tissue reaction is created.

The sutures available have a variety of swedged-on needles. Classification of needle types includes cutting, reverse cutting, taper, and spatula needles. In general, the needle diameters vary and are a three-eighths circle. The cutting needle is used for deep sutures and periosteal fixation, the taper or reverse-cutting needles are used for skin closure, and the spatula needle is used for suturing the tarsal plate.

The surgical instruments available should include a variety of fine-needle holders, tissue forceps, and scissors. Spring-type locking or nonlocking Castroviejo needle holders are commonly used with suture in the 4-0 to 7-0 size range. The Kalt and Webster needle holders can be used effectively with larger needles. Fine-tissue forceps with teeth should be used to minimize local tissue trauma. Adson tissue forceps are used for thick flaps and Bishop–Harmon forceps for handling of more delicate tissue. Lester forceps are similar to the Bishop–Harmon forceps and are available with fine and extrafine teeth. Fine-skin hooks, Blair retractors, and Tyrell–Iris hooks are used for atraumatic tissue retraction. The scissors most commonly used are the Iris scissors for skin-muscle flaps, and the Stevens tenotomy and Westcott spring-action scissors for finer tissue.

SUTURING TECHNIQUES

A traumatic wound should be properly prepared for closure in order to minimize the resultant scar. If the wound edges appear damaged or ragged, excision of the wound edges should be performed. All dirt and foreign material should be removed. Copious irrigation with an antibiotic solution should be performed to aid in mechanical debridement. At this point the wound is prepared with an antiseptic solution.

Accurate suturing techniques will ensure precise closure of a wound or surgical incision. In order to obtain a good functional and cosmetic result, wounds that penetrate deep in the subcutaneous tissue should be closed in layers (4). All dead space should be eliminated and the subcutaneous tissue reapproximated so that the skin edges are in apposition without tension or overlapping edges. Interrupted buried absorbable sutures are used to close the deep layers. Suturing the fascia and dermal layers is used to bring the subcutaneous tissue together, rather than suturing the subcutaneous tissue directly. Skin sutures will serve to approximate the skin loosely rather than to supply strength to the wound.

A key principle in wound closure is achieving good eversion of the skin edges. A prerequisite for good eversion is adequate closure of the deep tissue with minimal tension across the wound surface. In order to reduce tension, undermining of the subcutaneous tissue deep in the subdermal plexus can be performed with placement of inverted absorbable sutures at the level of the dermis. Eversion of the wound edge is created by placing a simple suture so that on cross-section a trapezoidal configuration is formed with the depth greater than the width (Fig. 3). This basic technique is accomplished by passing the needle obliquely away from the wound edge with inclusion of more subcutaneous tissue than skin to evert the margins. Proper alignment of skin height is achieved by suturing symmetric volumes of tissue, which will minimize shadow formation and scar visibility. When tied, the skin edges are forced outward. Other effective methods for eversion of wound edges are the use of the vertical mattress suture, the horizontal mattress suture, and the near–far/far–near suture (Fig. 4). These interrupted sutures are particularly useful for stellate wounds or wounds with moderate tension. Since wounds tend to contract vertically, margins should be slightly everted after skin closure or a depressed scar may result.

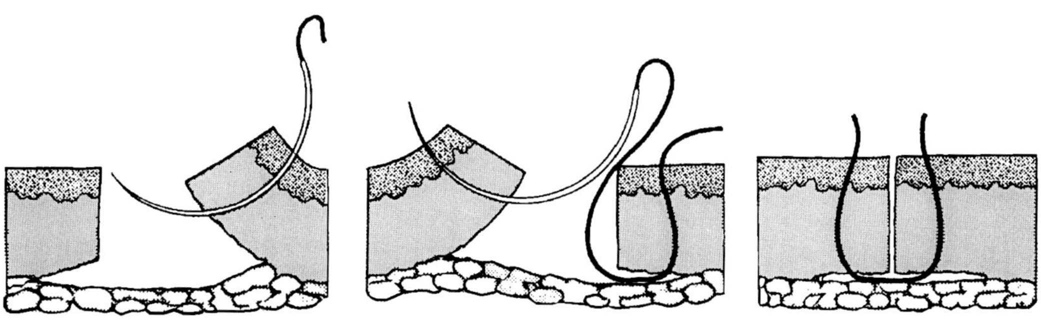

FIG. 3. Cross-sectional diagram demonstrates the eversion of skin edges with the inclusion of deeper tissue.

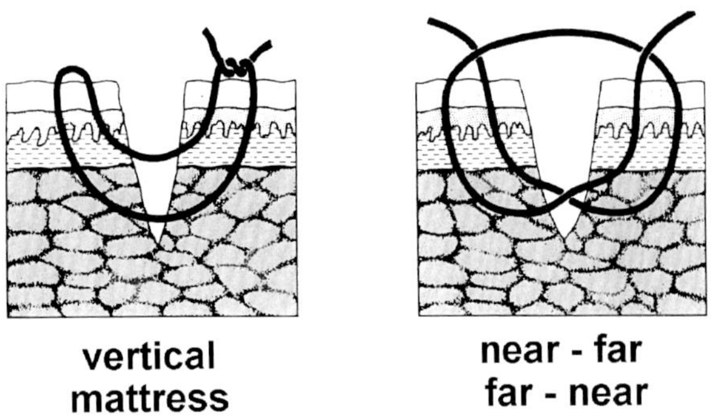

FIG. 4. Eversion of the wound edges with mattress suturing techniques prevents the formation of a depressed scar during wound healing.

Continuous suture techniques can be performed rapidly and are effective in select wounds, such as linear surgical incisions or wounds of unequal thickness. The continuous vertical mattress suture with the sutures placed in a criss-cross configuration is a very useful technique to distribute wound tension (Fig. 5). The deeper suture approximates the subcutaneous or muscle layer thereby reducing tension and the superficial suture approximates the skin edges. This method should be performed with a 6-0 or 7-0 suture. We prefer to use nylon or silk to close skin incisions. We have found that the continuous vertical mattress suture reduces scar visibility in the brow and forehead region and in wounds perpendicular to the lines of minimal tension (Fig. 6).

The next principle of wound closure relies on precise suture placement. Closure should begin on one side, rather than in the center, with sutures placed the same depth and distance on the opposite side. When there is more length on one side of the wound or when a circular defect is closed, a dog ear may be created at the end of the incision. This deformity is managed by excision of excess tissue on the side of the longer incision limb. A skin hook is used to retract the excess

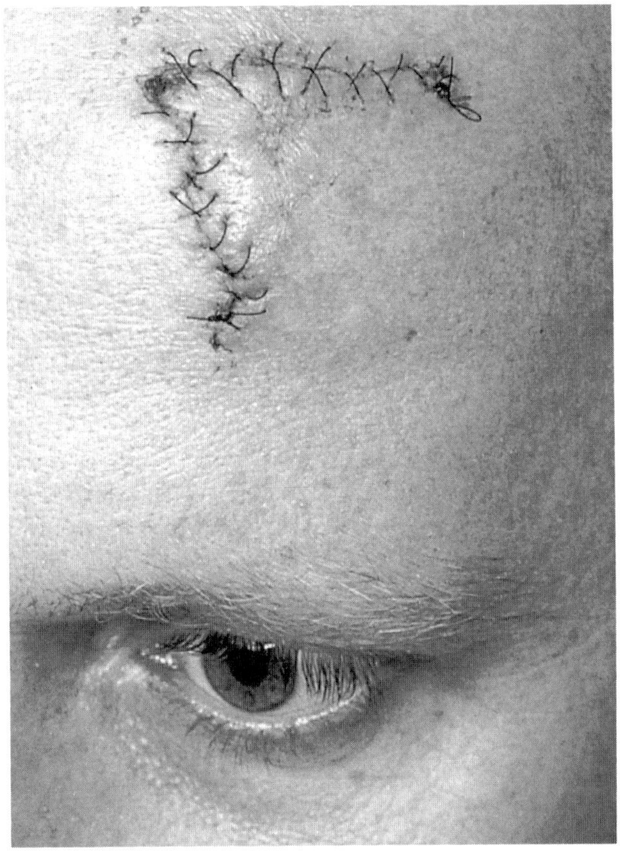

FIG. 6. Clinical example of the continuous vertical mattress suture for repair of a forehead laceration.

A

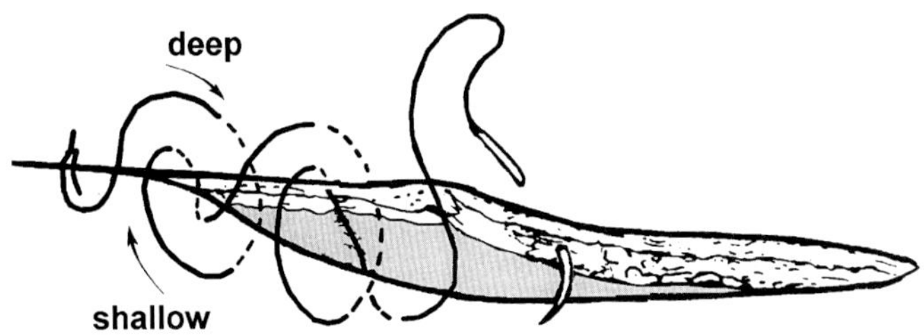

B

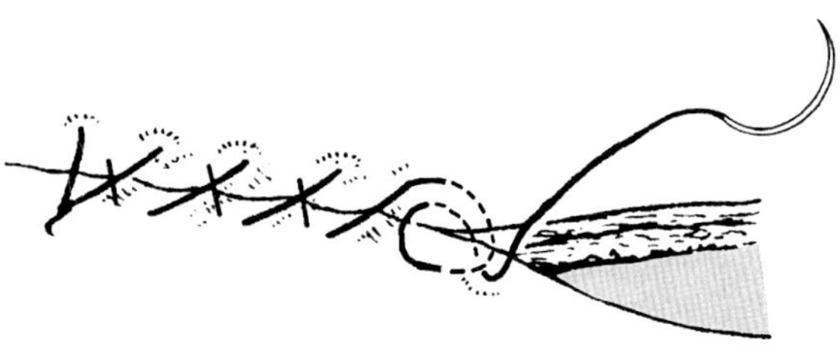

FIG. 5. The continuous vertical mattress suture is useful for the repair of linear wounds of differing depths that have a tendency to invert. **A:** Deep full-thickness sutures are alternated with shallow skin sutures. **B:** A criss-cross configuration is created when the suture is tightened.

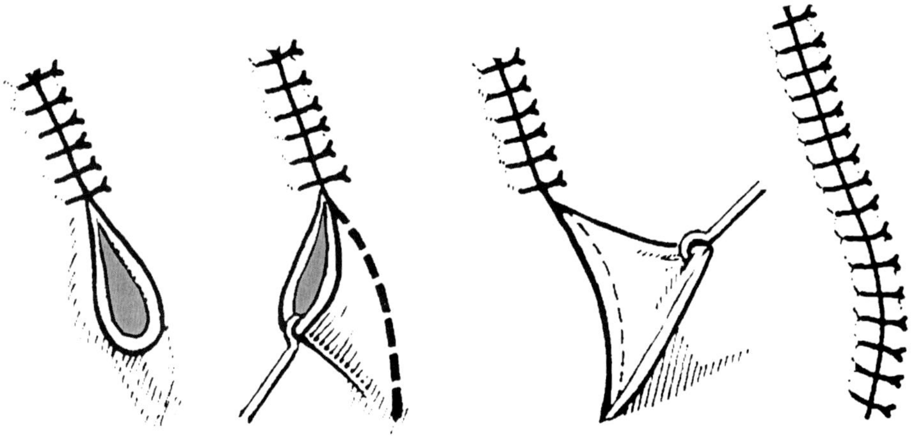

FIG. 7. Excess tissue at the end of an incision creates a dog ear deformity. The excess tissue is excised along the length of the incision and closure is completed.

tissue and define the extent of the dog ear. The skin is undermined and the incision extended angling toward the dog ear. The skin flap is advanced across the incision and resected (Fig. 7).

After suturing has been completed, proper placement of the postoperative dressing is the next integral part of the operative procedure. When an eyepatch is used to protect the wound, the dressing should not be taped tightly in order to avoid increasing the intraorbital pressure. Reports of blindness have been associated with increased intraorbital pressure causing central retinal artery occlusion following postoperative bleeding (5). Wound management recommendations following blepharoplasty include the application of antibiotic ointment on the incision site since dressings are generally not required. In contrast, a pressure dressing should be applied to the anophthalmic socket following enucleation or evisceration and left in place for 4–7 days in order to minimize postoperative swelling.

SUTURE REMOVAL

In order to prevent permanent scarring from suture marks on the skin surface, sutures should be removed within 7 days depending on the size and type of suture material. If sutures are left in too long, the suture tract may become epithelialized resulting in an inclusion cyst. If sutures are removed too early, the risk of wound disruption is increased. Although clinical impression should individualize timing of suture removal, as a general rule, 6-0 silk sutures are removed in 4–5 days, and nylon or prolene sutures in 6–7 days.

WOUND HEALING

A fundamental understanding of wound healing is important for an appreciation of both the normal healing process and abnormal healing, which may result in hypertrophic scars or keloids. Normal wound healing is generally divided into four categories: the inflammatory phase, the fibroblastic phase, the scar maturation phase, and the wound contraction phase (6).

The inflammatory phase of wound healing is often referred to as the latent or lag phase. Following a tissue wound created either surgically or traumatically, a complex cellular and humoral response to injury is initiated. Interleukins and a variety of chemotactic factors are stimulated that attract leukocytes, macrophages, fibroblasts, and other cells involved in wound healing. The wound is prepared for the fibroblastic phase with clearance of bacteria, debris, and necrotic tissue. If foreign material remains in the wound, chronic inflammation can result causing the formation of a suture granuloma. Epithelialization of the wound surface occurs during the inflammatory phase and is generally complete by 24 h.

After 4–6 days, the fibroblastic phase begins with the stimulation of fibroblasts that migrated into the wound during the inflammatory phase. Proliferating fibroblasts produce increasing amounts of collagen over a 2- to 4-week period. A dynamic equilibrium between collagen production and collagen degradation occurs during this phase. As the tensile strength of the wound increases, an early hypertrophic-appearing scar is produced.

During the second month of wound healing, the maturation phase begins, noted by a reduction in the density of fibroblasts. The tensile strength continues to increase and a plateau is reached by 12 weeks. Although the maturation phase continues for years, the tensile strength never reaches the strength of the tissue prior to surgery (7). The collagen fibrils become more organized and less bulky secondary to water loss resulting in a thinner appearing scar. Since the final scar appearance cannot be determined until a year after surgery, scar revision should generally not be performed until this period of healing has been complete.

Wound contraction overlaps the other phases of wound healing. Myofibroblasts are specialized fibroblasts with contractile properties that contribute to wound contraction. A surgical incision will undergo contraction perpendicular to the surface and along the scar length. An open would that heals by granulation will undergo centripetal contraction with migration from the periphery and intussusceptive growth of adjacent tissue.

HYPERTROPHIC SCARS AND KELOIDS

Abnormal wound healing can result in a red, thickened scar that gives rise to symptoms such as itching, burning, and tenderness. A hypertrophic scar presents as a raised, thickened scar and should be differentiated from a keloid. A hypertrophic scar remains within the tissue of the wound. In contrast, a keloid is more exuberant, proliferating similar to a tumor beyond the boundary of the wound edges invading normal surrounding issue (8). Although the precise cause of abnormal scarring has not been determined, gentle tissue manipulation and avoidance of tension may reduce scar formation.

Management of hypertrophic scars and keloids includes the use of pressure garments and massage as well as steroid injection. Although keloids are more common in black patients, their occurrence is not uncommon in white patients. Surgical excision of keloids is generally to be avoided since there is a high probability of recurrence. If excision is necessary, recurrence can be reduced with radiation treatment of 300–600 cGy to the wound immediately following surgery. When steroid injections are performed, triamcinolone should be injected into the substance of the scar under high pressure using a tuberculin syringe until the scar blanches. Injection can be repeated twice a week until flattening of the scar is achieved. Intradermal injection and injection into adjacent tissue should be avoided and can cause atrophy and depigmentation.

SCAR REVISION

Despite the utilization of methods aimed at minimizing scar formation, an unfavorable scar may require revision in order to improve its appearance. Although several techniques are available, scar revision should not be attempted prior to complete scar maturation.

Dermabrasion is a useful technique for the improvement of surface irregularities caused by scarring. Following infiltration with local anesthesia, mechanical abrasion of the scar is performed using a fine surgical burr. The goal is reduction of raised areas, which will minimize visible shadows. Dermabrasion is continued into the dermis, which heals by reepithelialization.

In addition to reducing surface irregularities, excision or redirection of more linear scars is a useful technique of scar revision. When complete elliptical excision is performed, incision should be oriented parallel to the relaxed skin tension lines. A linear scar can be converted to a less conspicuous broken scar by use of the Z-plasty procedure. The principle of the Z-plasty is to rely on the transposition of two triangular skin flaps. The technique increases the length of the tissue parallel to the scar with a change in the scar direction. Proper design can be used to redirect the scar toward the relaxed skin tension lines. A similar technique is the W-plasty, which relies on dividing a linear scar into multiple segments. An irregular scar can be excised with multiple triangular-shaped incisions made perpendicular to the axis of the scar. Closure is performed by advancement of the lateral adjacent tissue.

The dermal platform technique of scar revision may be used in patients prone to hypertrophic scar formation (9). A fusiform superficial excision of the cutaneous scar is performed. The underlying subcutaneous traction bands and dermal scarring are not excised. The adjacent skin is undermined and closed with advancement. The principle of this technique is to avoid restimulating dermal fibroblastic activity.

REFERENCES

1. Borges AF. *Elective incisions and scar revision*. Boston: Little, Brown; 1973.
2. Kraissl CJ. The selection of appropriate lines for elective surgical incisions. *Plast Reconstr Surg* 1951;8:1.
3. Siegel RJ, Vistnes LM, Iverson RE. Effective hemostasis with less epinephrine. *Plast Reconstr Surg* 1973;51:129.
4. McGregor IA. *Fundamental techniques of plastic surgery*. New York: Churchill Livingstone; 1989.
5. DeMere M, Wood T, Austin W. Eye complications with blepharoplasty or other eyelid surgery: a national survey. *Plast Reconstr Surg* 1974;53:634–637.
6. McCord CD, Tanenbaum M, Nunery WR. *Oculoplastic surgery* 3rd ed. New York: Raven Press; 1995.
7. Bucknall TE, Ellis H. *Wound healing for surgeons*. Philadelphia: Bailliere-Tindall; 1984.
8. Jukiewicz MJ, Krizek TJ, Mathes SJ, Ariyan S. *Plastic surgery: principles and practice*. St. Louis: CV Mosby; 1990.
9. Regnault P, Daniel PK. Depressed scars and soft tissues. *Ann Plast Surg* 1983;10:427–436.

CHAPTER 3

Free Tissue Grafts

Free tissue grafting techniques are an integral part of oculoplastic surgery particularly since in many patients large segments of soft tissue may be deficient or atrophic and cannot be replaced with flaps. Detailed use of free tissue grafts will be described in subsequent chapters and this chapter will serve as classification and summary of the grafts most commonly used in eyelid surgery.

The need for free grafts occurs commonly in eyelid reconstruction following tumor removal or trauma, but it also is present in many cases of atrophic, damaged, or contracted eyelids. Free tissue grafting must be used to rebuild or support the deficient anatomic area. Spacer or supporting material is needed in many cases to compensate for anticipated postoperative scar contracture or for needed supporting lid structures. The surgeon must understand the anatomic indications for using tissue grafts and be familiar with harvesting techniques. Grafts should be cosmetically or functionally matched, have little or no shrinkage or absorption, and have a very low rate of infection or rejection. Under most circumstances, autogenous tissue grafts can meet more of these criteria than can either homologous tissue grafts (e.g., eyebank-preserved sclera or preserved fascia lata) or alloplastic materials (e.g., Silastic, nylon, or Gore-tex). The following section discusses basic tissue harvesting techniques, including full-thickness skin grafts, split-thickness skin grafts, ear cartilage grafts, mucous membrane, nasal septal chondromucosal grafts, hard palate mucoperiosteal grafts, dermis fat grafts, fascia lata and temporalis fascia grafts.

SKIN GRAFTS

Full-Thickness Skin Grafts

A full-thickness skin graft contains both epidermal and dermal elements. For the eyelid, the best match of skin color and thickness is usually obtained from the contralateral upper eyelid but the amount of skin available may be insufficient in most cases. The retroauricular region and the supraclavicular regions provide good sources of donor skin, which can produce a good match. Donor sites that are second choices because they do not provide as good a match are the inner arm and the groin. All donor sites should be as hairless as possible to prevent trichiasis, although in many cases the dermal elements do not survive transplantation.

Contralateral Upper Lid

The skin match from this area is ideal but the amount is limited in supply and the potential for affecting the donor eye exists (Fig. 1A). A surgical marking pen is used to trace an outline of the area to be excised. A small amount of local anesthetic with epinephrine is used to diminish bleeding. The previously marked area is then incised, undermined, and excised freehand. The donor site can be closed directly. Excision of some of the underlying orbicularis fibers before closure can diminish tension on the skin and lagophthalmos.

Retroauricular Skin

The donor site is prepared with marking and injection (Fig. 1B). When excising the graft, one should try to remove as little subcutaneous tissue as possible along with the graft, but it is better to remove excess subcutaneous tissue than to buttonhole the graft. The graft is then inverted and placed on a single thickness of cotton gauze over the finger. Scissors are used to excise as much of the subcutaneous elements as possible so that the fine white color of the dermis with its associated rete pegs is visible. Some dermis removal can further thin the graft.

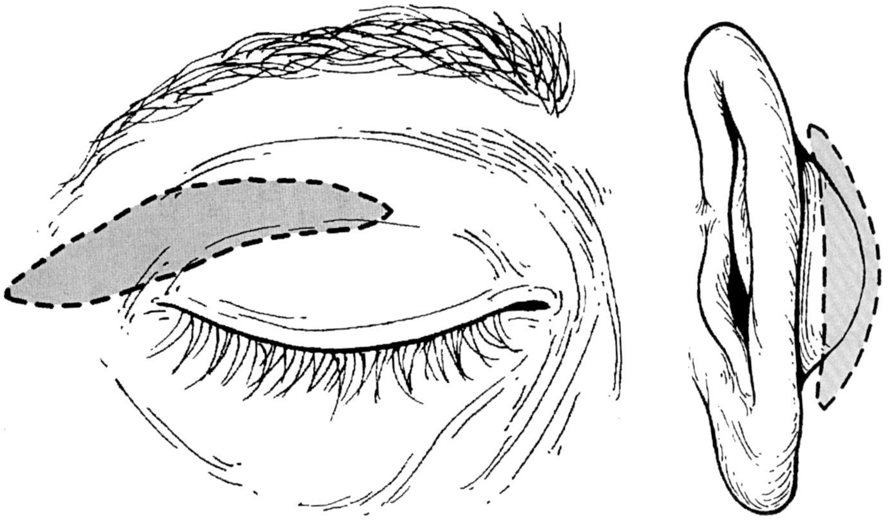

A B

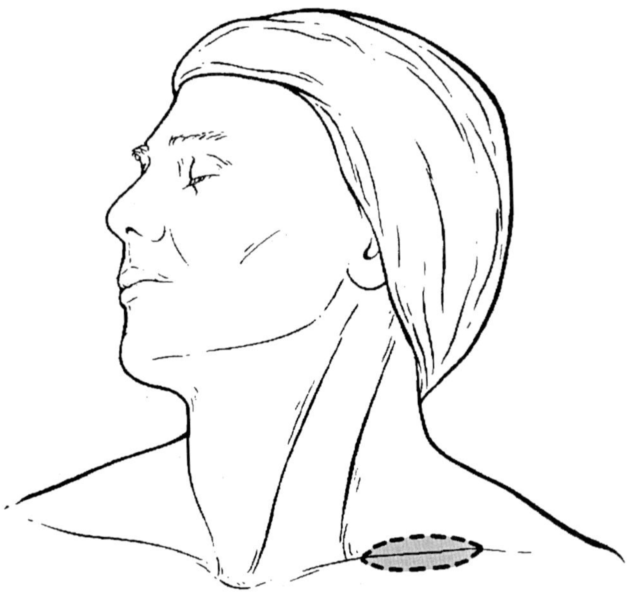

C

FIG. 1. A: Positioning of donor site of full-thickness skin graft from upper lid. This is the area of greatest laxity of skin in the upper lid and the area least likely to produce lagophthalmos. The area is infiltrated with red label xylocaine and marked. The skin is undermined from the underlying muscle with scissors and excised. **B:** Positioning of skin graft donor site in the retoauricular area. The graft generally straddles the posterior sulcus. There is a much thicker dermis in this area. Following removal of the graft, the graft is usually everted, stretched with tension, and the dermis trimmed from the undersurface. This thins the graft to prevent postoperative thickening and produce a better match. **C:** Donor site of graft from supraclavicular area. This is a common donor site location, particularly in the older age group. There is a very thick dermis underlying the skin. The skin should be peeled away from the underlying dermis with sharp dissection with a Bard-Parker blade, with an assistant tensing the area. The underlying dermis is then subsequently excised from the donor site so that closure of the supraclavicular area can be performed without tension on the skin edges. If performed in this manner, scarring is remarkably mild.

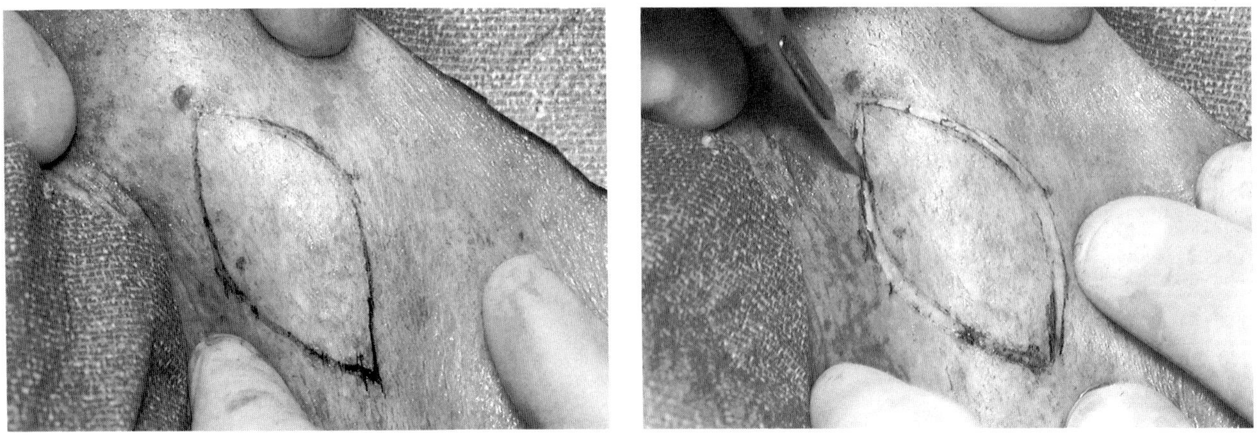

A B

FIG. 2. A: Outline of full-thickness skin graft to be taken from the supraclavicular area. **B:** Incision of the skin layer only with tension provided by assistant.

Supraclavicular Skin

The graft from the supraclavicular area is commonly used in the older patient (Fig. 1C) and is excised as shown in Fig. 2A–G. The graft is sutured into place on the host site using interrupted 6-0 silk sutures after graft bed hemostasis is assured. If the graft is very large, several tiny slits may be cut to drain any bleeding from the host site, preventing a hematoma from forming between graft and bed. After the full-thickness skin graft has been sutured into place (Fig. 3A), it is covered with a Telfa dressing. A sheet of softened dental wax is then molded over the Telfa dressing (Fig. 3B). The dental wax will conform to the shape of the tissue bed and prevent accumulation of fluids underneath the skin graft. A pressure dressing should be applied over the dental wax (Fig. 3C). The wound dressing and some of the sutures may be removed in 5 days. Antibiotic ointment is applied for several additional days, after which time the remaining skin sutures are removed. Postoperative compression of the graft produces a more even take of the graft and a smoother result.

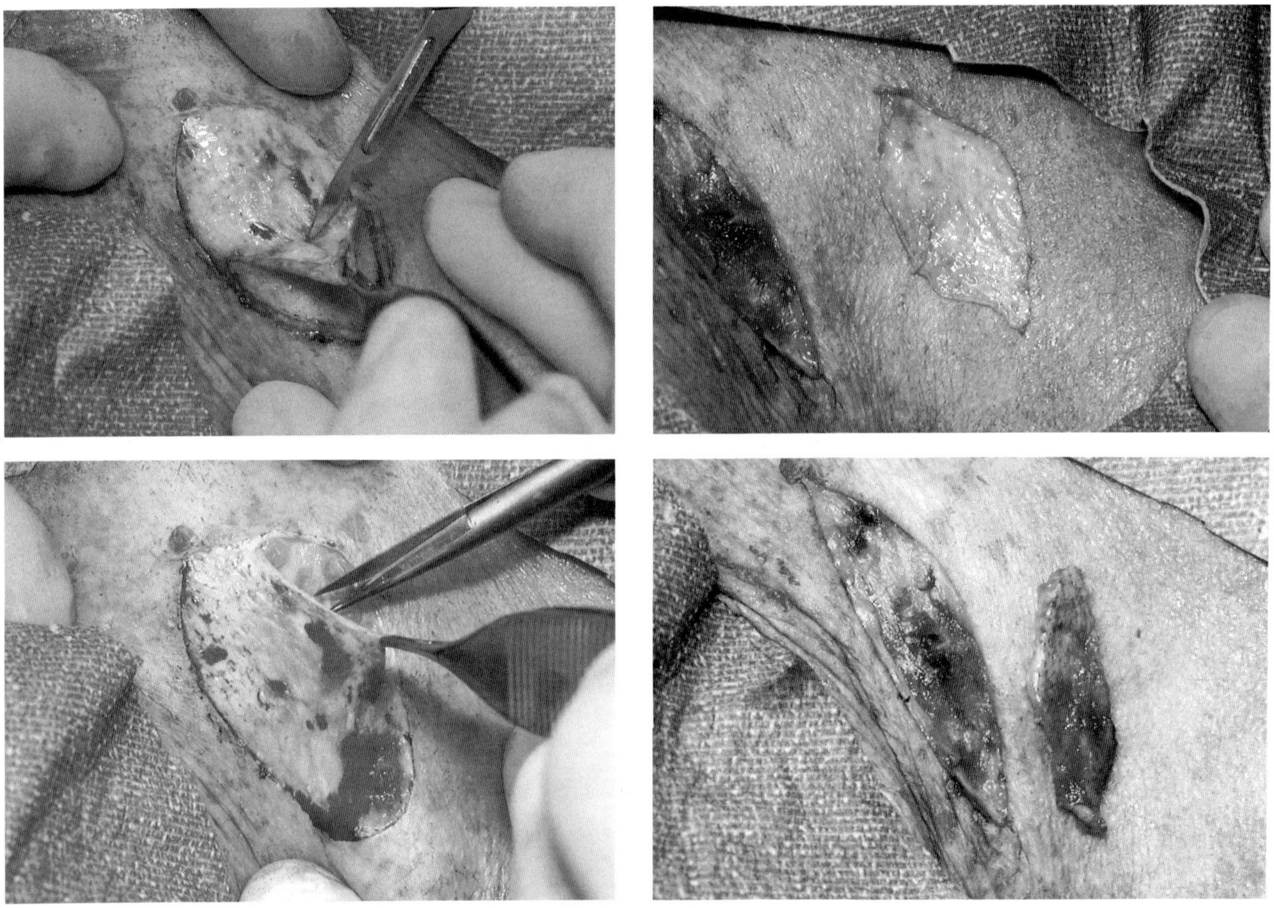

C D E F

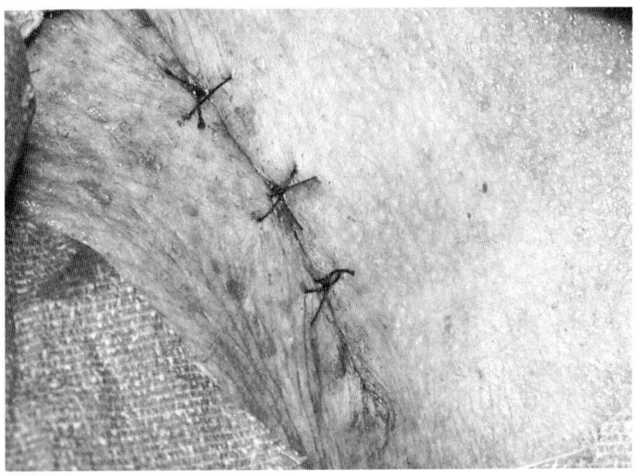

G

FIG. 2. *Continued.* **C:** Peeling of the skin from the underlying dermis with traction and dissection with a sharp blade. **D:** Undersurface of donor skin graft showing it free of dermis. **E:** Dissection of dermal layer from underlying fat and platysma muscle. **F:** Donor site following excision of dermis. The dermal graft is shown adjacent to the donor site and can be used if needed for filler. **G:** Closure of donor site with vertical mattress sutures and skin closure.

Split-Thickness Skin Grafts

The split-thickness skin graft is composed of epidermal elements only. A power-driven dermatome is used and the typical donor site is the anterior surface of the thigh. In general, split-thickness skin grafts have a poor texture, color-match to normal eyelid skin, and have a tendency to become pigmented. Their tendency to contract also mitigates against their use in routine eyelid and periocular reconstruction. The main use of split-thickness skin grafts in ophthalmic plastic and reconstructive surgery is for lining sockets and orbital cavities. However, in severe burn cases, there may be little or no full-thickness donor material available and the surgeon should be prepared to use split-thickness skin for eyelid coverage when there is no other choice.

The anterior surface of the thigh is prepped and draped in sterile fashion. If hair is excessive, it may be necessary to shave the anterior surface of the thigh. Both the anterior surface of the thigh and the dermatome are lubicated generously with sterile mineral oil. Following the insertion of a new blade, it is important to set the dermatome at the proper thickness, usually 12/1000 to 15/1000 of an inch. First the knob of the dermatome is turned clockwise until the zero mark is reached. At this point, the blade angle should be closed relative to the dermatome. The surgeon next turns the knob counterclockwise to the appropriate setting. The variable-width knob determining the width of the graft is set at the desired size. The assistant holds the lubricated thigh skin taut using two wooden tongue blades (Fig. 4A). The surgeon activates the dermatome and begins the steady advancement of the power-driven dermatome. Then the assistant picks up on the edges of the split-thickness skin graft with fine forceps as it comes out of the dermatome (Fig. 4B). When an adequate size split-thickness skin graft flap has been incised, the power of the dermatome is stopped. It is best to increase the width setting of the dermatome at this point so that it may easily be withdrawn with the graft sliding through still attached to the skin at the end of the graft. The surgeon excises the split-thickness

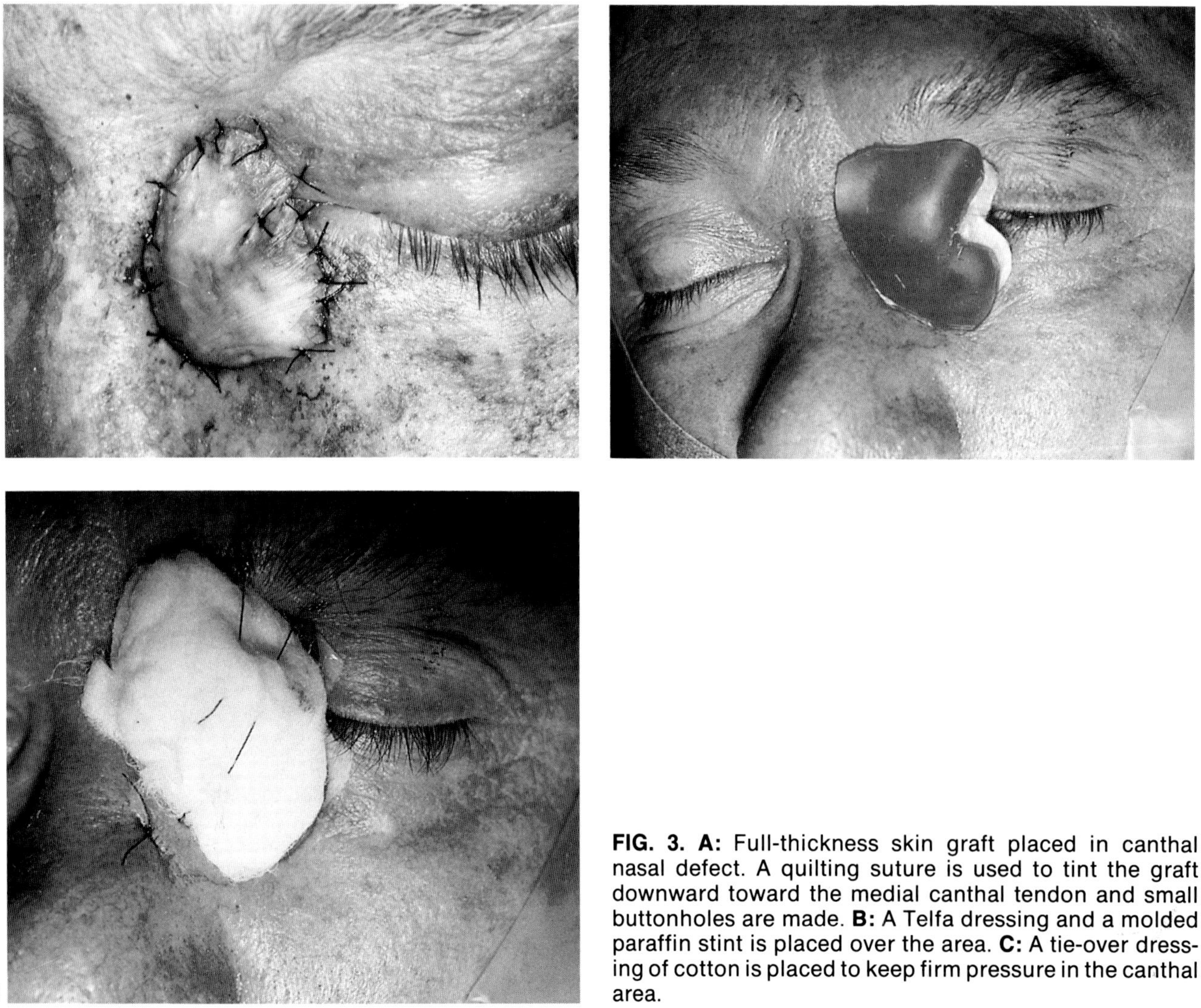

A B C

FIG. 3. A: Full-thickness skin graft placed in canthal nasal defect. A quilting suture is used to tint the graft downward toward the medial canthal tendon and small buttonholes are made. **B:** A Telfa dressing and a molded paraffin stint is placed over the area. **C:** A tie-over dressing of cotton is placed to keep firm pressure in the canthal area.

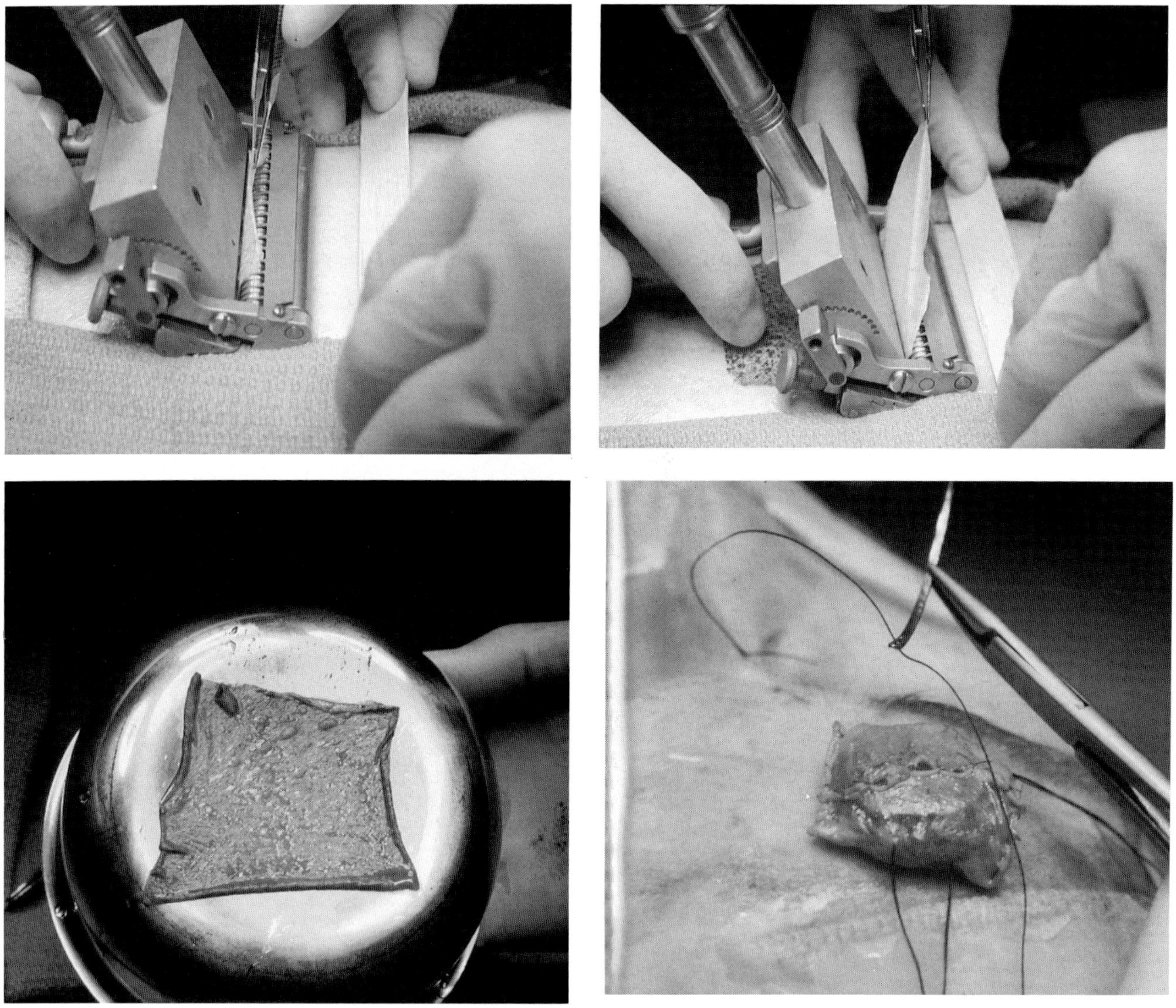

A B C D

FIG. 4. A: Split-thickness skin graft is taken from anterior thigh. The surface is lubricated with mineral oil and the skin surface preceding the dermatome head is kept flat with a tongue blade as the dermatome is advanced. **B:** As the dermatome is advanced, the skin graft, which exits through the top of the dermatome, is grasped and held under tension as it exits the dermatome. **C:** The graft is placed on a flat surface. **D:** In this instance the split skin graft is placed around a conformer for use in socket reconstruction. Split skin is not commonly used in eyelid surface repair but can be used as necessary in burn patients with loss of other donor areas.

skin graft from the donor site and places it on a surgical basin to maintain the correct orientation of the graft until it is placed in the desired location (Fig. 4C, D).

The anterior surface of the thigh should be wiped clean of mineral oil. A 4-in. × 4-in. gauze pad soaked in epinephrine is applied to the donor site and remains in place during the remainder of the procedure until final dressing of the donor site. Iodoform gauze covered with dry gauze pads is an adequate dressing for the donor site. The thigh can be gently wrapped in Kerlex gauze to maintain the dressings in place. Overly tight, constrictive bandages and tape should not be wrapped circumferentially around the thigh. Transparent wound dressings are also suitable for covering the split-thickness skin graft donor site, e.g., OpSite (Smith and Newton, Massillon, OH 04646), Uniflex (Pfizer).

EAR CARTILAGE GRAFTS

Successful eyelid reconstruction necessitates restoration of the posterior lamella of the eyelid. Freshly harvested autogenous ear cartilage is an excellent material for reconstruction of the posterior eyelid lamella (1). It furnishes rigid support and has the ability to become epithelialized over a period of several weeks. Ear

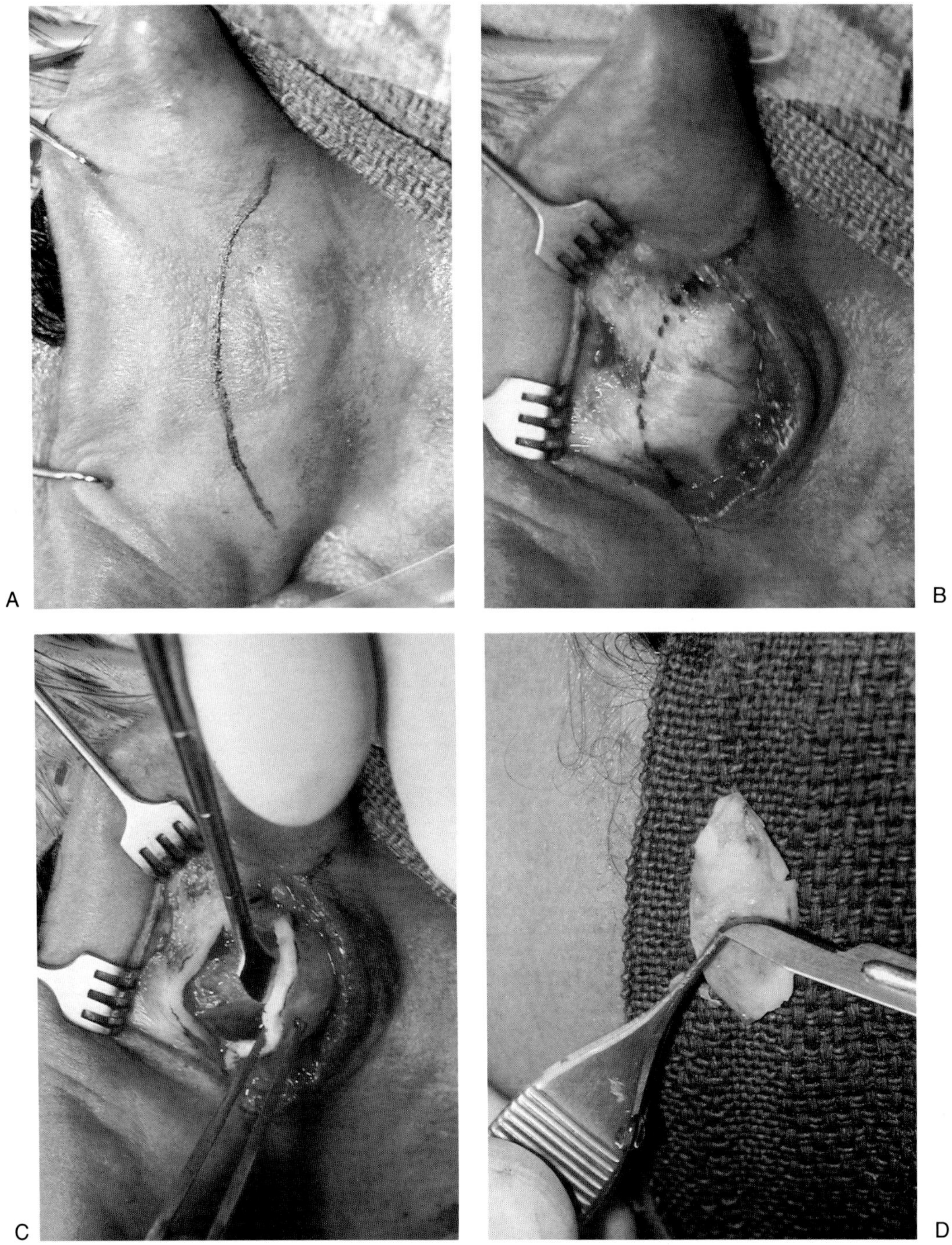

FIG. 5. Conchal cartilage graft. **A:** The ear has been everted and the proposed incision marked with methylene blue. **B:** The skin muscle subsutaneous tissue is elevated from the conchal portion of the ear. **C:** The conchal portion is dissected with blunt dissection from the anterior skin layer, which prevents buttonhole formation. **D:** The conchal cartilage, which is thicker than other areas, is trimmed of the extraneous surface tissue and thinned.

cartilage grafts are also useful to stabilize eyelids that have become structurally unsound such as complicated entropion of the upper or lower eyelid. The grafts' rigidity provides support to the eyelid and their ability to resist contraction postoperatively makes them an ideal spacer material for use within the lid or as posterior lamella substitute. The larger grafts when exposed to the conjunctiva can produce a temporary irritative conjunctivitis remedied with a cortisone-antibiotic ointment. The grafts are usually not used uncovered in the upper lid tarsus since they will be exposed directly to the corneal surface.

E

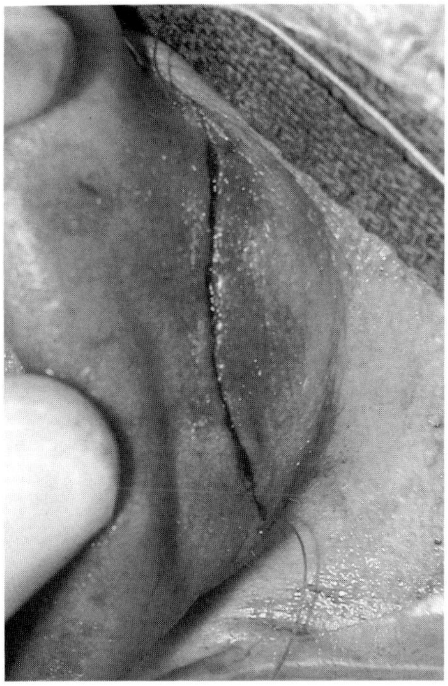

FIG. 5. *Continued.* **E:** Closure of the incision is accomplished with subcuticular 4-0 vicryl.

Conchal Cartilage

The grafts are excised as shown in Fig. 5A–C. The conchal ear cartilage grafts are thicker, with memory and a tendency to curl. Thinning of the graft is necessary and scoring one surface of the cartilage with a scalpel will help to flatten and relax the graft (Fig. 5D). Scoring a single surface of a cartilage graft with parallel lines will make that surface convex. When used for eyelid reconstruction, the concave surface of the cartilage should face the globe. Excessive passage of sutures through the grafts is to be avoided because they are brittle and will crumble with multiple attempts at suturing.

Scaphoid Area

This area provides cartilage that is most like tarsal plate in thickness and consistency. To obtain the graft, first the anterior and posterior skin of the scaphoid portion of the ear are infiltrated with local anesthetic with epinephrine and hyaluronidase. Skin hooks or sutures are used to reflect the ear to expose the posterior surface (Fig. 6A). A curvilinear line is marked parallel to the edge of the helix. This line should be 4 mm from the edge of the helix to avoid causing an ear deformity. The skin incision is made and then careful dissection is performed down to the level of ear cartilage exposing the posterior surface (Fig. 6B). The graft size is then marked with methylene blue on the exposed area (Fig. 6C). It is important to remain 4–5 mm from the edge of the ear to avoid producing a contour deformity. A scalpel is used to partially incise the cartilage and scissors are used to complete the incision through the full thickness of the cartilage avoiding penetration of the inner skin (Fig. 6D). A periosteal elevator is helpful in reflecting perichondrium and subcutaneous tissues off the anterior surface of the cartilage and scissors are then used to cut off the cartilage graft at its base. The scaphoid graft can also be scored if needed but it is usually not necessary (Fig. 6E). Good skin closure can be achieved with either a subcuticular 4-0 vicryl suture or a cutaneous silk suture closure (Fig. 6F). Cartilage may be stored in saline solution until needed later in the operation. If good hemostasis is achieved with electrocautery, only ice compresses are used post operatively.

MUCOUS MEMBRANE GRAFTS

For posterior lamella or eyelid margin resurfacing, it is necessary in most cases to use a mucous membrane graft. Mucous membrane is needed for reconstruction of the eyelid margin since the margin of the eyelid is the most intimate point of contact between the lid and the cornea and it is necessary to provide a smooth moist surface to the eyelid that will not produce corneal irritation (2). Buccal mucosa is the most ready supply of mucous membrane that can be grafted to the eyelid in these cases.

Full-Thickness Buccal Mucous Membrane

The graft donor site is usually the inner surface of the lower lip but additional grafts may be taken from

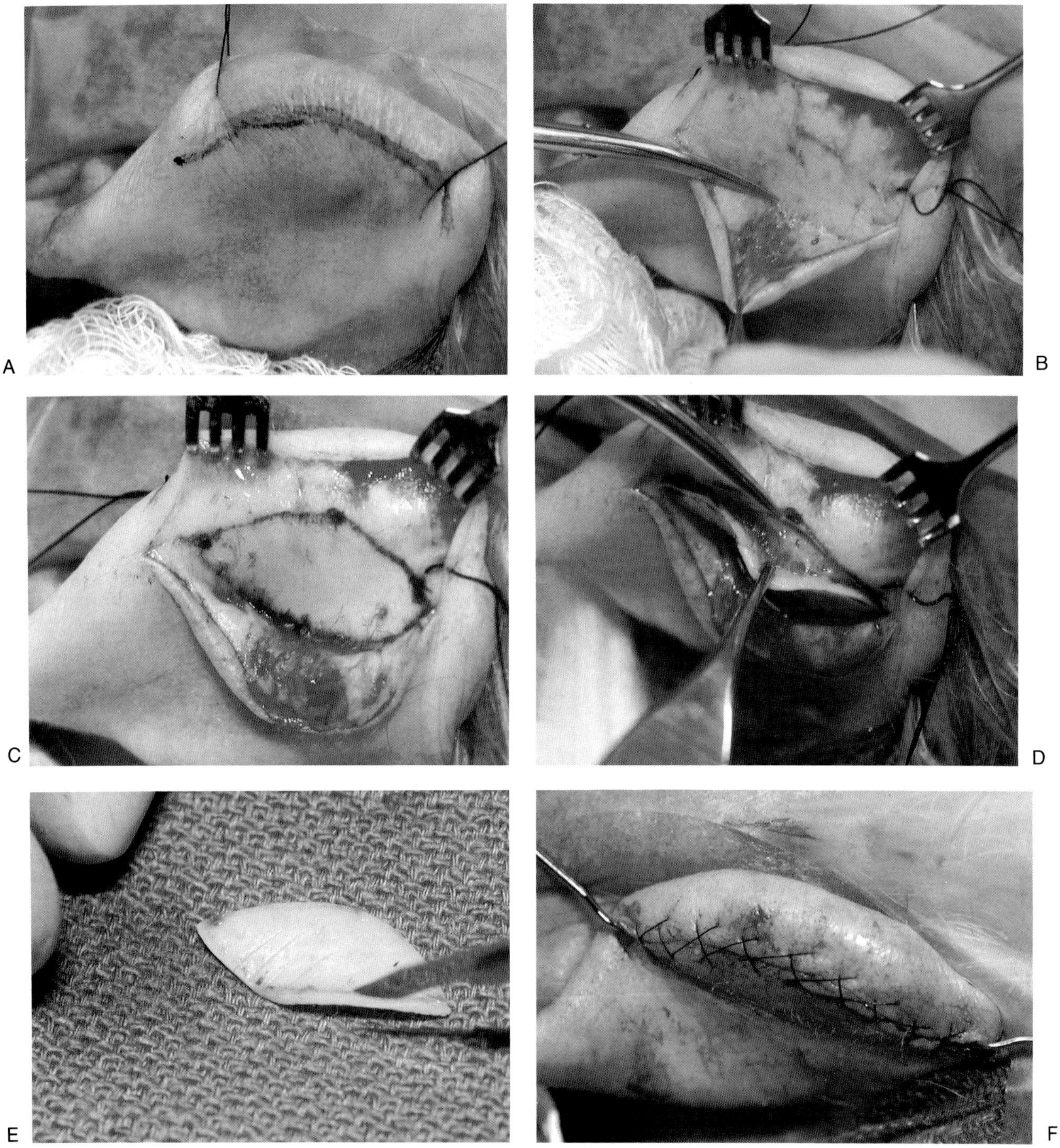

A B C D E F

FIG. 6. Scaphoid donor cartilage. **A:** The ear is everted with sutures or skin hooks and the incision line marked parallel to the curve of the ear. **B:** The skin muscle is elevated from the posterior surface of the scaphoid portion of the ear. **C:** The area of donor cartilage to be excised is marked with methylene blue. Care is taken to spare 4–5 mm of ear margin to prevent deformity. **D:** The cartilage is incised and with blunt dissection it is peeled away from the anterior skin muscle surface preserving perichondrium. **E:** The cartilage can be shaped and trimmed but is normally flat and pliable. **F:** The donor incision site is closed with mattress sutures of subcuticular vicryl.

the inner cheek or the upper lip if necessary. The graft should be outlined in such a way as to avoid the vermilion margin of the lips, the gum, and Stensen's duct (opposite the second upper molar). To diminish bleeding and obtain a dissection plane, the mucosa is infiltrated with lidocaine 2% with epinephrine 1:100,000 and hyaluronidase. The proposed graft is outlined with methylene blue (Fig. 7A) and then an incision is made with a number 15 blade (Fig. 7B). Because mucosal grafts tend to contract, they are usually made slightly

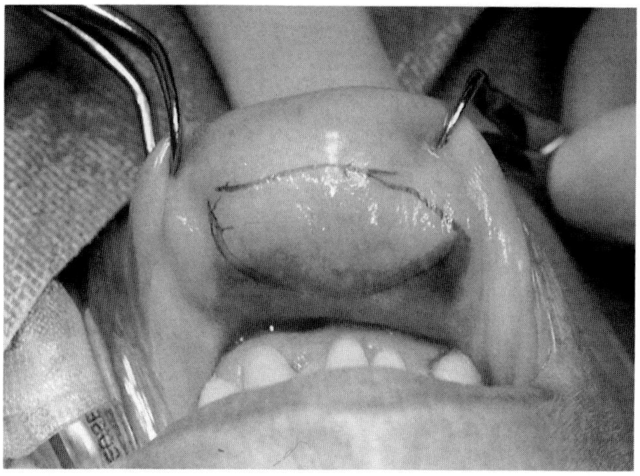
A

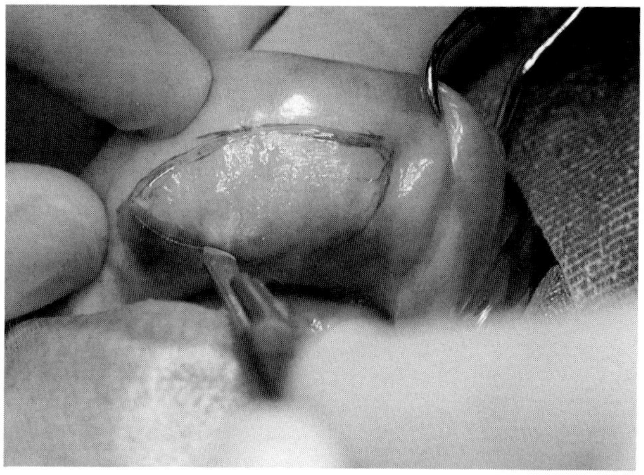
B

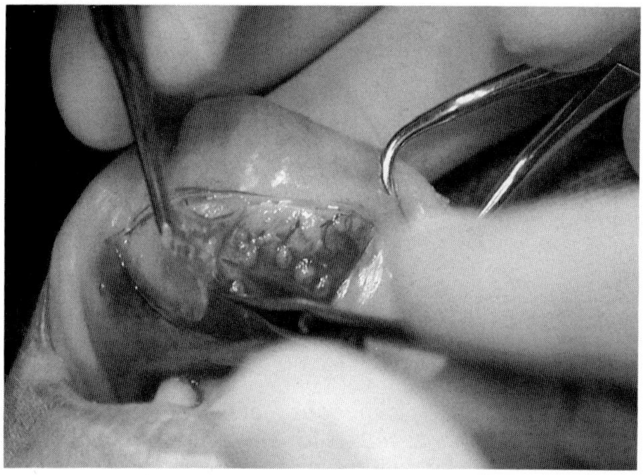
C

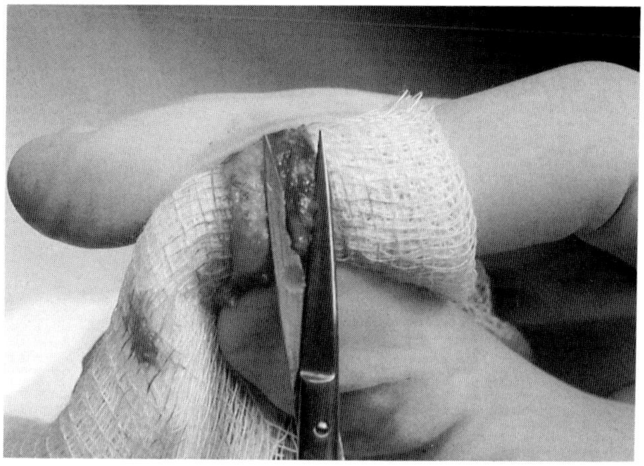
D

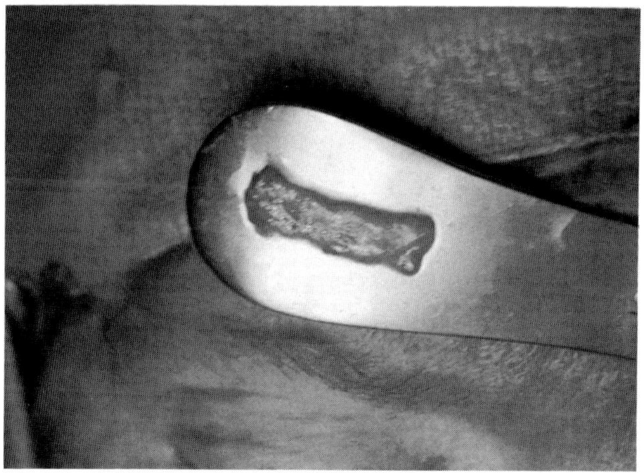
E

FIG. 7. Full-thickness buccal mucous membrane graft. This graft is usually taken from the inner surface of the lip or cheek. **A:** The lip is everted and the donor site, which has been infiltrated with red label xylocaine, has been marked. Anesthesia of the lower lid can be obtained by a mental block and local infiltration of the lip. A Castroviejo clamp or towel hooks can be used to evert the lower lip. **B:** The mucous membrane in the donor site is incised. **C:** The mucous membrane is undermined from the underlying tissue and salivary glands with scissors. Gelfoam is placed on the donor site. **D:** The graft is then placed on a flat surface. **E:** In many cases there is thickened redundant tissue that can be trimmed from the posterior surface of the graft to thin the graft. This is best accomplished when it is placed on stretch.

larger than the size of the proposed donor site. A full-thickness graft is removed with sharp and blunt scissor dissection (Fig. 7C). The graft is then thinned further removing submucosal tissue with scissors (Fig. 7D). Because the tissue graft is harvested from a nonsterile area, the oral cavity, the graft is placed in antibiotic solution, where it remains until needed later in the operation (Fig. 7E). Closure of the oral cavity donor site is not necessary. Electrocautery is to be used minimally since it makes the recovery period more painful for the patient. A dry gelfoam pad is placed over the donor site after harvesting the mucous membrane graft. The mucous membrane defect in the mouth will reepithelialize over several weeks. A dilute peroxide rinse and bacitracin oinment or petroleum jelly applied to the donor site can reduce postoperative discomfort. Ointment at night is particularly important to prevent the donor site from adhering to the teeth.

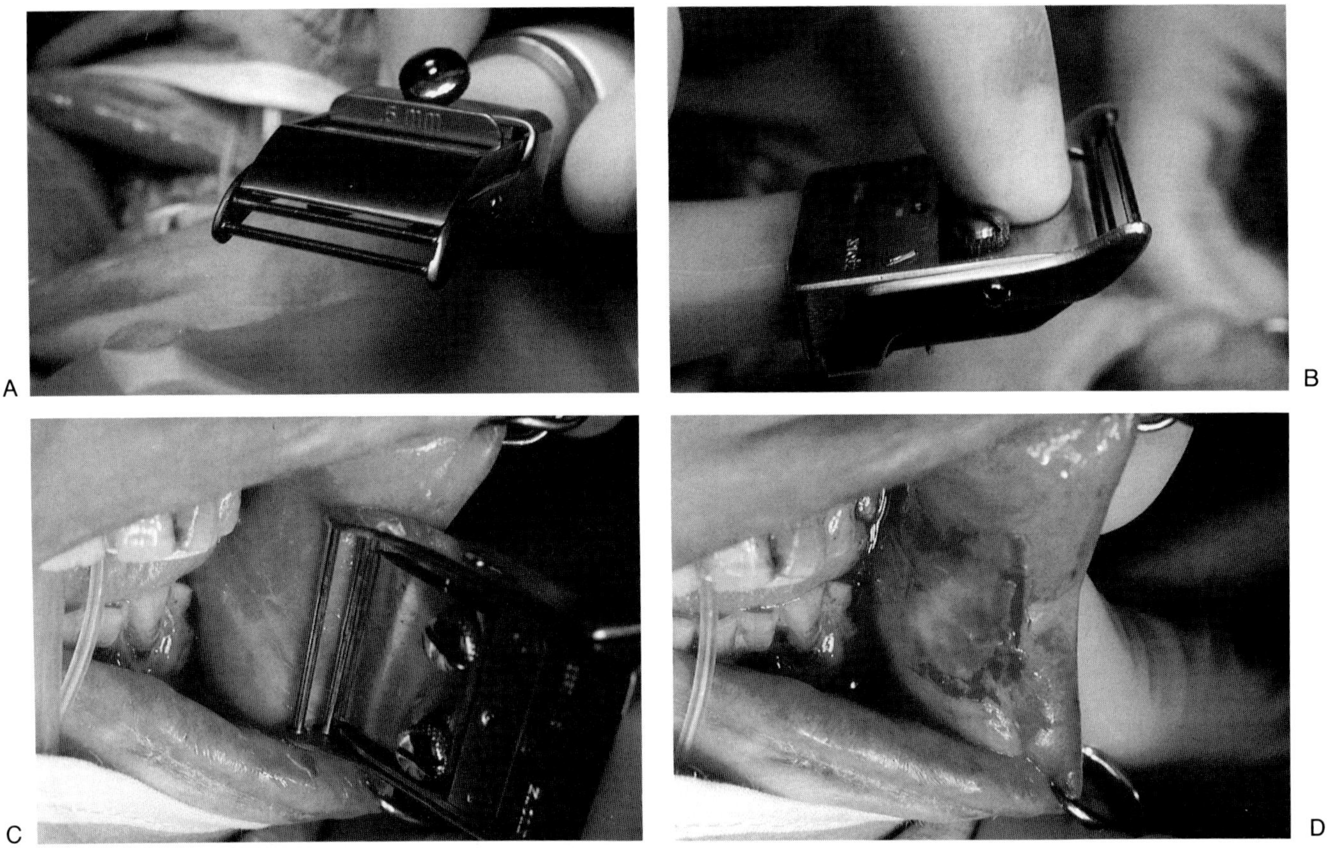

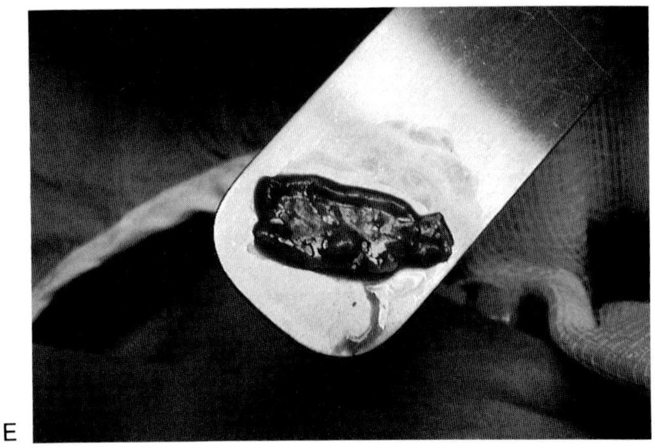

FIG. 8. Split-thickness mucous membrane grafts, thinner grafts 0.1–0.2 mm are used for ocular surface grafts but will shrink if placed on the eyelid margin or fornix. Thicker grafts of 0.5 mm can be taken with the mucotome for grafts to the lid margin. **A:** A Castroviejo mucotome with 0.5-mm shim in place. **B:** The mucotome must be oiled properly and resist loss of vibration with gentle finger pressure in order to ensure adequate cutting velocity. **C:** Flat tension must be created in the donor site for the mucotome to cut evenly. This can be accomplished with finger indentation and towel clips or the Castroviejo lip holder. **D:** The typical appearance of the donor site following excision of the split graft. **E:** Thin grafts can be confusing as to which is the epithelial side. The split graft is normally slid from the donor site with cut surface downward onto a smooth metal retractor to prevent disorientation of the cut surface.

Split-Thickness Buccal Mucous Membrane

Split-thickness mucous membrane grafts can be harvested with a Castroviejo mucotome with a 0.1- to 0.5-mm setting (Fig. 8A,B). The mucotome is prepared and the lip or cheek placed under tension, lubricated with mineral oil, and the appropriate thickness graft is excised in the same manner as a dermatome harvesting split skin grafts (Fig. 8C,D). The graft must be slid from the donor site, cut surface down, onto a smooth metal retractor to retain orientation of the surfaces (Fig. 8E). When applied to the eyelid or socket, the thinner grafts (0.1–0.3 mm) will tend to shrink and dry out over a period of time and very thin grafts should be reserved for use on the surface of the globe. Ideally grafts of 0.4–0.5 mm thickness should be used on the eyelid margin or posterior eyelid surface.

RIGID MUCOUS MEMBRANE–LINED GRAFTS

When reconstruction of both the mucosal surface and its supporting elements is necessary in the eyelid posterior lamella, a composite graft containing a rigid element with a mucous membrane lining is necessary. A rigid mucous membrane–lined graft can be obtained

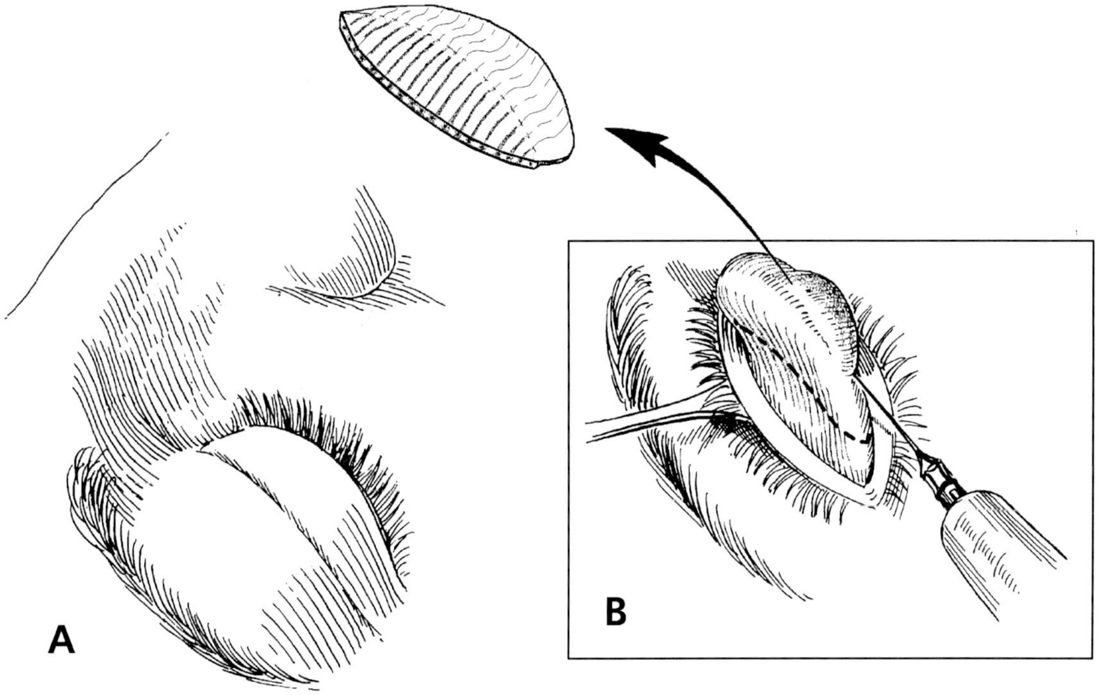

FIG. 9. Tarsoconjunctival graft from upper lid. **A:** The upper lid is everted over a Desmarr retractor and infiltrated with xylocaine. **B:** A full-thickness incision is made excising the superior 40% of the tarsal plate and dissection of the cuff of conjunctiva (free of Müller's muscle) of approximately 5 mm.

from tarsoconjunctiva from an upper lid, nasal chondral mucosa, or hard palate mucoperiosteum. There is an alternative to these composite grafts that necessitates a two-stage procedure. In the first stage, an appropriate-sized ear cartilage graft is harvested in the usual fashion. This cartilage graft is then inserted in a submucosal pocket in the cheek of the patient. Five to six weeks must elapse for adequate vascularization of the cartilage and overlying mucous membrane graft to occur. After this occurs, a composite cartilage–mucous membrane graft can be harvested in the second stage of the procedure for use in eyelid reconstruction.

Tarsoconjunctival Grafts

If the upper lids are intact, autogenous tarsoconjunctiva taken from the inner lamella of the upper lid is available to reconstruct the posterior lamella of an eyelid (3,4). The main limiting factor in the use of this graft is the reticence to use tissue for which there is only one opportunity for a graft at the donor site. The technique is performed with local anesthetic. The upper lid is infiltrated with anesthetic with adequate time allowed to elapse for hemostasis. A traction suture is placed through the upper lid margin so that the upper lid can be everted under tension (Fig. 9A,B). Additional local anesthetic can be infiltrated into the subconjunctival space at the everted exposed superior tarsal border. Methylene blue is used to mark the donor site along the upper lid tarsal plate (Fig. 11A). It is important to spare at least 4 mm of tarsus above the upper lid margin to maintain the proper shape and integrity of the upper lid postoperatively. The free tarsal conjunctival graft is harvested from the superior border of the tarsus (Fig. 10). A number 15 blade is used to

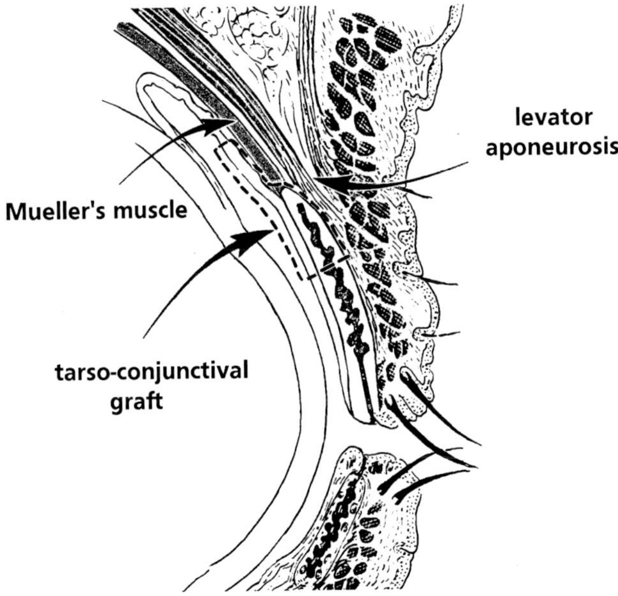

FIG. 10. Sagittal view showing the area of tarsoconjunctival tissue that is used as a free graft.

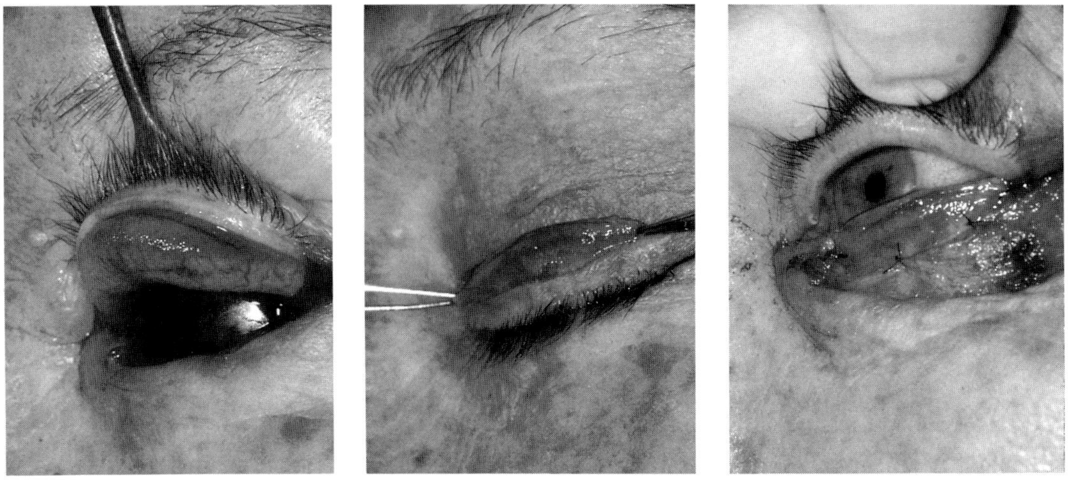

FIG. 11. A: Clinical slide showing the upper lid being everted and marked for excision of tarsoconjunctival graft. B: The tarsoconjunctival graft has been excised and the tarsoconjunctival cuff can be seen. C: The tarsoconjunctival graft has been placed in a lower lid defect to reconstruct the posterior lamella. The tarsal portion of the graft is sutured to the inferior portion of the defect.

make a partial thickness tarsoconjunctival incision on three sides. Sharp–Westcott scissors are then used to complete the incision of the tarsus and dissection and excision of the graft. The free graft is severed from the upper lid by incising the superior border conjunctival and Müller's muscle attachments. Bipolar wet-field cautery can be used to maintain good hemostasis. It is not necessary to close the donor site. Despite possible disinsertion of Müller's muscle at the superior tarsal border, ptosis is not usually seen postoperatively although some initial edema may be present. The tarsoconjunctival graft is most commonly used for lower lid reconstruction but can be used in any area requiring a rigid, mucous membrane–lined graft (see Fig. 11B,C).

Composite Eyelid-Margin Grafts

A full-thickness eyelid section from the upper or lower lid (Fig. 12A) can be used to replace a defect in the posterior lamella and margin of the eyelid. It is useful in correcting margin deformities and provides the possibility of eyelash replacement. The grafts are usually denuded of skin and muscle up to the lash follicles (Fig. 12B) to provide a suface for vascular ingrowth and are placed under a myocutaneous flap. The use of these grafts is discussed in the chapters on eyelid reconstruction. Retention of lashes in these grafts is a good bit less than 100% but the margin reconstruction is excellent.

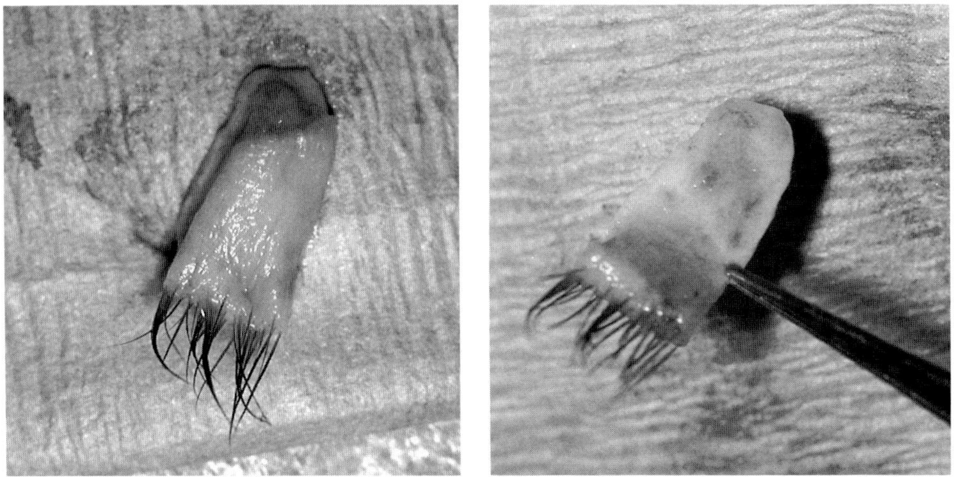

FIG. 12. Composite graft. A: Shows full-thickness section of eyelid with skin muscle, tarsoconjunctival layer, and margin intact. B: Composite graft with the skin muscle layer excised sparing the margin hair follicle. The bare tarsus area of the graft is placed under a myocutaneous flap in the recipient eyelid.

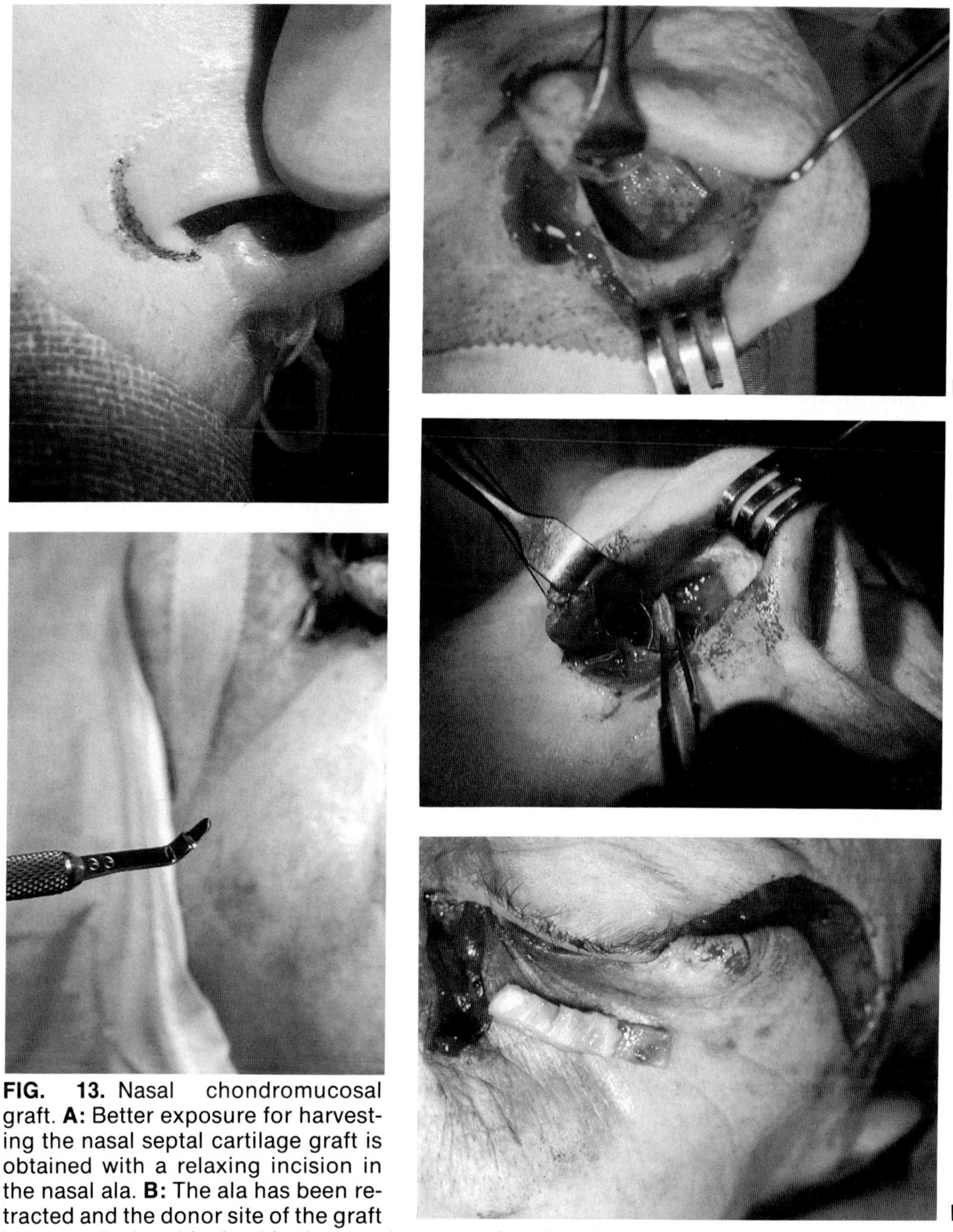

A

B

C

D

E

FIG. 13. Nasal chondromucosal graft. **A:** Better exposure for harvesting the nasal septal cartilage graft is obtained with a relaxing incision in the nasal ala. **B:** The ala has been retracted and the donor site of the graft been marked and incised in the nasal septum. Care is taken to incise only the mucosa on the nostril side and the cartilage, sparing the mucosa on the contralateral side. **C:** The dissection and incisions can be carried out with the angled Beaver blade. **D:** The cartilage can be grasped and dissected free from the opposing nasal mucous membrane with a blunt dissector. **E:** The nasal septal cartilage graft is most commonly used to reconstruct the posterior lamellar of the lower lid with a Mustarde flap. This shows the rotational flap in position with the donor graft on its surface before suturing it to the posterior surface of the flap.

Nasal Chondromucosal Grafts

As an alternative, the oculoplastic surgeon must be familiar with nasal chondromucosal harvesting techniques (5). Injection of nasal mucous membrane with lidocaine and packing with 4% cocaine provides hemostasis. A 4-0 silk retention suture is placed through the nasal ala and a flat, relaxing incision is made through the ala in the plane of the facial skin (Fig. 13A). Retraction of the nasal ala allows excellent exposure of the nasal septum. A rectangular strip of tissue, 10 × 5 mm, oriented parallel to the direction of the turbinates is outlined. The strip should include nasal mucosa and cartilage but should not penetrate nasal mucosa on the opposite side of the cartilage (Fig. 13B). A periosteal elevator may be inserted to protect the contralateral septal mucosa. The graft is elevated with a razor knife or number 64 Beaver blade. An angulated number 66 Beaver blade or Cottle knife is best for making the most posterior cut (Fig. 13C). A periosteal elevator can be used to dissect bluntly between cartilage and opposite mucosa, which is to be left behind in the donor site (Fig. 13D). The nasal ala is then resutured with interrupted 4-0 silk and the naris packed with petroleum jelly–impregnated gauze placed in the cut finger of a latex surgical glove (fingercot packing). The cartilage is trimmed with an iris scissors or scalpel to approximately one half the original width and thickness. The graft is sutured into place using interrupted 6-0 vicryl sutures, making certain that the mucosal side is in correct alignment (Fig. 13E). Since this is a free graft, it is necessary to appose it with a skin flap containing its own blood supply rather than with another graft such as a skin graft. Its most common use is in combination with a myocutaneous flap in lower lip reconstruction.

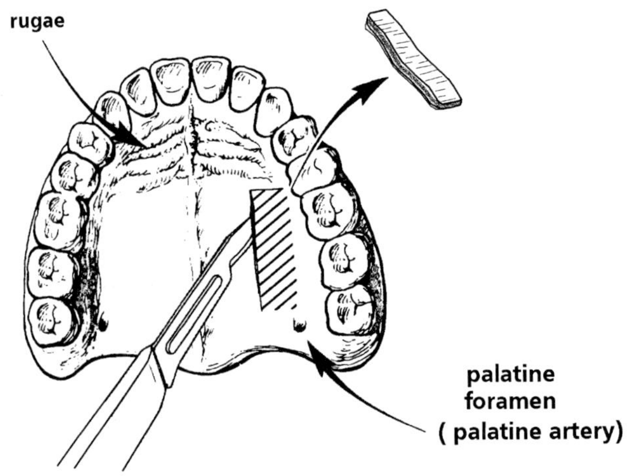

FIG. 14. Hard palate mucoperiosteal graft. This graft is commonly used to reconstruct the posterior lamella of the eyelid. It is rigid and has a mucous membrane lining. The thickness varies from 3 to 5 mm. When excising the graft from the hard palate, care is taken to avoid penetrating the palatine artery at its foramen in order to prevent excessive bleeding. Grafts can be taken from either side of the palate. A stint can be used postoperatively to protect the donor site from abrasions, which can produce discomfort in the postoperative period.

Hard Palate Mucosal Graft (Mucoperiosteum)

A hard palate mucosal graft is useful in reconstruction of the posterior lamella of the eyelid (6–8). These autogenous grafts are most useful in correcting lower eyelid retraction associated with dysthyroid orbitopathy, cicatricial lower lid entropion or retraction with deficient tarsus, and in reconstruction of eyelid tarsal defects. Hard palate mucosal grafts are stiff enough to bolster the posterior lamella of the eyelid yet are soft and pliable enough to conform readily to the curvature of the globe. The naturally keratinizing hard palate mucosa loses its keratin later when grafted into the ocular conjunctiva environment. This epithelial transition requires several weeks, such that these grafts should generally be avoided in upper lid reconstruction as they can be poorly tolerated by the cornea.

Harvesting the hard palate mucosal graft is performed after the hard palate donor site is infiltrated with a mixture of lidocaine 2%, marcaine 0.5%, epinephrine 1:100,000, and hyaluronidase. Adequate time is allowed to elapse for the hemostatic effect of the epinephrine. A headlight can illuminate the hard palate during harvesting of the graft. A suction apparatus must be available on the surgical field to aid visualization during the procedure and or remove blood and fluids from the patient's oropharynx. Methylene blue is used to mark the hard palate mucosa donor site. There is quite a lot of variation in size and shape of any given patient's hard palate, but in general hard palate mucosal graft taken will generally be 7–10 mm wide and 25–30 mm in length. The methylene blue marking is made between the alveolar ridge anteriorly and extends posteriorly to within 1–2 mm of the soft palate (see Fig. 14). The graft is harvested avoiding the midline and the foramen of the palatine artery is present at the junction of the hard and soft palates opposite the third molar. A number 15 blade is used to make two long parallel incisions that are the desired length of the graft. These incisions generally should not extend full thickness down through the level of mucoperiosteum. Once infiltrated with local anesthetic, the hard palate mucosa will be 3–5 mm thick, such that making a partial-thickness incision is not difficult if desired. A number 66 Beaver blade (right-angled blade) is helpful to undermine each side of the graft. If a full-thickness mucoperiosteal graft is desired, a sharp periosteal elevator is used to elevate the graft from the hard palate. Posteriorly, the surgeon must take care to avoid the hard palate–soft palate junction and the palatine artery foramen. Sharp–Wescott scissors can then be used to excise the entire graft. The graft should then be placed in appropriate antibiotic solution before being used in the eyelid recipient site. The hard palate should be inspected to verify that an intact layer of mucoperiosteum is present unless a full-thickness graft has been utilized. Cautery can be applied to help achieve good hemostasis. Gelfoam soaked in local anesthetic with epinephrine is applied to the hard palate site. In this manner the hemostasis will be maintained and the patient will remain comfortable throughout the remainder of the surgical procedure.

For patients with significant postoperative discomfort, topical viscous xylocaine jelly and/or periodontal paste may be of some use during the first 2–4 days following surgery. For very significant discomfort, an oral surgeon consultant can be used to fashion a temporary obturator plate to protect the raw hard palate. The donor site will partially fill in with granulation tissue and heal fully within 2–4 weeks.

DERMIS-FAT GRAFTS

The autogenous composite dermis-fat graft initially gained an importance in the management of the anophthalmic socket (9). This graft serves as an excellent replacement of the extruding implant and is a natural socket expander in anophthalmic states with inadequate mucous membranes. Subcutaneous defects in the upper lid, brow, and malar area can be well filled out with this dermis-fat graft. They also serve as an excellent tissue graft for facial soft tissue defects. The inclusion of the dermis with the fatty tissue increases early vascularization of the grafts, reducing absorption, and also allows a greater ease of positioning the grafts. A 25–30% absorption rate is expected.

Donor dermis and fat can be obtained easily from the iliac crest area, buttock, breast, or supraclavicular

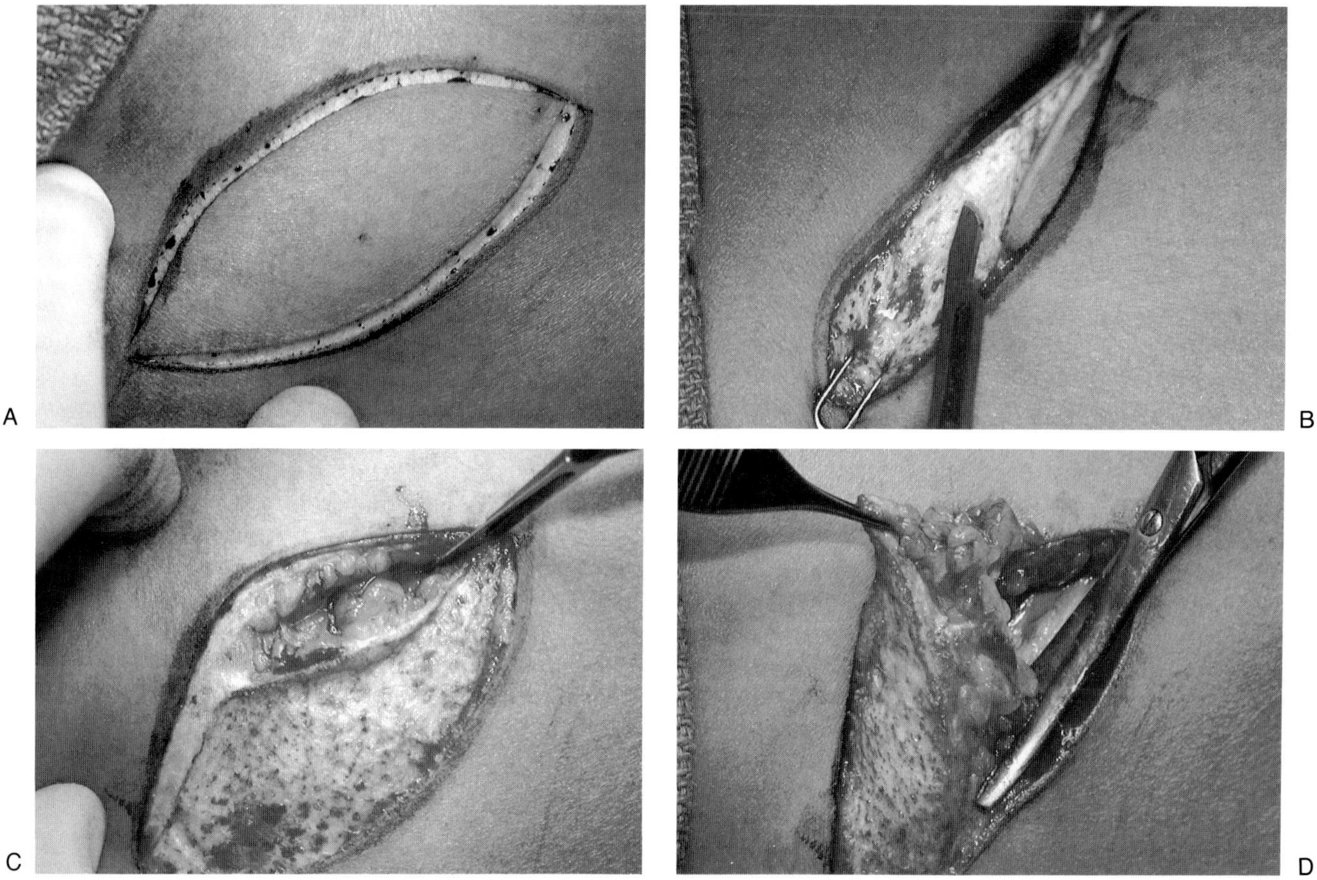

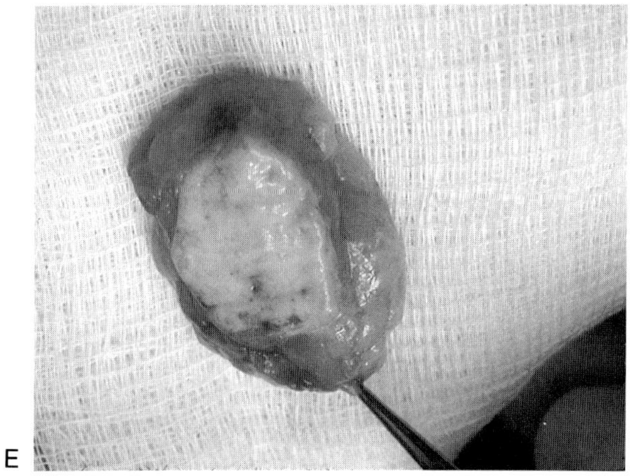

FIG. 15. Dermis-fat graft. The most common donor site is the roll of fat above the iliac crest. **A:** Outline of the donor site and incision through the skin. **B:** The skin is peeled away from the underlying dermis with sharp dissection. Tension on the edges is needed for smooth dissection. **C:** The dermis is then incised vertically throughout the entire outline of the graft into the fat. **D:** Scissors are used to excise dermis and attached fat from the underlying tissue. Square vertical edges are necessary for subsequent closure of the donor site. It is commonly necessary to trim additional fat to produce vertical edges in the donor site. The donor site must be closed with layers of deep sutures to prevent hematoma formation. **E:** Typical configuration of dermis-fat graft used for socket reconstruction. Elliptical grafts can be used for upper lid sulcus augmentation and other depressed areas in the lid-periorbital location.

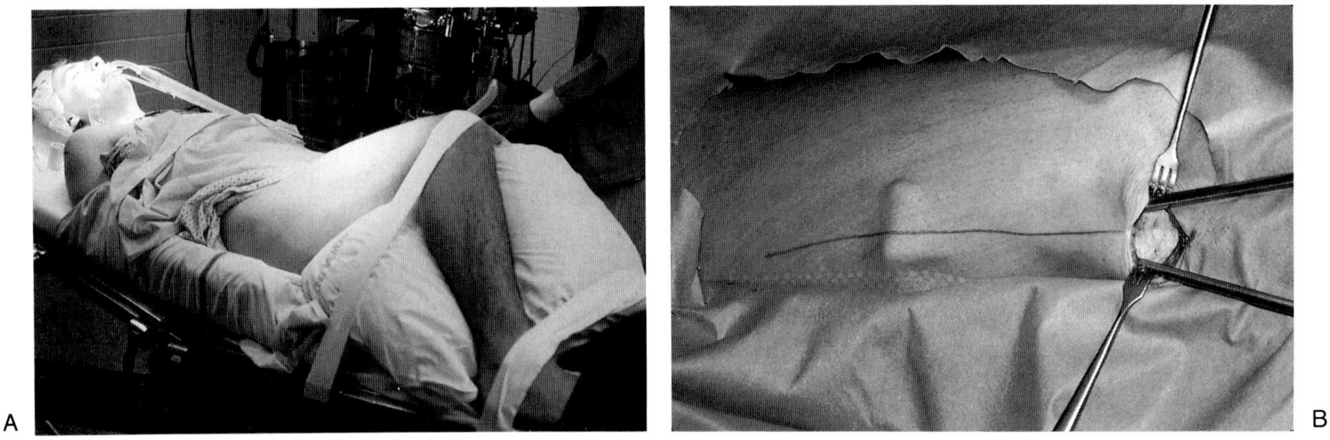

FIG. 16. Fascia lata graft. **A:** Figure shows proper positioning of the patient's leg to create tension on the fascia lata. The ideal position is for the leg to be flexed and intorted over a pillow, taping at the knee and ankle to the operative table. An alternative position is to have the leg extended with internal rotation of the foot. With either technique, adequate tension must be created on the fascia lata to allow the stripper to proceed smoothly. **B:** The skin overlying the fascia lata must be undermined. A line has been drawn from the incision site just above the knee laterally in a line that should parallel the fibers of the fascia lata. Undermining on the undersurface of the fascia is not needed.

area. The best donor site is usually the patient's lower abdominal quadrant or flank. This graft can be harvested with the patient in the usual supine position. This site is less prone to be tender, and is non–weight bearing, unlike the lateral portion of the thigh or buttock. The surgical site is locally infiltrated with lidocaine 2% with epinephrine 1:100,000 and hyaluronidase. An ellipse is next outlined on the skin. The ultimate diameter of the harvested dermis-fat graft should not exceed 25 mm and will usually be 20 mm or less. A skin incision is made with a number 15 blade (Fig. 15A). The epidermal layer is then sharply dissected off the dermis (Fig. 15B). This is important to prevent the subsequent formation of epidermal inclu-

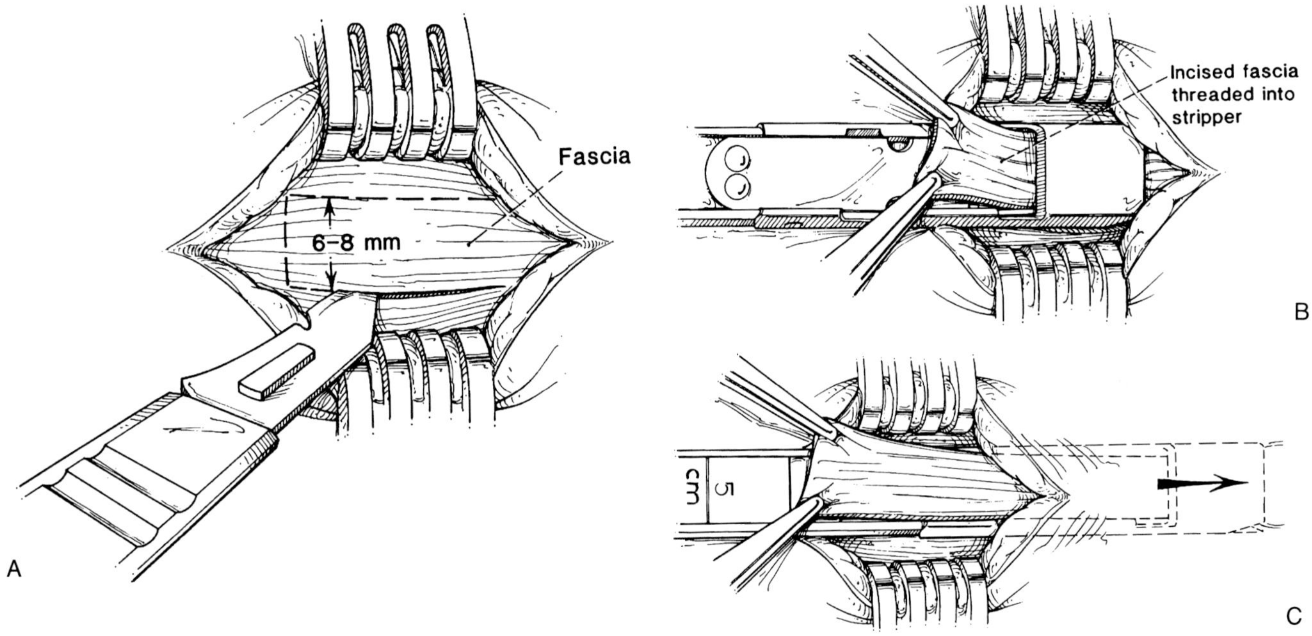

FIG. 17. A: The fascia is usually incised in two areas creating a strip of fascia 6–8 mm in width. **B:** A tab of fascia is elevated and threaded through the Crawford stripper. **C:** The fascial stripper is then advanced in the dissected plane with the side cutting edges, making incisions to create the fascial strip. If the Crawford separator has been used to precut the two longitudinal incisions, the side cutting edges are not needed and the stripper is simply advanced.

sion cysts. Holding the knife perpendicular to the dermal face, an incision is made through the dermis, following the outline of the ellipse (Fig. 15C). Holding the scalpel perpendicularly is important in harvesting an adequate-sized composite graft. Beveling of the blade will yield a cone-shaped graft with inadequate fatty tissue and cause difficulty in closure of the donor site. The entire plug of dermis and fat is held up and excised at its base with a scissors (Fig. 15D,E). Interrupted 3-0 chromic sutures with buried knots are used to close the fat layer and interrupted 4-0 prolene sutures with buried knots are used to close the dermis and subcutaneous tissues. It is this closure that will maintain the strength of the wound. Skin staples are used and provide excellent everting action of the skin edges. Staples are removed in 1 week. All patients in whom autogenous tissue grafts are used are placed on oral cephalosporins for 5–7 days.

FASCIA GRAFTS

Fascia grafts can be obtained from the lateral surface of the thigh (10,11) or from the overlying temporalis muscle (12). However, the temporal fascia is not as abundant or sturdy as fascia lata.

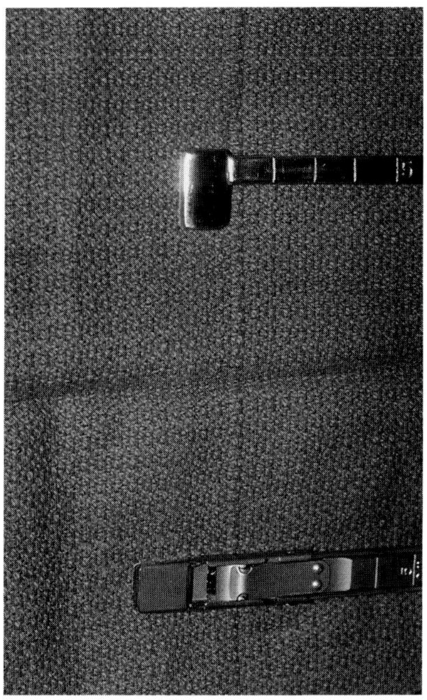

A

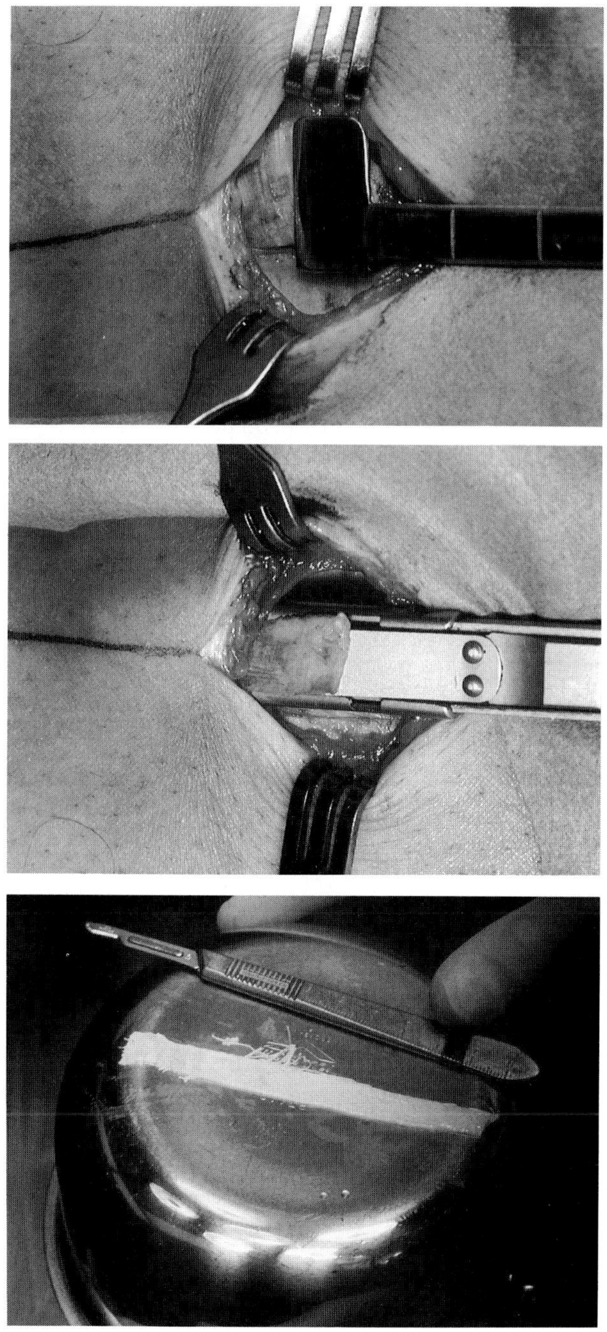

B

C

D

FIG. 18. Strip dissection with the Crawford separator and stripper. **A:** Since the side cutting mechanisms on the Crawford stripper can become dull, a separate Crawford separator device is used to create the long parallel incisions before using the stripper and its guillotine cutting device. The Crawford separator and stripper are shown. **B:** The Crawford separator is inserted through the initial parallel incisions and advanced in the leg creating two long parallel incisions before cutting the tab. **C:** The two long incisions have been made with the separator. The tab at the end has been cut and the fascia threaded through the Crawford stripper, which is then advanced. The side cutting edge of the stripper is not used, only the guillotine cutting device at the end. This seems to provide a more reliable method of fascia excision. **D:** This shows the usual amount of fascia lata obtained. The graft is then cut into 3-mm longitudinal strips.

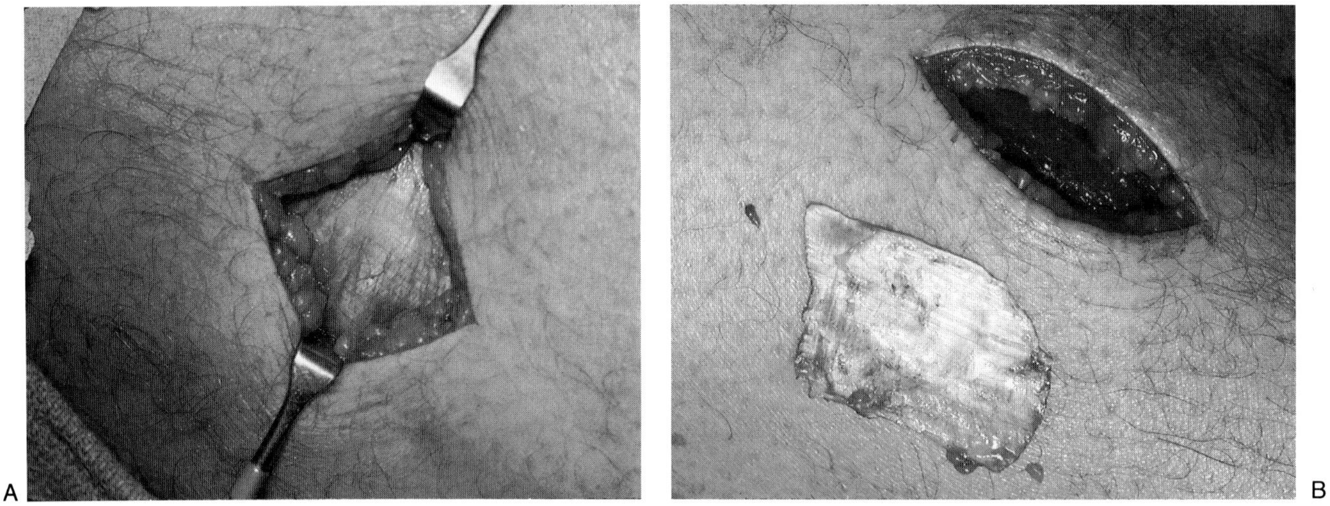

FIG. 19. Sheet fascia lata. **A:** A 5-cm incision is made on the lateral thigh exposing the fasica lata. The area is then undermined and incisions can be made in the fascia beyond the extent of the incision. **B:** Sheet of fascia obtained from the lateral thigh. Endoscopic visualization can also be used to make a fascial incision through a small incision and acquire a larger sheet of fascia.

Fascia Lata

Adequate amounts of fascia are quite easy to obtain in the adult but can be somewhat difficult in the child with a short thigh. For ease of stripping, the leg must be positioned to produce tension on the fascia lata (Fig. 16A). A skin incision 3–4 cm in length should be made in the lower lateral thigh just above the knee and along an imaginary line. The line between the head of the fibula and the anterior superior iliac crest is marked with methylene blue. Dissection through skin and subcutaneous fat will reveal the glistening white fascia lata, which can be easily exposed using a sponge wrapped around the index finger and sometimes using forceps and scissors to clean away the loose areolar tissue. The skin overlying and attached to the fascia is undermined with long, sturdy scissors (Fig. 16B).

Using a scalpel, parallel incisions are made in the fascia 6–8 mm apart at the inferior most aspect of the incision to initiate the dissection that will result in acquiring the fascia strips (Fig. 17A). Once parallel incisions have been made within the confines of the wound, longitudinal parallel cuts are made with the Crawford fascia separator (Fig. 18A,B). It is most helpful if the fascia stripper can be passed easily into the upper thigh without soft tissue obstruction. The fascia is incised to produce an end that is then threaded through the stripper mechanism and fixed (we prefer two Kocher clamps) while the cutting portion of the stripper is passed into the upper thigh within the tunnel created by the scissors (Fig. 17B,C, Fig. 18C). When the desired length of fascia is captured in the stripper (10 cm or more is usually desirable), the fascia is severed. Before dividing the fascia, one should wipe away the connective tissue that is invariably present (Fig. 18D). The fascia can be divided into the number of strips desired; usually, strips 2 mm in width are quite satisfactory, but the width can be smaller or larger if preferred. Fascial strips whose fibers are cut obliquely are to be avoided because they are weaker and more prone to breakage. Closure does not usually include closing the fascia defect; however, closure of subcutaneous tissue should be firm with 4-0 prolene. Skin staples are used to achieve good eversion of the wound edges. Healing is rarely a problem and ambulation can occur 12–24 h after surgery. Skin staples are removed in approximately 10 days.

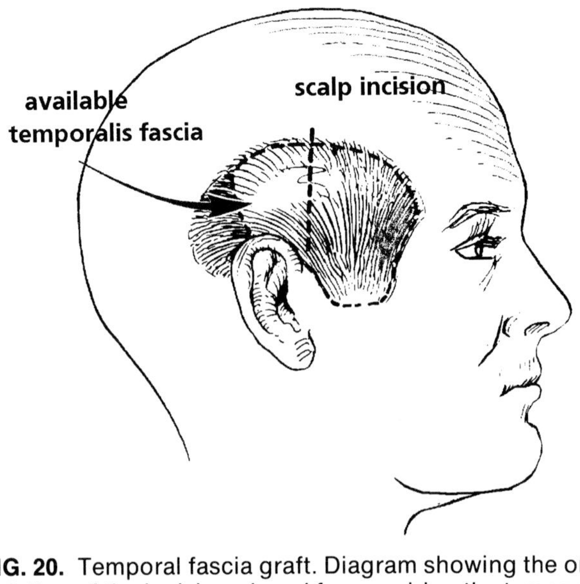

FIG. 20. Temporal fascia graft. Diagram showing the orientation of the incision placed for acquiring the temporal fascia and outline of available fascia in this area.

Fascia lata can be harvested as a rectangular patch of tissue (Fig. 19A,B). In this form it is useful as a patch graft or in socket reconstruction.

Deep Temporal Fascia (Temporalis Fascia)

An alternative donor site for fascia is that overlying the temporalis muscle. Temporal fascia may be harvested conveniently in conjunction with certain brow and eyelid procedures (e.g., reanimation procedures of the eyelids). It is a useful harvest site when broader pieces of fascia are necessary. The temporalis fascia covers the temporalis muscle, originating on the superior arch of the temporalis fossa and inserting on the zygomatic arch. To harvest it, a 4-cm vertical incision is made through the scalp above and anterior to the ear (Figs. 20 and 21A). Ultimately the scar will be hidden by the hairline. The temporalis fascia is exposed

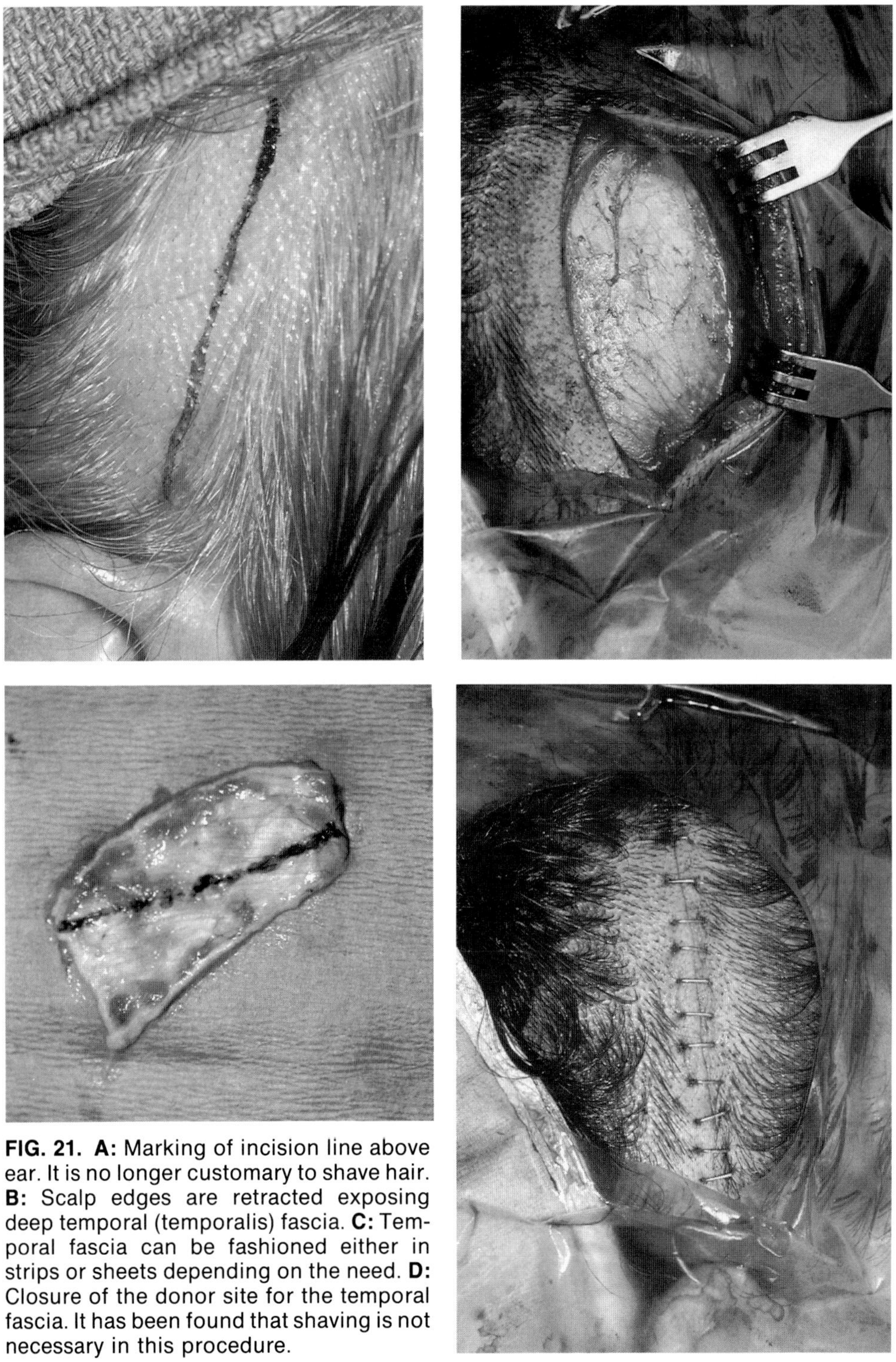

A B C D

FIG. 21. A: Marking of incision line above ear. It is no longer customary to shave hair. **B:** Scalp edges are retracted exposing deep temporal (temporalis) fascia. **C:** Temporal fascia can be fashioned either in strips or sheets depending on the need. **D:** Closure of the donor site for the temporal fascia. It has been found that shaving is not necessary in this procedure.

exactly as one would expose the fascia lata (Fig. 21B). The scalp edges are retracted and a number 15 blade is used to outline the graft. The graft can be divided into strips for sling procedures or remain in sheets for other purposes (Fig. 21C). Either skin staples or 6-0 silk sutures are used to close the skin incision (Fig. 21D). Temporal fascia is more fragile than fascia lata.

PRESERVED HOMOLOGOUS TISSUE

In virtually all aspects of oculoplastic surgery, autogenous grafts are superior to either fresh homologous or preserved homologous grafts. The autogeneous graft has the advantage of not inciting an immune reaction or foreign body reaction, not causing inflammation, having less shrinkage, and predictably surviving if an adequate blood supply is present. On the other hand, homologous grafts create an immune reaction, cause additional inflammation, and may shrink or even be totally absorbed. Despite these limitations, banked homologous tissue grafts can be useful in situations where the surgeon does not wish to disturb a donor site in the patient or situations in which sufficient autogenous donor tissue is not available. Banked sclera and fascia (Fig. 22) are among the most commonly used homologous tissue grafts in oculoplastic surgery (11,13). Homologous tarsus and cartilage are also used (14,15). In today's climate, the possibility of transmission of disease is of concern when using any banked homologous tissue grafts. Safeguards should be used to avoid this possibility. Strict donor selection criteria should be used to exclude any donor with known systemic infections, including human immunodeficiency virus (HIV), hepatitis, or other infectious agents (16).

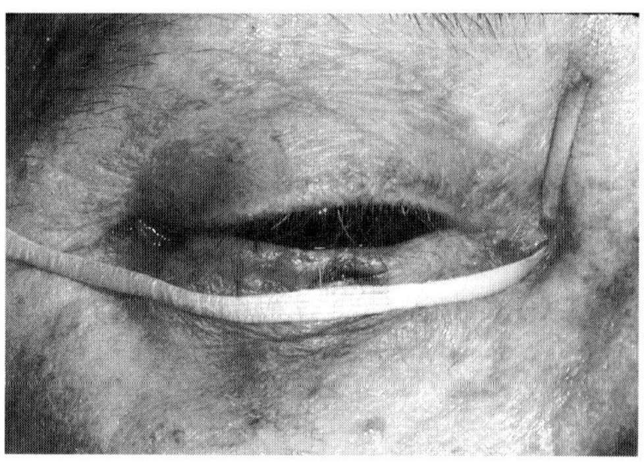

FIG. 22. Donor (homologous) fascia. Donor fascia can be obtained either in sheets or in strips. This illustration shows a strip for a lower lip sling. The fascia has been irradiated, dehydrated, and is free of infectious agents. It is normally rehydrated with antibiotic solution. The most recently used supplier of donor fascia is Pfrimmer Viggo, who produces a high-quality dehydrated human fascia lata for homotransplantation (distribution in the USA: Biodynamics Inc., 6611 Port West Drive, Suite 190, Houston, TX 77024, 713-862-6622).

Donors with a history of cancer, drug use, collagen vascular disease, or unknown cause of death should also be excluded. Donor blood should be tested to rule out antibody presence to HIV virus, hepatitis B antigens, and rapid plasma reagin. Beyond strict donor selection criteria, the donor tissue itself is treated to minimize any chance of transmission of communicable diseases. Heat treatment can be used to inactivate viruses. Cobalt-60 γ radiation is used for sterilization of donor tissue (e.g., irradiated fascia or cartilage). Eyebanks commonly supply glycerin- or alcohol-preserved sclera as donor tissue. Fresh homologous sclera will cause less inflammatory reaction than preserved sclera. It is appropriate to discuss the use of this tissue with the patient.

Alloplastic Material

A large variety of alloplastic implant materials are available for use in ophthalmic plastic surgery. Most of these materials are readily available. In later chapters, use of these alloplastic implants will be described in greater detail.

Several alloplastic materials are in common use for repair of eyelid problems. Solid silicone rod implants (Roger Klein, Ltd., Puerto Rico) have become the material of choice for frontalis muscle repair procedures in select problem ptosis patients (those with poor eye protective mechanisms) (17) and implants for eyelid closure in facial palsy. Medical grade gold weight implants (Meddev, P.O. Box 1352, Los Altos, CA, 415-948-1742) are used in facial paralysis patients with symptomatic lagophthalmos and exposure. The gold weights are implanted into the upper lid and sutured to the tarsal plate. The typical gold weight is approximately 1.0 g, although a variety of sizes (weights) are available. Polytetrafluoroethylene (Gore-tex, Gore and Associates, Flagstaff, AZ) is an autoclavable, readily available, biologically compatible material. Gore-tex implants were initially popularized by Steinkogler (18–20) for eyelid surgery and have been used successfully as spacer material in eyelid repair and for ptosis frontalis suspension in place of donor tissues or autogenous grafts. The micropore matrix of polytetrafluoroethylene allows for ingrowth of host fibrovascular tissue. Fibrovascular ingrowth occurs with minimal inflammation; thus the implant is well tolerated (21,22).

REFERENCES

1. Baylis HI, Rosen N, Neuhaus RW. Obtaining auricular cartilage for reconstructive surgery. *Am J Ophthalmol* 1982;93:709–712.
2. McCord CD, Chen WP. Tarsal polishing and mucous membrane grafting for cicatricial entropion, trichiasis, and epidermalization. *Ophth Surg* 1983;14:1021–1025.

3. Stephenson CM, Brown BZ. The use of tarsus as a free autogenous graft in eyelid surgery. *Ophth Plast Reconstr Surg* 1985; I:43–50.
4. Hawes MJ. Free autogenous grafts in eyelid tarsoconjunctival reconstruction. *Ophth Surg* 1987;9:37–41.
5. Millard DR Jr. Eyelid repairs with a chondromucosal graft. *Ophth Plast Reconstr Surg* 1962;30:267–272.
6. Kersten RC, Kulwin DR, Levartovsky S, Tiradellis H, Tse DT. Management of lower-lid retraction with hard-palate mucosa grafting. *Arch Ophthalmol* 1990;108:1339–1343.
7. Bartley GB, Kay PP. Posterior lamellar eyelid reconstruction with a hard palate mucosal graft. *Ophthalmology* 1989;107: 609–612.
8. Cohen MS, Shorr N. Eyelid reconstruction with hard palate mucosa grafts. *Ophth Plast Reconstr Surg* 1992;8:183–195.
9. Smith B, Petrelli R. Dermis-fat graft as a moveable implant within the muscle cone. *Am J Ophthalmol* 1978;85:62–66.
10. Crawford JS. Fascia lata: its nature and fate after implantation and its use in ophthalmic surgery. *Trans Am Ophthalmol Soc* 1968;66:673–745.
11. Beyer CK, Albert DM. The use and fate of fascia lata and sclera in ophthalmic plastic and reconstructive surgery. *Ophthalmology* 1981;88:869–886.
12. Holt JE, Holt GR. Use of temporalis fascia in eyelid reconstruction. *Ophthalmology* 1984;91:89–93.
13. Flanagan JC. Eyebank sclera in oculoplastic surgery. *Ophth Surg* 1974;5(3):45–53.
14. Brown BZ. The use of homologous tarsus as a donor graft in lid surgery. *Ophth Plast Reconstr Surg* 1985;1:91–95.
15. Schenk W, Linberg JV, McCormick S. Preserved irradiated homologous cartilage implants in canine eyelids. *Ophth Plast Reconstr Surg* 1985;I:267–272.
16. Bedrossian EH. HIV and banked fascia lata. *Ophth Plast Reconstr Surg* 1991;7(4):284–288.
17. McCord CD, Shore JW. Silicone rod frontalis suspension. *Adv Ophth Plast Reconstr Surg* 1982;1:213–219.
18. Steinkogler FJ, Kuchar A, Hubere A–M. Gore-Tex soft tissue patch frontalis suspension technique in congenital ptosis and in blepharophimosis-ptosis syndrome. *Plast Reconstr Surg* 1993; 92:1057–1060.
19. Steinkogler FJ. Ein neus Material fur die frontalisschlingenoperation bei kongenitaler Ptose. *Klin Monatsbl Augenheilk* 1987; 191:361.
20. Steinkogler FJ. A sandwich technique for full thickness reconstruction of the lower eyelid. *Orbit* 1989;8:37.
21. Karesh JW, Fabrega MA, Rodrigues MM, Ghlros DS. Polytetrafluoroethylene as an interpositional graft material for the correction of lower eyelid retraction. *Ophthalmology* 1989;96:419–423.
22. Levin PS, Dutton JJ. Polytef (polytetrafluoroethylene) alloplastic grafting as a substitute for mucous membrane. *Arch Ophthalmol* 1990;108:282–255.

CHAPTER 4

Reconstructive Flaps

Usually an extensive wound or surgical defect requires a flap for successful closure. A flap consists of a tissue segment that is moved from one part of the body to another with a vascular supply maintained by a pedicle or base attachment to adjacent tissue. Indications for flap coverage include defects that cannot adequately undergo primary closure. Because a properly designed flap has an independent blood supply, flaps are useful for the reconstruction of sites with poor vascularity that could not sustain a skin graft. In addition, a flap is useful to replace soft tissue deficiency in full-thickness defects when additonal tissue requirements are necessary to restore proper contour.

The most commonly used flaps in oculoplastic surgery are skin flaps from eyelid or periorbital skin (1). The blood supply to the skin flap is from the subdermal plexus of blood vessels. Most skin flaps are classified as random pattern flaps. The subdermal plexus derives vascular perfusion from deeper arteries that have perforating musculocutaneous branches to the skin. Since the blood supply is therefore random, flaps survive to approximately the same length independent of the width (Fig. 1) (2). In general, a random skin flap should be designed the length of which is no longer than four times the base width. Thinning of this flap should preserve a layer of subcutaneous tissue to protect the subdermal plexus. Eyelid skin flaps can be used to reconstruct full-thickness defects utilizing the skin flap to replace the anterior lamella and to function as the recipient blood supply for a posterior lamellar graft.

A standard classification system of flaps separates different flap designs according to the blood supply (Fig. 2). Axial pattern flaps contain a direct cutaneous artery or arteriole included in the flap design that provides additional blood supply. The safe length of an axial flap is therefore longer than a random flap and depends on the length of the cutaneous artery. Although axial pattern flaps are usually designed as a peninsula with continuity of adjacent skin over the base, the flap can be converted to an island pattern flap with division of adjacent skin and preservation of the cutaneous artery (3). A free flap requires division of the artery and vein supplying a flap with transfer to a distant site with microvascular attachment to vessels located at the recipient site. Microvascular free flaps can include the transfer of skin and subcutaneous tissue, fascia, muscle, musculocutaneous flaps, and vascularized bone (4). Although not commonly used in oculoplastic surgery, when adjacent tissue is inadequate for reconstruction, free flaps may be a useful alternative. Orbital exenteration often creates large soft tissue requirements that can only be satisfied with microvascular free flaps.

Local skin flaps usually provide the best match with respect to skin color, thickness, and texture by using adjacent tissue. Skin flaps are generally divided into two types according to the type of transfer movement used to relocate the tissue into the defect. Flaps that rotate about a pivot point are rotation and transposition flaps. Advancement and sliding flaps are moved directly into the defect without any lateral or rotational

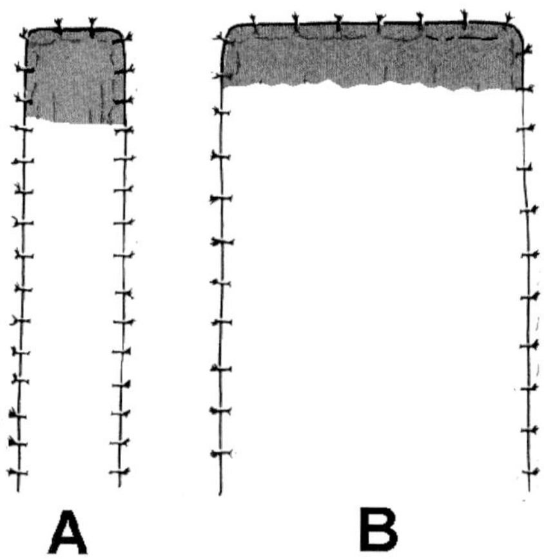

FIG. 1. The random pattern skin flap depends on blood flow from the subdermal plexus. The reliability of the length does not depend directly on the width of the flap.

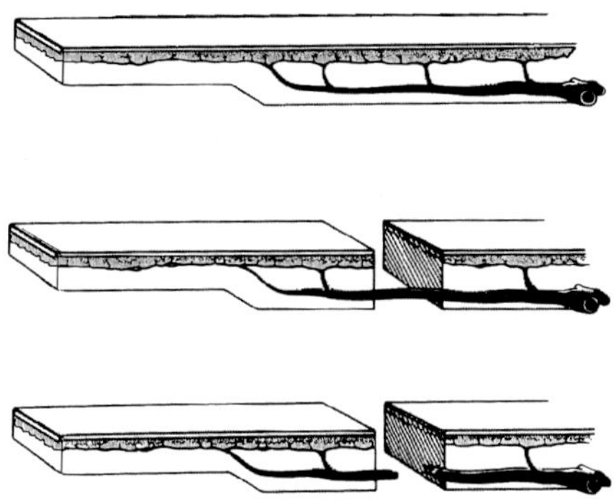

FIG. 2. The axial pattern skin flap contains a vessel deep to the subdermal plexus making the flap reliable as **(A)** a narrow peninsula, **(B)** an island flap connected by the vascular pedicle, and **(C)** a free flap using microvascular surgery.

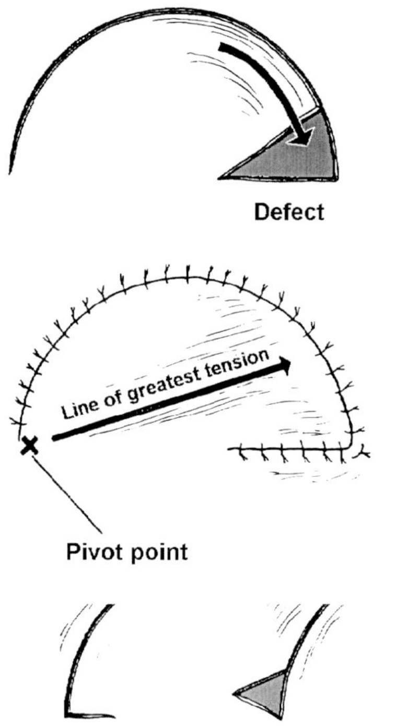

FIG. 3. The rotation flap utilizes adjacent tissue and a backcut or Burow's triangle to reduce tension at the pivot point.

movement. Careful preoperative planning of skin flaps helps in designing the flap to minimize tension and preserve blood supply.

ROTATION FLAPS

Rotation flaps are designed as a semicircular shape that rotates about a pivot point with the line of maximum tension along the radius of the arc of rotation (Fig. 3). A backcut or Burow's triangle can be used to reduce tension and gain additional rotation taking precaution not to compromise the blood supply to the flap (5). Rotation flaps are usually random pattern flaps, so that proper design should consider the length, base width, and degree of undermining. A rotation flap commonly used in eyelid reconstruction is the Tenzel semicircular flap, which can be used for upper and lower lateral eyelid rotation (6) (Fig. 4). The Mustarde cheek rotation flap is useful for lower eyelid and medial cheek reconstruction when a large defect requires closure.

TRANSPOSITION FLAPS

The transposition flap is usually an axial pattern flap that is transposed across normal tissue into a nonadjacent defect. The line of greatest tension extends from the pivot point (Fig. 5). As the arc of rotation increases, the effective length is reduced. This should be considered in the preoperative planning so that flap length design is sufficient. When the flap donor site cannot be primarily closed, the donor defect can be skin grafted or reconstructed with a bilobed flap (5). A bilobed flap utilizes a secondary transposition flap that

A 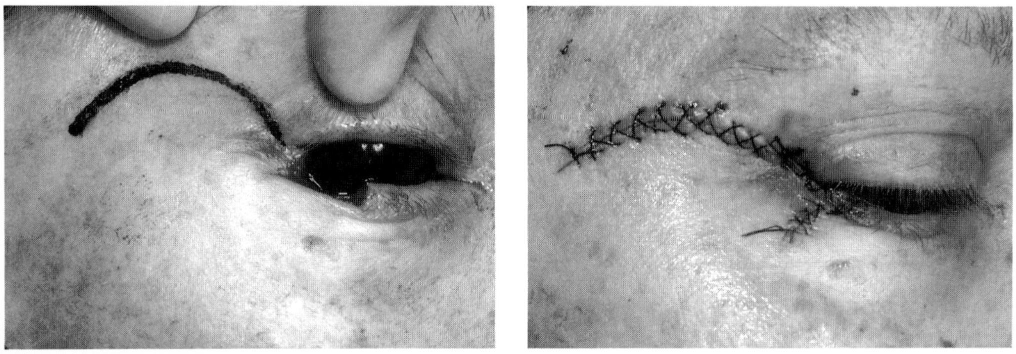 B

FIG. 4. The Tenzel rotation flap is used to close a lower eyelid defect.

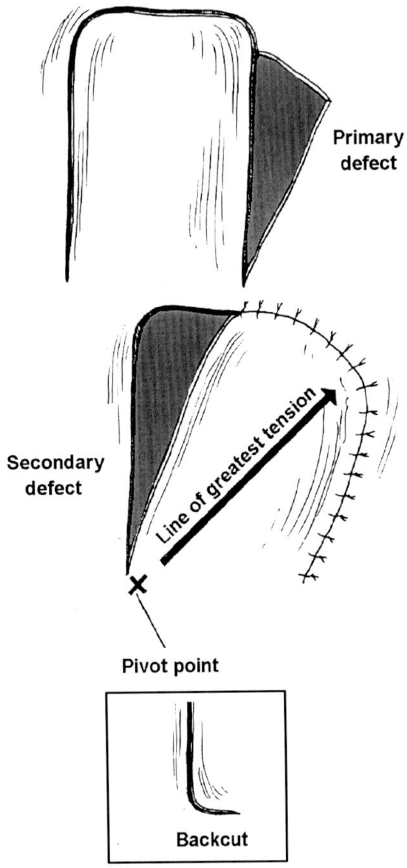

FIG. 5. The transposition flap crosses an adjacent tissue bridge and may create a secondary defect, which is often closed by a skin graft. A backcut is useful to reduce tension at the pivot point.

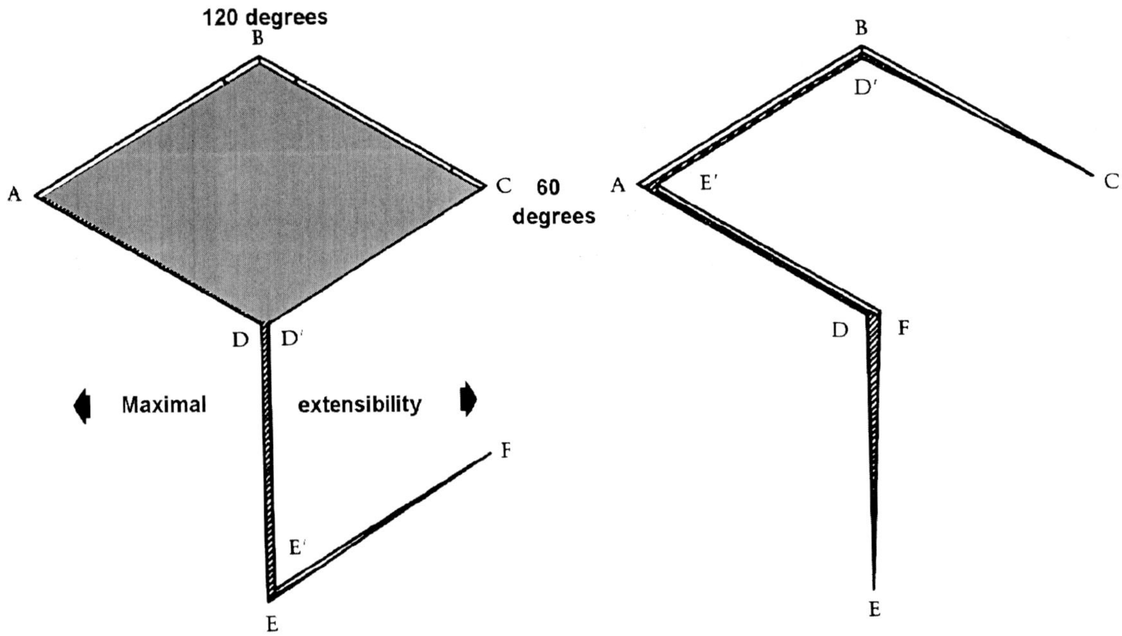

FIG. 6. The rhomboid flap should be designed with angles of 60° and 120°. Closure should be parallel to the lines of maximal extensibility.

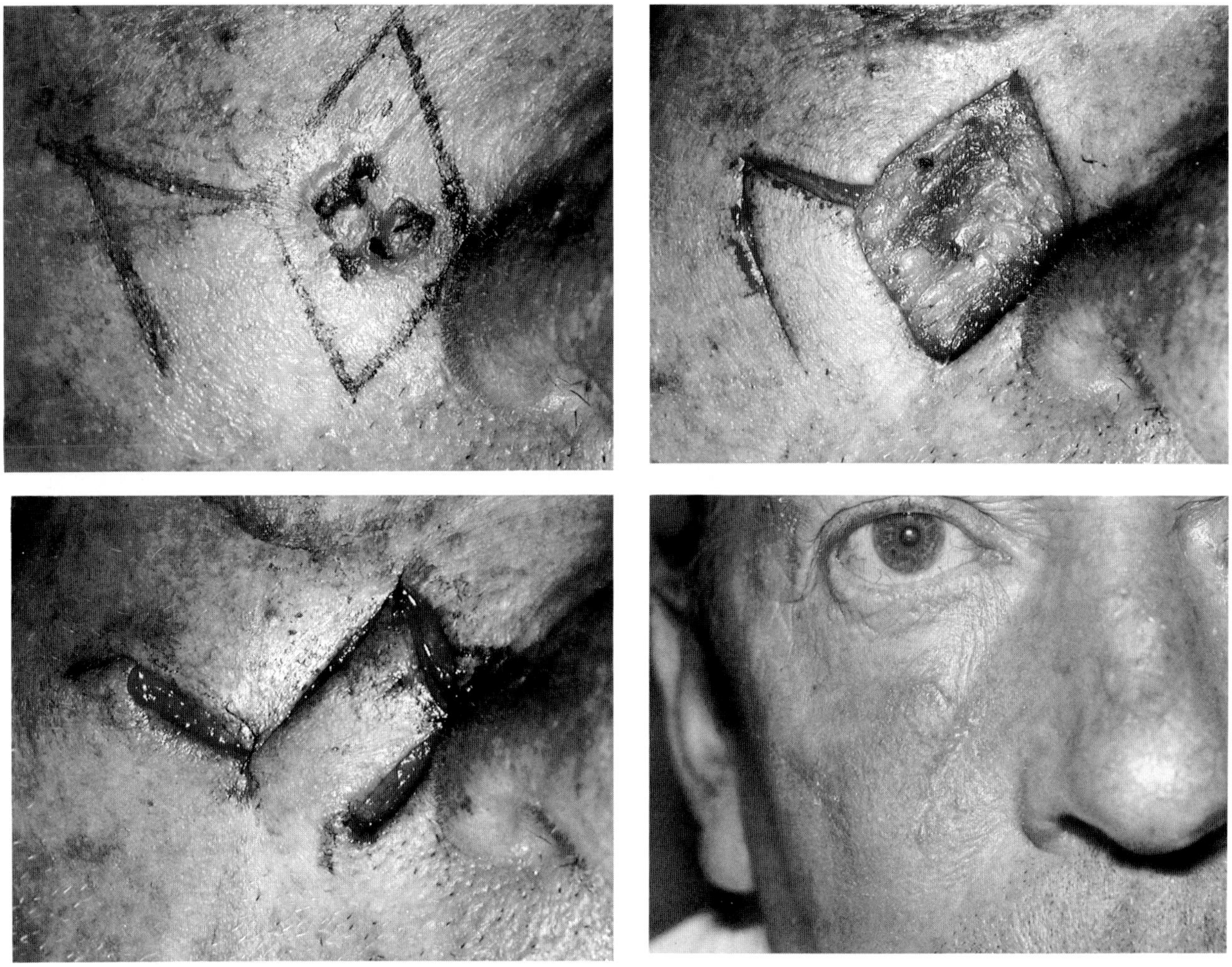

FIG. 7. The rhomboid flap. **(A)** Design of the excision and the flap. The defect following resection **(B)** and after flap transposition **(C)**. Postoperative result using the rhomboid flap **(D)**.

is half the diameter of the primary flap donor site. The Limberg flap is a commonly used transposition flap for closure of rhomboid shaped defects (7,8) (Fig. 6). There are four rhomboid flaps available to close any one defect. The ideal flap choice is designed from the adjacent area with maximal skin looseness (Fig. 7). Other examples of transposition flaps that are commonly used in more complex periocular reconstruction include the glabellar flap, the temporal forehead flap, and the forehead flap (Fig. 8).

Z-PLASTY

The Z-plasty is a simple transposition flap that utilizes two opposing triangular flaps of adjacent tissue. Indications for use of the Z-plasty include deformities that require additional length such as scar contractures, webs or folds, or rearrangement of tissue such as lateral canthal elevation. The standard Z-plasty incorporates two equal triangles that form a parallelogram. The limbs of the Z are generally equal in length and form an angle of 60° with the central limb (Fig. 9). The theoretical gain in length is obtained along the direction of the central limb and has been calculated as a 75% linear increase (9). In order to transpose the flaps of the Z-plasty, the random skin flaps must be undermined to the base, which should have sufficient elasticity.

ADVANCEMENT FLAPS

All advancement flaps depend on undermining and skin elasticity to directly move adjacent tissue into the defect without any lateral movement or rotation. The simplest example of a sliding flap is demonstrated by the adjacent undermining of tissue deep to the subder-

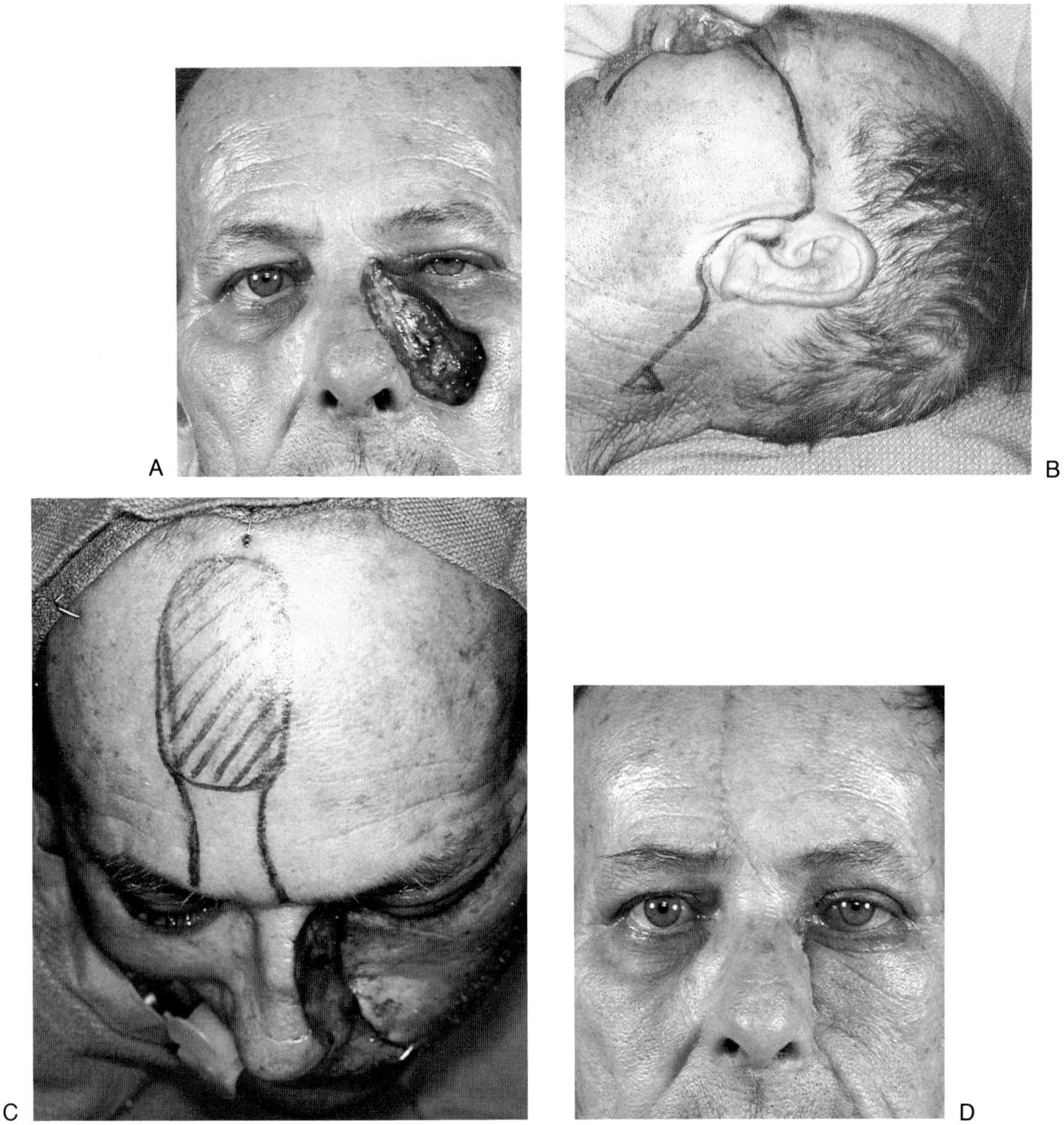

FIG. 8. **(A)** Complex defect following resection of a skin cancer adjacent to the medial canthus. Reconstruction with **(B)** an extended Mustarde cheek flap and **(C)** a paramedian forehead flap. Postoperative result 3 months after surgery **(D).**

mal plexus to permit primary closure. An advancement flap is a more complex form of a sliding flap utilizing a rectangular or square flap of skin and subcutaneous tissue elevated on three sides and advanced forward to close an adjacent defect (Fig. 10). Examples of advancement flaps used in eyelid reconstruction include the lateral canthotomy with advancement of the residual lateral lower eyelid and the Cutler–Beard advancement flap used in reconstruction of the upper eyelid (10). Excision of lateral Burow's triangles equalizes the flap length and lateral wound edge to avoid the creation of a dogear-type deformity. Another commonly used advancement technique is the V-Y advancement flap. A V-shaped incision is made adjacent to the defect and the incision closed as a Y-shape following advancement of adjacent skin (Fig. 11). The use of advancement flaps can be helpful in select periocular defects.

CIRCULAR DEFECTS

The excision of skin cancers on the face or periorbital region often results in a circular deformity that requires repair. Several methods of closing circular defects have been proposed because primary closure may result in dog ear deformities or scar depression (11). Techniques that utilize flaps from adjacent tissue have provided superior aesthetic results. Double rotation flaps can be used to convert a circular defect into a Z-shaped incision and closed as an O-Z-plasty (Fig. 12).

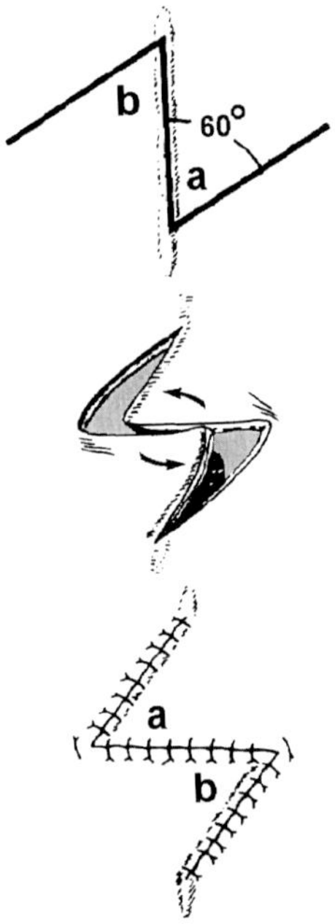

FIG. 9. The Z-plasty is designed with flaps at a 60° angle to the axis of the scar. Transposition of the flaps creates scar lengthening.

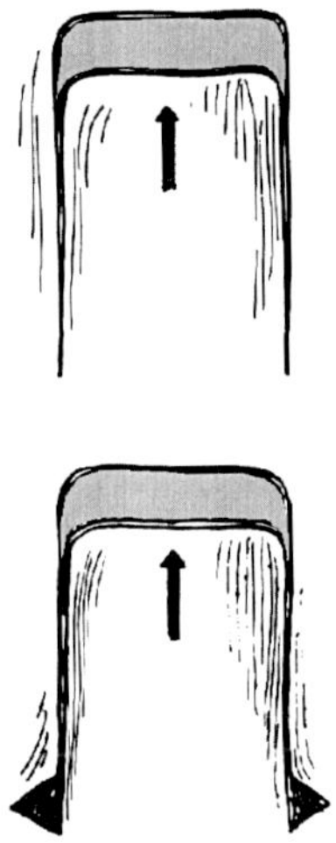

FIG. 10. The advancement flap moves forward adjacent tissue into the wound. The excision of Burow's triangles can be used to minimize tension along the base.

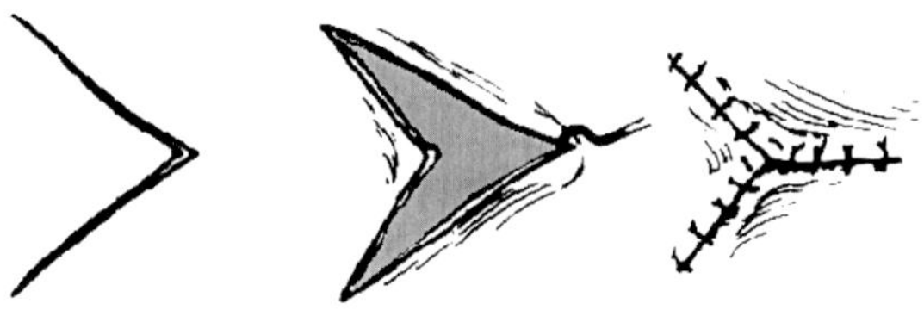

FIG. 11. The V-Y flap is a commonly used advancement flap.

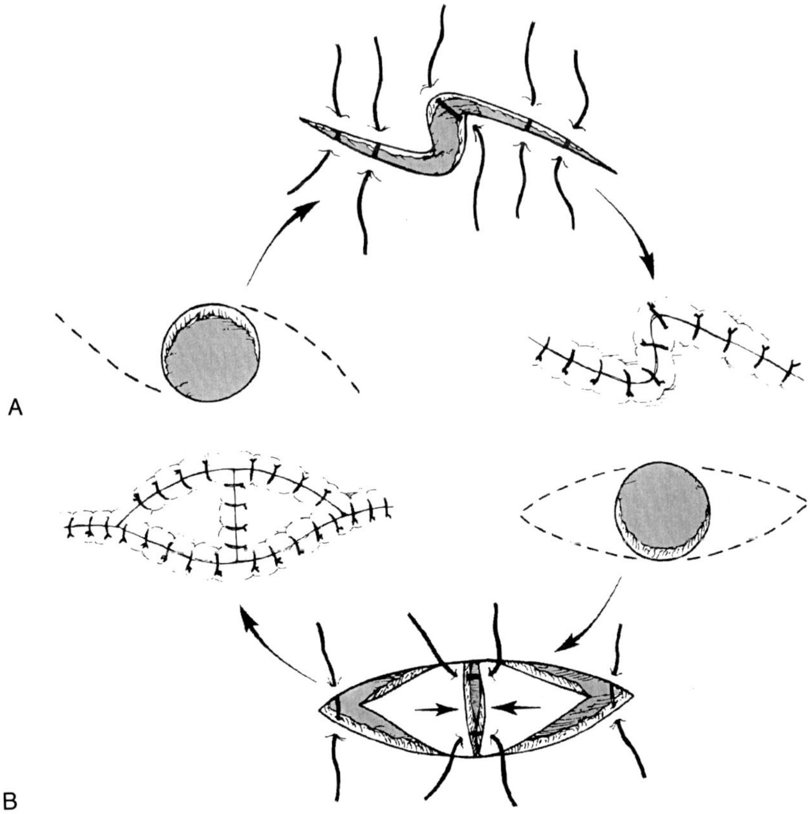

FIG. 12. Circular shaped defects can be closed with **(A)** double rotation flaps in an O-Z-plasty or with **(B)** double advancement flaps using bilateral V-Y flaps.

Double V-Y advancement flaps also provide excellent results with advancement parallel to the lines of minimal tension.

PITFALLS

Once a skin flap has been properly designed and transferred to reconstruct the deformity, several pitfalls should be avoided in order to maintain the blood supply and ensure flap survival. If a flap is stretched too tightly, excess tension may occur that can cause flap ischemia from lack of perfusion. A backcut or partial skin graft can be used to reduce tension. External pressure from a dressing or bolster can impair nutritive blood flow if capillary perfusion pressure is exceeded. Care should be taken to avoid tight pressure dressings. A hematoma can occur underneath a flap and contribute to flap failure. Early recognition and drainage of a hematoma will usually result in flap salvage. Studies have shown that cigarette smoking can adversely affect wound healing and contribute to loss of skin flaps (12). Patients should be asked to discontinue smoking for 2 weeks prior to elective surgery.

CONCLUSIONS

Overall the use of skin flaps is superior to that of skin grafts in the periocular and facial regions. Skin flaps maintain the original color and texture of the adjacent skin site providing a better match for the defect. The durability provides a distinct advantage over skin grafts with significantly less shrinkage and contracture formation. Flap growth in children, and characteristics of hair growth, sebaceous secretion, sensibility, and sweating are maintained in a similar fashion to the degree of the adjacent skin.

REFERENCES

1. Patrinely JR, Hector MM, Anderson RL. Skin flaps in periorbital reconstruction. *Surv Ophthalmol* 1987;31:249–261.
2. Milton SH. Pedicled skin flaps: the fallacy of length:width ratio. *Br J Surg* 1970;57:502.
3. Daniel RK, Taylor I. Distant transfer of an island flap by microvascular anastomoses. *Plast Reconstr Surg* 1973;52:111.
4. Mathes SJ, Nahai F. Clinical applications for muscle and musculocutaneous flaps. St. Louis: CV Mosby; 1979.
5. Smith JW, Aston SJ. *Plastic surgery*. 4th ed. Boston: Little, Brown; 1991.
6. McCord CD, Tanenbaum M, Nunery WR. *Oculoplastic surgery*. 3rd ed. New York: Raven Press; 1995.
7. Limberg AA. Design of local flaps. In: Gibson T, ed. *Modern trends in plastic surgery*. London: Butterworth; 1966;38–61.
8. Borges A. The rhombic flap. *Plast Reconstr Surg* 1981;67: 458–466.
9. Gibson T, Kenedi RM. Biomechanical properties of skin. *Surg Clin North Am* 1967;47:279.
10. Cutler N, Beard C. A method for partial and total upper lid reconstruction. *Am J Ophthalmol* 1955;39:1–7.
11. Golomb F. Closure of the circular defect with double rotation flaps and Z-plasties. *Plast Reconstr Surg* 1984;74:813–816.
12. Rees TD, Liverett DM, Guy CL. The effect of cigarette smoking on skin flap survival in the face lift patient. *Plast Reconstr Surg* 1984;54:585.

CHAPTER 5

Entropion and Related Conditions

Entropion is characterized by an inturning of the eyelid causing the margin, the lashes, and sometimes the external skin surface to turn inward, which results in corneal irritation and abrasions as well as general eye irritation. Some conditions simulate entropion, although they are not true entropion because the eyelid margin is not truly inturned. These include *epiblepharon*, an abnormal fold of skin occurring in young children that presses against the lower lid, turning the lashes inward; *epicanthal folds*, occurring in children and Asians, and producing the same effect as epiblepharon; *distichiasis*, in which extra rows of lashes are pointed inward abrading the cornea and eye; and *trichiasis*, in which the lid margin is normally positioned while the lashes or hairs grow inward against the cornea. There may be other cases with soft tissue *margin destruction* from a disease process causing a change in architecture, so that it is difficult to see if the margin is actually turning in or not. These damaged margins may nevertheless contain lashes or hairs, scar tissue, and epidermalized tissue that abrade the cornea. It is important to differentiate true entropion from some of these other conditions because the treatment may vary.

LOWER LID ENTROPIONS

Congenital Entropion

Congenital entropion is very rare and must be differentiated from epiblepharon. It may occur in the upper and lower lids, and spasm of the orbicularis muscle is a striking feature of this condition. It is felt that the underlying cause is hypertrophy of the pretarsal orbicularis fibers and a deficiency or absence of the tarsal plate. Congenital entropion may be accompanied by some epiblepharon. It has been treated by full-thickness mattress sutures to maintain eversion of the lid and by excision of the thickened pretarsal orbicularis fibers.

Transient Spastic Entropion

An acute swelling of the eyelid accompanied by orbicularis spasm can cause a temporary inturning of the eyelid. It frequently occurs after prolonged patching and inflammation of the eye. Although some underlying laxity of the eyelid may be present, often there is none. Temporary spastic entropion can occur in young persons. It generally resolves as the eyelid edema goes down. However, the physician should be aware that this type of entropion may be an early sign of a tendency to involutional entropion.

Involutional Laxity Entropion

Involutional or laxity entropion generally occurs at an advancing age. In the past, it has been called "senile" entropion, although it is not equated with senility. It has also been given the misnomer of "spastic" entropion because spasm is present, but true involutional entropion is not of a transient nature except perhaps in its early stage. There has been much study of the pathogenesis and biomechanics of involutional entropion (1–5).

Most patients with entropion will present with the eyelid margin rolled in and the orbicularis muscles in spasm, accompanied by a red, watery, scratchy eye (Fig. 1A). Occasionally a person will present with symptoms resembling entropion without the inturning. Entropion in its early stages may be intermittent, and incipient entropion can be elicited by asking the patient to squeeze the eyelids tightly and look downward; generally, this will precipitate entropion in those who have a strong tendency. When the lower eyelid margin rolls inward, the lower border of the tarsal plate swings outward. The preseptal orbicularis fibers migrate upward into the pretarsal area, forming a tight band of muscle tissue on the surface of the tarsus (Fig. 1B). This outward swinging of the lower tarsal border is what by

A

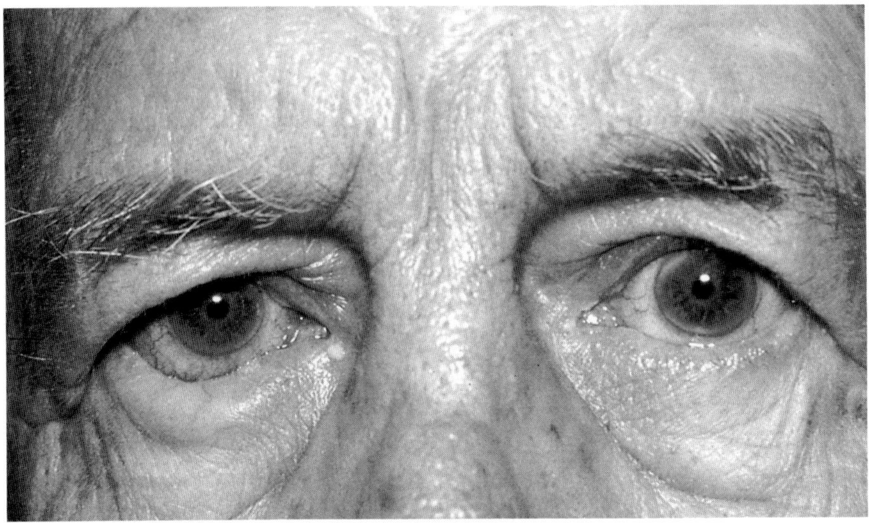

B

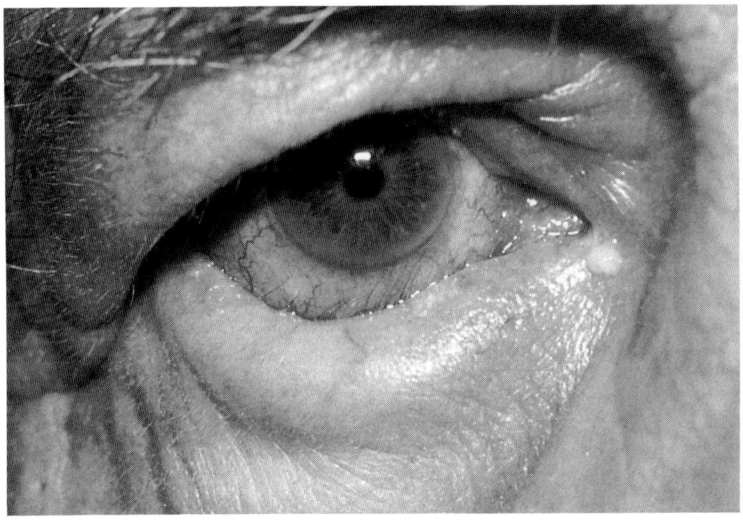

FIG. 1. A: Patient with involutional laxity entropion on the right with inturning of the eyelid margin. The patient demonstrates horizontal laxity of both lower lids. **B:** Close up of entropic eyelid showing inturning of the eyelid margin from spasm and migration of preseptal orbicularis fibers rotating the eyelid margin inward and buckling the lower border of the tarsal plate outward.

necessity causes an inward turning of the eyelid margin (Fig. 2A, B). The underlying anatomic defects that have been implicated in this process are horizontal lid laxity, with laxity of the tarsoligamentous sling, and laxity or disinsertion of the capsulopalpebral fascia in the lower lid (which can also be seen in ectropion) (Fig. 3A, B, Fig. 4). A factor that may cause an entropion rather than an ectropion in older patients with loose lids is hypertropied and vertically mobile preseptal orbicularis fibers. This occurs because of the loss of attachments of the fibers to the orbital septum. In entropion patients the preseptal orbicularis fibers bunch up and migrate superiorly and evert the lower border of the tarsus. Sisler and colleagues, in a histopathology study, demonstrated that patients with entropion usually have more hypertrophy of the orbicularis and Riolan's muscle and fewer ischemic changes than do patients with ectropion (6,7). Another factor that can aggravate an entropion is enophthalmos of an acquired or constitutional nature. Through the years there have been many approaches to the correction of involutional entropion to correct these anatomic problems (Table 1). Elements of all of these procedures as they affect the eyelid anatomy have been incorporated in the newer procedures.

TABLE 1. *Entropion procedures: principles of anatomic correction*

1. Horizontal lid tightening (emphasis at lower tarsal border)
2. Barricade or plication of preseptal orbicularis fibers
3. Plication of inferior retractors

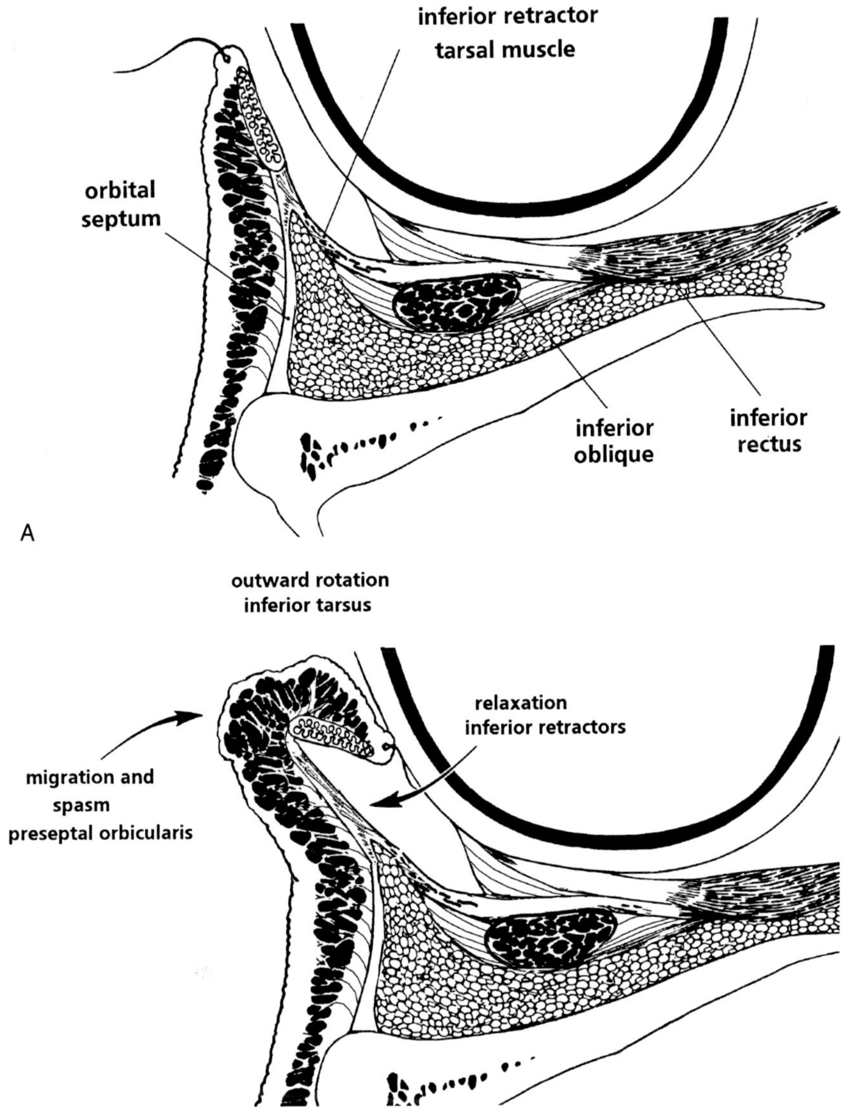

FIG. 2. A: Saggital view of eyelid and inferior orbit showing position of the support structures and retractors of the lower lid. **B:** Diagrammatic representation of lower lid with involutional entropion. There is an outward buckling of the lower tarsal border, relaxation of the inferior retractor tissue, and spasm and migration of the preseptal orbicularis fibers turning the margin of the eyelid inward.

Cicatricial Entropion

Cicatricial entropion is the inward turning of the eyelid margin caused by shortening of the internal lamella of the eyelid, forcing the margin of the eyelid and lashes to turn against the globe. It can occur in the upper and lower eyelids and can be caused by surgery, trauma, chemical injury, and inflammatory processes, including ocular pemphigoid and Stevens–Johnson syndrome. Usually accompanying these cicatricial processes is epidermalization of the mucosal surface of the inner eyelid margin and tarsoconjunctiva, causing chronic epithelial irritation of the cornea (4,8,9). The findings of scarring of the eyelid margin and internal surface combined with a clinical history are sufficient to make a diagnosis of cicatricial entropion. Many patients who have had surgical procedures for involutional laxity entropion can re-present with a recurrent entropion that has been converted from a laxity involutional type to a cicatricial type because of the previous surgical procedures. The eyelid margin architecture may be normal in these patients. It is very important to recognize this particular situation.

Entropion with Marginal Deformity and Trichiasis

Damage to the architecture of the eyelid margin can cause an abrasive effect on the cornea from scar tissue, inturning lashes and hairs and epidermalized tissue. This may occur in isolation from a true entropion of the lid but commonly is combined with a true entropion in many cicatrizing diseases such as Stevens–Johnson syndrome or following a burn. It also can result from chronic blepharoconjunctivitis, meibomitis, or rosacea. The techniques of correction or margin deformity will be discussed in the section on eyelid margin deformity and trichiasis.

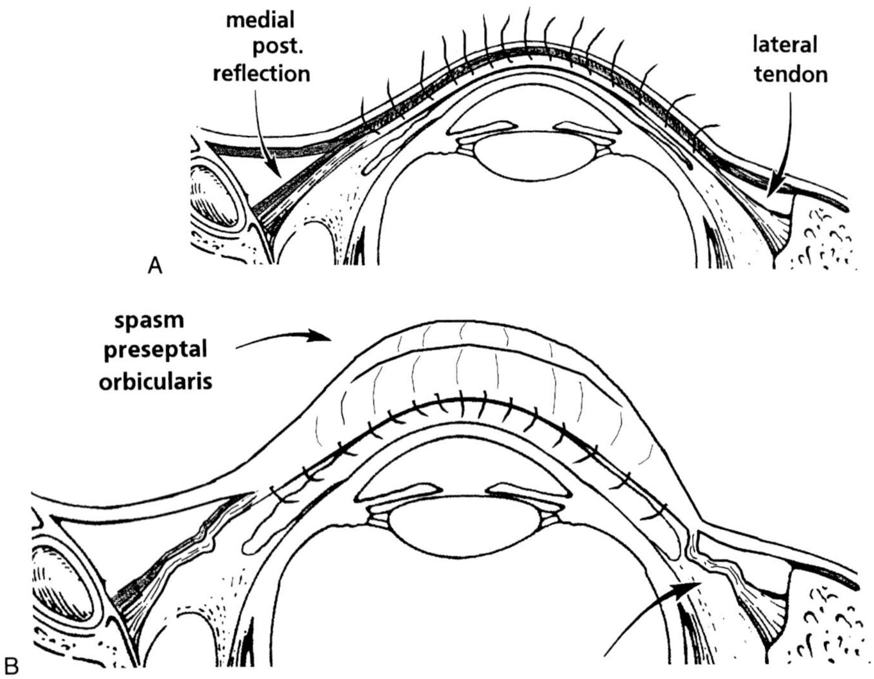

FIG. 3. A: Diagrammatic representation of the support structures of the lower lid tarsoligamental sling at the lateral and medial orbital walls. **B:** Diagrammatic representation of the entropic eyelid rotating inward showing the contribution of the laxity of the lateral and medial canthal tendons. The spasm of the preseptal orbicularis has rotated the lower border of the tarsus outward and the margin of the lid inward.

Complex Entropion

In damaged eyelids, complex situations can occur in which the entropion process is a combination of mechanisms. The elements of laxity or involutional entropion may be combined with those of cicatricial changes, particularly following previous surgery or multiple trauma to the eyelids. The eyelid structures may be fused or the retractor fascia attached in an unusual way to cause an entropic position that may require additional procedures for correction. It is important to recognize these complicating factors in entropion since it may be surgically unresponsive to a standard procedure.

Before considering surgical correction in a patient presenting with entropion, one must attempt to categorize the entropion into one of the above categories. Special attention must be given to "problem entropion" patients: those who have had previous surgery and had portions of tarsus excised, or have combined laxity and cicatricial components. The true entropion may be combined with trichiasis and epidermalization, and simple restoration of the eyelid margin to a normal position may not cure the patient's symptomatology. Patients who have coexistent severe enophthalmos may require correction of the enophthalmos before an entropion procedure can be successful. Other coexisting problems such as epiblepharon, epicanthal folds, and margin deformities following tarsorrhaphy must be noted. Unusual anatomic anomalies such as adhesions between the inferior rectus muscle and the capsulopalpebral fascia and the oblique muscle following inferior orbital trauma must be detected and corrected to prevent continued abnormal traction on lower lid structures.

Horizontal laxity of eyelid tissue—
lower tarsal border and canthus
+
Relaxation of inferior tarsal support structure
retractors (capsulopalpebral fascia)
+
Preseptal orbicularis spasm and migration of fibers
upward (loss of attachments to septum—hypertrophy)
+
enophthalmos
↘
Outward rotation of lower tarsal border
(inward rotation of eyelid margin)

FIG. 4. Laxity involutional entropion: anatomic causes.

SURGICAL PROCEDURES FOR THE CORRECTION OF LOWER LID ENTROPION

Congenital Entropion

Many cases of congenital entropion are temporary, can be managed with the use of adhesive tape or temporizing mattress sutures, and will resolve with time. Cases that are untreatable by temporizing procedures and involve more obviously thickened orbicularis fibers can be corrected by excision of the skin fold and pretarsal orbicularis fibers in combination with a transverse tarsotomy and rotation (Wies procedure), which will be described in a following section (10). Such a

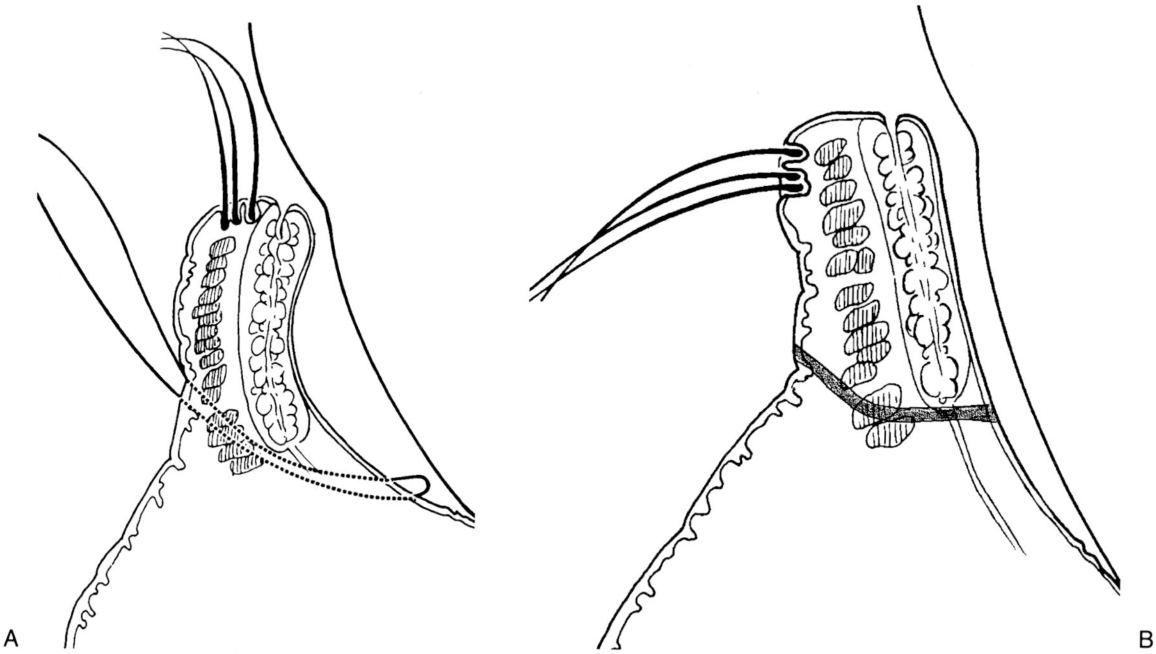

FIG. 5. A: Temporizing mattress suture correction of involutional entropion. The sutures pass from the conjunctival fornix beneath the inferior board of the tarsus transcutaneously and are tied and adjusted for rotational effect. **B:** Fibrous track formed from mattress suture placement for entropion showing stabilization of orbicularis muscle.

procedure can also be helpful in some cases of congenital epiblepharon.

Involutional Laxity Entropion

Temporary Taping

Until surgery, the patient can apply adhesive tape to the edge of the lower lid with the tape being brought downward to the cheek to temporarily hold the margin outturned until surgical correction.

Suture Techniques

In the suture technique (11,12), three 4-0 vicryl mattress sutures are placed full thickness starting inside the lid and brought through the lower lid at the lower border of the tarsus. In some cases the sutures can be placed deeper in the fornix (Fig. 5A, B). This procedure can be used in the office in cases of involutional laxity entropion as a temporizing procedure. In some milder cases the fibrous tracts formed by the sutures can stabilize the lid for a longer period.

Surgical Procedures

Many procedures described in the literature to correct an involutional entropion have addressed only one of the three major elements that combine to cause involutional entropion; horizontal laxity, stretching of the capsulopalpebral fascia (inferior retractors), and vertical mobility of the preseptal orbicularis fibers. Other procedures remedy at least two of those elements and have generally been most successful in terms of percentage of cure and absence of recurrence (2–5,13–16). To date there have probably been no procedures that are 100% successful in preventing a recurrence.

The following procedure is one that has stood the test of time in the authors' experience (4). This technique directs itself to the repair of two of the anatomic defects and possibly has a beneficial effect on the third. The procedure is a horizontal tightening procedure combined with plication of the preseptal orbicularis fibers. There also is probably some tightening of the capsulopalpebral fascia and septum. This effect is accomplished by tightening the tarsoligamentous sling and septal retractor tissue at the lower tarsal border.

Horizontal Tightening Technique

An incision is made in the subciliary area in the temporal one third of the lower lid and extended past the canthal angle. A canthotomy, i.e., cantholysis of the lower limb of the canthal tendon, is performed and after testing the amount of redundancy a full-thickness resection of the edge of the lid is carried out (Fig. 6A–D). For placement of sutures for the entropion re-

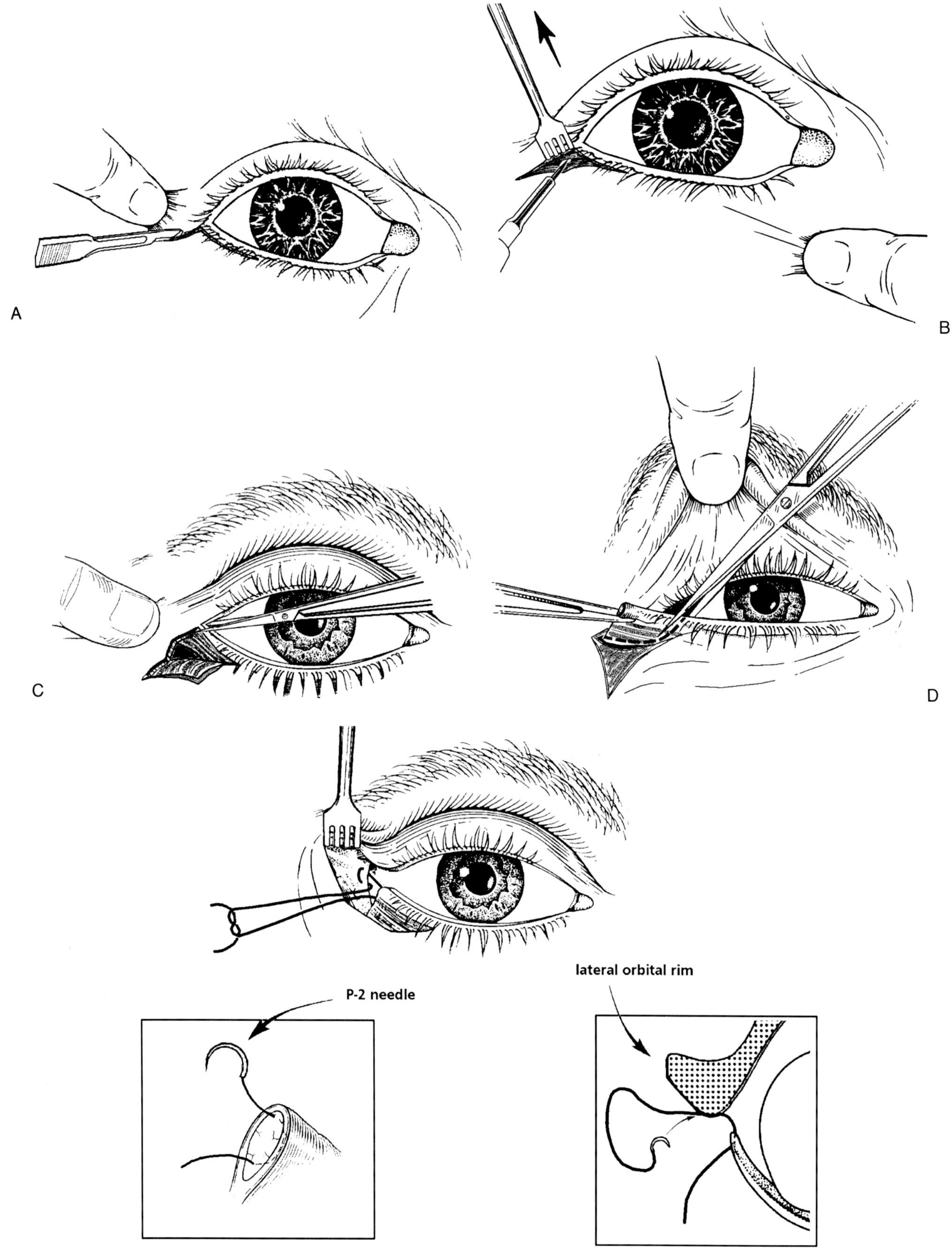
A
B
C
D
lateral orbital rim
P-2 needle

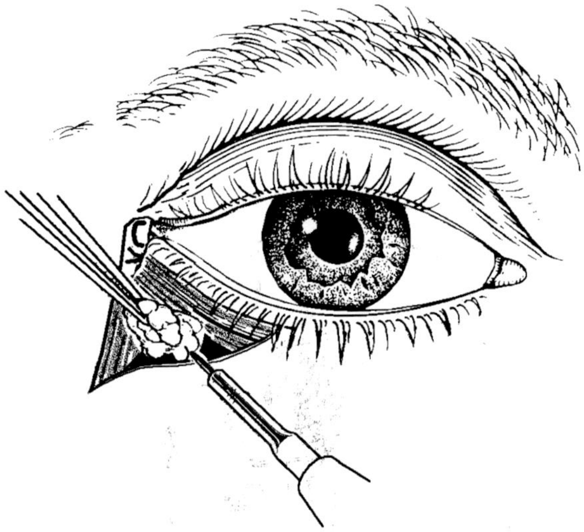

F

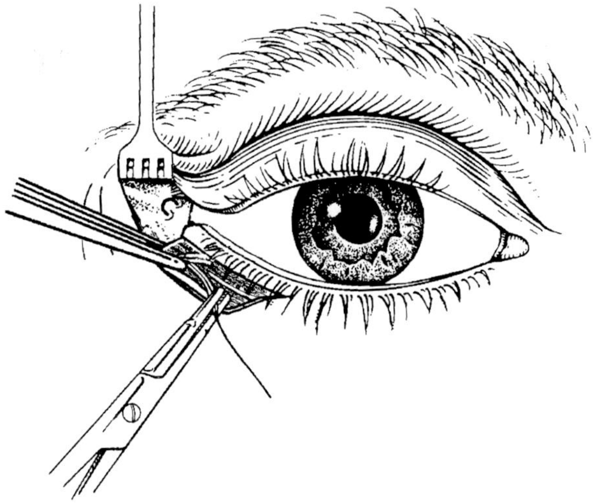

G

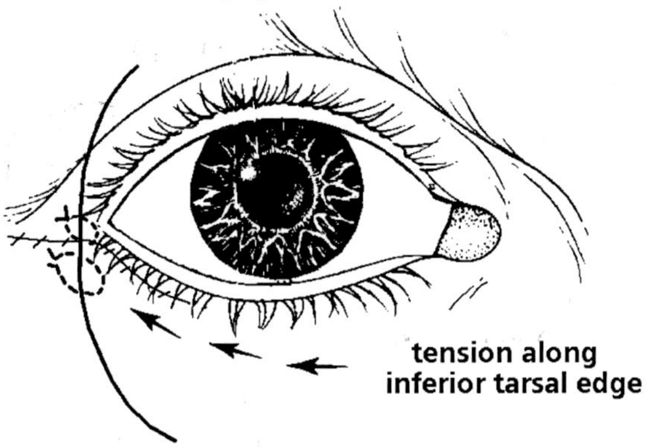

H

FIG. 6. The surgical correction of involutional laxity entropion. **A:** The subciliary skin incision is made in the temporal third of the lid and carried past the lateral canthal angle. **B:** Incision through the orbicularis layer allows development of a skin-muscle flap. **C:** The skin-muscle flap has been elevated exposing the lateral canthus. A canthotomy–canthal lysis of the lower limb of the lateral canthal tendon is performed at the exact canthal angle. **D:** After testing the horizontal redundancy of the lid against the lateral orbital rim, the portion of tarsoligamental sling that is felt to be redundant is excised. **E:** The lower tarsoligamental sling is then sutured to the lateral periosteum inside the orbital rim at the pupillary level. An intratarsal suture is placed and the suture inserted at the level of the orbital tubercle. A small half-circle (P2) needle is helpful. **F:** It is very common to have a protuberant lateral orbital fat pocket which, because of its bulk, interferes with tensing the tissue at the lower tarsal edge. It is excised. **G:** The tissue below the edge of the tarsal plate (septum, orbicularis) is grasped and tensed toward the lateral rim so that smoothing and tautness of the skin can be seen at the lower edge of the tarsal plate. This tissue is then sutured to the periosteum at the lateral orlbital rim. **H:** Final closure of entropion procedure showing the placement of the two horizontal tightening sutures and skin closure. Smoothing of the lower lid is seen.

pair, a double-armed 4-0 nonabsorbable suture (4-0 prolene with a P2 semicircular needle) is used to attach the lower lid in two places. The edge of the tarsal plate at its lower border and also the edge of the capsulopalpebral fascia is stretched and attached to the periosteum inside the lateral orbital rim. The half-circle needle enables one to introduce the suture inside the rim of the periosteum (Fig. 6E). The second suture is taken below the tarsal plate in the septum-capsulopalpebral fascia to tighten it to the lateral rim, which in turn stiffens the lower border of the tarsus. In most cases some excision of the lateral fat pad is necessary for debulking and for exposure for suture placement. The first suture is introduced into the lateral orbital rim at a horizontal level about on the plane of the mid-pupillary axis and then tightened. The second suture is placed and the skin is then closed (Fig. 6E–H). The lower edge of the skin may be somewhat redundant, and a small dog ear may be excised before closure. This procedure is used in most cases of involutional laxity entropion.

Horizontal Tightening with Inferior Retractor Plication

Some cases of entropion may be unusual in that there is not profound horizontal laxity present but spasm and entropion with outward rotation of the lower edge of the tarsal plate is present. In these cases a modification of the horizontal tightening procedure is used. The initial skin-muscle incision is extended further nasally. After the horizontal tightening is performed, 6-0 vicryl sutures are used to plicate the inferior retractors and septal tissue to the inferior tarsal border. Care is taken not to cause vertical lowering of the lower lid margin with scleral show.

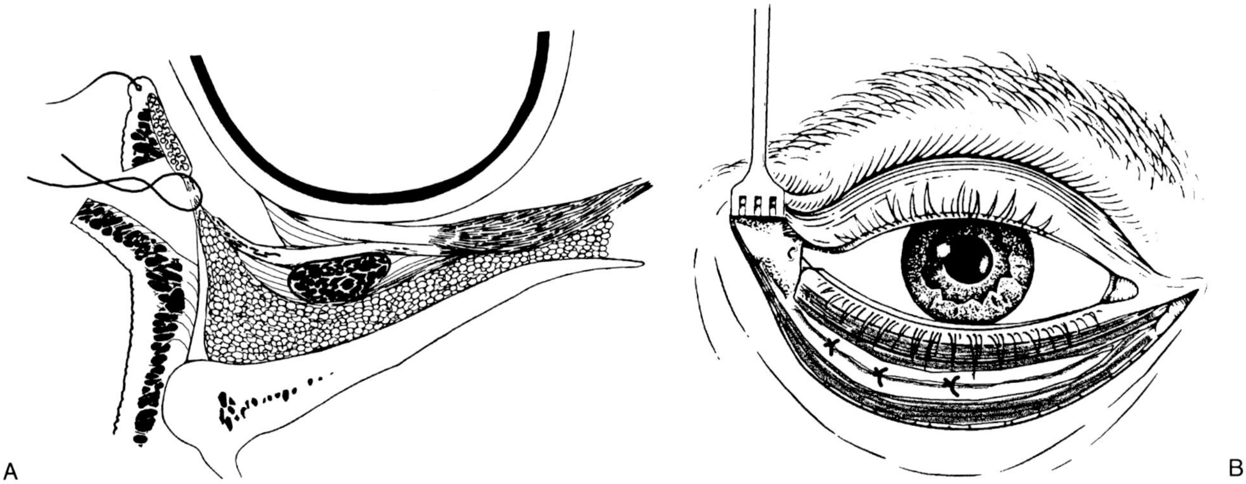

A B

FIG. 7. Repair of involutional and laxity entropion with combined horizontal tightening and plication of inferior retractor tissue. **A:** Sagittal view showing suture placement beneath the skin-muscle flap plicating the inferior tarsal edge to the inferior retractor. **B:** View showing the extension of the subciliary incision to expose the inferior retractors. Sutures have been placed from the inferior tarsal border to the retractors and tied. Care is taken not to cause vertical shortening of the lid with scleral show. The plication of the retractors is usually performed after the horizontal and tightening procedure is completed.

Cicatricial Entropion

The soundest surgical principle that one can use to correct cicatricial entropion from shortening of the posterior lamella is to replace the deficient tissue in the lid with a graft in the anatomic area of deficiency (Fig. 7A, B).

For mild cases (Fig. 8A, B) there are some valuable shortcut procedures that may be used to supplement one's armamentarium. The transverse tarsotomy and marginal rotation, or *Wies procedure,* has been used very frequently to correct mild cases of cicatricial entropion of the lower lids (10). The shortcoming of this procedure is that it produces a vertical shortening of

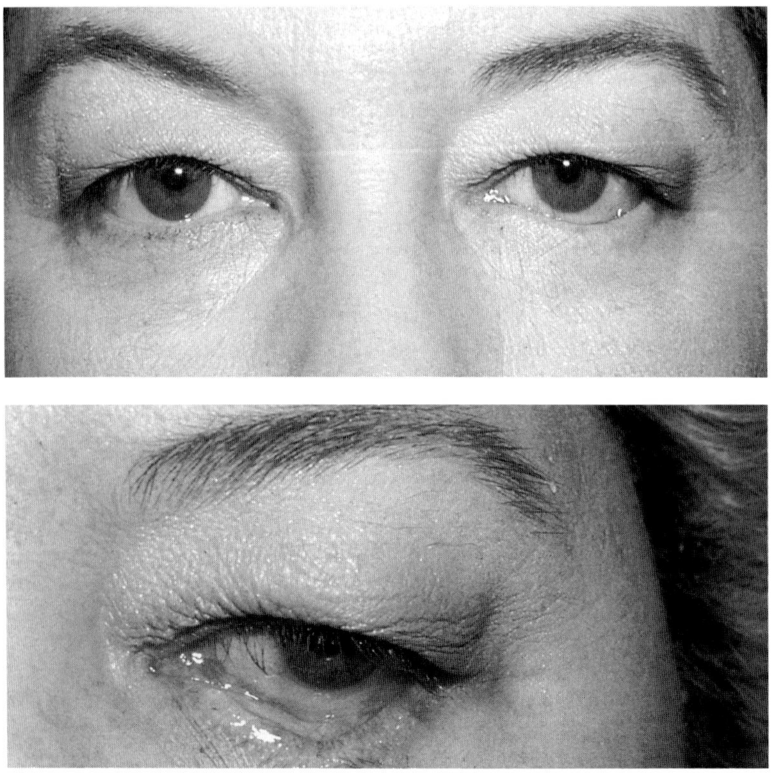

A B

FIG. 8. A: Patient with involutional laxity entropion with a cicatricial component. **B:** Eversion of lower lid shows scarring at the inferior tarsal border and conjunctiva buckling the tarsus inward. The patient had a previous tarsoconjunctival triangular resection for involutional laxity entropion. Since laxity was still present and the cicatricial elements were mild, it was felt that a combined horizontal tightening and Wies procedure would be appropriate.

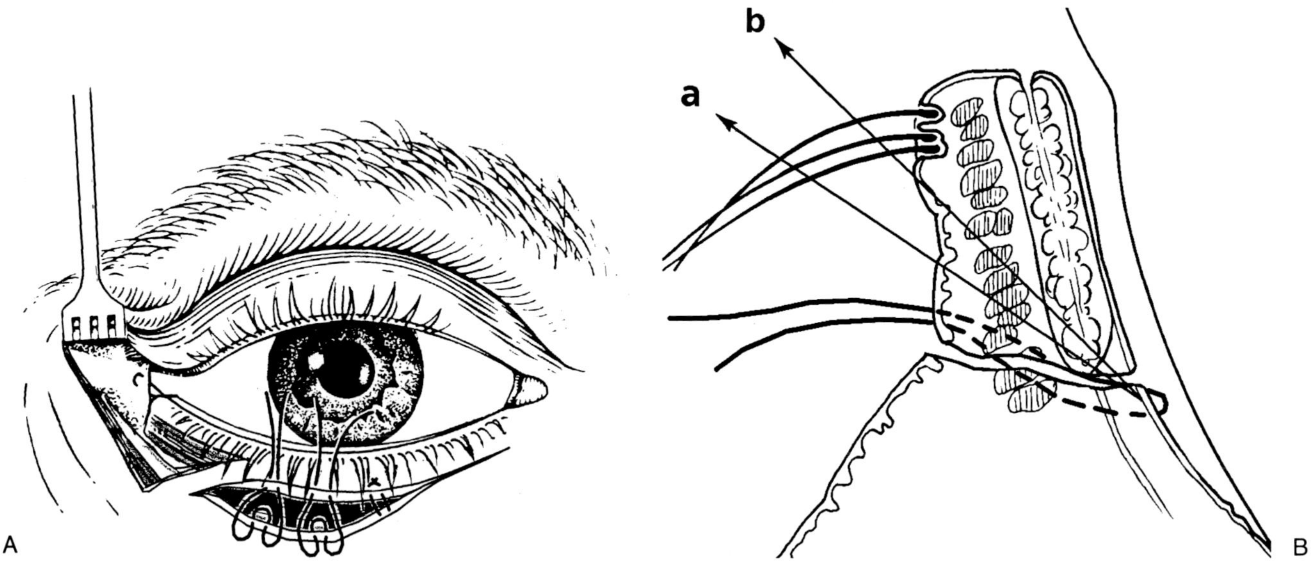

FIG. 9. Correction of involutional entropion. Combined horizontal tightening and Wies (transverse blepharotomy and marginal rotation) procedure. **A:** The horizontal tightening has been completed and a full-thickness transverse blepharotomy beneath the inferior edge of the tarsal border completed. Rotating sutures have been placed from the inferior edge of the tarsoconjunctival surface through the superior edge of the cutaneous incision to rotate the lid outward. **B:** Sagittal view showing suture placement for Wies procedure. An increasing rotational effect can be obtained by exiting the sutures higher above the transverse blepharotomy incision underneath the lashes. Placement B would give maximum outward rotation of the lid margin.

the lid, even though it can rotate the lashes satisfactorily. When considering corrective surgery, the surgeon must differentiate between patients with adequate tarsus and those who have deficient or unstable tarsus. The tarsotomy procedure makes the assumption that adequate tarsus is present. This is not always the case and the procedures will fail if the tarsus is unstable or deficient. In very severe cases with areas of deficient tissue, the entropion must be corrected with a graft (17). Sources of autogenous graft tissue include buccal mucous membrane, nasal chondromucosa, ear cartilage, and palatal mucoperichondrium. In upper lid entropion, since the tarsal plate is much wider than the lower lid, a rotational procedure can be used there for milder cases. However, severe cases must be corrected with grafting; commonly, in cases of margin destruction, a reconstructive procedure to the margin itself must be performed.

Wies Procedure (Transverse Tarsotomy, Marginal Rotation) with Horizontal Tightening

The authors do not use the transverse tarsotomy frequently as a stand alone procedure, but it is presented here for completeness. It is more commonly used in combination with a horizontal tightening procedure and in some cases of mixed laxity and cicatricial entropion. It was described initially for laxity entropion but has become widely used for mild cases of cicatricial entropion.

Technique

The horizontal tightening procedure is first performed to correct for any laxity component present. For a rotational effect to evert the lid margin in cases of mild residual inturning, a full-thickness horizontal blepharotomy incision is made below the inferior edge of the lower lid tarsal plate (best placed 4–5 mm from the margin). This is performed in a two-step manner with an external skin-muscle incision and then a buttonhole incision into the fornix, which is then enlarged with scissors. Sutures are passed from the lower edge of the inner incision to the superior edge of the external incision for a rotational effect. More eversion of the lid margin can be obtained by placing the sutures to the external surface at higher positions under the lashes (Fig. 9A, B).

Posterior Lamella Graft with Horizontal Tightening

In cases of severe cicatricial entropion, the posterior lamella of the eyelid (tarsoconjunctiva and the forniceal conjunctiva) is contracted and the only procedure that can be used for restoring lid position successfully is lengthening of the posterior lamella by grafted material (Fig. 10A, B). A Wies procedure generally will not correct the entropion and will only cause retraction of the lower lid. Figure 11A shows a patient with a severely contracted posterior lamella.

Technique

A canthotomy and cantholysis is performed and the lid is everted. On the posterior surface the tarsus is incised 3 mm below the eyelid margin and dissected until the lid assumes a normal position. The posterior lamella graft is then sutured in place. The available materials for posterior lamella grafts are ear cartilage, nasal chondromucosa, palatal mucoperichondrium, and full-thickness buccal mucous membrane; all have been used with success. Autogenous ear cartilage is most commonly used with good results, and the surface will completely epithelialize in 4–6 weeks. The use of steroid/antibiotic eye drops will reduce ocular irritation in the immediate postoperative period following ear cartilage grafting in which the internal surface is left bare. Nasochondromucosa can be used; however, because the nasal septal cartilage is very brittle and thick and the nasal mucous membrane is also very thick, there is exessive mucoid discharge. Palatal mucoperichondrium has provided excellent internal lamella replacement with a smooth mucous membrane surface and some ridigity.

Surgical views of the grafting technique used in lower lid surgery are shown in Fig. 11B–D. If severe lid atrophy is present, one may consider an eyelid reconstructive procedure as described in the chapter on lower lid reconstruction.

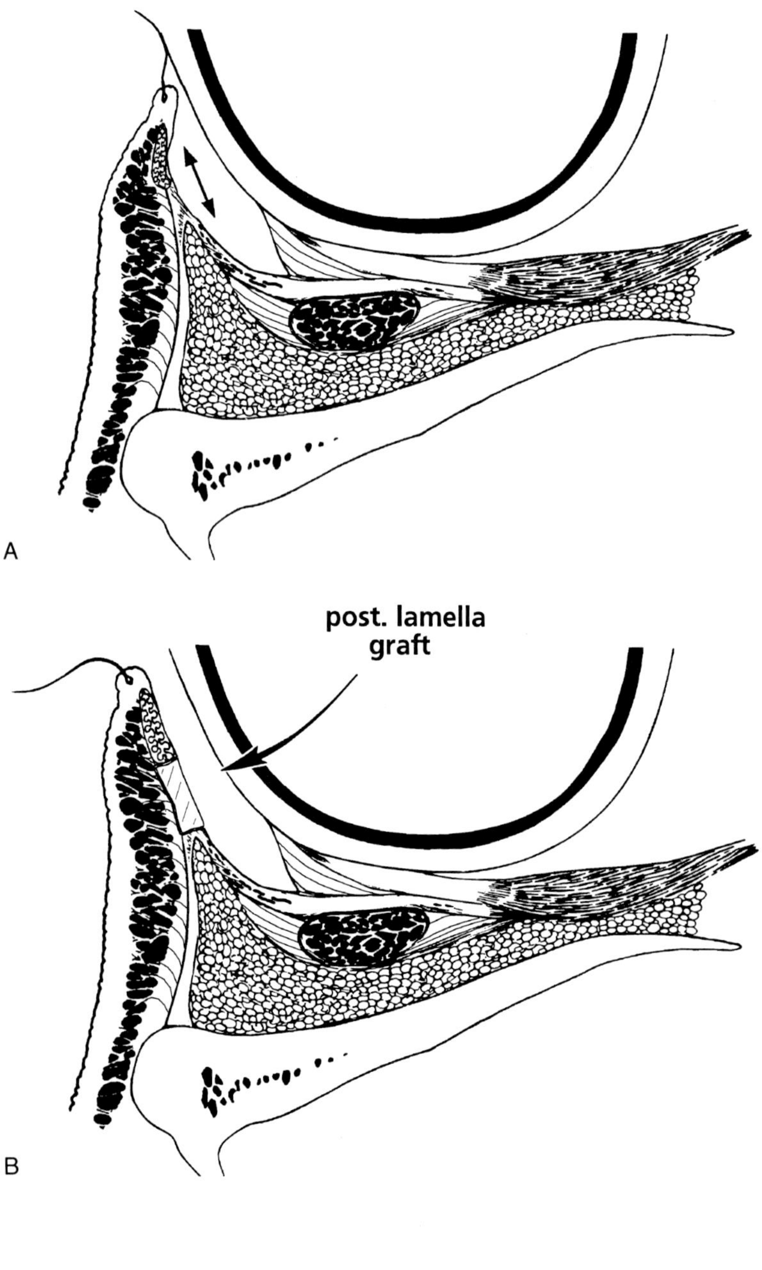

FIG. 10. Cicatricial entropion. **A:** Sagittal view showing scarring and shortening of the internal lamella of the eyelid causing an entropion. This can occur from any cicatrizing disease and commonly occurs following previous lower lid surgery. **B:** Correction of cicatricial entropion of the lower lid with posterior lamella graft. Tissue grafts available for the posterior lamella graft are autogenous ear cartilage, palatal mucoperichondrium, and buccal mucous membrane.

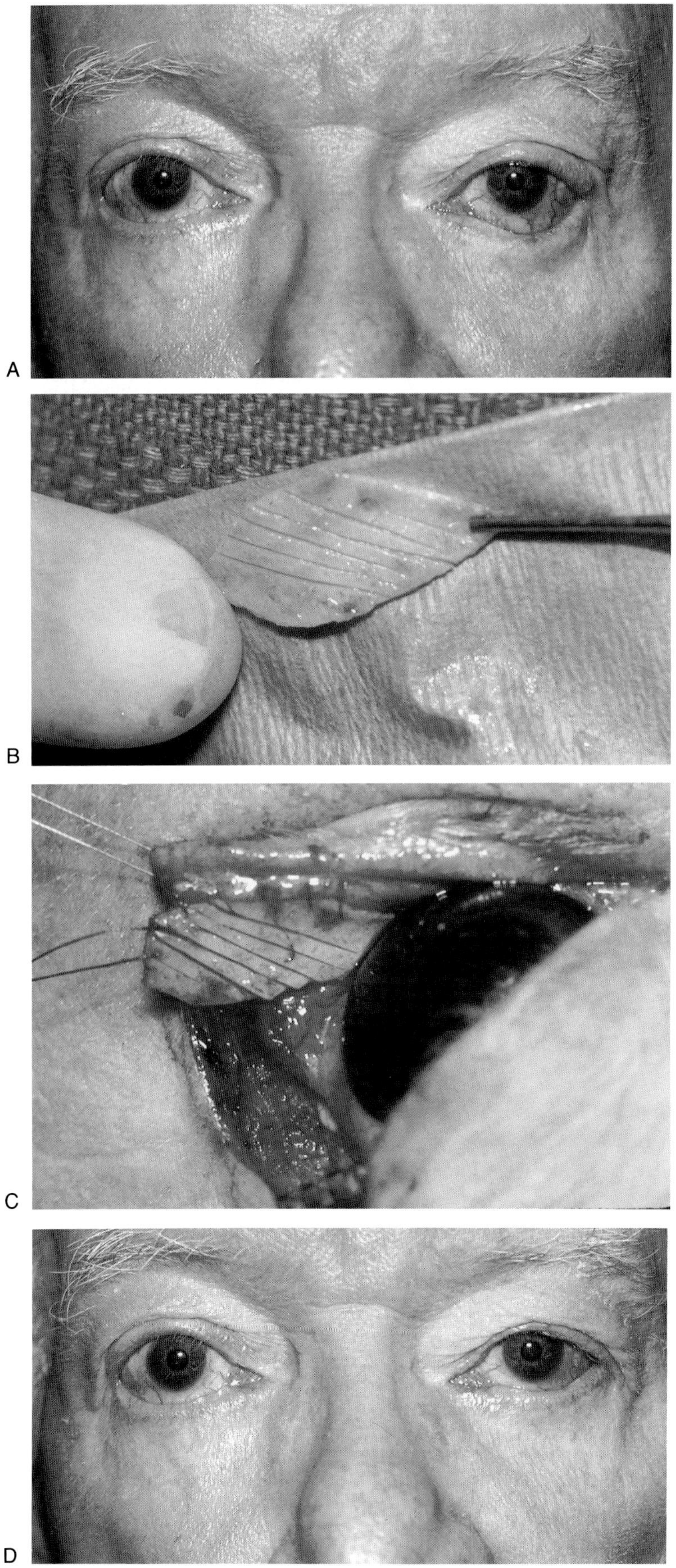

FIG. 11. A: Patient with cicatricial entropion in the left lower lid. The patient has had two previous entropion procedures that were unsuccessful. **B:** Posterior lamella graft of autogenous ear cartilage. The graft has been "diced" to flatten the graft. **C:** Removal of the scar tissue in the posterior lamella has been performed and the graft been positioned to lengthen the posterior lamella. A horizontal tightening procedure is also being performed. **D:** The same patient postoperatively following placement of a posterior lamella graft and horizontal tightening.

UPPER LID ENTROPIONS

Upper lid entropion is usually the result of a scarring process. Worldwide the most common cause is trachoma; however, in the United States the most common causes are scarring from chronic blepharoconjunctivitis, Stevens–Johnson syndrome, or burns (18) (Table 2). Some conditions may produce or mimic an entropion variant but behave differently from the true entropion. Floppy lid syndrome (19–23), congenital tarsal kink (24), and epicanthal folds, congenital or otherwise, may produce an entropion-like situation.

Congenital Tarsal Kink Syndrome

Congenital tarsal kink syndrome is a condition that is recognized shortly after birth and may present as a corneal ulceration. On examination is noted an inturning of the upper lid and marked blepharospasm. There is an inward kink in the upper tarsal plate encompassing the entire horizontal length with resultant inversion of the lid margin abrading the cornea. A tarsal fracture procedure and rotation of the tarsal plate as subsequently described can be used as a corrective procedure (24).

Acquired Entropion of the Upper Lid

The large majority of cases of upper lid entropion are on a cicatricial basis and the upper lid entropion may be accompanied by destructive disease of the margin with changes that also requires specific procedures. In the more severe cases, the deficient posterior lamella must be restored with a posterior lamella graft.

Tarsal Fracture with Margin Rotation (Tenzel Procedure)

A procedure to rotate the upper lid margin without grafts was described by Tenzel et al. (25). It can be used in milder cases in which the tarsal plate is healthy and relatively unaffected by the scarring process. Some lid retraction can occur with this procedure. It should not be used in severe cases of cicatricial entropion because in these cases the margin cannot be fully rotated and it will produce significant vertical shortening of the eyelid.

Technique

A lid crease incision is made with elevation of the musculocutaneous layer from the tarsal plate. A trough or wedge is cut in the tarsal plate; try not to make a full-thickness incision (Fig. 12A, B). An incision is also made in the margin separating the skin and muscle from

TABLE 2. *Etiology of upper lid entropion (after Collin)*

Trachoma
Chronic blepharoconjunctivitis
Erythema multiforme
Chemical/radiant injury
Postsurgical
Pemphigoid
Mechanical
Postenucleation socket syndrome
Herpes zoster
Vernal conjunctivitis
Graves' disease

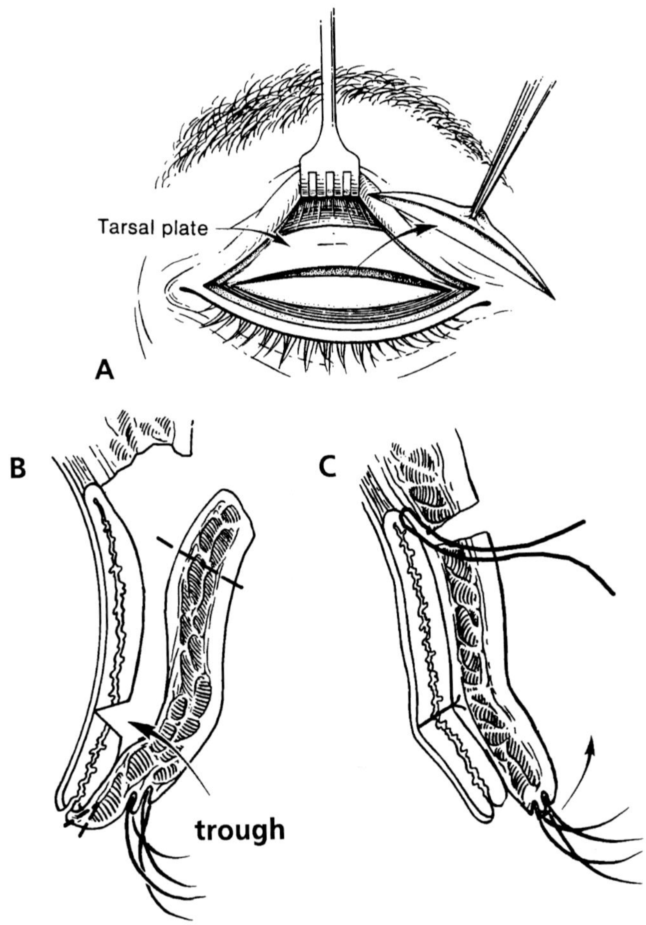

FIG. 12. Mild entropion of the upper lid. Correction by tarsal fracture procedure (Tenzel). **A:** An eyelid crease incision with exposure of the tarsal plate has been performed. A wedge of tarsus has been excised above the lash line. **B:** Sagittal view of procedure showing wedge excision, excision of redundant skin, and incision at the eyelid margin separating the anterior and posterior lamella. **C:** A suture has been placed in the tarsal plate buckling the tarsal plate outward for partial correction of the entropion. Tensing sutures in the pretarsal skin-muscle layer have also been placed rotating the lashes outward.

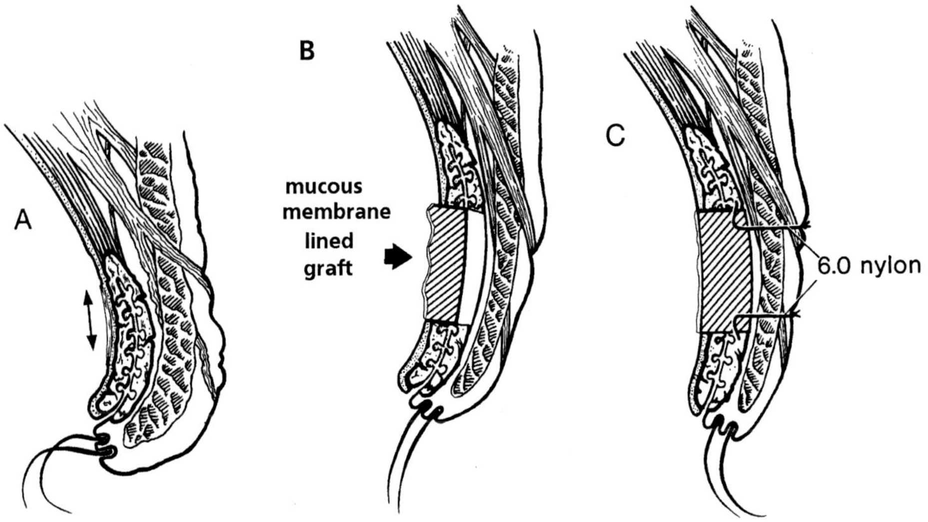

FIG. 13. Severe cicatricial entropion of the upper lid. **A:** Saggittal view showing cicatricial entropion of the upper lid with shrinkage of the tarsus and conjunctival layer. **B:** Relaxing incision has been made in the residual tarsus allowing outward rotation of the lashes and a posterior lamellar mucous membrane–lined graft has been inserted. Tissue that can be used for this can be palatal mucoperichondrium, full-thickness buccal mucous membrane, or nasal chondromucosa. **C:** Placement of the graft in the recipient site with sutures brought externally to the skin surface to avoid exposure to the cornea with possible abrasions.

the tarsal plate in that area. Some redundant skin and muscle is excised from the upper edge of the skin incision. Although the thinness of the upper lid tarsus may prevent it, closure of the tarsal trough with fine sutures can be attempted. Transcutaneous 6-0 vicryl sutures are placed through the musculocutaneous flap and into the levator aponeurosis, everting the margin and rotating the lashes. Separate sutures may be placed for musculocutaneous closure. This procedure is a tarsal fracture and rotation of the upper lid margin, which can be used in mild cases of cicatricial entropion of the upper lid (Fig. 12C).

Posterior Lamella Grafting

Many cases of cicatricial entropion of the lids cannot be treated with the other described procedure because of a tarsal shortage. When the posterior lamella of the eyelid, the tarsoconjunctiva, and the forniceal conjunctiva are contracted (Fig. 13A), the only procedure that can be used successfully is lengthening of the posterior lamella with grafted material. Replacement of the contracted posterior lamella can be performed by itself if the margin of the eyelid is normal. Commonly, however, the margin is affected by the destructive process and posterior lamella grafting must be accompanied by a reconstructive procedure for the margin. Figure 13B and C shows correction of cicatricial entropion of upper lid, with loss of tarsoconjunctiva requiring replacement. In these cases a graft must be placed on the posterior lamella of the eyelid. A transverse incision throughout the entire width of the lid and the dissection are carried out, creating space in which to put the graft. The graft is then fixed in position with sutures that are brought externally through the lid and tied on the anterior surface. The available materials are ear cartilage, nasochondromucosa, full-thickness buccal mucous membrane, and palatal mucoperichondrium. Autogenous ear cartilage may be used in certain cases with good results and the surface will completely epithelialize in 4–6 weeks; however, if directly exposed to the cornea it may cause corneal abrasions. Any graft not lined with mucosa has the potential of abrading the cornea in the early postoperative period. Nasochondromucosa can be used; however, because the nasal septal cartilage is very brittle and thick and the nasal mucous membrane is also very thick, there is excessive mucoid discharge. Palatal mucochondrium has provided excellent internal lamella replacement with a smooth mucous membrane surface and some ridigity. If a severely damaged tarsal plate is a problem with the cicatricial entropion in the upper lid, one may consider an eyelid reconstructive procedure.

Floppy Upper Lid Syndrome

The floppy upper lid syndrome was defined as a condition usually seen in obese, middle-aged males with degenerative changes and loss of elasticity in the tarsal plate in the upper lid (19–23). The patients characteris-

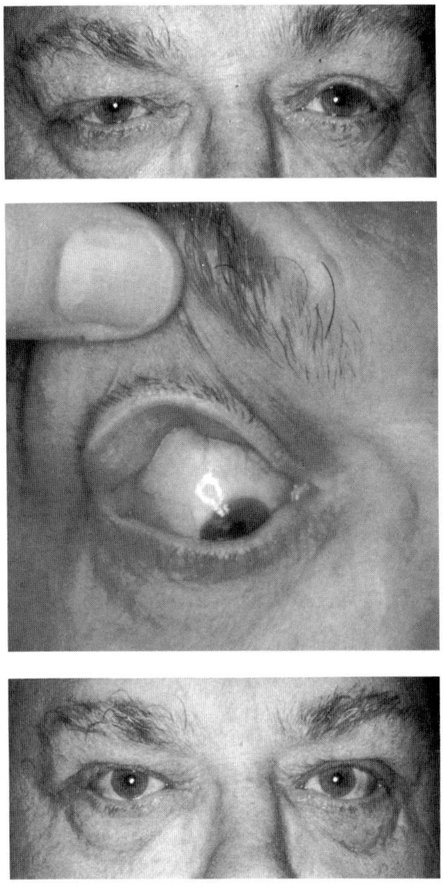

FIG. 14. Floppy eyelid syndrome. **A:** Patient with bilateral floppy upper lid syndrome with recurrent corneal irritation, chronic conjunctivitis, and intermittent entropion of the upper lid with lash dystrophy. **B:** Right upper lid is everted showing loss of elasticity of the superior torsal plate, redundancy of the upper lid tissue, and chronic conjunctivitis. **C:** Same patient following the lateral canthoplasty, lid resection with periosteal flaps, and aponeurotic repair, bilaterally.

tically have a very distensible upper lid and suffer from chronic irritation of the lid and eye from malposition. The malposition can occur during sleep with lid eversion causing exposure and an overlapping of the upper lid over the lower lid has been described. The authors have seen patients with the described changes who also have episodes of upper lid entropion and many are seen to have a dystrophy of the lashes with a downward turning (Fig. 14A, B). Although with this condition the upper lid undergoes periodic eversion, for the purpose of convenience the condition is listed with upper lid entropion since it may also occur. The underlying etiology is unknown.

Technique of Correction

Simple full-thickness resection of the lids and tightening at the lateral canthus can help. Because in these cases the canthal tissue has severe atrophy and loss of integrity, recurrence is common. Canthal resection and reconstruction with periosteal flaps combined with levator plication can give a more definitive correction (see Fig. 15A–C for surgical steps). Figure 13C shows the same patient shown in the previous figures after correction by this technique.

EYELID MARGIN DEFORMITY AND TRICHIASIS

Marginal destruction together with trichiasis is a variant of cicatricial entropion in which the disease process has primarily affected the eyelid margin, causing destruction of marginal architecture and inturning of the margin with abrasion of the cornea from normal and abnormal cilia and epidermalized tissue.

Disorders of the margin of the eyelid arise from a variety of causes, including inflammation, trauma, and surgery. Regardless of the etiology or the specific anatomic changes, any change in the eyelid margin has significant impact on the integrity of the cornea because of the constant movement of the eyelid margin against its surface. Three basic processes can occur pathologically in the eyelid margin that have adverse effects on the cornea: trichiasis, margin destruction and entropion with trichiasis, and epidermalization of the margin and palpebral conjunctiva. Some patients will manifest all three of these changes, whereas in others one aspect will predominate. It is useful to try to group these patients in this manner for treatment. Insofar as possible, one must determine clinically the specific underlying problem and treat it accordingly.

Trichiasis

Trichiasis refers to the misalignment of lashes, with their direction inward against the conjunctiva and cornea. If these lashes impinge on the conjunctiva, a foreign body sensation occurs and conjunctival infection may result. However, if the lashes are directed against the cornea, pain, corneal epithelial irregularities, and even corneal ulceration may occur. Although it would seem that these lashes could be easily destroyed, management of trichiasis requires a systematic and persistent approach. Patients and physicians are frequently annoyed by the recalcitrant nature of this problem.

Classification and Etiology

The eitiology of trichiasis is varied. The classifications include trichiasis resulting from the following situations: (a) mechanical disruption of the eyelid margin, (b) cicatricial changes in the eyelid that produce an inversion of the lid margin with or without metaplastic

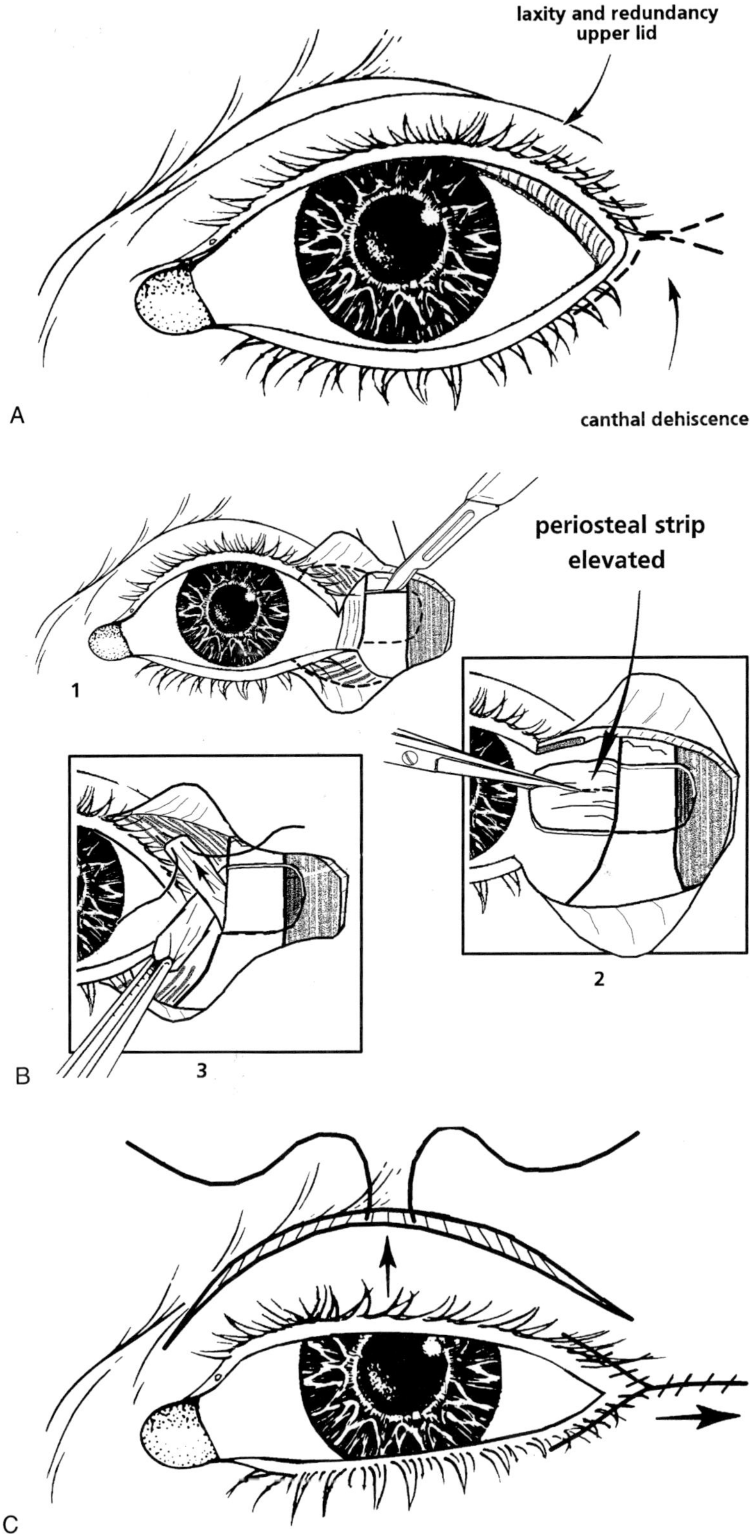

FIG. 15. Corrective procedure for floppy upper lid syndrome. **A:** Incisions are made at the lateral canthus to create an upper and lower lid flap to expose the canthal angle. **B:** Steps in the procedure of lateral canthoplasty with periosteal flaps. (1) A canthotomy and canthal lysis of the upper and lower limb of the canthal tendon has been performed. A periosteal strip is elevated from the lateral orbital rim. (2) The periosteal strip is brought inward and divided. (3) The upper periosteal strip is brought downward toward the lower lid edge and sutured and the lower periosteal strip is brought upward to the upper lid edge and sutured. They are adjusted to create the desired tension in the upper and lower lid to cause the lids to oppose the globe. Further details of the procedure can be found in the chapter on lateral canthal reconstruction. **C:** Following the canthoplasty, the upper lid is normally pulled downward creating a ptosis. An aponeurotic repair is then performed in the upper lid. Details of this procedure can be found in the chapter on levator surgery.

changes of the meibomian glands, (c) congenital misdirected lashes (distichiasis), and (d) idiopathic. This classification is effective in conveying an appreciation of the etiology of trichiasis; however, treatment considerations are based on physical features of trichiasis (see Table 3).

Mechanical disruption of the eyelid margin may produce trichiasis. Laceration of the eyelid margin requires careful repair. Faulty approximation of the wound edges may result in notching of the eyelid and trichiasis. Block resections of the eyelid for tumor excision or lid-shortening procedures may also produce

TABLE 3. *Trichiasis classification and etiology*

Segmental
- Idiopathic aberrant lashes
- Misdirected normal lashes
- Posttrauma lid laceration
- Postoperative tarsorraphy-chalazion

Generalized
- without margin epidermalization
  - Congenital
  - Distichiasis
- margin epidermalization usually present
  - Chronic blepharoconjunctivitis
  - Pemphigoid
  - Erythema multiforme
  - Trachoma
  - Chemical injury
  - Chronic glaucoma drop use

notching and trichiasis. Even with careful anatomic reapproximation, trichiasis may result from disruption of follicles. Trichiasis may be observed following shave excision of nevi of the eyelid margin or may result from the mechanical disruption of the tumor itself. Multiple fine lanugo hairs may be the result of eyelid reconstructions such as the Mustarde cheek rotation. Diffuse trichiasis is more apt to be present in the latter conditions.

Cicatricial changes of the eyelids may be a manifestation of chronic inflammatory conditions, including cicatricial pemphigoid ("benign" ocular pemphigoid), erythema multiforme (Stevens–Johnson syndrome), chemical injury, trachoma, chronic blepharitis, acne rosacea, and chronic allergic reactions. Chronic use of glaucoma drops can produce cicatricial changes. These conditions have a common feature in that a chronic inflammatory infiltrate produces cicatricial changes in the eyelid. The posterior lamella of the eyelid, consisting of the tarsus and conjunctiva, is shortened, causing inversion of the eyelid margin to produce a cicatricial entropion of varying degrees. In addition, the chronic inflammatory changes of the meibomian glands produce a metaplasia of the glands and fine hairs emerge from the orifices of the gland. There may be an associated irritating epidermalization of the conjunctiva. These abnormal lashes and cicatricial changes of the eyelid aggravate the inflammation of the eyelid tissues. A cycle is then created. Trichiasis persists and even worsens, causing more inflammation and scarring. Trichiasis may be the initial complaint of patients with cicatricial pemphigoid. A slit-lamp examination may reveal blunting of the cul-de-sacs and symblepharon to confirm this diagnosis.

Congenital trichiasis may be associated with distichiasis, epiblepharon, or tarsal kink. Distichiasis is an extra one or two rows of lashes and is usually a dominant congenital anomaly. The accessory row of lashes comes from the meibomian gland openings. These accessory cilia may produce irritation. Epiblepharon consists of lashes rolled against the cornea by an infralash fold of skin. This defect frequently occurs in Asians or is associated with epicanthal folds.

Trichiasis that does not have apparent etiology is termed idiopathic. Idiopathic aberrant lashes are usually localized in nature but may affect the entire eyelid margin. These patients may sometimes represent an early manifestation of cicatricial pemphigoid. Sullivan et al. (29) reported 72 patients with trichiasis. The most common single class of trichiasis encountered was idiopathic aberrant lashes, accounting for approximately 30% of cases encountered.

Treatment

Multiple treatment modalities are employed for the management of trichiasis. Management is based on the diagnosis, degree, and extent of the abnormal lash involvement. The surgical approach to trichiasis should be tailored to the individual and clinical situation and will vary based on its localized or generalized nature. A localized area of abnormal lashes following eyelid laceration would be approached differently from a trichiasis associated with cicatricial pemphigoid. Fine lanugo hairs are more difficult to erradicate than normal-appearing cilia, so their presence should be noted. Associated ocular features characteristic of inflammation or cicatrization should be observed.

Cicatricial pemphigoid may have progressive scarring of the eyelids and mucous membranes of the eyelid. The resulting dry eye syndrome produced by obliteration of goblet cells (mucin secretion), meibomian glands (lipin secretion), and accessory lacrimal glands (Krause, Wolfring) accelerates the damaging effects of trichiasis. All attempts at the correction of this condition may be futile in that approximately 30% of eyes affected with this condition become blind (8).

Epilation

One or several lashes may be epilated on a repetitive basis, but persistent recurrences should be treated with a more permanent method if progressive or corneal changes occur.

Electrolysis

Electrolysis has a success rate of 30–50%. A local anesthetic agent may be used. The lash follicle is impaled with the electrolysis needle. Current is applied until bubbles exude from the follicle. Approximately 15–20 s of treatment is required for each lash. All the lashes in a localized area are treated. If lashes are effectively treated, they can easily be extracted from their follicle. Fine lanugo hairs respond poorly to treatment with electrolysis. It should be noted that electrolysis does produce localized scarring of the eyelid and may accentuate entropion. Therefore, it should be used with caution because of the cicatricial and metaplastic changes it may produce.

Lid Resection

Localized trichiasis associated with notching or scarring or involving a localized segment of the eyelid are ideally treated by removing a pentagonal block of the affected eyelid margin as described in the chapters on eyelid reconstruction.

Cryotherapy

If widespread trichiasis or fine lanugo hairs are present, local resection is not possible. If trichiasis is diffuse, entropion is not present, the tear film is adequate, and there is no soft tissue damage, cryotherapy can be used (28–30). It should be noted that cryotherapy of the upper eyelid may produce a total loss of lashes and may be cosmetically undesirable. Additionally, loss of pigment is to be expected. Cryotherapy has been utilized in diffuse trichiasis resulting from inflammatory or cicatricial eyelid disorders, including postsurgical problems. Lash follicles are destroyed at temperatures of −20°C. Fortunately, the tarsus and lacrimal outflow system are relatively resistant to freezing and require tissue temperatures of −40 to −70°C before destruction occurs. Because of this discrepancy in sensitivity to cryotherapy, the larger eyelid structures usually display little sequelae of treatment. Cicatricial changes of the eyelids, particularly in pemphigoid, may be aggravated by cryotherapy, thus causing signficant progression of damage to the lids and the eye. Therefore, we are very reluctant to freeze pemphigoid lids unless it is absolutely necessary because of lack of a better procedure. In these cases, repeated treatments at −10°C are safer than those at −20°C in our experience. Figure 16A and B shows the application of ointment for conduction and freezing using the above technique. Once the freeze time for a particular freezing unit to produce the desired temperature in the tissue has been determined, the thermocouple need not be used in subsequent freezes.

Complications are minimized by correct freezing techniques. Monitoring of tissue temperatures with a thermocouple ensures a correctly applied freeze to maximize the destruction of lashes and minimize the damage to the eyelid. Double freeze–thaw cycles may produce considerable postoperative pain and edema. Dermal melanocytes are sensitive to temperatures ranging from −15° to −20°C. A localized area of depigmentation results from treatment and may persist. Cryotherapy should therefore be used with reservation in darkly pigmented individuals. Eyelid sloughing has been reported following therapy. Most individuals do have some thinning and alteration of eyelid thickness with the use of cryotherapy. In summary, the complications of lid cryopexy are tissue shrinkage, acceleration of pemphigoid, alteration of tear film (ablation of tarsal and mucin glands), and depigmentation.

Laser Ablation

Argon laser thermal ablation may be a suitable alternative to electrolysis or cryotherapy in selected cases

A

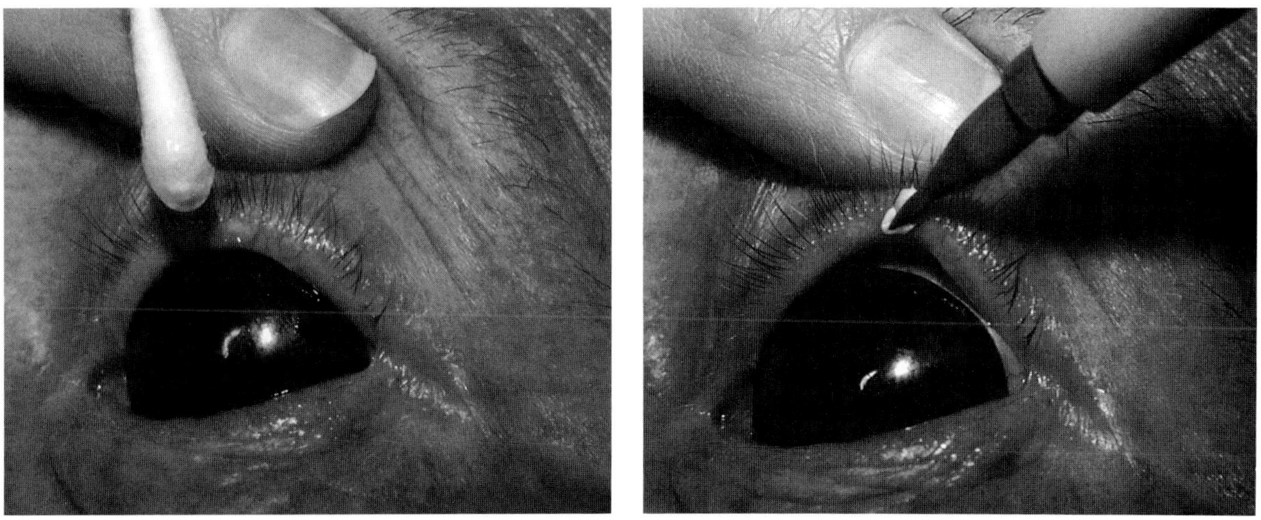

B

FIG. 16. Cryopexy for trichiasis of the eyelid. **A:** To enhance thermal transfer and freezing, K-Y jelly is applied to the area of the lid to be frozen. **B:** The cryoprobe is applied to the localized area of trichiasis with the freeze-thaw, freeze-thaw technique.

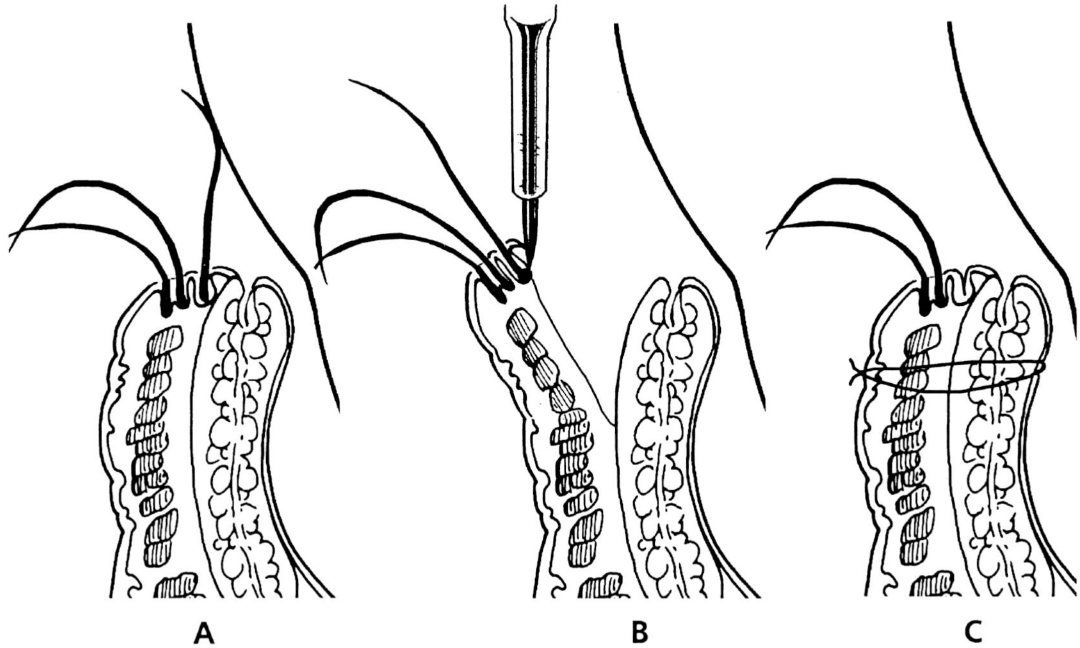

FIG. 17. Direct removal of lash follicles with incision and cautery. **A:** An incision is made separating the anterior and posterior lamella in the eyelid to expose the lash follicles. **B:** The lash follicles are seen in the inner surface of the external lamella as black globules. With magnification they can be selectively cauterized with a bipolar cautery. The lash is then removed with light pulling. If the follicle has been destroyed, the lash can be easily lifted from the tissue. **C:** Closure of the anterior and posterior lamella with a mattress suture tied on the external surface. This procedure can be performed successfully in lids with reasonably normal architecture of the margin.

of trichiasis. Argon laser application will produce focal destruction of lash follicles with mild to moderate soft tissue inflammation. The argon blue–green laser is used and a spot size of 50 μm, 300 mW power, and 0.5-s duration is the standard setting. Marking dye seems to enhance the results. Retreatment is usually needed in 50% of cases (31,32).

Direct Follicle Ablation with Margin Incision

Offending lash follicles can be excised or ablated with electrocautery, sparing the soft tissue damage associated with electrolysis involing direct incision into the eyelid margin splitting the anterior and posterior lamella. With magnification, the black, globular lash follicles can be directly cauterized with the bipolar or needle cautery (Fig. 17A–C). Closure is accomplished with simple mattress sutures. Tissue damage is minimal with this technique (33,34).

ARCHITECTURAL DEFORMITY OF THE EYELID MARGIN

Metaplasia and Epidermalization

Some patients will manifest scarring and metaplasia of the eyelid margin following traumatic and inflammatory changes that do not produce either abnormal hairs or destruction of margin architecture. These patients will have a metaplasia of the posterior lid margin edge and palpebral conjunctiva, which produces a roughened surface and will abrade the cornea and produce punctate keratitis and vascularization in the absence of trichiasis.

Margin Dermabrasion with Mucous Membrane Grafting

The treatment of isolated epidermalization of the margin has been very gratifying. It consists of a technique of abrasion of the margin of the eyelid, with removal of the scar tissue and metaplastic epithelium, and overgrafting of the abraded area with a full-thickness buccal mucous membrane graft (35). This can be used on the margin itself or for larger areas that include the margin and palpebral conjunctiva. The ability to graft on an intact tarsus is far superior to the excisional methods of repair and those that damage the tarsus or cause it to lose its integrity in some manner, thereby decreasing the stability of the eyelid. Figure 19A and B shows the everted lids of a patient with Stevens–Johnson syndrome with epidermalization of the posterior edge of the eyelid causing cornea vascularization, although very few trichiatic hairs are present.

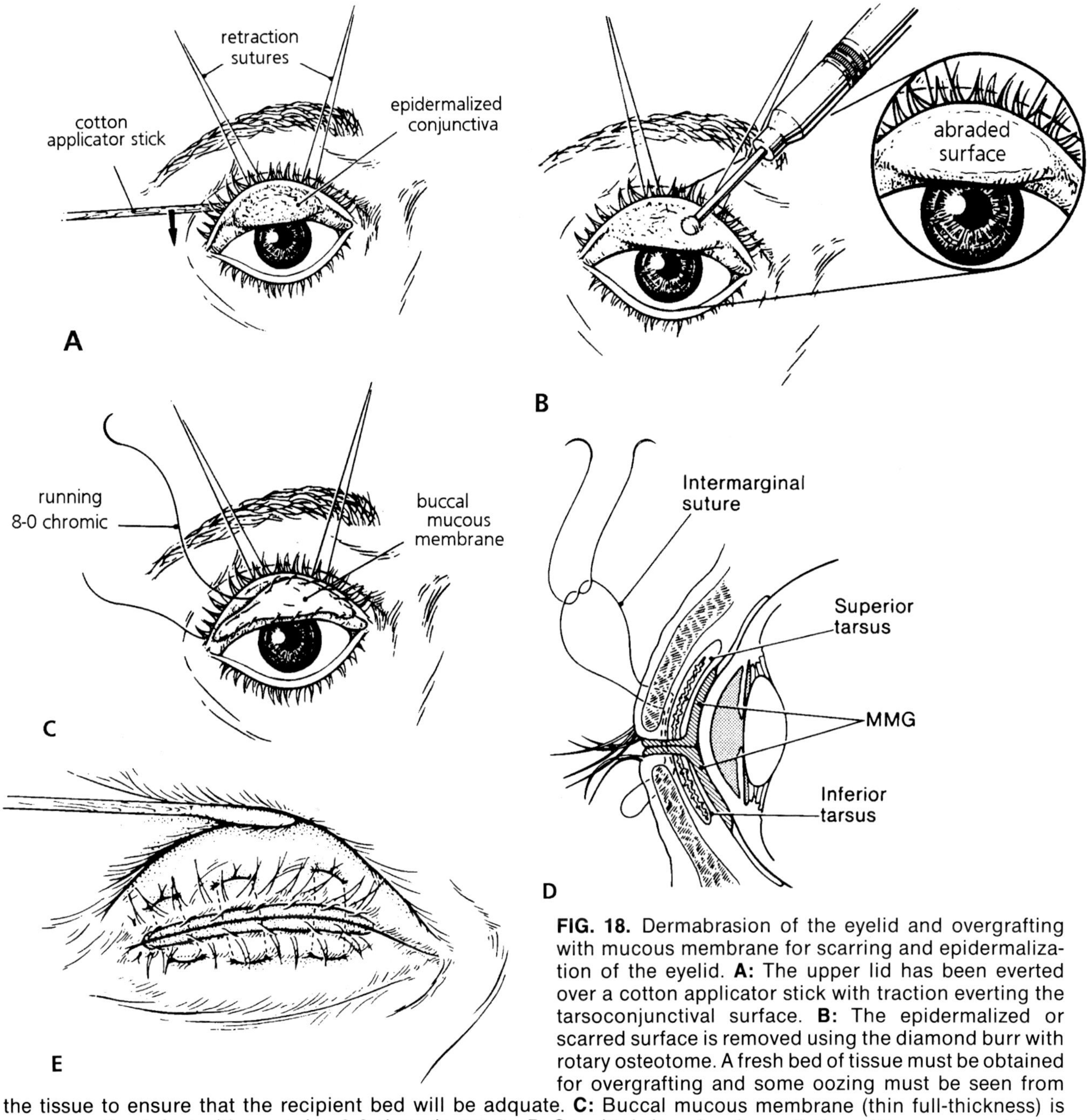

FIG. 18. Dermabrasion of the eyelid and overgrafting with mucous membrane for scarring and epidermalization of the eyelid. **A:** The upper lid has been everted over a cotton applicator stick with traction everting the tarsoconjunctival surface. **B:** The epidermalized or scarred surface is removed using the diamond burr with rotary osteotome. A fresh bed of tissue must be obtained for overgrafting and some oozing must be seen from the tissue to ensure that the recipient bed will be adquate. **C:** Buccal mucous membrane (thin full-thickness) is sutured to the defect with a running 8-0 chromic suture. **D:** Saggittal view showing splinting of the upper and lower lids to stabilize the mucous membrane graft with an intermarginal suture. **E:** External view showing inner marginal sutures stabilizing the eyelids for one week.

A full-thickness buccal mucous membrane graft is harvested in the usual manner, as described in Chapter 3 (split-thickness grafts have been found to be inadequate to resurface the margin and palpebral conjunctiva). One must measure the width of the eyelid and the area to be covered before harvesting the graft. One should remember that after excision of a full-thickness buccal mucous membrane graft from the lip, the graft will contract to a much smaller size and therefore stretching must be used for it to fit the intended recipient site. Epidermalization can also manifest itself together with trichiasis and margin destruction in many cases.

The lid is everted with traction sutures over a cotton-tipped swab and tensed (Fig. 18A). A 3-mm diamond burr on a microrotary osteotome is used to abrade the entire edge of the eyelid and the palpebral conjuctiva that is epidermalized and scarred. If good vasoconstriction has been obtained, there will be very little oozing in some cases (Fig. 18B). The buccal mucous

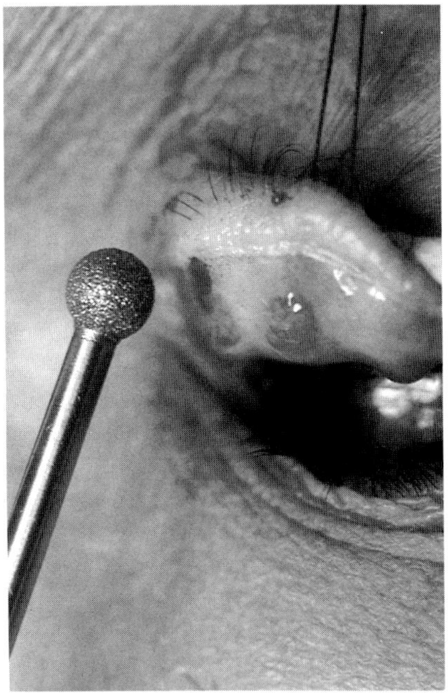

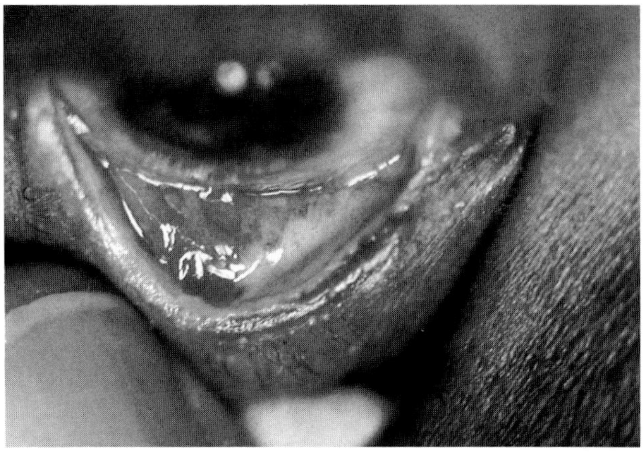

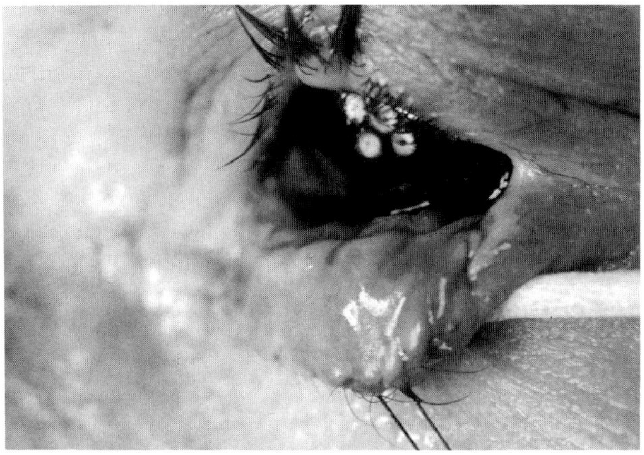

FIG. 19. Surgical views of dermabrasion and mucous membrane overgrafting. **A:** The upper lid has been everted exposing the scarred epidermalized tarsoconjunctiva. The diamond burr will be used to remove the scar tissue. **B:** Lower lid in the same patient showing epidermalization and scarring of the eyelid margin. **C:** The scar tissue has been dermabraded from the lid margin and fornix and overgrafting with a full-thickness buccal mucous membrane has been performed.

membrane graft is tailored to fit the defect and the graft is then positioned with an 8-0 chromic running suture. The suture is introduced from the cutaneous surface, sewn in a continuous running manner around the entire graft, and tied on the external surface of the lid (Fig. 18C). Figure 19C shows a surgical view of a graft sutured into position.

The lid is then sutured together in a slightly everted position with intramarginal sutures for one week (Fig. 18D and E). It has been found that almost 100% take of the graft occurs if this eyelid splinting is performed. The graft may take without intramarginal sutures, but in many cases a good bit of shrinkage will occur. Grafts may still have a bluish tinge at the end of a week but

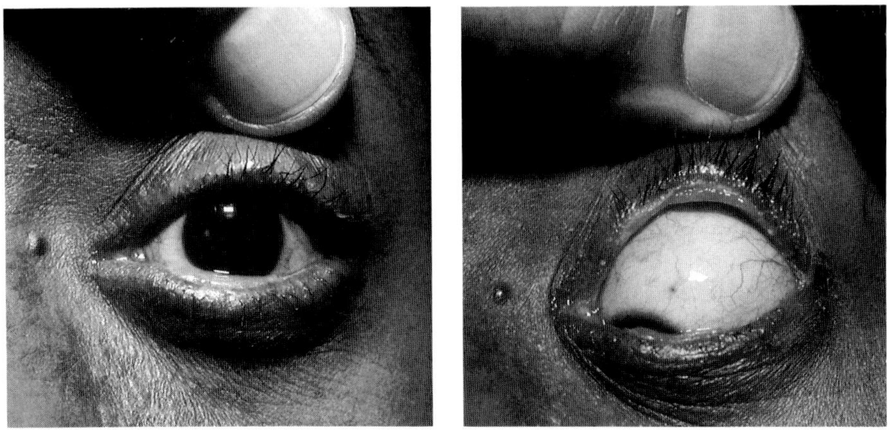

FIG. 20. A: Patient postoperatively from dermabrasion and mucous membrane grafting of the lid margin showing the lower lid graft in position. **B:** After dermabrasion and mucous membrane grafting showing graft in position of the upper lid.

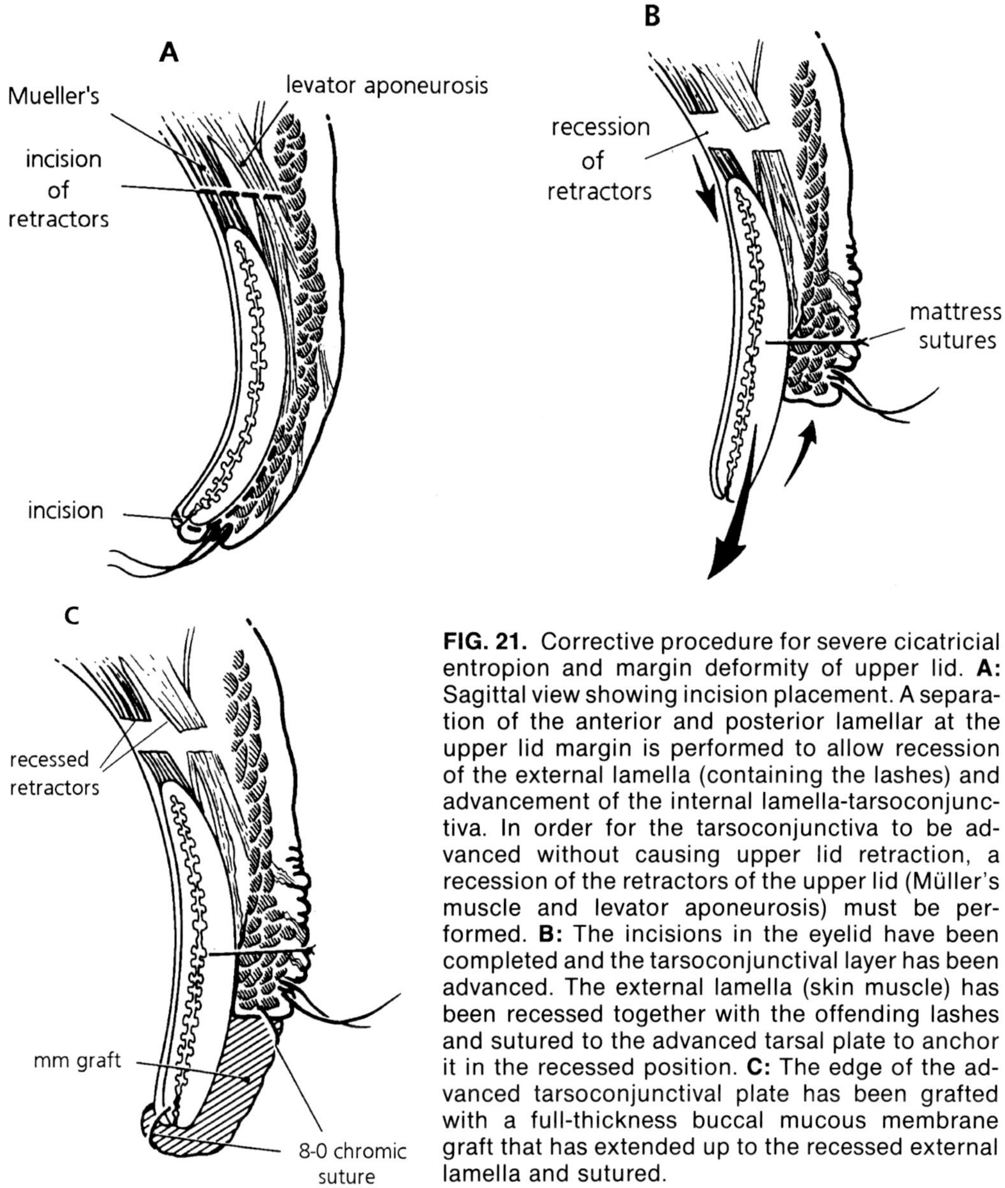

FIG. 21. Corrective procedure for severe cicatricial entropion and margin deformity of upper lid. **A:** Sagittal view showing incision placement. A separation of the anterior and posterior lamellar at the upper lid margin is performed to allow recession of the external lamella (containing the lashes) and advancement of the internal lamella-tarsoconjunctiva. In order for the tarsoconjunctiva to be advanced without causing upper lid retraction, a recession of the retractors of the upper lid (Müller's muscle and levator aponeurosis) must be performed. **B:** The incisions in the eyelid have been completed and the tarsoconjunctival layer has been advanced. The external lamella (skin muscle) has been recessed together with the offending lashes and sutured to the advanced tarsal plate to anchor it in the recessed position. **C:** The edge of the advanced tarsoconjunctival plate has been grafted with a full-thickness buccal mucous membrane graft that has extended up to the recessed external lamella and sutured.

generally will "pink up" over the next week. Figure 20A and B shows the lid edges of a patient with Stevens–Johnson syndrome following mucous membrane overgrafting.

The improvement noted in patients is largely due to the mechanical effect of the smooth eyelid margin on the cornea. Other possibilities are restoration of the goblet cells and increased corneal oxygenation from healthy mucous membrane opposed to the cornea.

Severe Margin Deformity with Trichiasis

Increasing degrees of damage to the eyelid margin from inflammatory causes such as Stevens–Johnson syndrome, burns, or postsurgical or traumatic etiologies will not only cause aberrant lash formation and scarring but loss of the architecture of the edge of the eyelid. This margin destruction when combined with trichiasis may not respond to cryopexy alone, and reconstruction procedures must be employed to restore the integrity of the eyelid margin.

The technique of tarsal advancement with recession of the lash line and buccal mucous membrane grafting has been used quite successfully over the years (14,16,23,24). The techniques do presume that there is adequate tarsus present to advance. If one is faced with a patient with damaged tarsus to the point that the lid is unstable, then one must employ a formal eyelid reconstructive procedure to correct the problem. (See Chapters 20 and 21.)

Margin Reconstruction with Mucous Membrane Grafting

Incisions are made through the eyelid margin, and the tarsoconjunctiva is advanced in the upper and

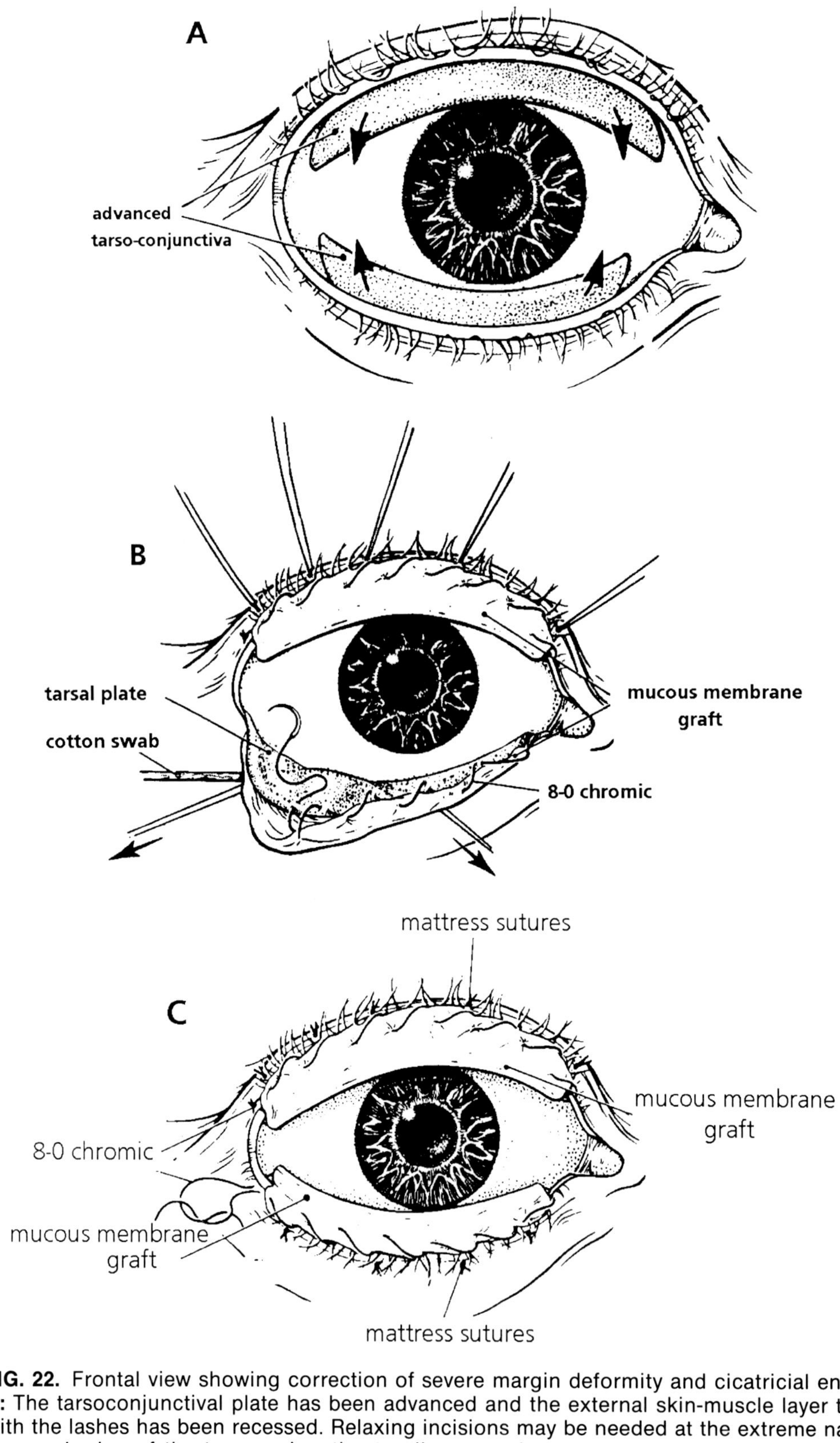

FIG. 22. Frontal view showing correction of severe margin deformity and cicatricial entropion. **A:** The tarsoconjunctival plate has been advanced and the external skin-muscle layer together with the lashes has been recessed. Relaxing incisions may be needed at the extreme nasal and temporal edge of the tarsoconjunctiva to allow complete advancement. **B:** The full-thickness buccal mucous membrane graft has been sutured to cover the advanced edge of the tarsoconjunctiva and extend up to the recessed anterior lamella. The lid must be everted with retraction sutures and cotton applicators to allow direct visualization for suturing. **C:** Final positioning of the mucous membrane grafts over the advanced tarsoconjunctival edge.

lower lid (Fig. 21A,B). It is important to make relaxing incisions at the ends of the tarsoconjunctiva so that the tarsal plate will slide forward (Fig. 22A). Full-thickness buccal mucous membrane graft is sutured to the raw surface of the advanced edge of the tarsoconjunctiva. An 8-0 chromic suture is then introduced from the skin surface and brought in a continuous running manner to close the graft on the anterior and posterior incision (Figs. 21C and 22B).

Having been completely sutured around, the graft is then brought back out through the skin in order that it can be tied externally in such a way that the ends of the stitches will not rub against the cornea (Fig. 22C). It is important to close the eyelid with intermarginal sutures during this period in order for the graft to take.

Formal Eyelid Reconstruction

In entropic eyelids severely damaged from destructive disease or multiple surgeries, there may be deficiency in the tissue (tarsus, supporting tissue) such that the above procedure will be inadequate. In this situation the surgeon should consider the lid to be damaged to the point that a formal reconstructive procedure must be utilized as described in Chapters 20 and 21 on eyelid reconstruction.

REFERENCES

1. Sisler HA. A biochemical and physiologic approach to corrective surgery for senile entropion. *Ann Ophthalmol* 1973;5:483.
2. Jones LT. The anatomy of the lower eyelid and its relationship to the cause and cure of entropion. *Am J Ophthalmol* 1960;49: 29.
3. Dryden RM, Leibsohn J, Wobig J. Senile entropion: pathogenesis and treatment. *Arch Ophthalmol* 1978;96:1183.
4. McCord CD Jr. Surgery of the eyelids. In: Duane TD, Jaeger EA, eds. *Clinical ophthalmology*. vol 5, New York: Harper and Row; 1985:1–54.
5. Collin JRO, Rathbun JE. Involutional entropin. *Arch Ophthalmol* 1978;96:1058.
6. Dalgleish R, Smith JLS. Mechanics and histology of senile ectropin. *Br J Ophthalmol* 1966;50:79.
7. Sisler HA, Lebay GR, Finlay JR. Senile ectropion and entropion: a compared and histopathologic study. *Ann Ophthalmol* 1976;8:319.
8. Hardy K, Perry H, Kirby T. Benign mucous membrane pemphigoid. *Arch Dermatol* 1971;104:467.
9. Maumenee AE. Keratinization of the conjunctiva. *Trans Am Ophthalmol Soc* 1979;77:133.
10. Wies FA. Surgical treatment of entropion. *J Int Coll Surg* 1954; 21:758.
11. Feldstein M. A method of correction of entropion in aged persons. *Eye Ear Nose Throat Month* 1960;39:730–731.
12. Quickert MH, Rathbun E. Suture repair of entropion. *Arch Ophthalmol* 1971;85:304–305.
13. Bick MW. Surgical management of orbital tarsal disparity. *Arch Ophthalmol* 1966;75:386.
14. Hornblass A, Bercovici S, Smith B. Senile entropion. *Ophth Surg* 1977;8:47.
15. Dresner S, Karesh JW. Transconjunctival entropion repair. *Arch Ophthalmol* 1993;111:1144–1148.
16. Wesley RE, Collin JW. Combined procedure for senile entropion. *Ophth Surg* 1983;14:401–406.
17. Leone CR. Mucous membrane grafting for cicatricial entropion. *Ophth Surg* 1974;5:24.
18. Collin JRO, Kemp EG. Upper lid entropion: a review of over 200 cases. *Ophth Plast Reconstr Surg* 1986;23:50–51.
19. Goldberg R, Seiff S, McFarland J, Simons K, Shorr N. Floppy eyelid syndrome and blepharochalasis. *Am J Ophthalmol* 1986; 2:376–391.
20. Karesh JW, et al. Eyelid imbrication. *Ophthalmology* 1993;100: 883–889.
21. Dutton JJ. Surgical management of floppy eyelid syndrome. *Am J Ophthalmol* 1985;99:557–560.
22. Culbertson WW, Ostler HB. The floppy eyelid syndrome. *Am J Ophthalmol* 1981;92:568–575.
23. Netland PA, et al. Histopathologic features of the floppy eyelid syndrome. *Ophthalmology* 1994;101:174–181.
24. Biglan AW, Bueger GF. Congenital horizontal tarsal kink. *Am J Ophthalmol* 1980;89:522–524.
25. Tenzel RR, Miller GR, Rubnzik R. Cicatricial upper lid entropion treated with bank scleral graft. *Arch Ophthalmol* 1975;93: 999.
26. Callahan A. Correction of entropion from Stevens–Johnson syndrome, use of nasal septum and mucosa for severely cicatrized eyelid entropion. *Arch Ophthalmol* 1976;94:1154.
27. Hoschni R, Faruk J. Repair of trichomatous cicatricial entropion using a mucous membrane graft. *Arch Ophthalmol* 1974;91:49.
28. Fraunfelder FT, Peterson GL. The use of liquid nitrogen cryospray for the treatment of trichiasis. *Ophth Surg* 1979;10:42–46.
29. Sullivan JH, Beard C, Bullock JD. Cryosurgery for the treatment of trichiasis. *Am J Ophthalmol* 1976;82:117–121.
30. Wilkes TDL, Fraunfelder FT. Principles of cryosurgery. *Ophth Surg* 1979;10:21–30.
31. Bartley GB, Bullock JD, et al. An experimental study to compare methods of eyelash ablation. *Ophthalmology* 1987;94: 1286–1289.
32. Huneke JW. Argon laser treatment for trichiasis. *Ophth Plast Reconst Surg* 1992;8:50–56.
33. Dortzbach RK, Butera RT. Excision of distinchiasis eyelashes through a tarsoconjunctival trapdoor. *Arch Ophthalmol* 1978; 96:111–112.
34. Wojno TH. Lid splitting with lash resection for cicatricial entropion and trichiasis. *Ophth Plast Reconst Surg* 1992;8:287–289.
35. McCord CD, Chen WP. Tarsal polishing and mucous membrane grafting for cicatricial entropion, trichiasis and epidermalization. *Ophth Surg* 1983;14:1021–1025.

CHAPTER 6

Ectropion and Related Conditions

ECTROPION AND RELATED CONDITIONS

Ectropion of the eyelid is characterized by an outturning of the eyelid margin and separation of the eyelid from the globe. It can occur as a result of a variety of mechanical reasons: laxity of the tarsoligamentous sling, loss of inferior tarsal support, mechanical changes in the tarsus itself, shortening of the musculocutaneous layer of the lid, and loss of tone of the orbicularis muscle due to denervation or atrophy.

Classifying the types of ectropion on an anatomic basis is important so that a specific anatomic cause can be assigned. This allows a more specific anatomic correction of the malposition. The classification shown in Table 1 has served this purpose.

LAXITY OR INVOLUTIONAL ECTROPION

Involutional ectropion is caused by laxity of the tarsoligamentous sling and generalized loss of elastin. The supportive orbicularis fibers have also been found to be atrophic (1,2). The onset may be gradual and the laxity may first cause a mild sagging of the lid which over time can progress to eversion of the lid; in most cases this process begins medially and is subcategorized as medial ectropion with eversion of the punctum eversion (Fig. 1A). Tears cannot enter the punctum and patients with normal tear flow become symptomatic from epiphora. Patients who have deficient tearing may not complain of epiphora but have exposure symptoms and the exposed conjunctival surface of the lid margin becomes epidermalized. The punctum itself may become atretic. As the condition progresses further the lid turns outward more (Fig. 1B) and exposure causes a generalized thickening of the eyelid margin with conjunctival hypertrophy. A paradoxical inversion of the lashes may occur (Fig. 2A, B).

Figure 3 presents the commonly seen stages in the anatomic progression of laxity or involutional ectropion. As the ectropion progresses, the conjunctiva becomes chronically exposed producing prominent inflammatory changes within the eyelid tissues and the patient may complain of eye redness and irritation. Inflammatory changes of the eyelid and chronic exposure produce metaplastic changes of the goblet cells that contain stratified squamous epithelium of the conjunctiva and keratinization, results that can produce considerable irritation to the globe. If the eyelids are unable to close adequately, exposure can produce corneal epithelial breakdown and subsequent keratitis.

In considering corrective surgery, it should be recognized that the tarsal plate is the most stable part of the lid and it is the ligamentous sling at the canthal angles that is the most abnormal. Therefore, whenever possible, the surgeon should avoid excising healthy tarsal plate. Horizontal tightening performed at the lateral canthal angle has become the procedure of choice and has many variations (3–12). Tightening the lid at the lateral canthus will reposition the eyelid margin and in many cases, even with mild medial ectropion, restore the punctum to a reasonably normal position. With extreme tightening of the lid, however, the punctum can be displaced temporally.

Lateral Horizontal Tightening

Lateral horizontal tightening (LHT) is the most effective method of repositioning the lax involutional eyelid. A skin-muscle flap is developed at the temporal third of lid and canthal angle (Fig. 4A). A canthotomy, cantholysis, and resection of the tarsal plate edge is performed. The amount of resection is determined by stretching the edge of the lid to the lateral rim and determining the overlap when the desired lid position and tension is obtained (Fig. 4B, C). A 4-0 prolene suture (special order Ethicon P2 needle) is placed through edge of tarsus (Fig. 4D). The P2 needle is then inserted inside the edge of lateral rim periosteum at

TABLE 1. *Classification of ectropian types*

Type	Features
Involutional Laxity Ectropion	laxity of tarsoligamentous sling
(Medial Ectropion)	orbicularis atrophy
	loss of tarsal elastin
Tarsal Ectropion	inferior retractor dehiscence
Laxity-Dehiscence Syndromes	loss of elastic-connective tissue
Floppy Lid Syndrome	laxity of tarsoligamentous sling
Blepharochalasis Syndrome	
Idiopathic Lateral Dehiscence	
Cicatricial Ectropion—	external Skin (muscle) Shortage
Complex Ectropion—	external Skin (muscle) Shortage
	internal septal scarring
	bony adhesions
Paralytic Ectropion	loss of orbicularis tone
	horizontal laxity (older patients)
Congenital Ectropion—	septal anomaly
Bent Tarsus—Upper Lid Eversion	skin—connective tissue shortage
Euryblepharon	anomalous tarsoligamentous sling
	bony hypoplasia, skin shortage
Blepharophimosis Syndrome	
Treacher Collins Syndrome	

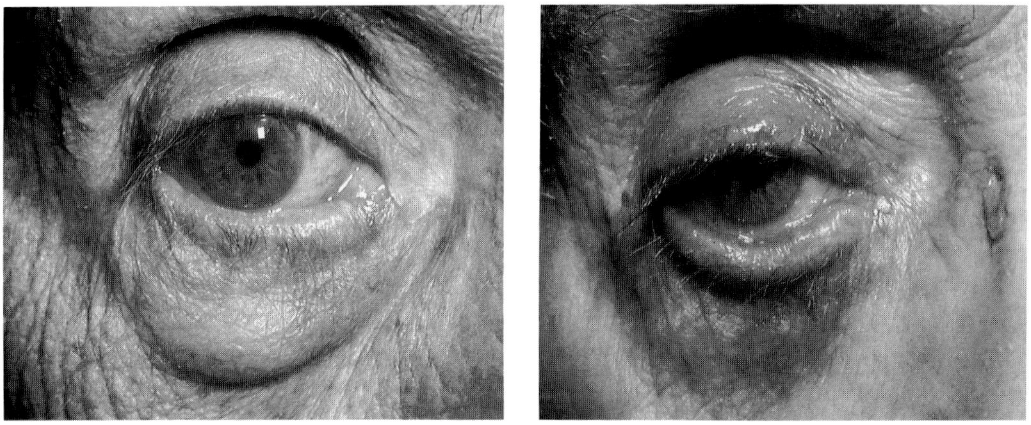

A B

FIG. 1. Involutional laxity ectropion. **A:** Early stage with medial ectropion and punctal eversion. **B:** More advanced stage with laxity extending to central portion of the lid with outturning.

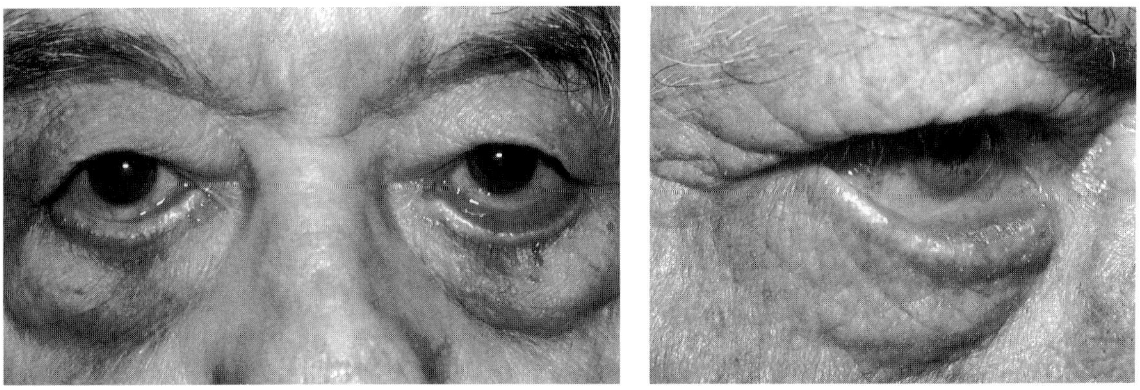

A B

FIG. 2. Laxity involutional ectropion. **A:** Shows patient with advanced laxity ectropion on the right side and less advanced laxity ectropion on the left. **B:** Keratinization and thickening of eyelid margin and conjunctiva from chronic exposure.

Laxity of the tarsoligamentous sling
orbicularis atrophy
Usually medially first
↘
Medial ectropion punctal eversion
Tearing
↘
Generalized ectropion
Conjunctival hypertrophy-keratinization

FIG. 3. Involutional ectropion progressive changes.

pupillary level (Fig. 4E). The second bite on the outside of the rim is taken to produce mattress effect and the eyelid is tightened to the lateral rim (Fig. 4F, G). An additional suture may be placed in the septum or the muscle flap as well as in the lateral periosteum for added lift (14,15). The upper and lower lid margin is aligned with 6-0 nylon and closure is completed.

Transverse Blepharotomy with Rotational Sutures

Transverse blepharotomy with rotational sutures supplements the horizontal tightening in patients who have severe deformity in the tarsus and eyelid margin.

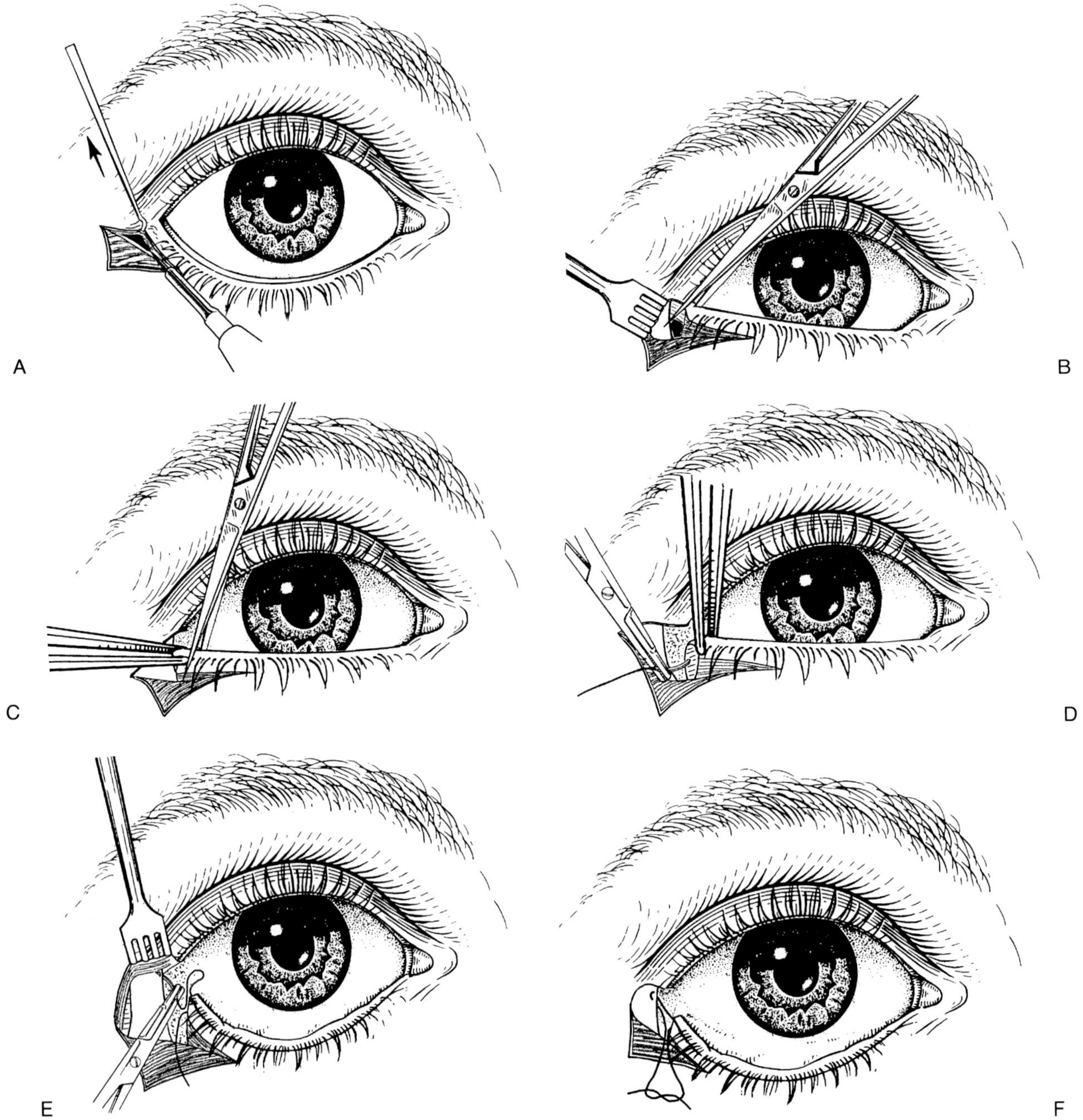

FIG. 4. See legend at top of next page.

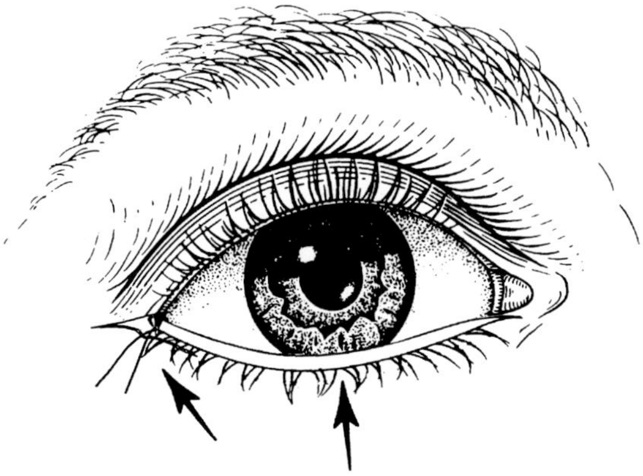

G

FIG. 4. Horizontal tightening of the lid at the lateral canthus for laxity ectropion. **A:** Skin-muscle flap is elevated with a subciliary incision at the lateral canthus. **B:** Canthotomy and cantholysis is performed. **C:** Resection of the edge of the lid including a portion of the tarsus and margin. The amount of resection is determined by stretching the lid toward the orbital rim to determine redundancy. **D:** Insertion of suture into edge of tarsal plate (4.0 prolene with a P2 needle). **E:** Suture is then placed in periosteum inside the lateral orbital rim at the level of the pupil. **F:** Suture is then passed in a mattress-like manner to complete the mattress suture at the lateral rim. **G:** Suture is tightened laterally tensing the lid and elevating the margin to the lower limbus or above.

Thickening and deformity in the tarsus may cause residual margin eversion in spite of adequate tightening and an added rotational effect is obtained (Fig. 5A–C).

Fascial Sling

Some cases of laxity involutional ectropion are so severe as to resist full correction with lateral horizontal tightening because of extreme loss of tarsoligamentous integrity. In these extreme cases the author has used the fascia sling with good results. This procedure is described later in the chapter for the correction of mild to moderate cicatricial ectropion (16,17).

MEDIAL ECTROPION

Medial ectropion may be the first stage of a generalized laxity ectropion, but it also may occur in isolation

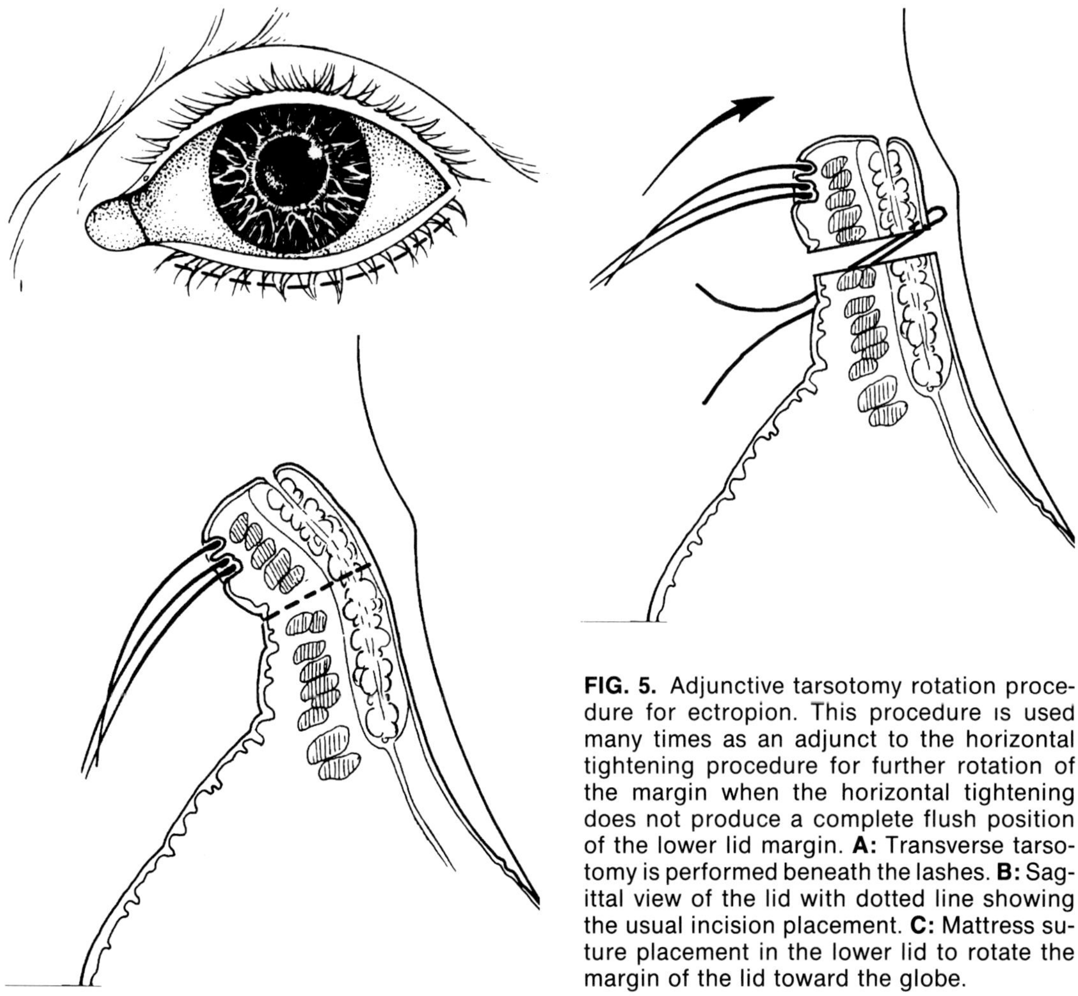

A B C

FIG. 5. Adjunctive tarsotomy rotation procedure for ectropion. This procedure is used many times as an adjunct to the horizontal tightening procedure for further rotation of the margin when the horizontal tightening does not produce a complete flush position of the lower lid margin. **A:** Transverse tarsotomy is performed beneath the lashes. **B:** Sagittal view of the lid with dotted line showing the usual incision placement. **C:** Mattress suture placement in the lower lid to rotate the margin of the lid toward the globe.

and be severe enough to warrant a separate repair. There are different useful procedures available (18,19). The indications for different procedures are on the basis of whether lacrimal drainage with epiphora is a problem to the patient or not. Some patients may have a dry eye syndrome with exposure as the primary problem. The needed medial ectropion procedures may be performed by themselves but are usually combined with lateral horizontal tightening.

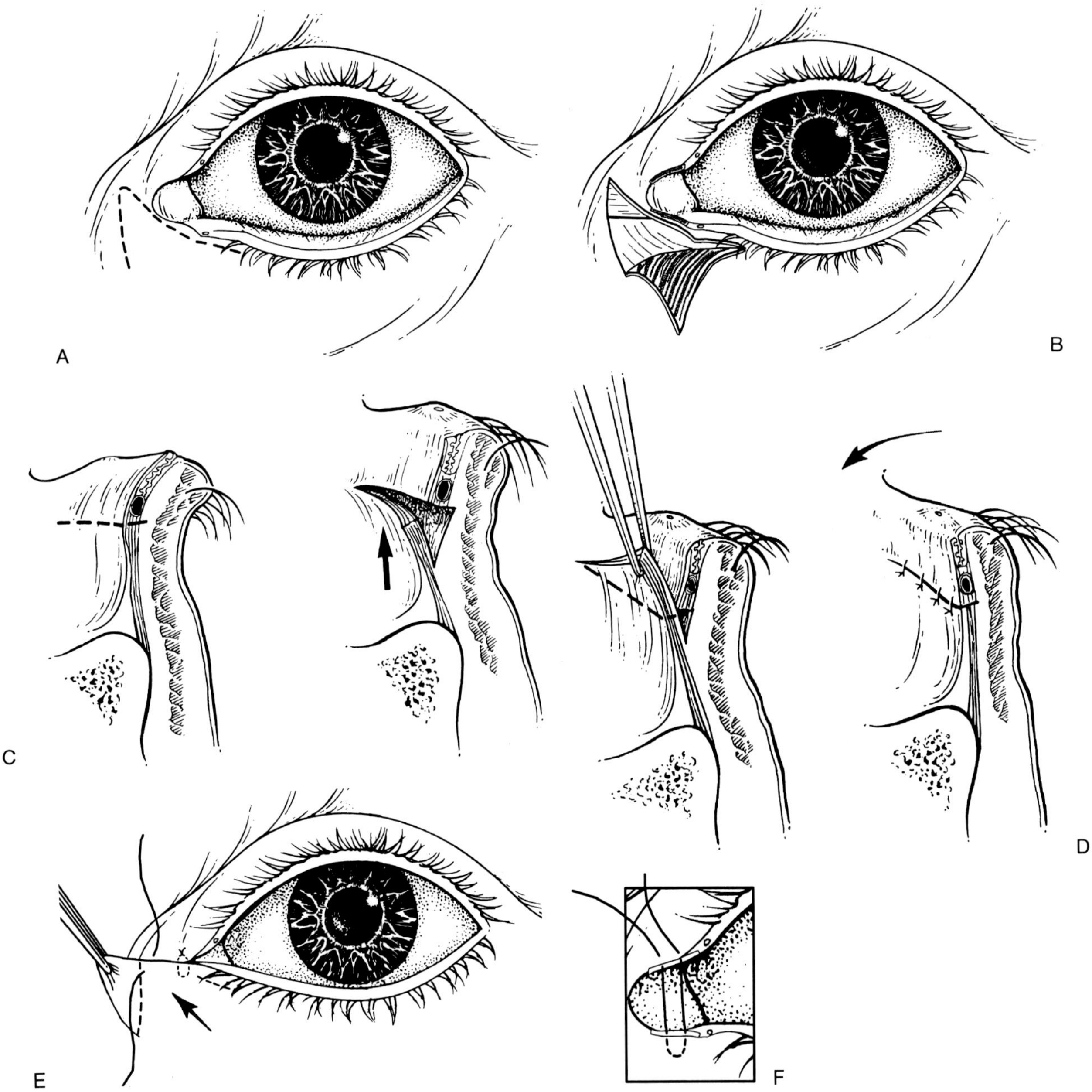

FIG. 6. Medial canthoplasty ectropion procedure. **A:** Skin-muscle flap is elevated from the medial canthus and the incision extends above the level of the medial canthal tendon. **B:** Flap is elevated and the medial canthal tendon is exposed. The margin of the lid nasal to the punctum has been denuded of epithelium for placement of sutures. Lower lid is also everted to facilitate performance of a posterior resection of the internal lid inferior to the punctum. **C:** Incision in the posterior lamella of the lid below the ampulla and canaliculus and elevation of a flap upward. **D:** Flap is elevated and resected so that suturing the posterior lamella will cause an internal rotation of the punctum. **E:** Denuded spaces on the margin are then sutured together to form an adhesion of the lid nasal to the punctum. **F:** Skin-muscle flap nasally is then advanced tensing the lid toward the medial canthal tendon. The advanced flap is then sutured to the tendon to create tension on the lid for elevation of the canthal angle. The redundant skin marked with the dotted line is excised.

Medial Skin-Muscle Flap and Internal Resection

A skin-muscle flap is marked to extend above medial canthal tendon and then incised (Fig. 6A). The skin-muscle flap is developed with cutting Bovie exposing anterior reflection of medial canthal tendon (MCT) (Fig. 6B). The lower lid is everted and methylene blue should outline an ellipse to be excised to rotate the punctum inward. With the lid on stretch, the marked area is excised with cutting Bovie avoiding ampulla. The palpebral artery may need cautery. In addition to simple closure, inverting sutures from superior cut edge to outside skin may also be placed to cause maximum inward rotation (Fig. 6C, D). The nasal skin-muscle flap is then stretched to the MCT causing a redundant triangle that is resected. The flap is then sutured to the MCT with 6-0 nylon (Fig. 6E). With sharp scissors, the epithelial edge of the upper and lower lids at the inner canthus is excised sparing the canaliculi. This area is then sutured together with mattress 6-0 vicryl to create a nasal canthorrhaphy (Fig. 6F). Figure 7A and B shows a patient before and after the procedure.

Medial Full-Thickness Resection

In patients who have a tear deficiency and in whom the main problem is exposure, a full-thickness resection of the medial portion of the eyelid including portions of the lower canaliculus can be performed to reposition the medial portion of the eyelid. The resected edge of the nasal eyelid must be attached to the posterior reflection of the MCT for the lid to be repositioned flush with the globe. This technique is the same as described in the next section with canalicular intubation and canaliculostomy omitted. Lower canalicular drainage is not needed in patients who have a tear deficiency or in whom the punctal malposition has not caused symptomatic tearing.

Medial Full-Thickness Resection with Posterior Tendon Plication and Canaliculostomy

In patients with medial ectropion who have a normal tear flow or who already suffer from epiphora because of poor lacrimal drainage from eyelid malposition, medial resection must include reestablishment of drainage from the lower canaliculus.

A full-thickness resection of lid starting just lateral to punctum is performed (Fig. 8A, B). The caruncle is excised if it is prominent. Intubation with Crawford tubes is performed and the inferior canalicular stump is dissected out from the surrounding tissue (Fig. 8C). The nasal cut edge of lid is sutured to the posterior reflection of the MCT with 4-0 prolene with half-circle needle (P2) (Fig. 8D, E). The exposure for this step is

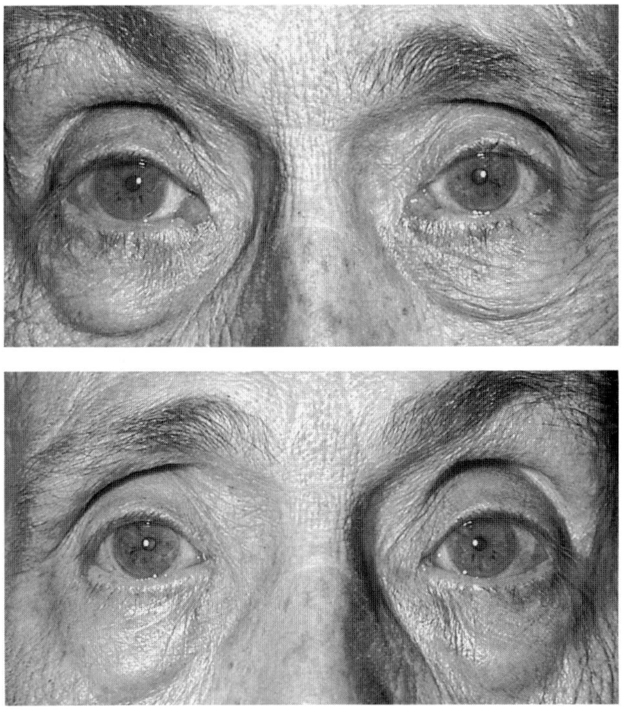

A

B

FIG. 7. Patient with bilateral medial ectropion. **A:** Patient prior to medial canthoplasty, medial ectropion procedure. **B:** Same patient following medial canthoplasty, medial ectropion procedure.

obtained by retraction of the nasal skin with small rakes and depression of the orbital fat with cotton applicators. A bite with needle is taken in the lid edge from below to margin then in post-MCT from below to above. This prevents the placement of the suture from being too high resulting in supraplacement of the canthal angle. If canalicular intubation has been performed, the suture must be placed lower in the lid edge in such a way as to prevent compression of the canaliculus, which will travel above the suture to the edge of the lid. The suture and the canaliculus criss-cross at different levels. The suture is tightened and the canaliculus sutured to the posterior edge of the lid. A groove is cut in the posterior edge to receive the canaliculus (Fig. 8F).

LAXITY-DEHISCENCE SYNDROMES

Floppy Eyelid Syndrome

Floppy eyelid syndrome is characterized by a rubbery and easily everted upper eyelid associated with chronic papillary conjunctivitis and nonspecific irritative symptoms (22). Ectropion and entropion have been reported in this condition. Although common in obese men, this syndrome may also occur in women. Histologically there is marked decrease in the amount

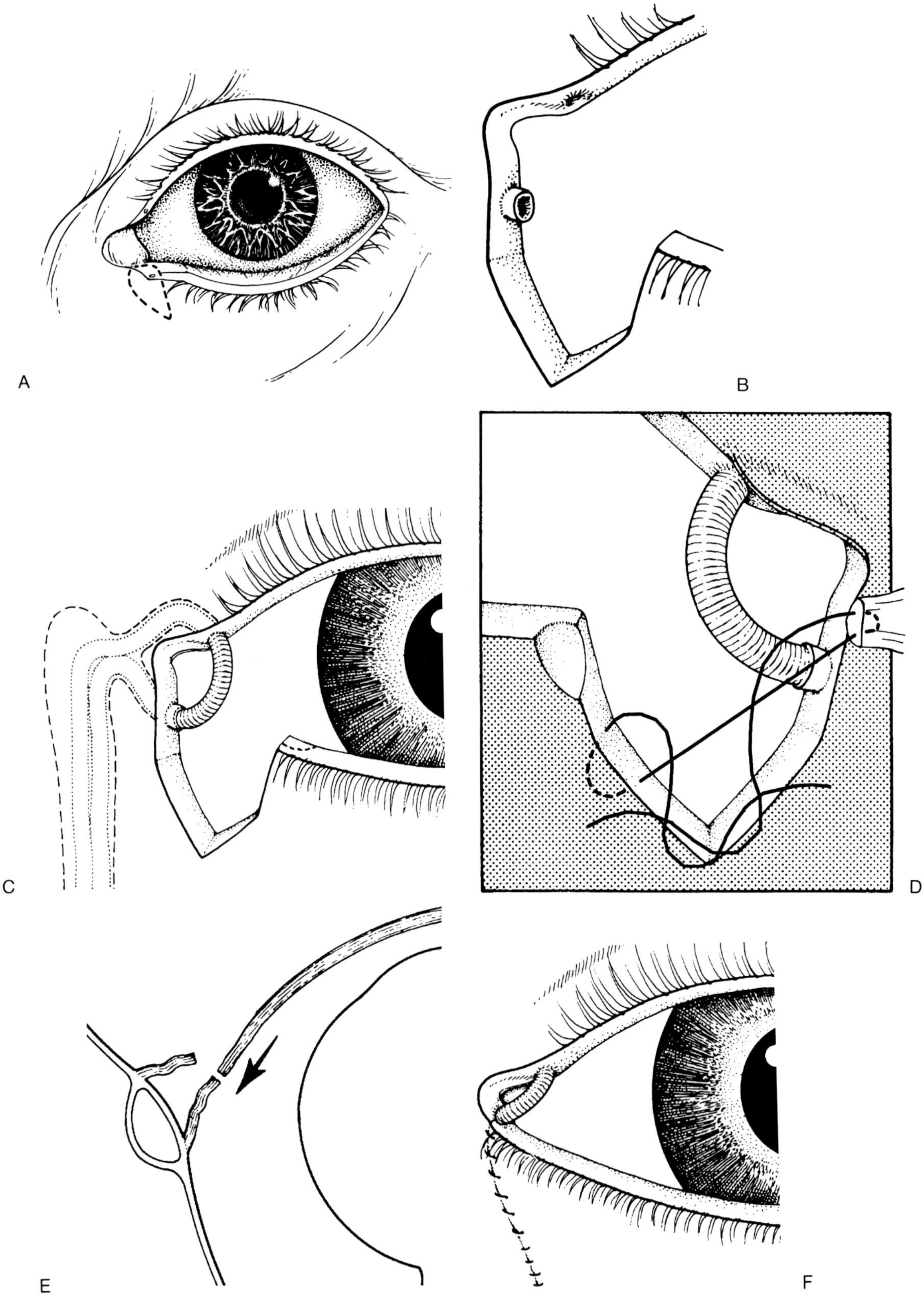

FIG. 8. Correction of medial ectropion and punctal eversion in patient with tearing with resection of lid and tightening. **A:** Outline of area of lax lid to be resected including punctum and ampulla and full-thickness eyelid. **B:** Defect created following resection of lax everted area. **C:** Intubation of residual lower canaliculus and upper canaliculus with silicone tubing. Resection of notch in posterior edge of temporal lid to receive edge of canaliculus to be advanced. **D:** Tightening of lower lid to posterior reflection of medial canthal tendon (4.0 prolene with P2 needle is used).

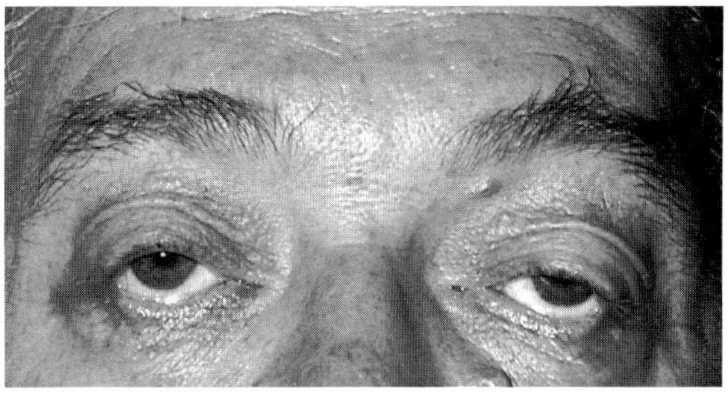

FIG. 9. Canthal dehiscence syndrome with lower lid retraction. This patient had idiopathic canthal dehiscence. An identical situation can be seen with the blepharochalasis syndrome from repeated inflammatory edema.

of elastin fibers in tarsus from patients with floppy eyelid syndrome compared with controls. Floppy lid syndrome more commonly results in entropion; however, because of laxity, eyelid eversion may occur. The author has seen entropion and ectropion in the lower lid in these patients. (Correction is discussed in Chapter 5.)

Blepharochalasis Syndrome

Blepharochalasis is a rare condition, most common in young females, characterized by recurrent, nonpainful, nonerythematous episodes of eyelid edema. Multiple attacks of eyelid edema result in thinning, stretching, and atrophy of eyelid tissues (20–24). The eyelid skin becomes redundant, discolored, and atrophic, resembling wrinkled cigarette paper. The upper eyelids are more commonly affected but the lower eyelids may also be involved. Laxity of the lateral canthal tendon results in rounding of the lateral canthal angle, ectropion, and phimosis. Other deformities are ptosis and pseudoepicanthal folds, formed by atrophy of the superior nasal fat pads.

Idiopathic Dehiscence

The changes in this condition are similar to the blepharochalasis syndrome, but a history of swelling cannot be elicited and changes may not be as severe. It most commonly affects the lateral canthus with ectropion (Fig. 9).

The ectropion and canthal deformity seen with these dehiscence syndromes can be improved (albeit temporarily) with a lateral horizontal tightening procedure. In most cases the tissue atrophy is so severe that reconstruction of the lateral canthal angle must be performed with the use of periosteal strips as described in the chapter on lateral canthal reconstruction.

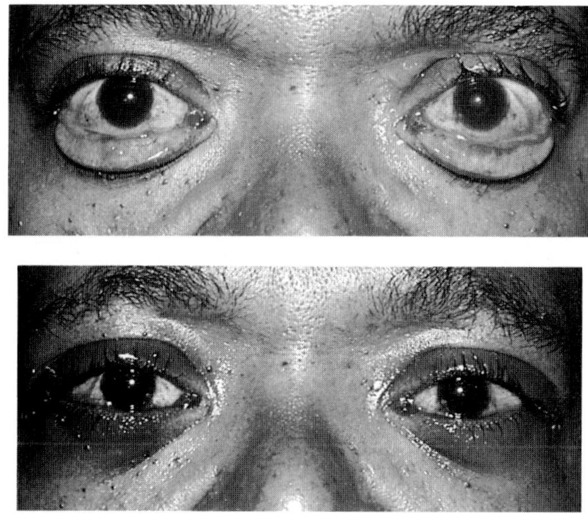

A

B

FIG. 10. Patient with bilateral tarsal ectropion with dehiscence of inferior retractors. **A:** Preoperatively. **B:** Same patient postoperatively with posterior lamellar resection and repair of inferior retractors and horizontal tightening at the lateral canthus.

TARSAL ECTROPION

The term *tarsal ectropion* was originally used to describe an unusual form of ectropion that is not due to horizontal laxity of the tarsoligamentous sling (Fig. 10A). In these patients, the lower lid is completely everted, with the lower border of the tarsus rotated outward. This type of ectropion has been attributed to dehiscence or stretching of the capsulopalpebral fascia at the inferior tarsal border (25–28). In these patients tarsoligamentous laxity may be present but is not striking. Tarsal ectropion may occur in younger people. Repair of the lower lid retractors from an internal eyelid approach has been used successfully in these patients. This repair corrects the lower tarsal eversion; however, it is generally recommended that a horizontal tightening procedure be combined with it for correction of any existing horizontal lid laxity.

A fold of internal lamellar tissue consisting of conjunctiva and remnants of the inferior retractors beneath

FIG. 8. *Continued.* Figure shows view from inside left eyelid. The placement should be lower in the cut edge of the lid than the notch to receive the canaliculus so as not to crimp the canaliculus when the defect is closed. **E:** Diagrammatic representation showing proper direction of pull of the edge of the lower lid towards the posterior reflection of the canthal tendon at the posterior retinaculum behind the lacrimal sac in the nasal orbit. **F:** Position of tubing and canaliculostomy following closure of defect with correction of medial ectropion and tightening of the lid.

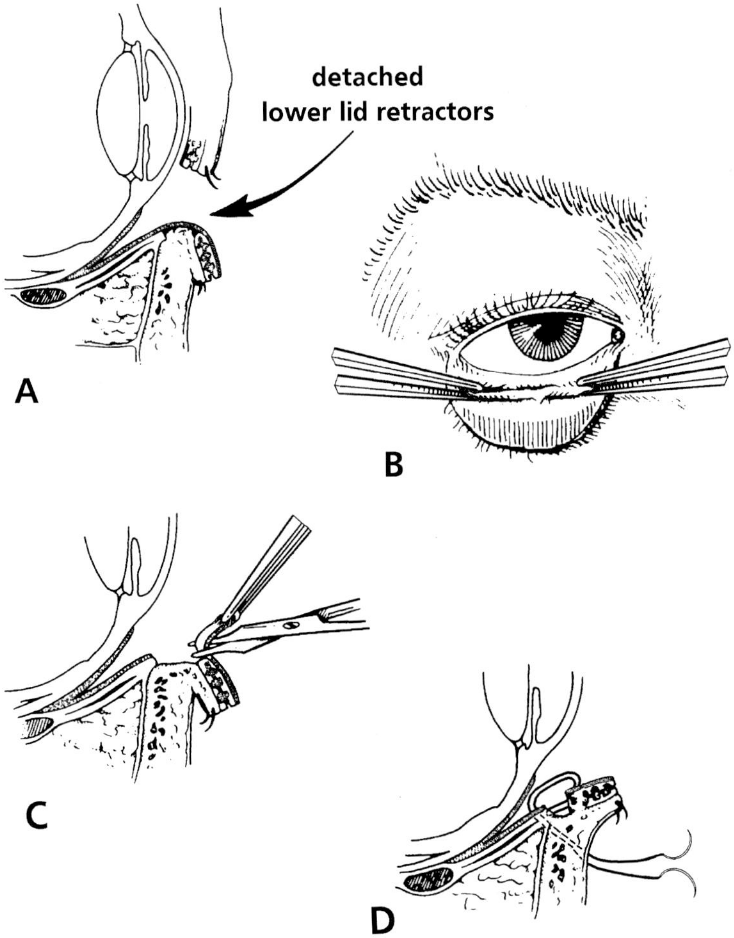

FIG. 11. Correction of tarsal ectropion with dehiscence of inferior retractors. A: Cross-section of eyelid and inferior orbits showing eversion of the lid. B: Grasping of internal lamella of the lid with redundant conjunctiva and approximating inferior retractors. C: Resection of portion of inferior retractors and conjunctiva. D: Repair of resected area with inverting mattress suture.

the inferior tarsal edge are grasped with forceps and excised (Fig. 11A, B). The posterior lamellar defect created is closed with inverting mattress sutures reapproximating the inferior tarsal edge to the inferior retractors (Fig. 10C, D). Nonabsorbable sutures can be used but slowly absorbing sutures may create a firmer adhesion. Many patients will require a lateral canthal tightening procedure following the resection.

CICATRICIAL ECTROPION

Cicatricial ectropion is caused by a shortage of the eyelid skin from actinic changes, trauma, burns, resection of lesions, inflammatory changes, or blepharoplasty (Figs. 12 and 13). Shortening of both skin and muscle may occur as a result of burns, irradiation, or an inflammatory condition. Ectropion caused by internal septal or posterior lamellar scarring, as well as skin shortage, is considered to be complex ectropion. Morpheaform basal cell carcinomas can cause epidermal shrinkage and may actually present as a cicatricial ectropion (Fig. 14). When ectropion is caused by significant shortage of the skin layer, skin must be replaced to correct the deformity.

Although skin grafts can in most cases be placed in the lid so as to produce an acceptable cosmetic result, most patients perceive it as an involved, disfiguring operation. This can be a significant obstacle in certain patients, particularly those acquiring ectropion following blepharoplasty.

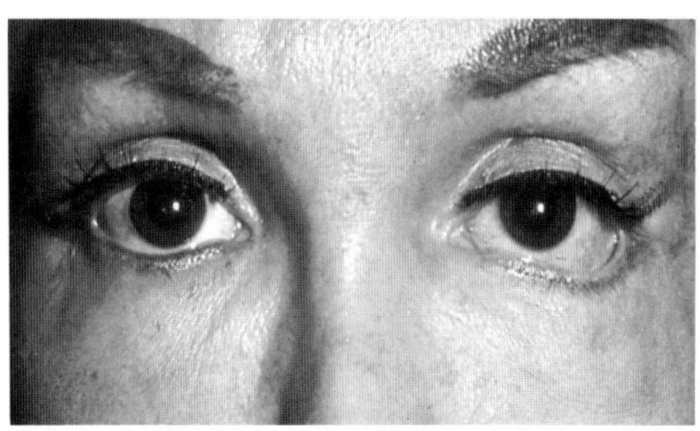

FIG. 12. Skin shortage cicatricial ectropion secondary to cosmetic blepharoplasty.

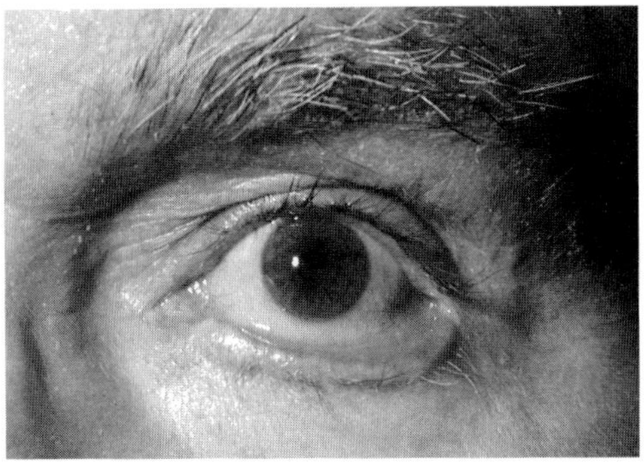

FIG. 13. Skin shortage cicatricial ectropion from actinic skin shrinkage. No surgery or injury had occurred.

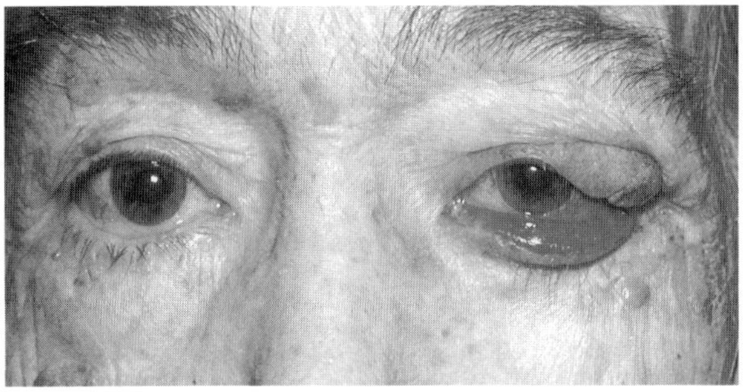

FIG. 14. Cicatricial ectropion. The patient was initially diagnosed as probable actinic shrinkage until a biopsy performed revealed a sclerosing basal cell carcinoma.

In some of the less severe cases of cicatricial ectropion or retraction, other procedures can be used instead of a skin graft that are more acceptable to the patient.

Horizontal Tightening

In older patients and, frequently, in younger patients, a horizontal tightening procedure with supraplacement of the tendon can overcome ectropion with cicatricial elements. Care must be taken, however, not to overcompensate with horizontal tightening to avoid a lateral displacement of the punctum, which can occur if the lid is overstretched.

Spacer Cartilage Graft to Posterior Lamellar

In cases of tighter vertical skin shortage, particularly those with predominant retraction, a spacer graft can be used in the posterior eyelid lamella, combined with a lateral horizontal tightening, to avoid an externally visible skin graft. Flat ear cartilage from the scaphoid fossa is preferred.

A canthotomy and cantholysis is first performed for exposure. An incision can be made beneath the inferior tarsus separating the conjunctiva and inferior retractors from the tarsus. Placement and suturing of the ear cartilage in the defect created can allow the lid margin to be elevated and repositioned when it is combined, tightening and supraplacement of the lateral canthal tendon overcoming the downward pull of skin shortage (Fig. 15A, B). Figure 16A and B shows a patient with tight skin before and after a posterior lamella spacer implant with tightening of the lateral canthal tendon.

Fascial Sling

Increased support of the lower lid with an internal sling can in some cases override shortage in the skin layer and correct a milder ectropion or retraction. The procedure has the advantage of repositioning the edge of the lid with little distortion. The skin is marked with a curvilinear line in the inner canthus (temporal portion of MCT), central lid, and lateral canthus (Fig. 17A). Incisions are made in the skin nasally; then the skin is retracted to expose the MCT using a rake retractor

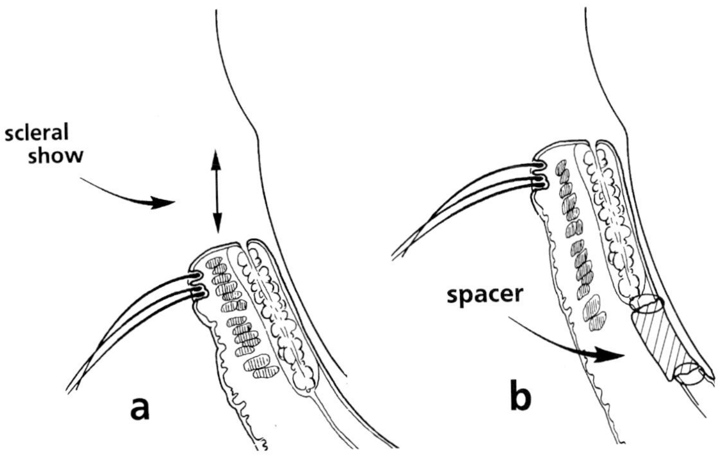

FIG. 15. Correction of lower lid retraction (scleral show) with spacer material implant. **A:** Lower lid retraction exposing conjunctiva and sclera beneath the limbus. **B:** Lid has been elevated to the limbus with posterior lamellar spacer implant, usually autogenous ear cartilage.

A 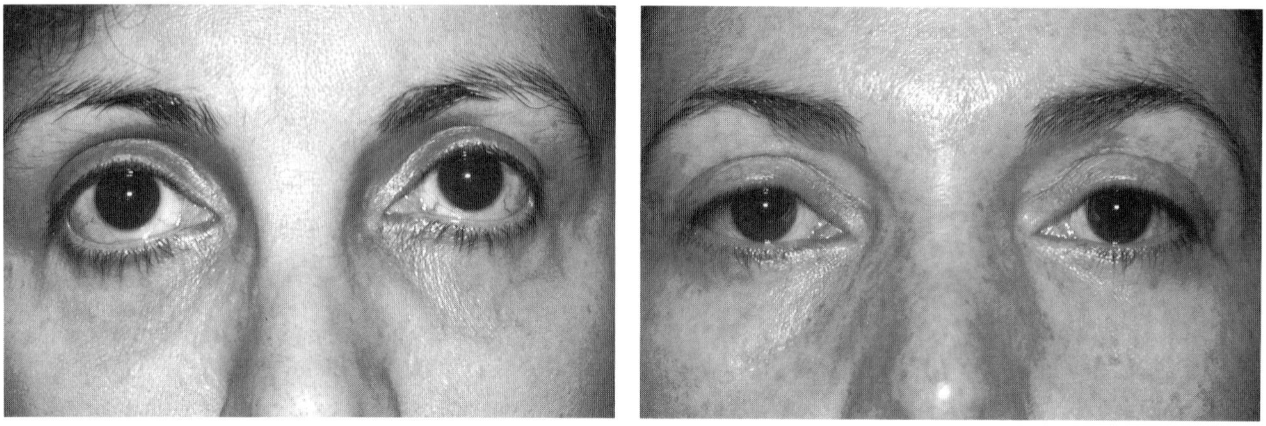 B

FIG. 16. A: Patient with lower lid retraction and scleral show following a four-lid blepharoplasty. The patient was experiencing severe exposure symptoms and was unhappy with the rounding appearance. The patient did not wish skin grafting and the amount of retraction was felt to be more than could be corrected with simple horizontal tightening. **B:** Same patient following posterior lamellar spacer implants of autogenous ear cartilage and horizontal tightening of the lateral canthal tendon with correction of the retraction.

A 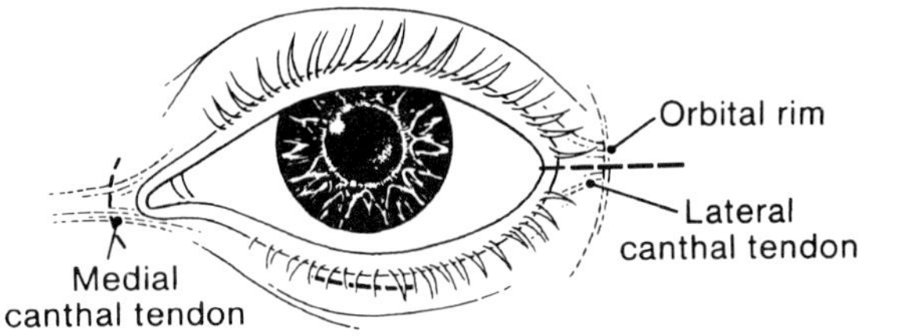

B

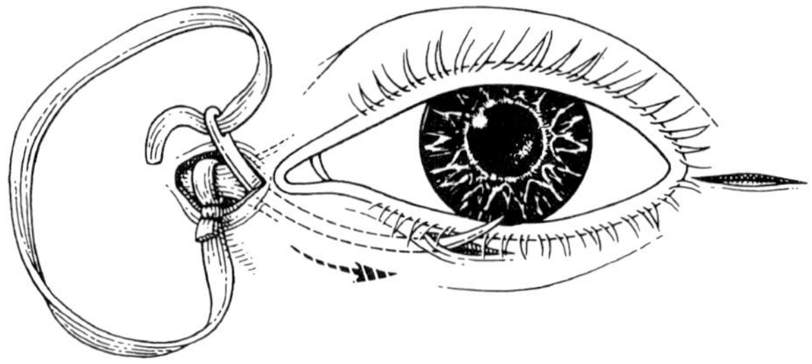

C

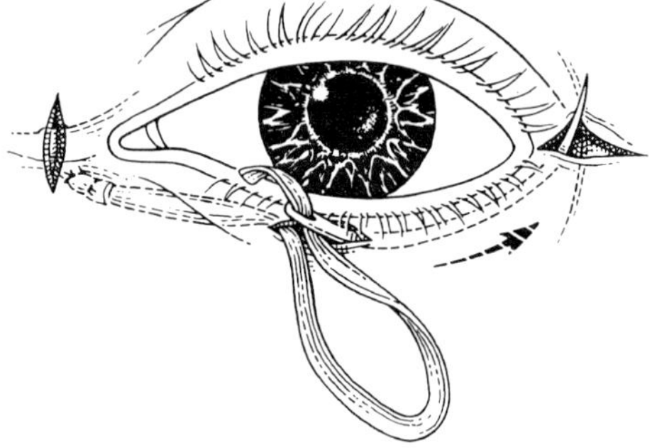

D

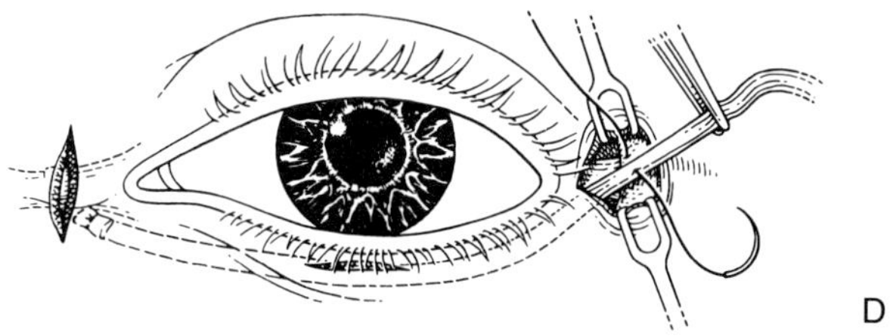

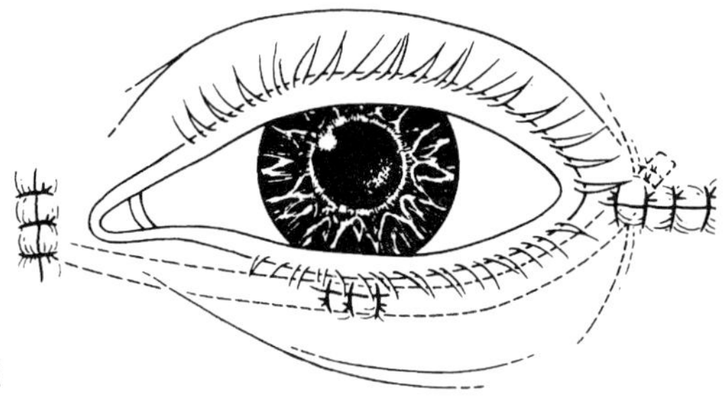

E

FIG. 17. Fascia sling to the lower lid for lower lid retraction. **A:** Diagram representing lower lid retraction and scleral show with labeling of anatomic landmarks. Skin incisions are made over the medial canthal tendon and the central portion of the lid in the subciliary area, and a canthotomy and cantholysis is performed laterally exposing the lateral periosteum. **B:** A fascia strip has been threaded beneath the anterior reflection of the medial canthal tendon and sutured to itself and the tendon. The fascia is being passed from the medial incision to the central incision beneath the lashes. **C:** The fascia is being passed from the central incision to the lateral canthal incision. A Wright fascia needle or a curved general closure needle with a large eyelet is used. **D:** The fascia is sutured to the lateral orbital rim. Before this step, usually a horizontal tightening of the tarsal ligamental sling to the internal periosteum is performed. **E:** All the skin incisions are closed with 6.0 nylon suture, the lower lid having been elevated to the inferior corneal limbus or higher.

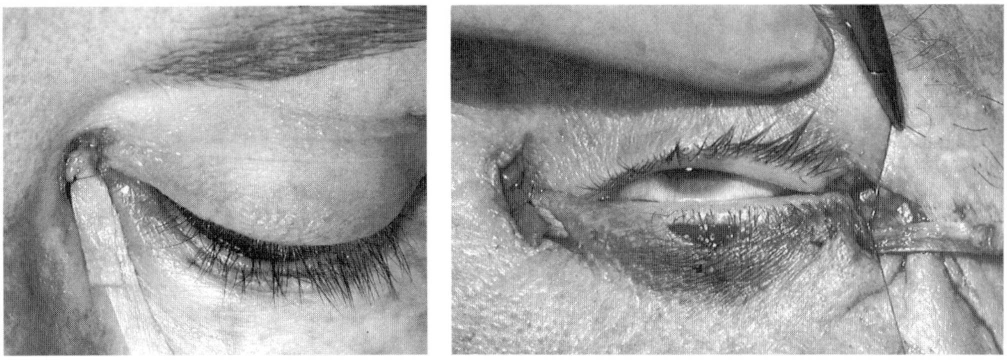

A B

FIG. 18. A: View at surgery of the preserved fascia strip having been looped around the anterior reflection of the medial canthal tendon and sutured to itself. **B:** Fascia strip has been threaded in the submuscular and pretarsal plain in the lower lid to the lateral periosteum where it has been sutured to the rim and tightened. A horizontal tightening procedure of the tarsal ligamental sling has also been performed.

and cotton applicator stick. The cutting Bovie needle is used to incise orbicularis above and below the MCT. The MCT is undermined with sharp Wescotts and a mosquito hemostat inserted under the tendon.

Autogenous fascia may be used but preserved fascia has been found to be very satisfactory for the lower lid. The preserved fascia (if used) is rehydrated or soaked in an antibiotic solution and then trimmed to the desired width.

The fascia is threaded into the hemostat with small forceps (the fascia may have to be divided into thinner strips) and pulled under the MCT, and the loop sutured to itself and to the tendon. The central incision is made with the lid on stretch undermining the orbicularis with sharp Wescott scissors.

A lateral canthotomy, cantholysis, and then a trim of the edge of the tarsal plate is performed followed by some undermining of orbicularis laterally in the pretarsal plane. With the lid on stretch (using heavy forceps) the fascia is threaded in the submuscular plane in front of the lower lid tarsal plate between the incisions. A straightened Wright fascia needle or a straightened closure needle can be used (Fig. 17B, C). It is important that the fascia be placed in the pretarsal plane above the inferior edge of the tarsus in order not to buckle the tarsus outward. The fascia should be deep to the muscle to avoid visibility through the skin.

The horizontal tightening mattress sutures are placed from the edge of the tarsal plate to the orbital rim periosteum. The skin incision is closed nasally prior to completion of the horizontal tightening.

The fascia strip is stretched laterally to position the lower lid margin with the desired tension and 4-0 prolene sutures are placed in the lateral rim periosteum. The fascia is stretched to overlap the area and then the suture is passed through the fascia strip and tied (Fig. 17D). Another suture is taken through the periosteum at the edge of the rim, looped around the fascia, and tied. The skin incisions can be closed.

Figure 18A and B shows surgical views of important steps in the procedure. Figure 19A and B shows a patient before and after the procedure.

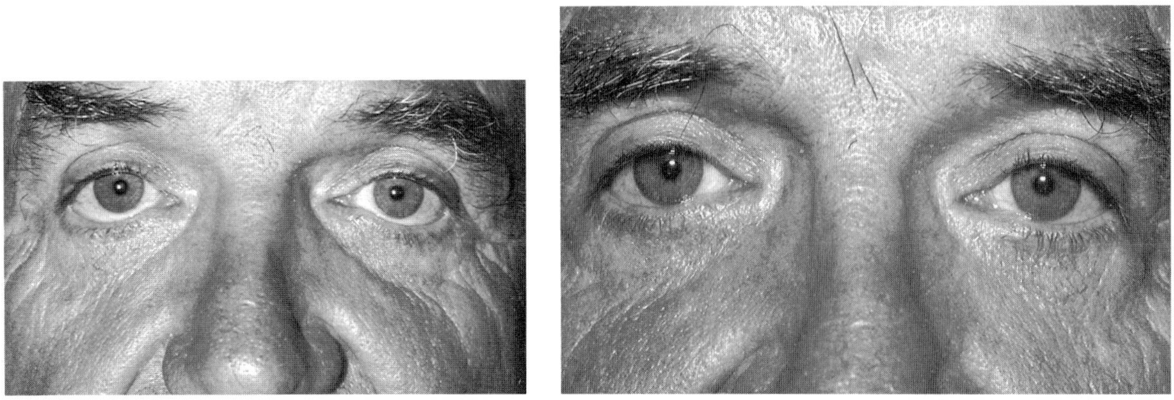

A B

FIG. 19. Patient who has had a lower lid blepharoplasty with some skin shortage causing lower lid retraction and scleral show. Patient did not want skin grafting or any autogenous grafting. **A:** Preoperative before fascia sling. **B:** Postoperative after fascia slings to lower lids correcting lower lid malposition.

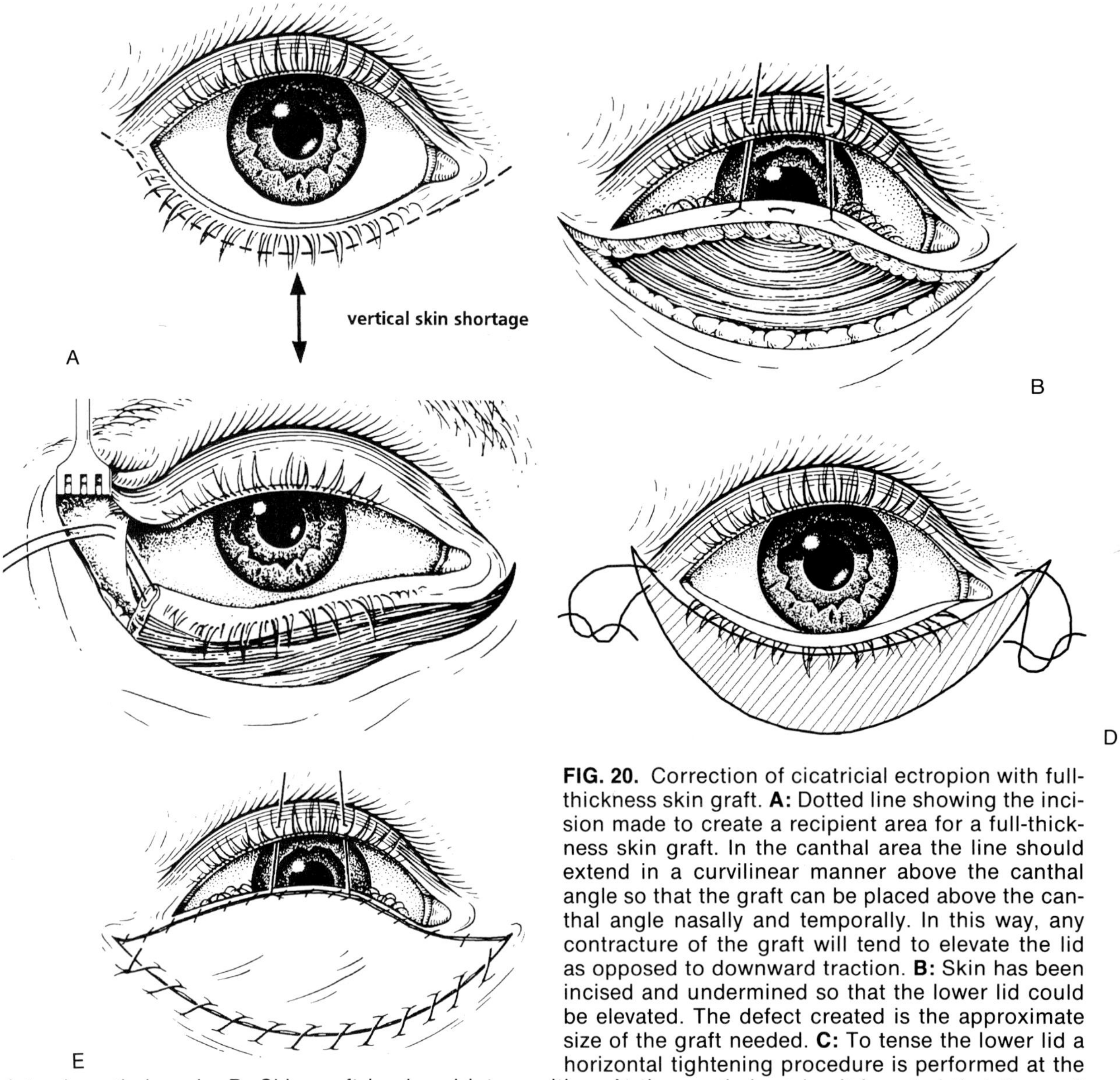

FIG. 20. Correction of cicatricial ectropion with full-thickness skin graft. **A:** Dotted line showing the incision made to create a recipient area for a full-thickness skin graft. In the canthal area the line should extend in a curvilinear manner above the canthal angle so that the graft can be placed above the canthal angle nasally and temporally. In this way, any contracture of the graft will tend to elevate the lid as opposed to downward traction. **B:** Skin has been incised and undermined so that the lower lid could be elevated. The defect created is the approximate size of the graft needed. **C:** To tense the lower lid a horizontal tightening procedure is performed at the lateral canthal angle. **D:** Skin graft is placed into position. At the canthal angles it is noted that the graft extends above the level of the canthal angle. At the medial canthal angle the graft is sutured to the medial canthal tendon. At the lateral canthal angle it is sutured to the lateral periosteum. **E:** The lower lid is usually put on upward traction during the healing.

Full-Thickness Skin Grafts

In many cases of skin shortage ectropion, repositioning of the lower lid will require an external skin graft. Proper placement of the graft is important to produce the best cosmetic result. Proper positioning is also important to ensure that when some of the inevitable postoperative contraction occurs the retracting forces will not pull the lid downward. The grafts should be placed as high as possible under the lashes to hide the interface. The grafts should also be positioned to turn the corner above the canthal angle, so that when contraction occurs postoperatively it will cause an upward not a downward pull. Whenever possible the graft in the canthal angles should be anchored to the medial canthal tendon nasally or the lateral rim periosteum laterally.

Skin Replacement Technique

A subciliary incision is made in the contracted area extending above the canthal angle if possible (only a skin is needed if just skin shortage is present; a skin-muscle incision is needed if skin-muscle contracture is present) (Fig. 20A, B). Dissection is carried out until the lid can be elevated with normal stretchability. A lateral lid tightening as previously described is per-

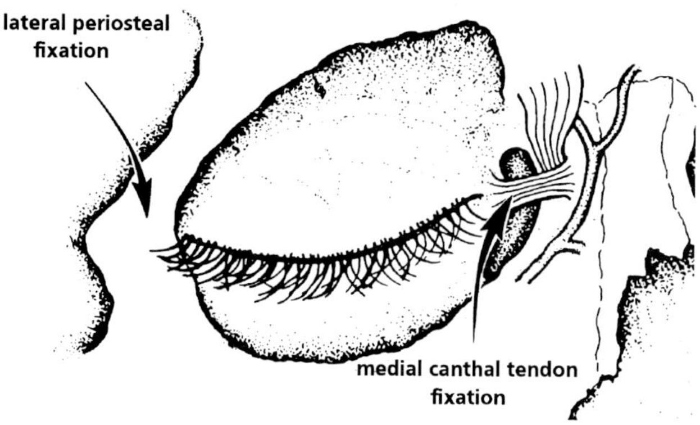

A

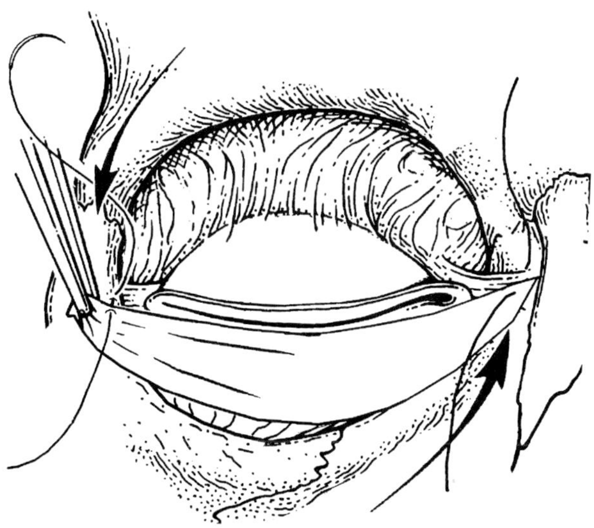

B

FIG. 21. A: Anatomic landmarks for fixation of a large skin graft to the lower lid or smaller skin grafts that span only one canthal angle. **B:** Large "hammock" skin graft applied to the lower lid to fill the defect and fixated to the medial canthal tendon and lateral periosteum to act as a sling for the ectropic lid.

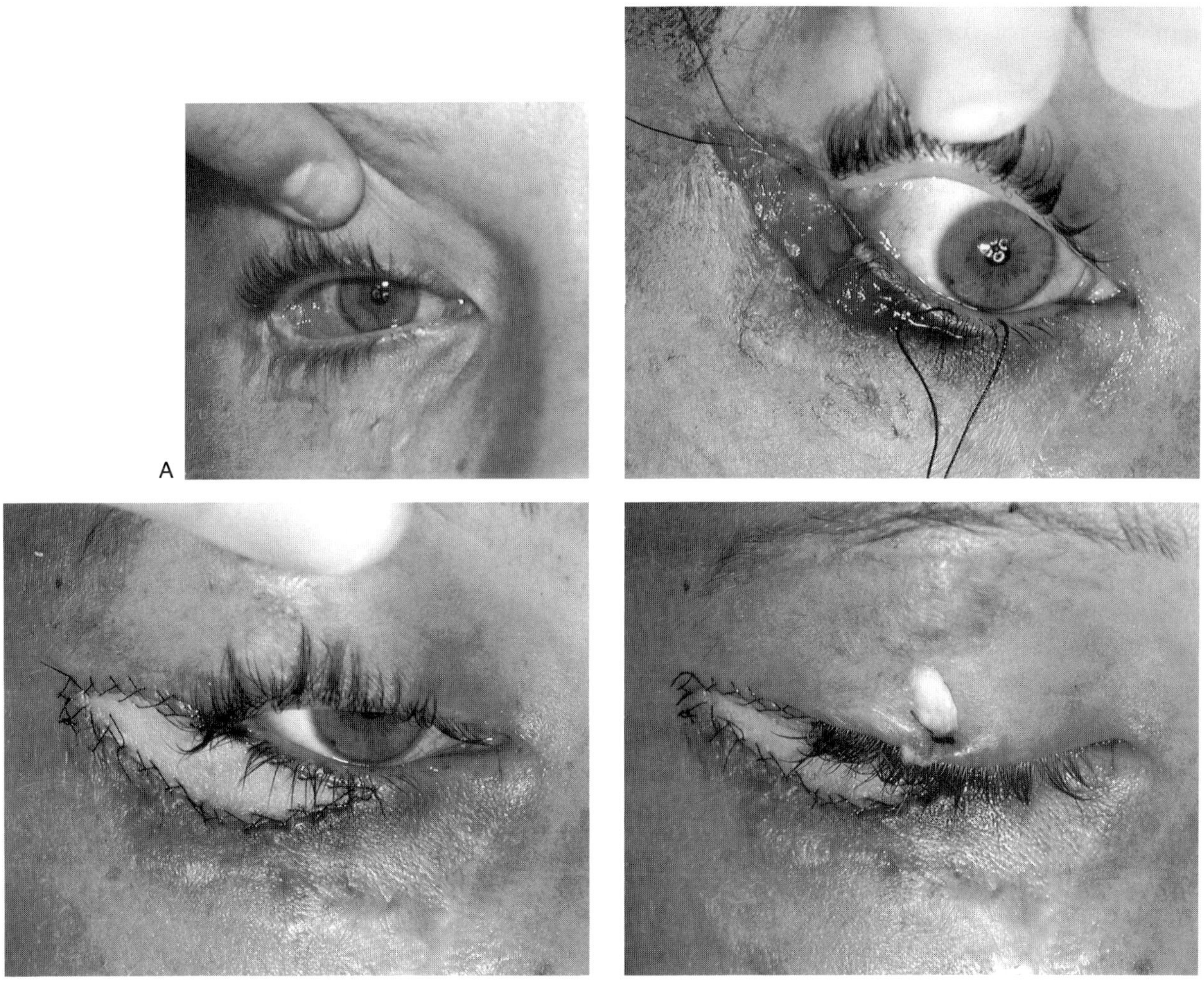

A B C D

FIG. 22. Cicatricial ectropion surgical views. **A:** Patient with posttraumatic scarring and cicatricial ectropion of the right lower lid. **B:** The subciliary incision has been made extending around the canthal angle and the skin allowed to retract so the lower lid can be elevated. A horizontal tightening suture has been placed through the periosteum. **C:** The lower lid has been tightened and the skin graft sutured in a position to fill in the defect. **D:** Intermarginal suture between the lower lid and upper lid causing upward traction is placed during the healing.

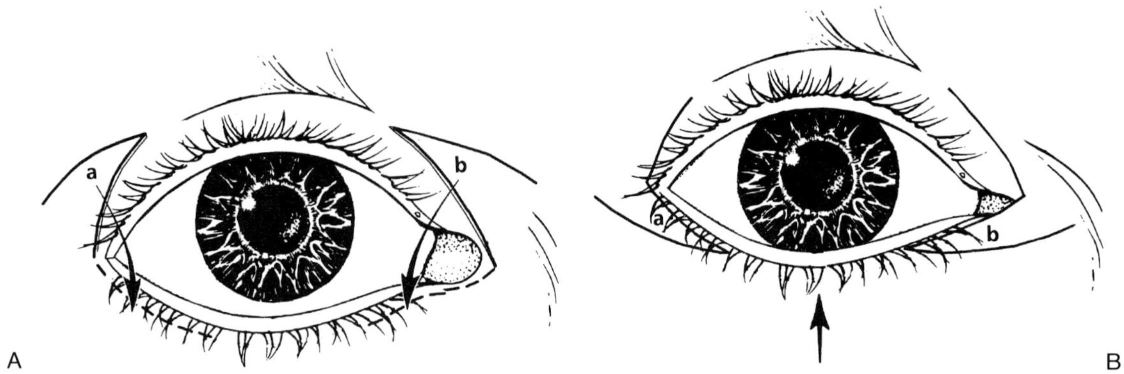

FIG. 23. Cicatricial ectropion. Transposition skin flaps from upper to lower lid. This technique can be used by itself in patients who have lax upper lid skin and moderate shortage of skin particularly in the canthal angles in the lower lid. It also can be used to supplement the full-thickness skin graft to the lower lid. **A:** Design of flaps based at the canthal angle to be transposed to the lower lid. **B:** Transposition of the flaps to the lower lid in defects elevating the lid margin. A horizontal tightening procedure can be performed as well with this technique.

formed with 4-0 prolene (Fig. 20C). The skin graft is placed in the defect and fixated to the periosteum laterally or the MCT nasally (Fig. 20D). Intermarginal sutures are placed for extra splinting if necessary (Fig. 20E).

"Sling" Skin Graft to Lower Lid

For severe cases with extensive skin shortage, particularly those cases with severe horizontal laxity, the skin graft can be made into a supporting "sling." A large subciliary incision extending past and above the MCT and the lateral orbital rim periosteum is made. A lateral horizontal tightening is performed. A lengthy skin graft (usually a supraclavicular donor site is needed) is taken and centered in the defect. One edge of the graft is sutured to the MCT. The graft is tensed and sutured beneath the lashes. The temporal end of the graft is sutured to the lateral periosteum, positioning and tensing the lower lid (Fig. 21A, B). Surgical views of placement of a full skin graft are shown in Fig. 22A–D.

Transposition Flap Skin Replacement

Some canthal support and skin replacement can be obtained with transposition flaps from the upper lid. In many cases they must be supplemented with a free skin graft in the central area. Usually horizontal tightening is also performed.

"V" flaps based at the canthus in the upper lid are outlined after subciliary incisions have been made in the lower lid. Horizontal tightening is then performed if needed. The flaps are transposed and sutured. An intermarginal suture may be needed postoperatively (Fig. 23A, B).

SURGICAL PLANNING FOR THE PATIENT WITH LOWER LID RETRACTION AND SKIN SHORTAGE

Lower lid retraction with lesser amounts of skin shortage (e.g., postblepharoplasty patients) can be corrected in many cases without grafting. Preoperative decisions in planning the corrective surgical procedure

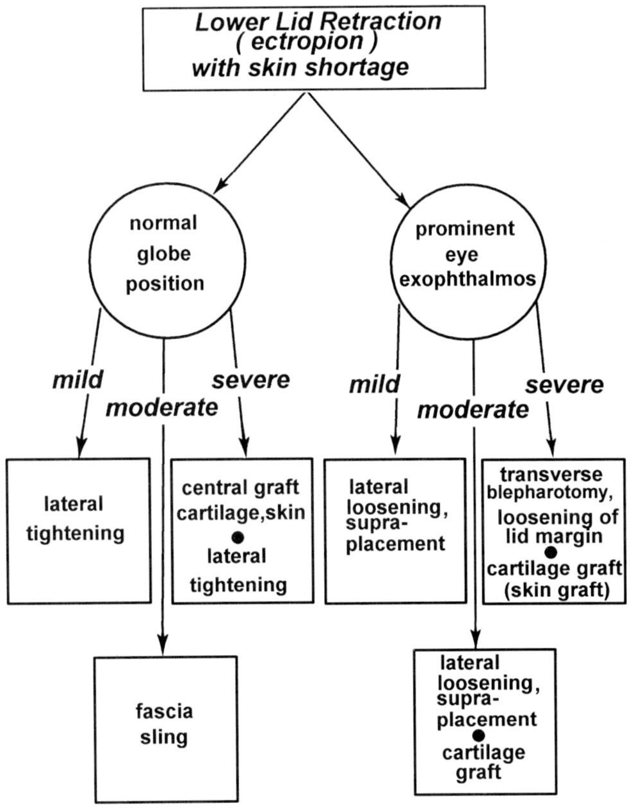

FIG. 24. Skin shortage and eye prominence in ectropion and related conditions.

for patients with lower lid retraction must take into consideration the severity of the skin shortage and the amount of globe prominence in these patients. Milder amounts of skin shortage can be overcome without skin grafts with stiffening of the tarsoligamentous sling using a lateral, horizontal tightening procedure or a fascia lata sling as previously described. In more severe cases, autogeneous grafting with ear cartilage spacer or full-thickness skin must be used.

The presence of increasingly prominent globe position or exophthalmos can affect the ease of correction. In patients with increasing amounts of exophthalmos, tightening or stiffening of the lower lid by the methods described above will produce a "clothes lining" effect on the lid, and when the lower lid is tensed at the lateral canthus it will tend to slide under the globe worsening the lower lid malposition in these patients. This problem is also addressed in the chapters on lower lid blepharoplasty and Graves' disease in which procedures for elevating the lid by supraplacing the lateral tendon combined with lid loosening are described. The severest amount of exophthalmos is be found in patients with Graves' disease and a procedure that employs loosening of the lower lid margin with a full-thickness transverse blepharotomy, canthotomy, and small spacer graft is described in detail. This transverse blepharotomy procedure, although originally used only in patients with Graves' disease, has also been used successfully in postblepharoplasty patients with lower lid retraction who have very prominent eyes.

It is helpful to organize the surgical approaches needed in these patients logically according to the amount of skin shortage present and prominence of the eye (Fig. 24).

COMPLEX ECTROPION

Following severe eyelid lacerations, scarring in the eyelid from repeated surgery, or other unusual situations, many anatomic components of the eyelid may be contracted and scarred causing ectropion. Layers may be fused together, so that the ectropion cannot be blamed entirely on skin-muscle shortage, horizontal laxity, or any other single component. These complex cases of ectropion can be seen commonly following multiple surgical procedures for orbital eyelid trauma and in certain congenital situations.

Scarring of the orbital septum and capsulopalpebral fascia is often an important factor in the pathogenesis of complex cicatricial ectropion. Adhesions to the inferior orbital rim may further complicate the picture (Fig. 25A, B).

In many cases, the lower lid malposition can be corrected only with grafting of the external and internal lamella and, often, separation of fibrous adhesions from the orbital rim if they exist. The grafting may have to be done at separate stages.

Split Level Graft

Vertical lengthening of the lid to correct full-thickness contracture can be accomplished with grafts to each layer placed at different levels. Combined grafting with skin and spacer material placed at the same operative setting must be done in such a way that the grafts not overlap, which allows each graft to obtain enough blood supply for survival.

If adequate muscle is present then it can be interposed between the grafts to provide blood supply. If not then the grafts must be placed in a split level manner so as not to be back-to-back.

A canthotomy and cantholysis with dissection of adhesions can be performed with placement of the 4-0 prolene tightening suture. A posterior incision is made at the inferior tarsal edge with dissection of adhesions involving upward retraction with retractors. The inferior incision should be below the inferior marginal artery leaving the nasal blood supply intact to ensure survival of the margin. Placement of the graft at the inferior tarsal edge can then be performed (ear cartilage, palatal mucosa).

An incision can then be made across the subciliary

A B

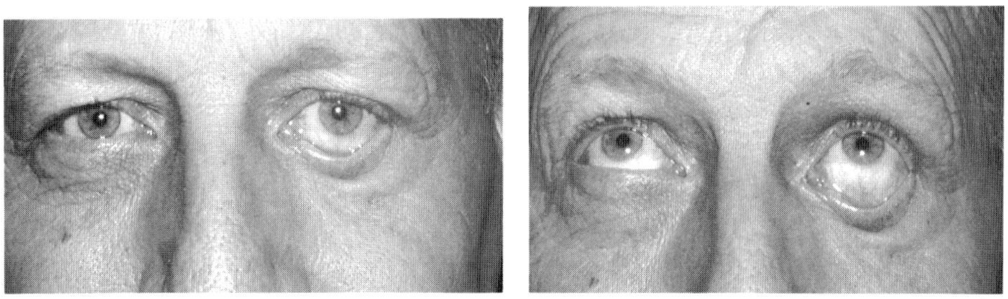

FIG. 25. Patient with complex ectropion with external skin shortage and internal lamellar shortage with adhesions to septum and bone. **A:** Patient had orbital fracture with transcutaneous orbital exploration resulting in septal scarring and complex ectropion. **B:** Patient in upgaze with complete immobility of lower lid and binding down to the septum and bone.

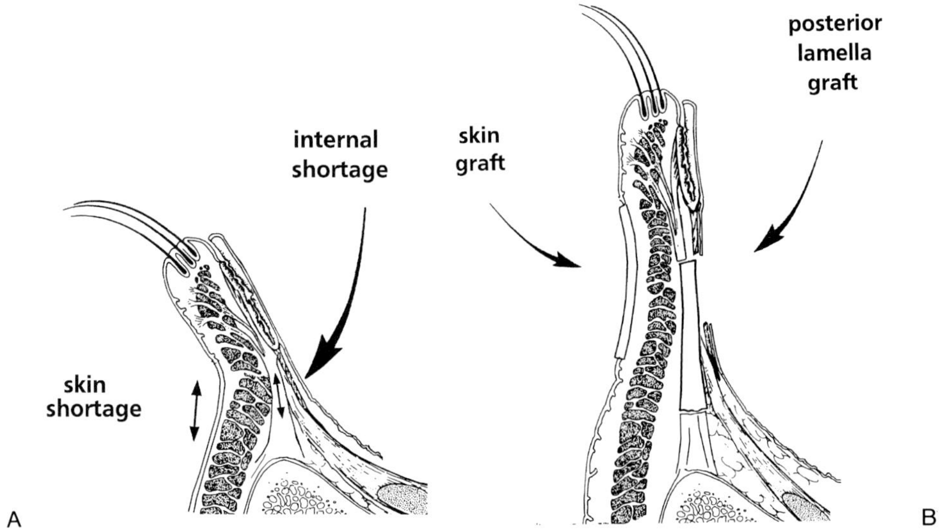

FIG. 26. Correction of complex ectropion with interior and posterior lamellar shortage. "Split level" grafting to lower lid. **A:** Diagram showing lower lid retraction and ectropion from skin shortage externally and internal scarring binding the tarsal plate to the septum and inferior orbital rim. **B:** Elevation of the same eyelid by placement of an external full-thickness skin graft and a posterior lamellar graft freeing the tarsal plate from the retraction to the orbital rim. The grafts are placed at different levels so as not to overlap if possible. Interposing muscle will, however, provide blood supply if this is not possible.

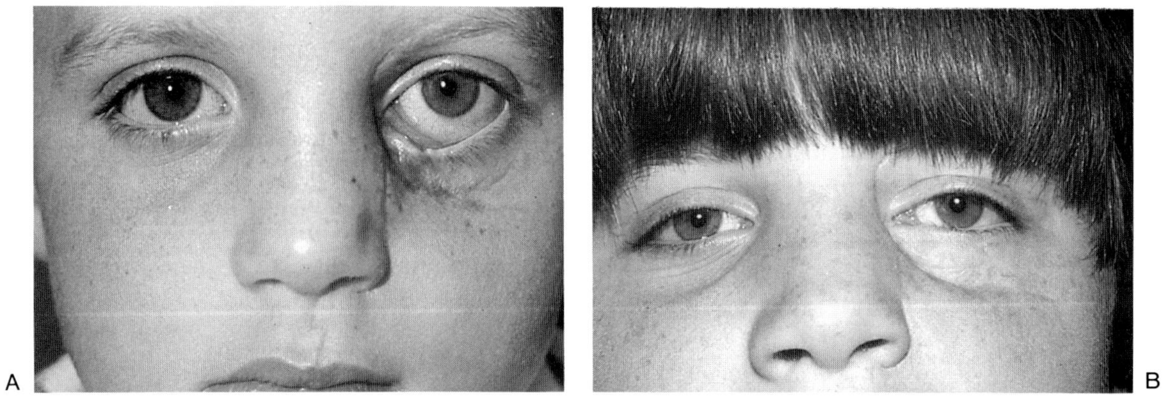

FIG. 27. Complex ectropion and retraction of the lower lid with interior and posterior lamellar shortening. **A:** Young patient who has had a Weber–Ferguson incision with resection of a portion of the maxilla and sinus for a childhood tumor with resulting lower lid retraction. **B:** Same patient following split level grafting to the external surface of the lid and spacer implants correcting the internal retraction. The patient required more than one procedure to arrive at a full correction.

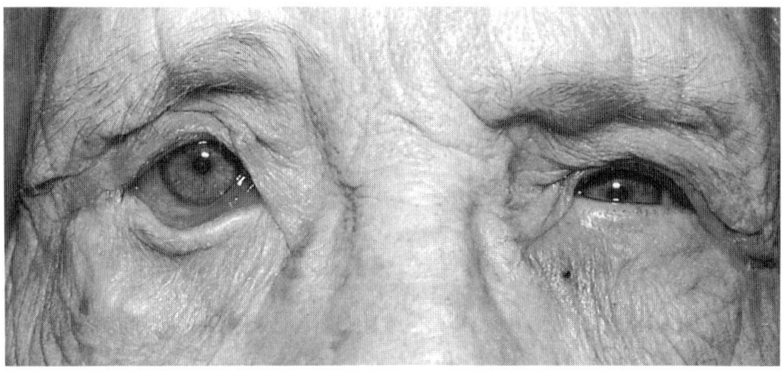

FIG. 28. Paralytic ectropion in patient with Bell's palsy showing more central than medial laxity.

area with dissection of skin or skin-muscle flap away from lid. The skin graft is then placed in this area and fixated laterally to the periosteum or nasally to the MCT depending on the location of the skin defect (Fig. 26A, B). A patient with complex ectropion and retraction before and after repair is shown in Fig. 27A and B.

PARALYTIC ECTROPION

Paralytic ectropion is a type of laxity ectropion that results from the denervation of orbicularis muscle (eyelid protractors) because of a seventh nerve palsy. In many cases it can be aggravated by laxity of the tarsoligamentous sling and it is a condition that can be striking in older persons (Fig. 28). In younger people, innervation to the orbicularis fibers can often be lost without as severe an ectropion if there is adequate elasticity of the sling. The treatment of seventh nerve will be discussed in Chapter 27. Lower lid laxity can be improved by a lateral horizontal tightening, fascia sling, or a temporalis muscle transfer. The silicone implant is not felt to give a lasting satisfactory result.

CONGENITAL ECTROPION

Euryblepharon-Megaloblepharon (29) (Fig. 29)

These patients are born with an elongated eyelid margin in relationship to the fissure width—a blepharoorbital disparity—causing an eversion of the eyelid margin. Skin shortage is also present in these patients adding an everting force to the eyelid margin.

Treacher–Collins Syndrome: Cleft Defects

With the congenital cleft deformities eyelid notch formation occurs because of tissue agenesis and skin shortage. Retraction and eversion of the lid edge can be a prominent component.

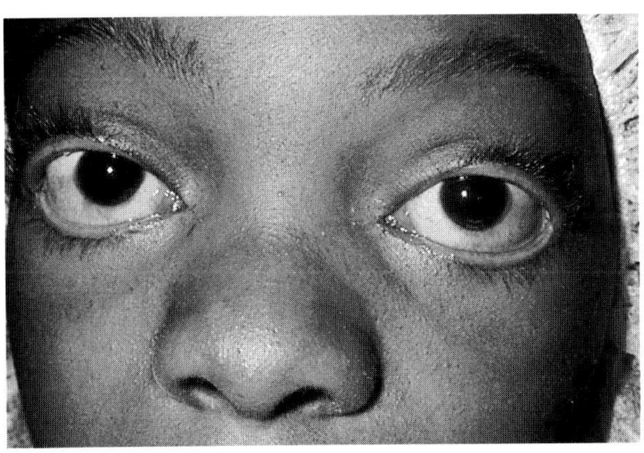

FIG. 29. Patient with congenital euryblepharon. There is an abnormal increased horizontal width to the eyelid combined with skin shortage resulting in eversion of the lids. A similar situation occurs in megaloblepharon.

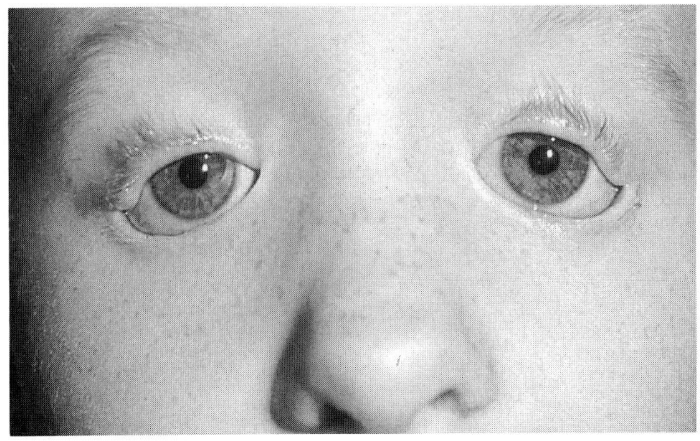

FIG. 30. Congenital ectropion associated with blepharophimosis syndrome. This type of lower lid deformity can be seen apart from the blepharophimosis syndrome.

Blepharophimosis Syndrome

Lower lid retraction and a euryblepharon type of disparity can commonly occur in patients with the blepharophimosis syndrome and its variants. The ectropion and retraction is due to skin shortage in these patients and may require grafting for correction (Fig. 30).

Congenital Upper Lid Eversion: "Tarsal Kink" Syndrome

In these patients a dramatic eversion of the upper lid occurring at birth occurs and usually requires early surgical intervention. With the eversion of the upper lid, conjunctival prolapse occurs, which tends to progress because of irritation from drying. This is usually corrected by fornix-imbricating sutures but some conjunctival resection may also be necessary (30).

REFERENCES

1. Sisler HA, Labay GR, Finlay JR. Senile ectropion and entropion: a comparative histopathological study. *Ann Ophthalmol* 1976;8:319–322.
2. Stefanyszyn MA, Hidayat AA, Flanagan JC. The histopathology of involutional ectropion. *Ophthalmology* 1985;92:120–127.
3. Shore JW. Changes in lower eyelid resting position, movement, and tone with age. *Am J Ophthalmol* 1985;99:414–423.
4. Bick MW. Surgical management of orbital tarsal disparity. *Arch Ophthalmol* 1966;75:386–389.
5. Tenzel RR. Treatment of lagophthalmos of the lower lid. *Arch Ophthalmol* 1969;81:366–368.
6. Tenzel RR, Buffam FV, Miller GR. The use of the "lateral canthal sling" in ectropion repair. *Can J Ophthalmol* 1977;12: 199–202.

7. Leone CR. The treatment of entropion and ectropion. *Ophth Forum* 1983;1(5):16–24.
8. Anderson RL, Gordy DD. The tarsal strip procedure. *Arch Ophthalmol* 1979;97:2192–2196.
9. Ousterhout DK, Weil RB. The role of the lateral canthal tendon in lower eyelid laxity. *Plast Reconstr Surg* 1982;59:620–622.
10. McCord CD, Shore JW. Avoidance of complications in lower blepharoplasty. *Ophthalmology* 1983;90:1039–1046.
11. McCord CD, Moses JL. Exposure of the inferior orbit with fornix incision and lateral eanthotomy. *Ophth Surg* 1979;10(6): 53–63.
12. Jordan DR, Anderson RL. The lateral tarsal strip revisited: the enhanced tarsal strip. *Arch Ophthalmol* 1989;107:604–606.
13. Tenzel RR. Treatment of lagophthalmos of the lower lid. *Arch Ophthalmol* 1969;81:366–368.
14. Small RG, Scott M. The tight retracted lower lid. *Arch Ophthamol* 1990;108:438–444.
15. Baylis H, Nelson ER, Goldberg RA. Lower lid retraction following blepharoplasty. *Ophth Plast Reconstr Surg* 1992;8:170–175.
16. Vistnes LM, Iverson RE, Laub DR. The anophthalmic orbit: surgical correction of lower eyelid ptosis. *Plast Reconstr Surg* 1973;52:346.
17. McCord CD, Ellis DS. The correction of lower lid malposition following lower lid blepharoplasty. *Plast Reconstr Surg* 1993; 92:1068–1072.
18. Lee OS. An operation for the correction of everted lacrimal Puncta. *Am J Ophthalmol* 1951;34:575–578.
19. Smith B. The ''lazy-T'' correction of ectropion of the lower punctum. *Arch Ophthalmol* 1976;94:1149–1152.
20. Tenzel RR, Stewart WB. Blepharo-confusion: blepharochalasis or dermatochalasis? *Arch Ophthalmol* 1978;96:911–912.
21. Custer PL, Tenzel RR, Kowalczyk AP. Blepharochalasis syndrome. *Am J Ophthalmol* 1985;99:424–428.
22. Goldberg R, Seiff S, McFarland J, Simons K, Shorr N. Floppy eyelid syndrome and blepharochalasis. *Am J Ophthalmol* 1986; 102:376–391.
23. Collin JRO, Beard C, Stern WH, Schoengarth D. Blepharochalasis. *Br J Ophthalmol* 1979;63:542–546.
24. Bergin DJ, McCord CD, Berger T, Friedberg H. Blepharochalasis *Br J Ophthalmol* 1988;72:863–867.
25. Wesley RE. Tarsal ectropion from detachment of the lower eyelid retractors. *Am J Ophthalmol* 1982;93:491–495.
26. Hawes MJ, Dortzbach RK. The microscopic anatomy of the lower eyelid retractors. *Arch Ophthalmol* 1982;100:1313–1318.
27. Putterman AM. Ectropion of the lower eyelid secondary to Muller's muscle-capsulopalpebral fascia detachment. *Am J Ophthalmol* 1978;85:814–817.
28. Tse D, Kronish JW, Buus D. Surgical correction of lower eyelid tarsal ectropion by reinsertion of the retractors. *Arch Ophthalmol* 1991;109:427–432.
29. McCord CD, Chappell J, Pollard ZF. Congenital euryblepharon. *Ann Ophthalmol* 1979;11:1217–1224.
30. Blechman B, Isenberg S. An anatomic etiology of congenital eyelid eversion. *Ophth Surg* 1984;15:111–114.

CHAPTER 7

Evaluation of the Ptosis Patient

In recent years there have been advancements in the surgical technique of ptosis repair (1–4). However, there remains some unpredictability in the management of patients. This chapter will present techniques that in the author's hands have produced the most consistently predictable methods of correction, but the surgeon must always be aware that there will be a need for postoperative revisions in some ptosis patients. It is emphasized that there is no single "formula" for the correction of ptosis in all patients and many patients require intraoperative adjustments and postoperative modification (5).

Patients should be grouped preoperatively into appropriate subgroups, usually into categories reflecting similar behavior in their response to a surgical procedure. In this way, the surgeon can develop a quantitative surgical approach to ptosis. It is also emphasized that although the correction of lid droopiness is the primary goal in ptosis surgery, there are important related issues. The protection and health of the eyes must remain of utmost concern, as well as the identification of any underlying pathologic process that may need diagnosis and treatment.

Ptosis may seem to lend itself to a cookbook approach. If one wishes optimum results, the surgeon must always be prepared to perform revisional surgery. Formulas are only a starting point for each surgeon to develop his or her own individual technique to obtain the best and most predictable ptosis correction.

DIFFERENTIAL DIAGNOSIS OF PTOSIS

Ptosis of the upper lid is the drooping of the upper lid margin to a position lower than it normally would be. There is a wide range of "normal positions" of the upper lid margin. Ptosis itself may be relative to the position of the opposing eyelid but the upper lid margin does not normally encroach on the pupillary aperture.

There are many conditions that mimic ptosis that are not true ptosis and should be differentiated from it (Table 1). *Retraction of the opposite lid* from Graves' disease, in many cases, may simulate ptosis (Fig. 1A, B). A downward rotation of the globe, *hypotropia,* with accompanying lid movement may present as ptosis (Fig. 2A, B). *Enophthalmos* may simulate a true ptosis because the globe is recessed and the upper lid migrates downward to a lower position (Fig. 3A, B). A *contralateral exophthalmos* may also cause an upward movement of the lid that will produce a relative enophthalmos and ptosis on the opposite side. Any *mechanical pressure on the lid,* such as heavy skin folds, eyelid edema, or tumor, can produce a downward position of the lid margin and in many cases may be difficult to differentiate from a true ptosis (Fig. 4A, B). *Guarding or squinting of the eye* in the presence of an irritative phenomenon may also simulate ptosis. Spasm may occur with aberrant regeneration of a seventh nerve palsy, hemifacial spasm, or benign essential blepharospasm (Fig. 5A, B). *Retraction syndromes* (e.g., Duane's syndrome) with extraocular muscle fibrosis may cause the lid to fall as the globe is retracted backward with eye movement.

TABLE 1. *Causes of pseudoptosis*

Contralateral lid retraction
Hypotropia
Enophthalmos
Contralateral exophthalmos
Upper lid pressure (swelling, tumor, or redundant skin)
Guarding
Duane's retraction syndrome (enophthalmos)
Aberrant seventh regeneration (Marin–Amat) syndrome
Essential blepharospasm
Hemifacial spasm

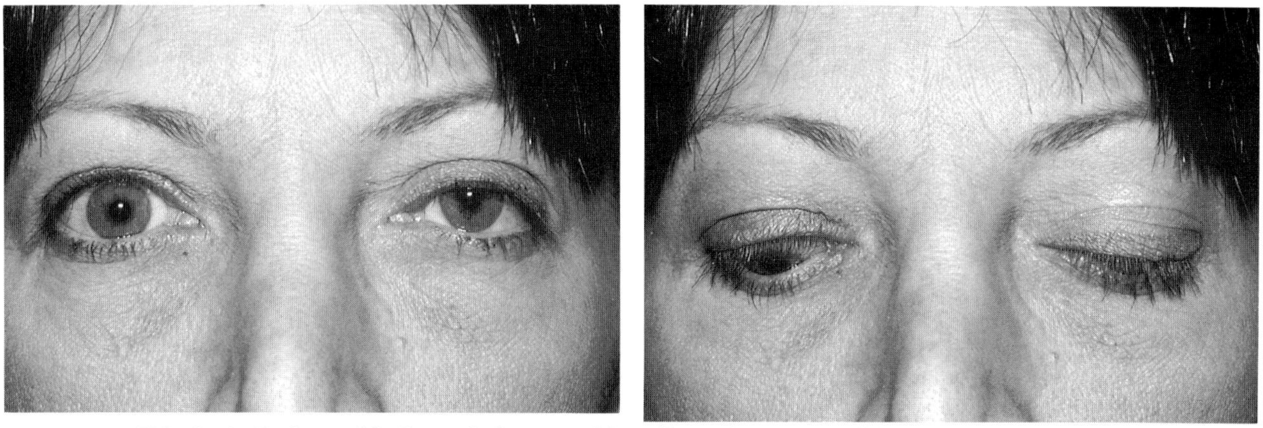

A B

FIG. 1. A: Patient with Graves' disease with unilateral upper eyelid retraction on the right side and pseudoptosis on the left. **B:** Lagophthalmos of the right upper eyelid in downgaze consistent with Graves' disease.

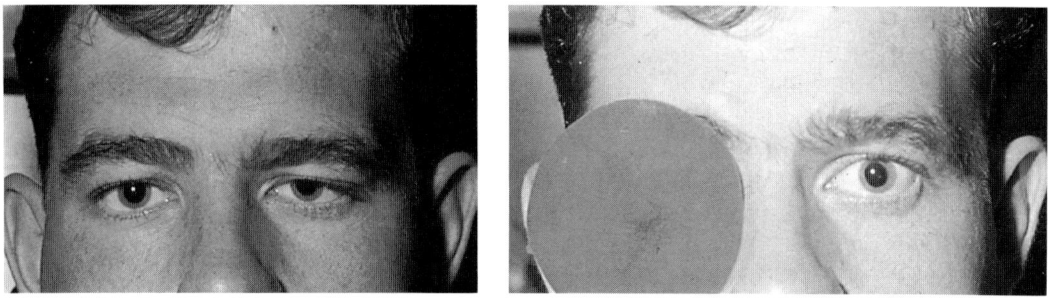

A B

FIG. 2. A: Patient with a left hypotrophia and pseudoptosis as the eyelid follows the globe in downgaze. **B:** Patient fixating with hypotrophic eye in the primary position with elevation of the pseudoptotic lid.

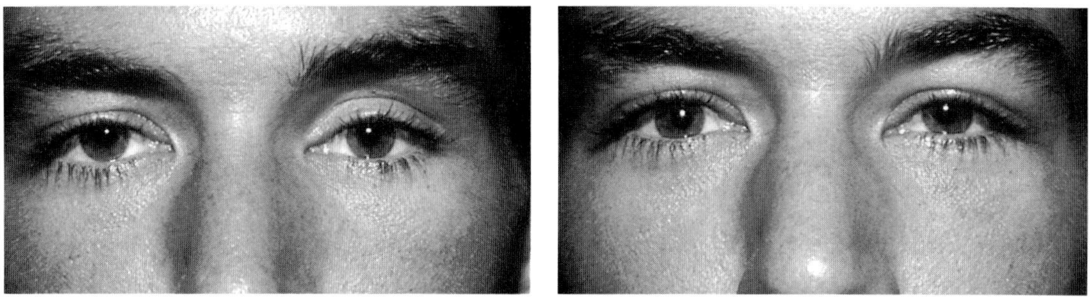

A B

FIG. 3. A: Patient with enophthalmos on the left following an orbital fracture with a high lid crease and pseudoptosis. **B:** Same patient following augmentation of orbital volume correcting deep sulcus and pseudoptosis.

CLASSIFICATION OF PTOSIS

It has been traditional to group ptosis patients according to those who have ptosis at birth *(congenital)* and those who acquire ptosis later *(acquired)*. This grouping has a very practical significance in that congenital and acquired ptosis usually behave differently in their response to surgical procedures. In the acquired category, many patients will require diagnostic testing to rule out underlying neurologic or neuromuscular conditions.

Congenital Ptosis

True congenital ptosis is a developmental dystrophy present in the levator muscle. The word "congenital"

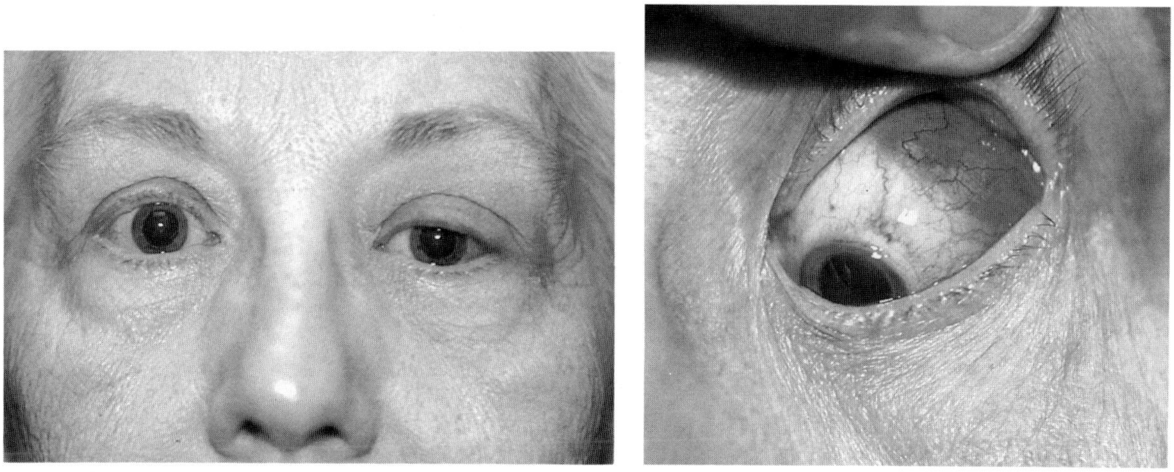

A B

FIG. 4. A: Patient with ptosis of the left upper lid presenting for corrective surgery. **B:** Eversion of the left upper lid showing subconjunctival mass in lacrimal gland area consistent with lymphoma.

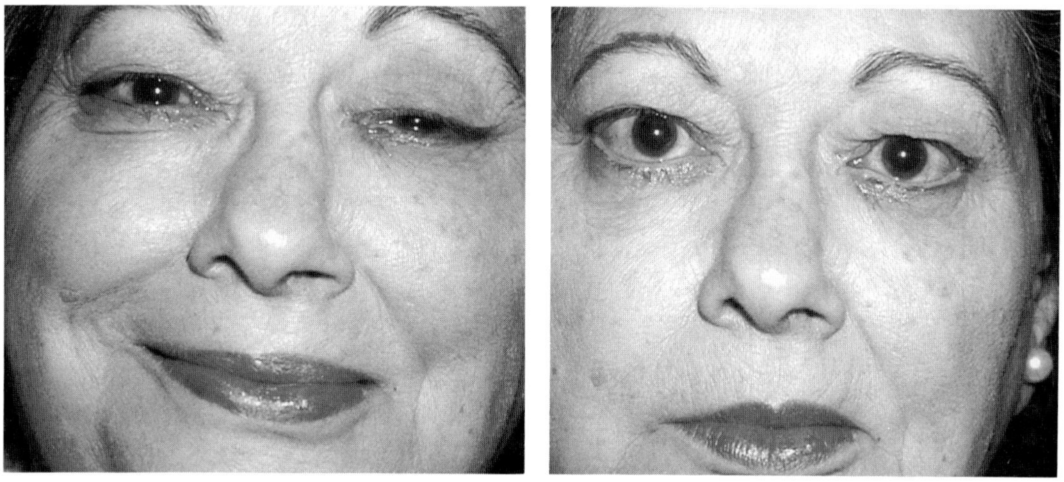

A B

FIG. 5. A: Patient with a narrowing of the right fissure with lower facial muscle contraction. The patient had aberrant regeneration of a seventh nerve palsy. **B:** Same patient with lower fascial muscles relaxed and opening of eyelid.

implies that the ptosis is present from birth; however, ptosis may exist at birth from other causes such as birth injuries or congenital third nerve paralysis. These patients should be grouped with those acquiring ptosis because the levator in these patients is usually not dystrophic in nature. Patients with congenital ptosis have a lack of differentiation of the levator muscle at birth. Embryologically, the levator complex develops from the superior rectus muscle but does not reach normal position until the fourth fetal month. Failure or aberration in its development will result in ptosis. Levator muscle biopsies performed in a series of congenital ptosis patients showed an absence of striated muscle fibers with fibrosis, a histologic picture similar to muscular dystrophy (6).

In these patients, the levator muscle is "stiff," which has important clinical significance in that the stiff muscle does not respond as well to resection as in those patients with acquired ptosis, who have a more contractive, elastic muscle. In addition, the stiffness of the lid helps diagnostically in the recognition of congenital ptosis in that there is lagophthalmos in downgaze (Fig. 6A–C). This lagophthalmos in downgaze can be an important diagnostic aid in the absence of history, when one wishes to differentiate congenital from acquired ptosis. Ptosis occurring at birth usually has a familial basis but may be associated with birth trauma. Levator dehiscence can occur at birth or in the neonatal period, and in these cases the droopy lid does not have this stiffness and will not have a lagophthalmos in downgaze (7).

Recent series have shown that the number of patients with congenital ptosis and acquired ptosis are equally divided in the patient population. In most cases

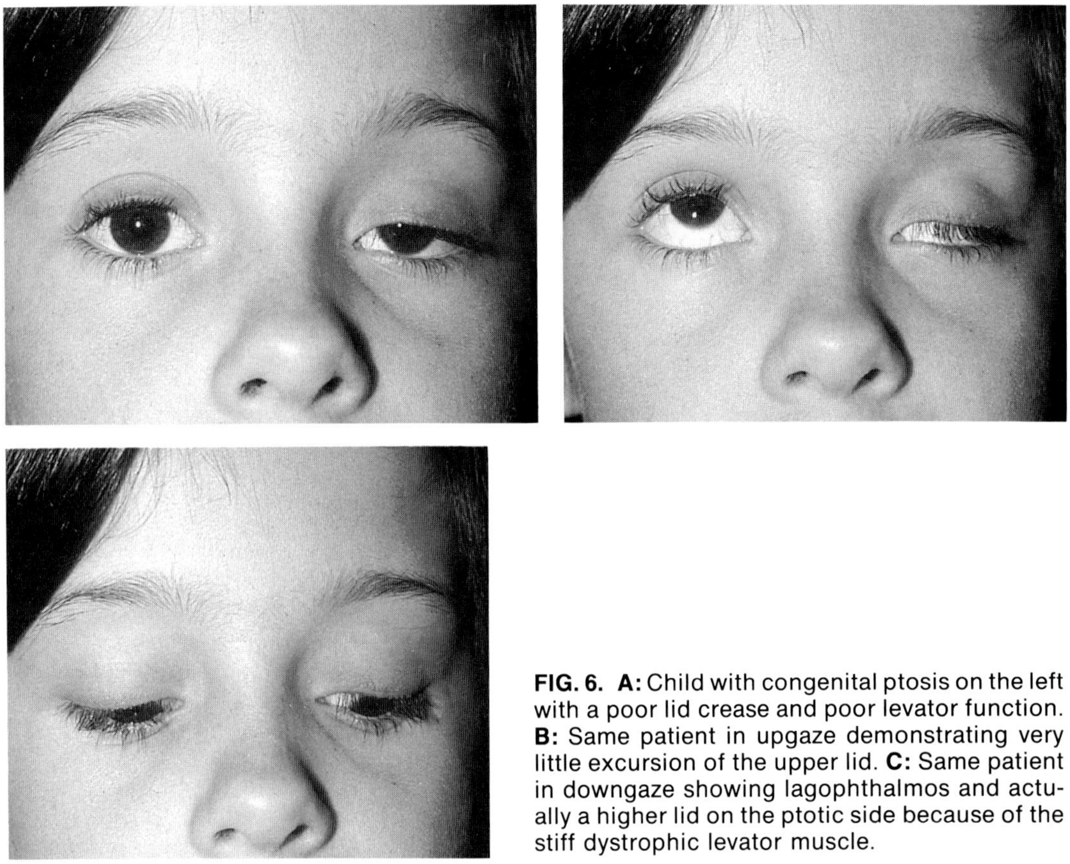

FIG. 6. A: Child with congenital ptosis on the left with a poor lid crease and poor levator function. **B:** Same patient in upgaze demonstrating very little excursion of the upper lid. **C:** Same patient in downgaze showing lagophthalmos and actually a higher lid on the ptotic side because of the stiff dystrophic levator muscle.

of congenital ptosis, there is some family history of ptosis.

Associated Ocular Anomalies, Coexistent Strabismus and Amblyopia

In the past childhood ptosis was thought to be benign with regard to visual development if the child could be observed to "peek under the lid." This has been shown to be untrue and occlusion amblyopia can occur even in children who do not have a complete ptosis. In addition, several reports have indicated a high incidence of coexistent strabismus, amblyopia, and anisometropia in children with congenital ptosis.

Decisions to intervene and correct the ptosis with a surgical procedure are usually related to the extent of visual blockage and its effect on the development of visual and motor skills. Bilateral ptosis can impair a child's ability to learn motor skills such as walking. If the ptosis is unilateral, the child will use the nonptotic eye for sight and motor skills. The lack of use of the ptotic eye can impair visual development because of occlusion amblyopia or the induced astigmatism from eyelid pressure. If amblyopia is a concern, then some type of eyelid elevation is indicated as soon as is feasible. Surgery before the age of 4 years has been shown to reduce astigmatism. Children with ptosis have a high incidence (29–36%) of coexistent strabismus and a high incidence of amblyopia on that basis (8–12). These children at risk should have visual evaluation and indicated visual treatment by an appropriate professional trained in visual care.

Current information suggests that childhood ptosis has a greater influence on vision than formerly thought and early surgical correction should be performed.

Marcus–Gunn Jaw Winking Syndrome

Synkinetic movement of the upper lid is present with chewing in patients with congenital ptosis in approximately 2–6% of the cases, the result of abnormal neural connections in the central nervous system between the levator and the external pterygoid portion of the fifth cranial nerve (13). This condition should be identified because the winking anomaly must be dealt with separately. There is also a higher incidence of superior rectus muscle weakness in these patients (Fig. 7A, B).

Blepharophimosis Syndrome

The blepharophimosis syndrome classically has been described as a triad of ptosis of the upper lids, telecanthus, and phimosis of the eyelid fissure (Fig. 8).

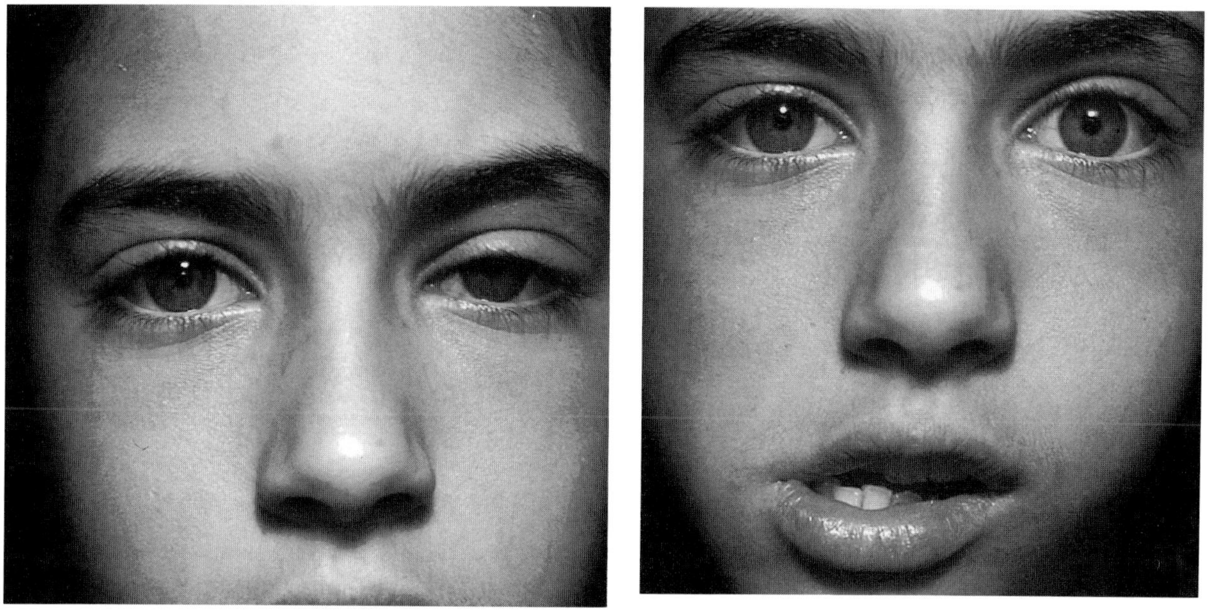

FIG. 7. A: Child with congenital Marcus–Gunn jaw winking syndrome with ptosis on the right side with the jaw relaxed. **B:** Same patient with lower jaw movement to the contralateral side showing retraction of the ptotic eyelid.

Other anomalies may be present, such as epicanthus inversus, skin shortage in the upper and lower lid, congenital ectropion, and flattening of the glabellar area. Usually, the lids are hypoplastic with deficient tarsi, adding to the complexity of the reconstruction. This is commonly a hereditary condition and autosomal dominant once established. Many cases are forme fruste with no family history of the condition. All children with the syndrome seem to have normal or above average intelligence.

Congenital Anophthalmos-Microphthalmos

Agenesis and absence of the globe occurs as a birth defect. Ptosis is an accompanying abnormality in patients with this syndrome and in many cases coexistent hypoplasia of the lids and orbital bones is present.

Coexistent Eyelid Hamartomas

Hamartomatous tissue occurring at birth is often unrecognized because of its subtlety; however, it may present a problem in the initial diagnosis and correction of ptosis.

Congenital Neurofibromatosis

Congenital neurofibromatosis may not be readily diagnosed if there is an absence of cafe-au-lait spots or other stigmata; however, the presence of a thickened, puffy, S-shaped lid is a characteristic finding (Fig. 9A, B).

Capillary Hemangiomas

These lesions usually present at birth and appear as an obvious mass in the eyelid or periocular tissue, pinkish and bluish in color, and may have a florid red cutaneous component. Their natural growth history is that they tend to enlarge and progress for the first year and then undergo varying degrees of involution. In some children the lesions may involute enough that the remnants may be barely detectable by the time they reach

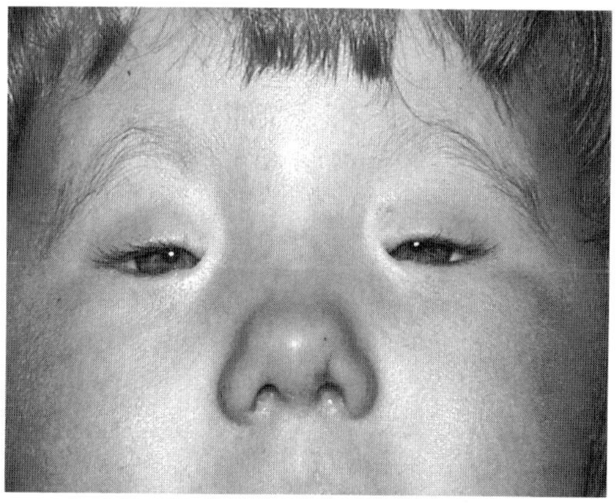

FIG. 8. Child with blepharophimosis syndrome with ptosis of the upper lids, telecanthus, epicanthus inversus, and phimosis of the eyelid fissures.

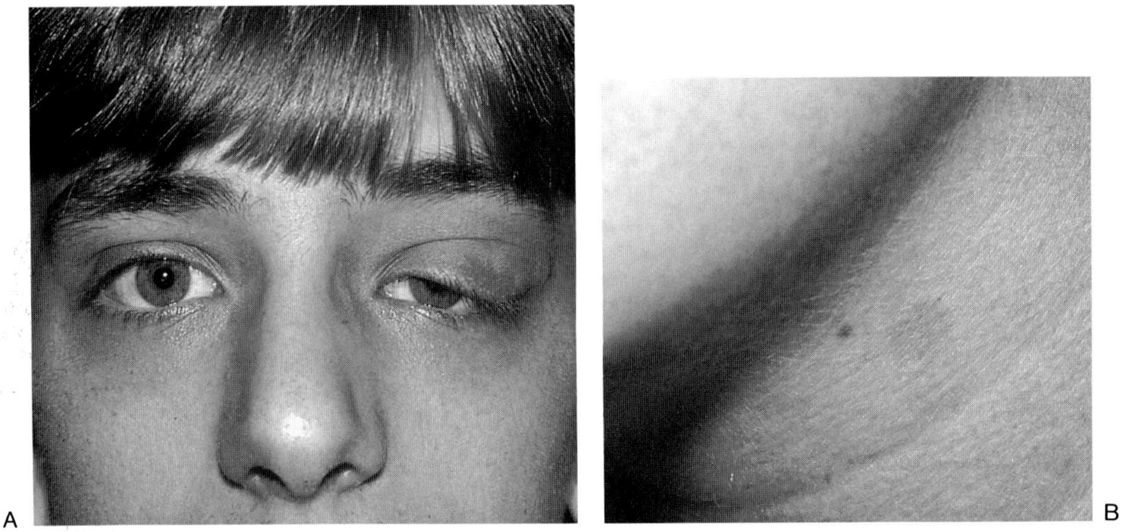

FIG. 9. A: Young male with neurofibromatosis of the left upper lid. Mild ptosis was noticed at birth but the ptosis progresses through adolescence. **B:** Cafe-au-lait spot on the patient's neck.

adolescence. Some may have large venous components, some may be more cellular, and some may have characteristics of an arteriovenous malformation. All have the same mode of progression.

Reasons to intervene and try to speed up the course of involution are *visual blockage* that may lead to amblyopia or *unusual growth* with acceleration of the extent of the lesion. Visual impairment can occur as the result of occlusion amblyopia from sensory deprivation when the lesion actually covers the pupil. Amblyopia can also occur from a change in the shape of the eye from local pressure causing astigmatism and refractive amblyopia. Despite treatment, many of these children will develop a significant refractive error, usually myopia astigmatism, and some amblyopia.

Interventional treatment for these capillary hemangiomas takes the form of surgical excision, localized irradiation, and injections with deposteroids (the last is the most popular). The use of sclerosing agents has been abandoned.

Systemic steroids or locally injected steroids (triamcinolone, betamethasone) can speed up the involution of the hemangiomas but both can cause adrenal suppression with retardation of growth and other side effects. None of the modes of treatment for capillary hemangiomas are without side effects or shortcomings, and these must be balanced against the visual threat or other needs of the patient.

Lymphangioma

Lymphangioma occurs at birth. The involvement of the periocular tissue causes eyelid swelling and thickening. Lymphangiomas do not involute but may progressively enlarge through adolescence. Acute swelling with upper respiratory infections and trauma may occur. Acute blood cyst formation may occur with trauma causing rapid dramatic swelling requiring decompression. Surgical excision or debulking of the lymphangioma with the CO_2 laser can be helpful but not curative.

Acquired Ptosis

Acquired ptosis consists of a heterogeneous group of disorders that are not easily placed in a simple classification. Because there may be mixed physiologic elements of the ptosis, it is sometimes difficult to place them in the classic grouping of (a) neurogenic, (b) myogenic, (6) traumatic, and (d) mechanical. More practically, cases of acquired ptosis can be grouped by frequency as per cause (Table 2). A review of studies on ptosis patients over the years shows that the large majority of patients with acquired ptosis who present to the surgeon will be either involutional or posttraumatic (13). In most series, approximately 40–50% are of the involutional type and 30% are posttraumatic.

TABLE 2. *Causes of acquired ptosis*

Involutional
Trauma
Chronic progressive external ophthalmoplegia (myopathic)
Third nerve palsy
Mechanical changes with anophthalmos
Horner's syndrome
Myasthenia gravis
Upper lid tumors

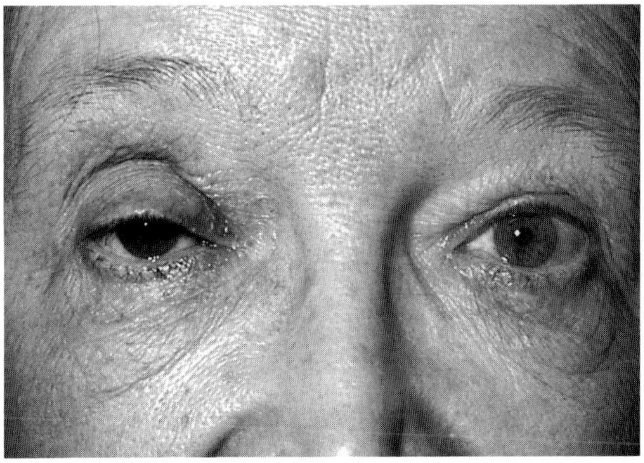

FIG. 10. Patient with involutional ptosis and levator dehiscence on the right side showing ptosis of the eyelid, a high lid crease, and thinning of the lid above the tarsal plate. The patient had previous cataract surgery on that side.

Recognizing a ptosis as "noncongenital" is important because in many cases there is a need for diagnostic testing to rule out neurologic or myopathic disease. In all acquired cases of ptosis, the levator at one time was "normal" and does respond to surgery differently than in the congenital case. In practical terms, there is more lift per millimeter in a levator resection procedure for acquired ptosis.

Involutional Ptosis

The most common type of acquired ptosis is involutional ptosis. In the majority of cases, it is due to an abnormality or defect of the levator allowing a thinning and stretching in the aponeurosis and a downward shift of the tarsal plate (4). Characteristically, there is significant ptosis, good to excellent levator function, a high lid crease, and thinning of the eyelid tissues above the tarsal plate (Fig. 10). The rarification of the aponeurosis and some atrophy of the horns can cause very characteristic anatomic changes in patients with involutional ptosis. A schematic of upper eyelid anatomy is shown in Fig. 11. The three major attachments of the levator complex are demonstrated; (1) Müller's muscle, inserting into the upper tarsal border; (2) the anterior tarsal attachments of the aponeurosis, inserting into the lower third of the anterior tarsus; and (3) the aponeurotic bands that penetrate the orbicularis mus-

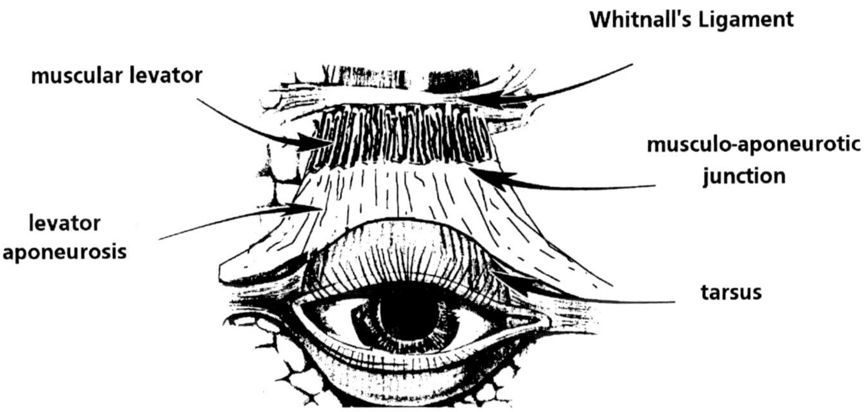

FIG. 11. A diagrammatic representation of landmarks in the retractor layer of the upper lid.

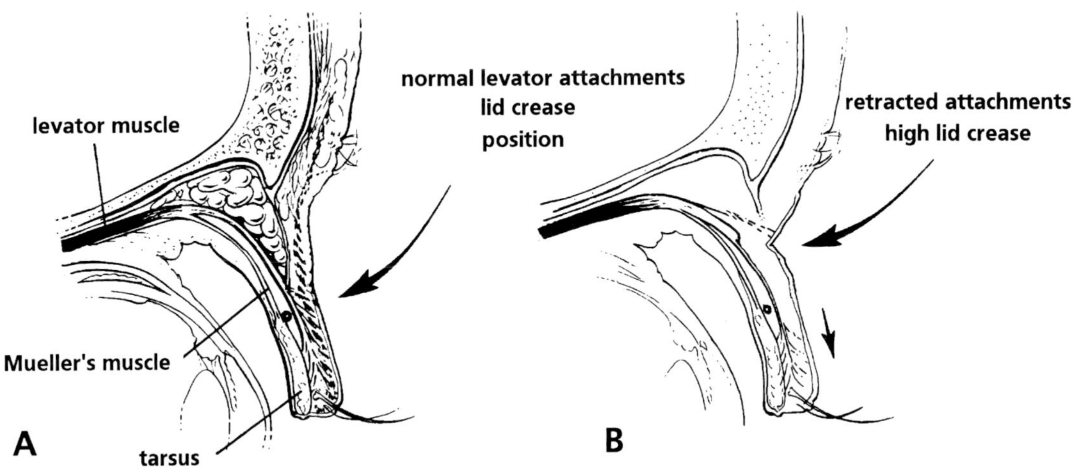

FIG. 12. Cross-section of upper lid. **A:** Normal structure showing attachment of Müller's muscle and levator aponeurosis in position of lid crease. **B:** Diagrammatic representation of aponeurotic dehiscence with retraction of the lid crease.

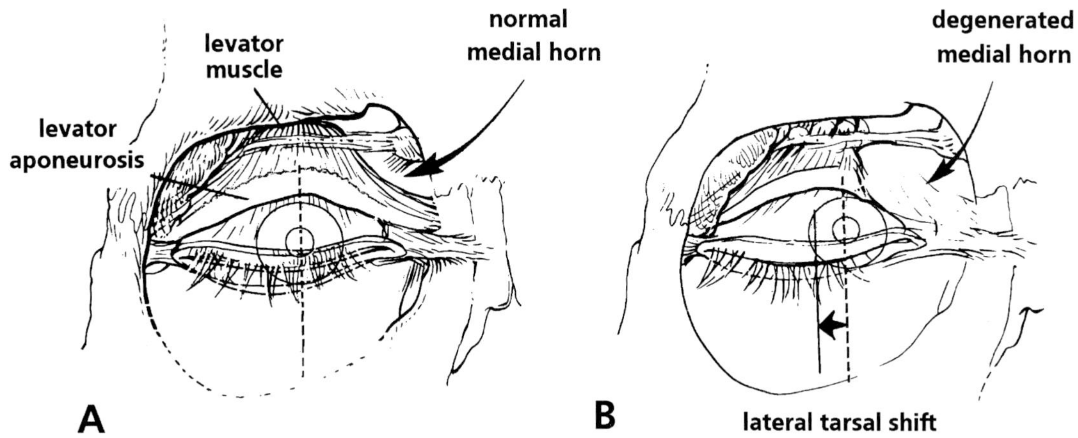

FIG. 13. Diagrammatic representation of the eyelid in the frontal view. **A:** Normal structures and landmarks. **B:** Lateral shift of the tarsal plate because of atrophy and dehiscence of the medial horn and supportive structures of the upper lid.

cle, inserting into the skin, creating the lid crease. In the patient with involutional ptosis, the anterior tarsal attachments of the aponeurosis are defective because of stretching and disinsertion, thus causing lengthening of the lid and ptosis (Fig. 12) (15). The medial horn of the levator has often lost its support, causing a lateral shift of the tarsal plate (Figs. 13–15). The lid crease attachments of the aponeurosis tend to remain intact, and this preservation of the attachments to the skin allows the migration of the lid crease to a higher level. The levator function is characteristically good to excellent in these patients.

In some involutional patients, ptosis may be caused by levator weakening from a fatty degeneration of the levator muscle rather than an aponeurotic thinning. This is not as common as aponeurotic defects and is thought to represent another subgroup within the etiologies of involutional ptosis.

Posttraumatic Ptosis

In this subcategory, all mechanisms—neurologic, myogenic, and mechanical—may be present. In the acute situation, damage to the levator complex can be

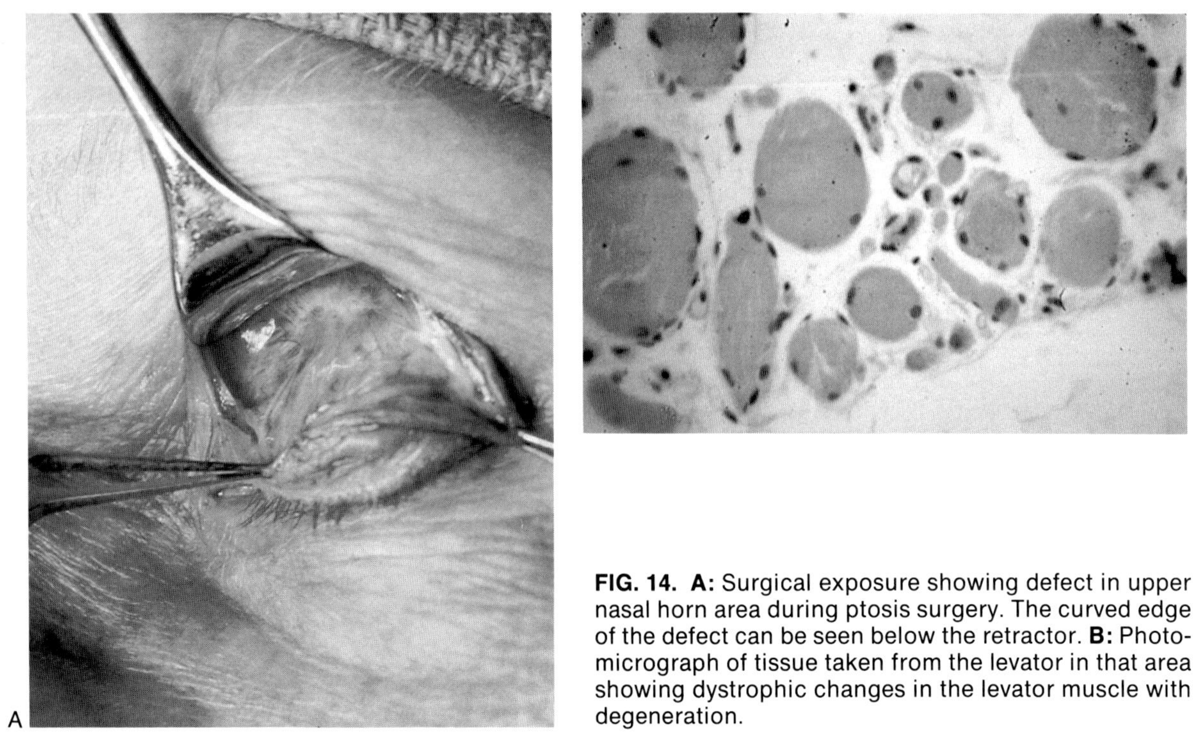

FIG. 14. A: Surgical exposure showing defect in upper nasal horn area during ptosis surgery. The curved edge of the defect can be seen below the retractor. **B:** Photomicrograph of tissue taken from the levator in that area showing dystrophic changes in the levator muscle with degeneration.

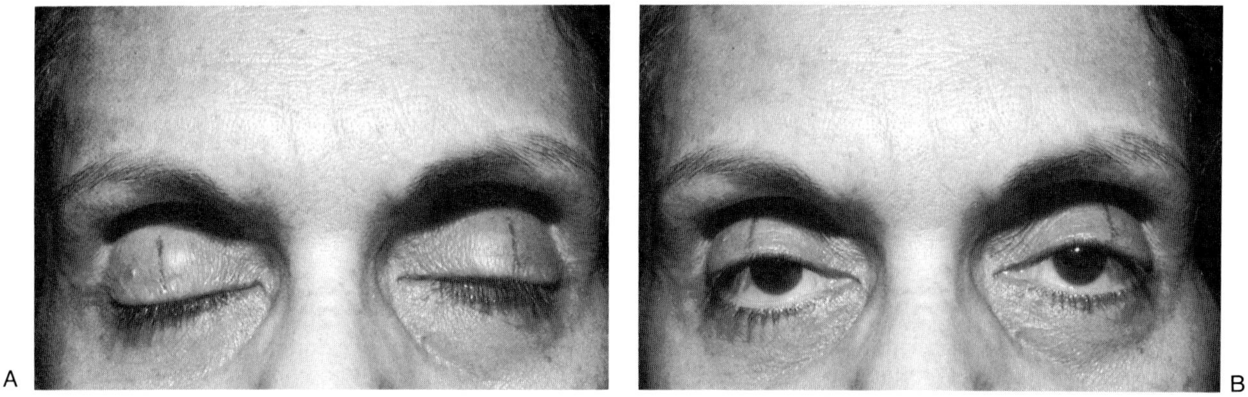

FIG. 15. **A:** Patient with involutional ptosis with eyelid closure with markings placed on eyelid in line with the peak of the tarsal plate superiorly. **B:** Same patient with eyelids open showing the lateral displacement of the peak of the tarsal plate because of degeneration of the medial horns.

masked by edema. Following trauma, it is very important to allow adequate time for possible recovery of any myoneural dysfunction, the resolution of edema, and the softening of scar tissue before attempting ptosis repair.

Chronic, Progressive External Ophthalmoplegia

This condition is a progressive muscular dystrophy that principally affects the extraocular muscles including the levator muscle. Its onset can be subtle and it may begin in childhood or adolescence, with gradual development of ptosis. The facial or oropharyngeal muscles may also be involved in 25% of these patients. The diagnosis can be confirmed by muscle biopsy. Even though there is impairment in ocular motility, the patients do not usually complain of diplopia. Because of a poor Bell's phenomenon, postoperative corneal exposure may be a problem (16–20) (Fig. 16A, B).

Myasthenia Gravis

This disease primarily affects young women and old men. It is extremely rare in children. The extraocular muscle manifestations may be the initial findings in the majority of patients, with presentation with unilateral or bilateral asymmetric ptosis and/or diplopia (21). Both of these become worse with fatigue. The extraocular weakness may vary on multiple testing and alerts the examiner to the possibility of this condition. Injection of neostigmine or edrophonium chloride can make the ptosis less noticeable and is used as a confirmatory test for ocular myasthenia gravis. Serum antibodies may also be measured (Fig. 17A, B).

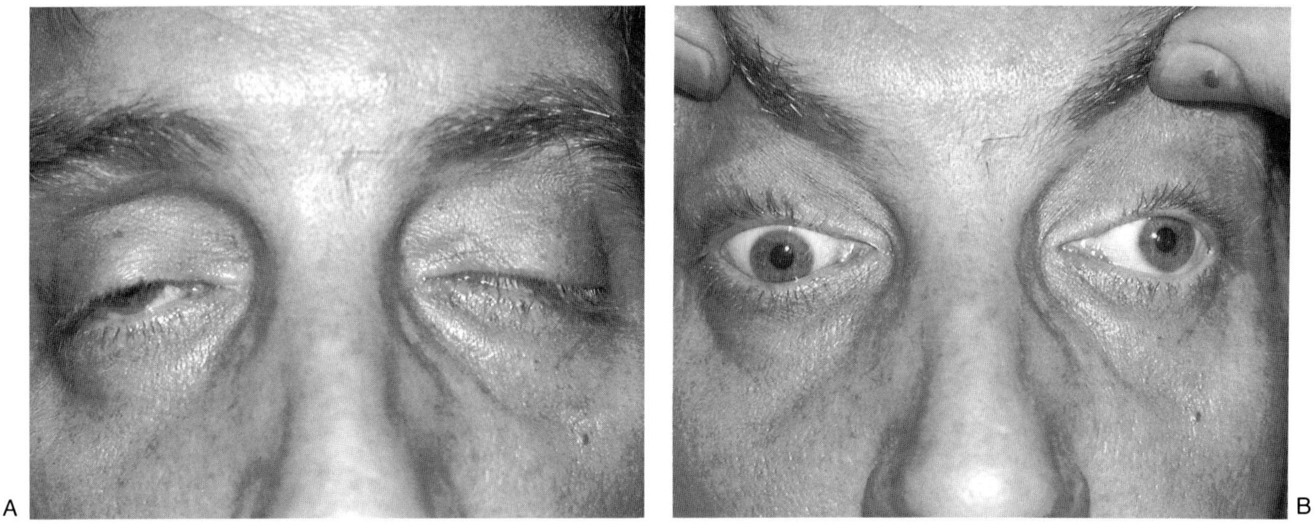

FIG. 16. **A:** Patient with chronic progressive external ophthalmoplegia (CPEO) at an advanced stage. **B:** Same patient with lids elevated. Patient has extremely poor levator function and very poor ocular motility.

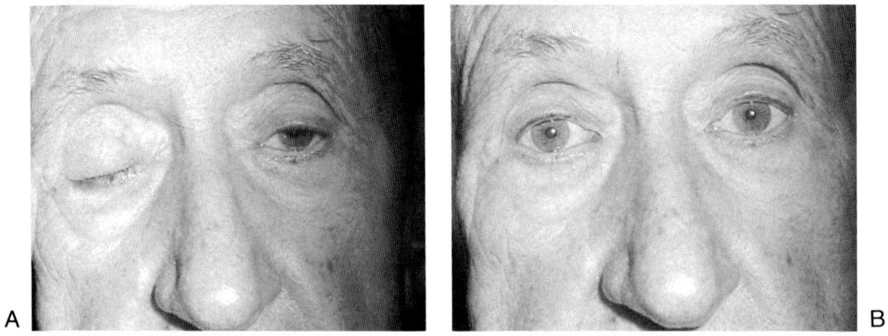

FIG. 17. **A:** Patient with myasthenia gravis who was referred unknowingly for ptosis repair. Patient had also a history of difficulty swallowing. **B:** Same patient following 10 mg iv of edrophonium chloride (Tensilon) with complete resolution of ptosis and weakness.

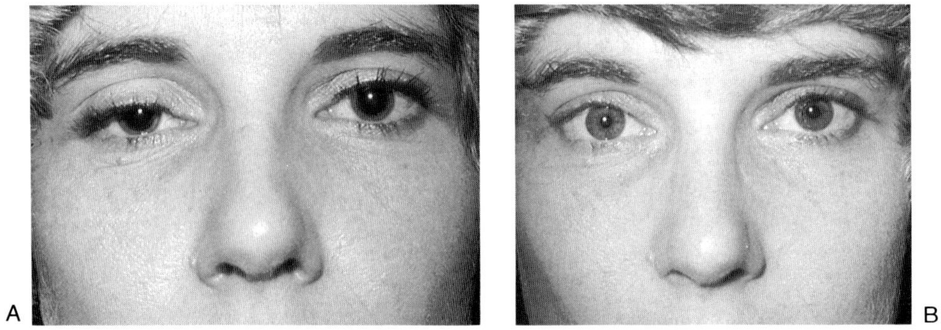

FIG. 18. **A:** Patient who had cervical sympathectomy with Horner's syndrome on the right side. Pupils had been dilated for ophthalmic exam. **B:** Patient with Horner's syndrome following aponeurotic surgery for correction showing the myotic pupil on the right.

Horner's Syndrome

Ptosis associated with miosis and failure of the pupil to dilate in dark should suggest the possibility of Horner's syndrome from sympathetic denervation. The diagnosis of sympathetic denervation sensitivity can be confirmed with pharmacologic testing with 10% cocaine, 1% hydroxyamphetamine drops, or pupillography. If the cause of denervation is apparent, such as that occurring postsurgically or posttrauma, no neurologic workup is needed (22–24). Horner's can be the presenting sign of an occult neoplasm or vascular disease, and thorough workup is needed in some patients presenting with the syndrome (Fig. 18A, B).

EVALUATION OF THE PTOSIS PATIENT

Determination of Cause

The differentiation of the patients with acquired and congenital ptosis has great practical significance because the two respond to surgery differently. Furthermore, additional diagnostic testing may be indicated in acquired cases. If the patient cannot be determined to have had a congenital onset of ptosis, then one should determine other possible etiologies. The surgeon should specifically ask for a history of trauma, medications, severe eyelid swelling, bee stings, or a family history of ptosis. Neurologic symptomatology, such as double vision or difficulty in swallowing, should be evaluated. Old photographs may sometimes reveal an unrecognized ptosis at an earlier age. In the absence of any history or old photographs, the dynamic behavior of the lid may give a clue as to the etiology. If the lid is indeed "stiff" with lagophthalmos on downgaze in the ptotic eye, a congenital etiology is very likely. Levator muscles that have been scarred by trauma, inflammation, or previous surgery may also be stiff and lagophthalmos in downgaze may be present in these patients.

Levator Function

Determination of the strength of function (range of motion) of the levator muscle is essential information that one must have to determine which surgical procedure will best correct the ptosis. Levator function (the excursion of the lid from downgaze to upgaze) is measured in millimeters. The measurement of the excursion spans the distance from extreme downgaze to ex-

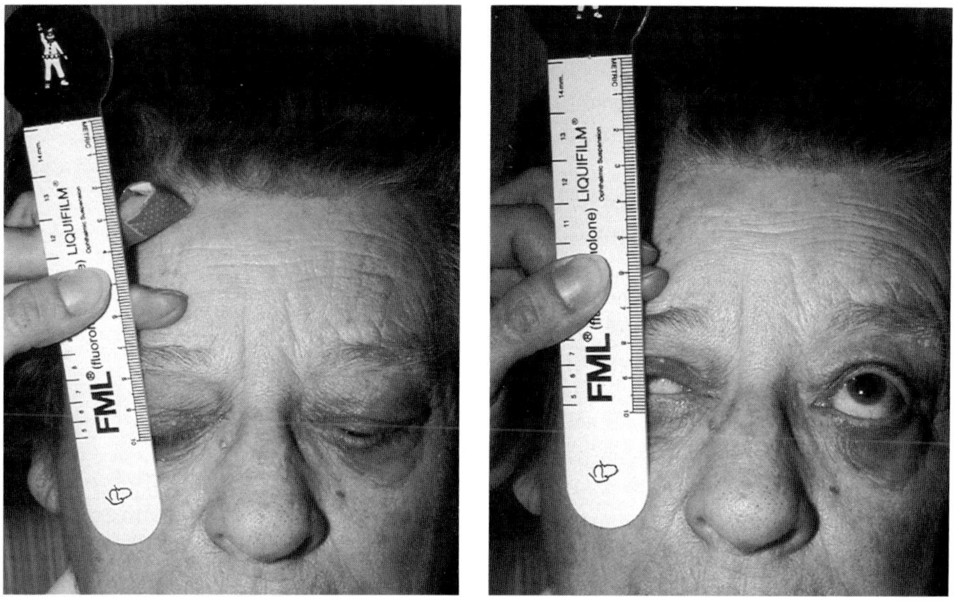

A B

FIG. 19. Measurement of levator function. **A:** The patient has the eyebrow splinted and has eyes turned in extreme downgaze with zeroing of the scale at the edge of the lid. **B:** The patient is asked to look upward measuring the excursion of the lid from down- to upgaze.

treme upgaze with the eyebrow firmly splinted by the examiner's thumb to eliminate any contribution by the brow-to-lid elevation. A millimeter rule may be placed vertically in front of the eyelid to accomplish the measurement (Fig. 19A, B). In most cases, levator function can be determined more precisely if one measures on multiple times. The assignment of the terminology "good," "fair," or "poor" to levator function is somewhat arbitrary; however, in general, if the excursion of the lid is less than 5 mm, the function is poor; 5–10 mm, fair; and 10 mm or more, good.

Eye Protective Mechanisms

In almost all cases, ptosis procedures produce some postoperative stiffness and lagophthalmos of the upper lid and in many cases some gapping of the eyelids at night. If the eye retains its moisture and has an adequate tear film with good protective eye movements, the patient will tolerate this postoperative lagophthalmos well. If the patient has an impairment of eye protective mechanisms (Table 3), exposure problems and visually threatening situations may develop. Each patient should be examined preoperatively with basic secretion tear test and evaluation of motility including an assessment of Bell's phenomenon. Additional deficiencies, such as decreased corneal sensation or facial nerve weakness, may introduce problems of unacceptable postoperative exposure. All of these protective mechanisms must be present to be sure of a safe postoperative course. With the loss of one or more eye protective mechanisms, one should reconsider the use of any surgical procedure. The patient should be informed that special lubrication may be necessary and that in some situations it may be necessary to reverse the ptosis procedure if the cornea does not tolerate the raising of the eyelid.

Extent of Ptosis

The position of the upper lid margin is relative in all people, with a range of "normal" position from just above the pupil to just below the upper limbus. In cases of unilateral ptosis, the amount of ptosis present would relate to its position compared to the opposite "normal eyelid." In bilateral cases, one must come to an agreement with the patient as to where to position the lid for ptosis surgery. It is not uncommon for severe ptosis on one side to mask a lesser degree of ptosis on the other side.

TABLE 3. *Conditions with poor eye protective mechanisms*

Neuroparalytic keratitis
Third nerve palsy
Chronic progressive external ophthalmoplegia
Myasthenia gravis
Orbital fibrosis syndromes
Seventh nerve paresis
Severe keratoconjunctivitis sicca
Double elevator palsy
Syndromes with deficient precorneal tear film

Abnormal Eyelid Movement

Anamolous innervation of the eyelid causing abnormal retraction of the eyelid can coexist with eyelid ptosis with the congenital Marcus–Gunn "jaw winking" phenomenon. Usual synkinetic movement with the jaw muscles (external pterygoids) causes the eyelid to retract when the lower jaw moves to the opposite side and to become ptotic when the jaw is moved to the same side. When the child chews, the eyelid flutters. Synkinetic retraction can also occur in acquired post-trauma cases following aberrant regeneration of third nerve palsies. If the synkinetic movement is mild, one may simply ignore it and perform the indicated ptosis procedure. To rid the eyelid of the more severe synkinetic movement and correct the ptosis may require levator muscle excision followed by frontalis suspensions (25,26).

Abnormal closure of the eyelid may occur with regeneration of the seventh nerve following palsy or paresis. This is seen as eyelid closure when the patient smiles or contracts his or her lower facial muscles, and it can be misinterpreted as ptosis. Benign essential blepharospasm or hemifacial spasm will also cause abnormal eyelid closure.

Lid Contour and Lid Crease

It is important to have a symmetric contour of the edge and lash line of the eyelid and of the position of the upper lid crease between the two upper lids. With unilateral cases, the opposite or "normal" side is the reference point. This judgment is best determined in the preoperative exam documented with photographs. The lid crease position is very important in that even if the surgeon doesn't produce a perfect ptosis correction, improvement in the lid crease symmetry can result in considerable patient satisfaction. Conversely, the surgeon may have an excellent correction of ptosis and elevation of the lid but a poor or asymmetric lid crease, which can result in a dissatisfied patient. The upper lid crease is formed by extensions of the levator to the skin. There are a wide variety of lid crease positions, from the extremely high lid crease in the patient with levator dehiscence to possible absence of a visible lid crease in the Asian patient.

Ocular Examination

It is important preoperatively to perform a thorough eye examination in the ptosis patient to document any preexisting ocular or eyelid disease and to identify any potential problems that may occur. The measurement of the visual field in ptosis patients has now become standard in the documentation for insurance purposes to represent the ptosis as functional in nature. Most insurance companies require a visual field with the lid in the ptotic position and a visual field with the lid elevated.

TABLE 4. *Special problems encountered in candidates for ptosis surgery*

Poor eye protective mechanisms
Previous ptosis-eyelid surgery
Deficient tarsus
Paralytic/immobile brow
Eyelid hamartoma
Floppy upper lid syndrome
Tarsal shift with involutional ptosis
Coexistent ocular eyelid anomalies
Asymmetric ptosis
Chronic brow elevation
Blepharochalasis syndrome
Canthal dehiscence

Problem Patients

Special situations exist in the ptosis patient population that must be identified because their management poses special difficulties. As the surgeon gains experience with larger numbers of patients, this identification process gets easier (Table 4).

As previously mentioned, patients with *poor eye protective mechanisms* should be identified before surgery and warned of the possibility of corneal exposure. These are the most important problem patients to identify because of the possibility of permanent visual loss (Fig. 20).

Many patients encountered will have an unstable upper lid because of a *deficient tarsal plate*. There is a problem in correction of ptosis in these patients because the purchase of the ptosis procedure on the eyelid will be uneven and in most cases cause rotation of the lid. This situation occurs following surgery in which the tarsus has been removed (e.g., Fasanella proce-

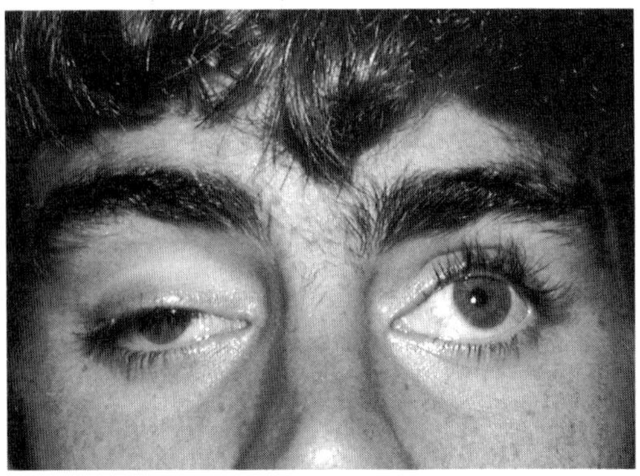

FIG. 20. Patient with poor eye protective mechanisms of reduced ocular motility from congenital orbital fibrosis syndrome.

dure), in cases of congenital anophthalmos, or in the blepharophimosis syndrome, in which patients have a hypoplastic tarsal plate. Adjunctive reconstructive procedures may be necessary. Patients who have had *previous ptosis surgery* in some cases can pose severe problems because of a deficient tarsus and ill-defined tissue planes due to fibrosis and adhesions. These patients may require a classical Berke levator dissection to be able to dissect out the levator properly.

An *akinetic or paralytic eyebrow,* or an eyebrow that has been immobilized from scar tissue, causes difficulty in achieving full correction with the frontalis suspension procedure.

Hamartomatous tissue such as neurofibromas or lymphangiomas creates great difficulty in ptosis correction, with recurrence of the ptosis as the tissue progressively grows over the years. It may be expeditious to resect the hamartomatous portion of the lid and reconstruct it before ptosis surgery is undertaken.

Older patients may have a loose and *floppy upper lid syndrome* that presents difficulties in the correction for contour because of the instability of the lid (27). This is usually more of a problem when using the frontalis suspension procedure. A horizontal tightening procedure to stabilize the upper lid should be performed prior to the specific ptosis surgical procedure.

In many patients with involutional ptosis, dehiscence of the medial horn of the levator causes outward migration and a *lateral shift of the tarsal plate*. The peak of the tarsal plate, which is normally centered above the pupil, may be shifted temporally. If one performs surgery on the levator so that the maximum pull is at the tarsal peak, then one will get consistent temporal overcorrections and "flare." This problem must be identified and the sutures must be moved nasally to acquire proper contour.

The *blepharophimosis syndrome* has additional anomalies that must be corrected to produce a satisfactory result.

Asymmetric ptosis, in which a more severely ptotic lid can mask a lesser ptosis in the older eye, is common. Preoperatively, voluntary effort on the patient's part will cause a normalization of the less ptotic lid, leaving only the more ptotic lid to appear to require correction. Postoperatively, if correction is performed only on the more ptotic lid, the voluntary effort will cease and the ptosis will appear on the nonoperated side. It is important to recognize this asymmetry and compensatory effort preoperatively by alternately covering and uncovering the eyes. Bilateral surgery is often required to correct this situation.

Patients with longstanding ptosis may continue to have *chronic brow elevation* despite a successful correction of the ptosis. This is probably from habit; however, it will produce a persistent asymmetric appearance with a higher lid crease.

The *blepharochalasis syndrome* is a rare condition occurring in young people with recurrent idiopathic edema of the eyelids. The recurrent severe swelling results in stretching of the skin, levator aponeurosis, and the lateral canthal tendon, and occasionally in atrophy of the nasal fat pad (Fig. 21) (28). These patients are surgically correctable but usually require staged procedures including blepharoplasty, dermal fat grafting, and plication of the canthal tendon. The acquired dehiscence syndrome also has some of the above changes without the history of episodes of edema (Fig. 22). *Anomalous eyelid movement* from symkinetic retraction in the Marcus–Gunn syndrome or abnormal closure in the spasm syndromes may present problems in diagnosis and treatment.

CHOICE OF SURGICAL PROCEDURE

The single factor that determines the proper ptosis procedure to utilize is the amount of levator function

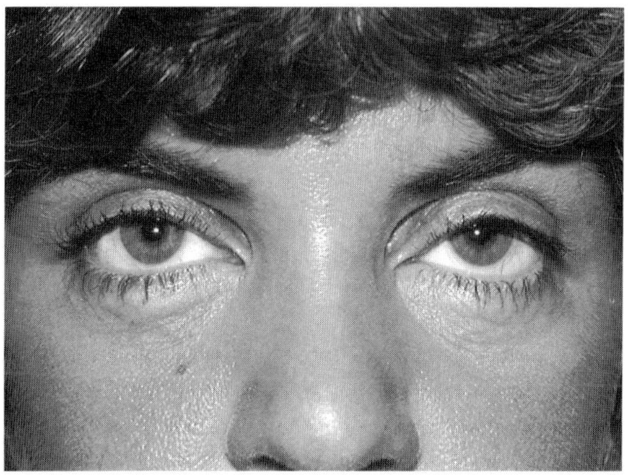

FIG. 21. Young female with the tissue changes resulting from the blepharochalasis syndrome. The young woman had repeated bouts of inflammatory edema during childhood resulting in loss of elastic tissue dehiscence of the levator, loss of the nasal fat pad, lateral canthal dehiscence, and crepe skin changes.

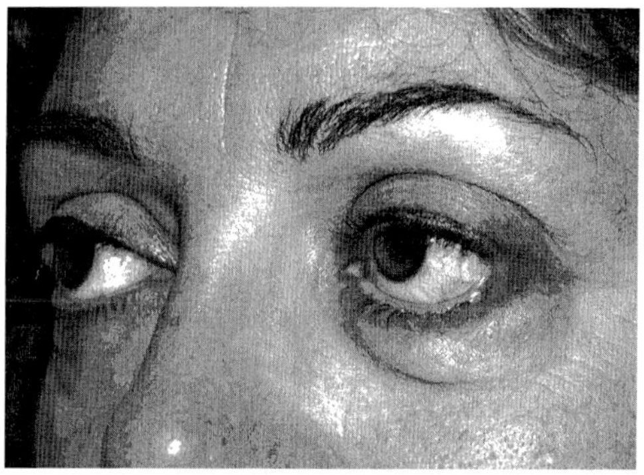

FIG. 22. Patient with idiopathic canthal dehiscence syndrome. Patient was referred because of "skin growing between upper and lower lid." Patient also has levator dehiscence in addition to canthal dehiscence.

TABLE 5. *Choice of ptosis procedure with regard to levator function*

Levator function	Procedure
0–5 mm (poor)	Frontalis suspension
6–10 mm (moderate)	Levator resection (extensive dissection)
10+ mm (excellent)	Aponeurotic surgery

present. In patients with very poor levator function, a suspension-type procedure must be used. In those patients who have better levator function, the levator itself can be surgically shortened to elevate the lid (Table 5). One modifying factor that must be considered in selecting a ptosis procedure is the adequacy of eye protective mechanisms. The surgeon may choose to use a more "reversible" procedure in the presence of poor eye protective mechanisms if the eye cannot tolerate the surgery.

The three basic procedures for ptosis repair are *frontalis suspension,* used in those patients with poor levator function; *resection of the levator with extensive dissection* (as popularized by Berke), used in those patients with fair levator function; and *aponeurotic surgery* surgery on the distal portion of the levator (aponeurosis), used in those patients with good to normal levator function. The ptosis surgeon can fare well with almost all patients utilizing only these procedures. Other procedures have been described that have been used successfully.

Other procedures that have been used are Putterman's müllerectomy (29) and the Fasanella tarsomüllerectomy (30). Although not used by the author, the Putterman procedure is well accepted as safe and predictable in certain patients.

The Fasanella–Servat procedure is still used by some experienced surgeons; however, it does involve excision of a portion of the tarsal plate. It is considered somewhat nonanatomic in nature; corneal complications may occur with this procedure and any needed reoperations are rendered much more difficult. It has been largely replaced by the newer, more anatomic, aponeurotic approach to ptosis surgery in patients with good to excellent levator function.

The Fasanella procedure, although workable in some patients, is nonanatomic and can produce problems and unwanted results because of the excision part of the tarsal plate.

REFERENCES

1. Beard C. The surgical treatment of blepharoptosis: a quantitative approach. *Trans Am Ophthalmol Soc* 1966;64:401–487.
2. McCord CD. The evaluation and management of the patient with ptosis. In: Jelks GW, ed. *Clinics in plastic surgery.* Philadelphia: WB Saunders; 1988.
3. McCord CD Jr, Tanenbaum M, eds. *Oculoplastic surgery.* 2nd ed. New York: Raven Press; 1987.
4. Jones LT, Quickert MH, Wobig JL. The cure of ptosis by aponeurotic repair. *Arch Ophthalmol* 1975;93:629–634.
5. Shore JW, Bergin DJ, Garrett SW. Results of blepharoptosis surgery with early postoperative adjustment. *Ophthalmology* 1990;97:1502–1511.
6. Berke RN, Wadsworth JAC. Histology of the levator muscle in congenital and acquired ptosis. *Arch Ophthalmol* 1955;53: 413–428.
7. Anderson RL, Gordy DD. Aponeurotic defects in congenital ptosis. *Ophthalmology* 1979;86:1493–1499.
8. Merriam WW, Ellis FD, Helveston EH. Congenital blepharoptosis, anisometropia, and amblyopia. *Am J Ophthalmol* 1980;89:401–407.
9. Anderson RA, et al. Strabismus in ptosis. *Arch Ophthalmol* 1980;98:1062–1067.
10. Anderson RL, et al. Amblyopia in ptosis. *Arch Ophthalmol* 1980;98:1068–1069.
11. Cadera W, et al. Changes in astigmatism after surgery for congenital ptosis. *J Pediatr Ophthalmol Strabismus* 1992;29:85–88.
12. Hoyt CS, Stone RD, Fromer C, Billson FA. Monocular axial myopia associated with neonatal eyelid closure in human infants. *Am J Ophthalmol* 1981;91:197–200.
13. Smith B, McCord CD, Baylis HL. Surgical treatment of blepharoptosis. *Am J Ophthalmol* 1969;68:92–99.
14. Kohn R, Romano PE. Blepharoptosis, blepharophimosis, epicanthus inversus, and telecanthus—a syndrome with no name. *Am J Ophthalmol* 1971;72:625.
15. Shore JW, McCord CD. Anatomic changes in involutional blepharoptosis. *Am J Ophthalmol* 1984;98:211–227.
16. Walsh FB, Hoyt WF. Progressive muscular dystrophy principally affecting extraocular muscles: chronic progressive external ophthalmoplegia. In: Walsh FB, Hoyt WF, eds. *Clinical neuro-ophthalmology.* 3rd ed. Baltimore: Williams and Wilkins; 1969.
17. Moses L, Heller GL. Ocular myopathy. *Am J Ophthalmol* 1965; 59:1051–1057.
18. Drachman DA. Ophthalmoplegia plus: the neurodegenerative disorders associated with progressive external ophthalmoplegia. *Arch Neurol* 1968;18:654–674.
19. Keams TP. External ophthalmoplegia, pigmentary degeneration of the retina and cardiomyopathy: a newly recognized syndrome. *Trans Am Ophthalmol Soc* 1965;63:559–625.
20. Burian HM, Burns CA. Ocular changes in myotonic dystrophy. *Am J Ophthalmol* 1967;63:22–34.
21. Cogan DG. Myasthenia gravis: a review of the disease and a description of lid twitch as a characteristic sign. *Arch Ophthalmol* 1965;74:217–221.
22. Kardon RH, Denison CE, Brown MS, Thompson ST. Critical evaluation of the cocaine test in the diagnosis of Horner's syndrome. *Arch Ophthalmol* 1990;108:384–387.
23. Weinstein TN, Zweifel TJ, Thompson ST. Congenital Horner's syndrome. *Arch Ophthalmol* 1980;98:1074–1078.
24. Maloney WF, Younge BR, Moyer NJ. Evaluation of the causes and accuracy of pharmacologic localization in Horner's syndrome. *Am J Ophthalmol* 1980;90:394–402.
25. Beard C. *Ptosis.* 2nd ed. St Louis: CV Mosby; 1976.
26. Dillman DR, Anderson RL. Levator myectomy in synkinetic ptosis. *Arch Ophthalmol* 1984;102:422–423.
27. Goldberg R, Seiff S, McFarland J, Simons K, Shorr N. Floppy eyelid syndrome and blepharochalasis. *Am J Ophthalmol* 1986; 102:376–391.
28. Bergin DJ, McCord CD, Berger T, Friedberg H. Blepharochalasis. *Br J Ophthalmol* 1988;72:863–867.
29. Putterman AM, Urist MJ. Mueller's muscle–conjunctival resection. *Arch Ophthalmol* 1975;93:619–623.
30. Fasanella RM, Servat J. Levator resection for minimal ptosis, another simplified procedure. *Arch Ophthalmol* 1961;65: 493–496.

CHAPTER 8

Levator Surgery

This chapter discusses standard aponeurotic surgery, levator resection, and levator excision for synkinetic movement. Certain other procedures that have been used successfully by other authors but are not routinely used by the present author will not be included. Such procedures include "supramaximal" levator resection, Whitnall's sling, and the Fasanella procedure (1–3).

APONEUROTIC SURGERY

Patients undergoing aponeurotic surgery have, by selection, excellent levator function and commonly are involutional patients with an aponeurotic defect or dehiscence. Aponeurotic defects can also occur congenitally and in younger patients who have had repeated lid edema or trauma. They can also result from chronic hard contact lens wear as well as from cataract or ocular surgery. Aponeurotic surgery can be used in patients with normal aponeurosis but who need ptosis surgery if they have mild ptosis and good levator function (i.e., Horner's syndrome) (4–7).

SURGICAL TECHNIQUE

Anesthesia

Ideally quantitation aponeurotic repair is performed intraoperatively by having the patient voluntarily open his or her eyelids and having the surgeon adjust until the eyelids have reached the desired levels. This requires that there be no paresis of the levator from the local anesthetic. This type of anesthesia is achieved with a frontal nerve block for the lid and infiltration of the eyelid crease area (0.50–0.75 cm^3 of short-acting infiltrative anesthetic placed along the site of the intended lid crease, just beneath the skin with a minimal amount in the nasal lid). In most cases anesthesia is achieved without loss of levator function.

Technique

A lid crease incision is made at the desired level, usually at the upper border of the tarsal plate (approx. 9–10 mm above the lash line). A strip of skin and muscle above the crease may be removed (Fig. 1). Separation of the orbicularis fibers will expose the orbital septum and a portion of the levator aponeurosis beneath the orbicularis fibers. In some cases, the levator aponeurosis may be relatively intact; however, usually it is rarefied and stretched with Müller's muscle and the superior vascular arcade visible through the tissue at the superior edge of the tarsus. The skin-muscle edge at the superior portion of the wound is retracted, and the orbital septum is incised horizontally, exposing the preaponeurotic fat, which is retracted. The aponeurosis is marked at the superior tarsal border (Fig. 2) and incised just inside the superior edge of the tarsal plate (Fig. 3). With aponeurotic surgery, it is not necessary to disturb Müller's muscle or the superior vascular arcade, thus reducing the amount of bleeding during the procedure (Figs. 4 and 5).

After the levator has been dissected free from Müller's muscle and exposed by retraction of the preaponeurotic fat, a 6-0 caliber suture, with a small cutting needle, is introduced half-thickness near the upper

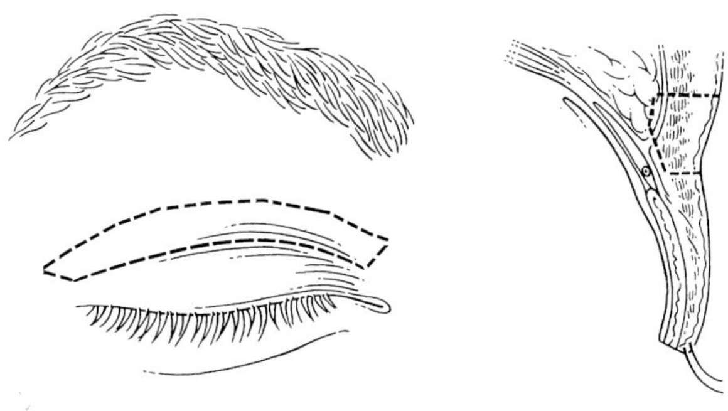

FIG. 1. Aponeurotic surgery. Skin marking and tissue excision outlined.

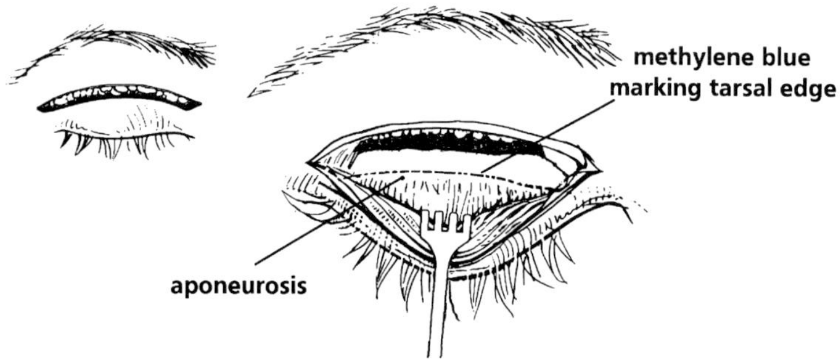

FIG. 2. Aponeurotic surgery. The levator aponeurosis is marked at the superior tarsal border with methylene blue.

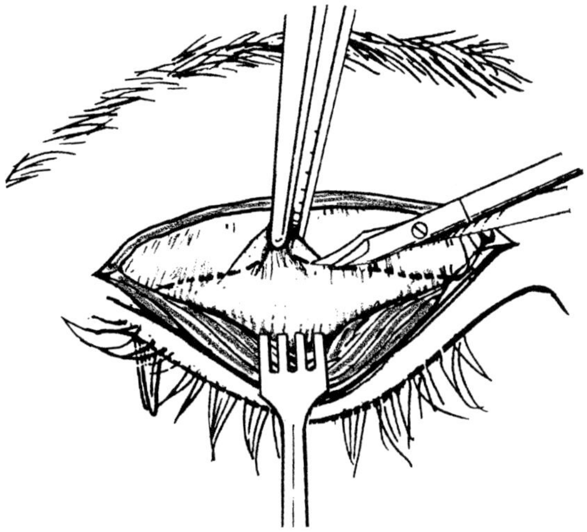

FIG. 3. Aponeurotic surgery. The aponeurosis is tinted up just over the superior tarsus, a buttonhole incision is made, and incision across the marked line is completed.

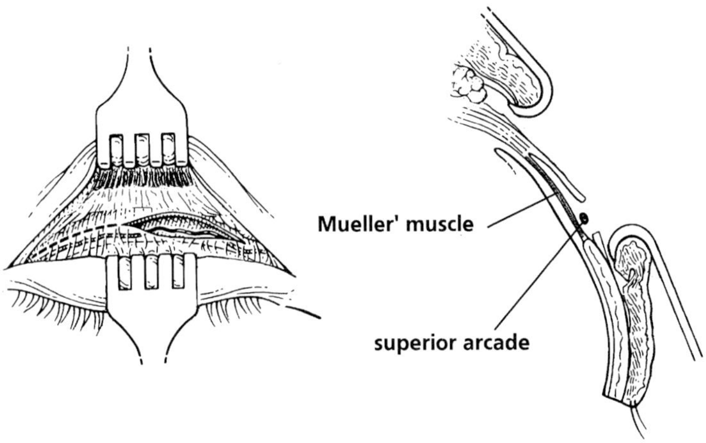

FIG. 4. Aponeurotic surgery. Frontal and sagittal view of the incision in the aponeurosis.

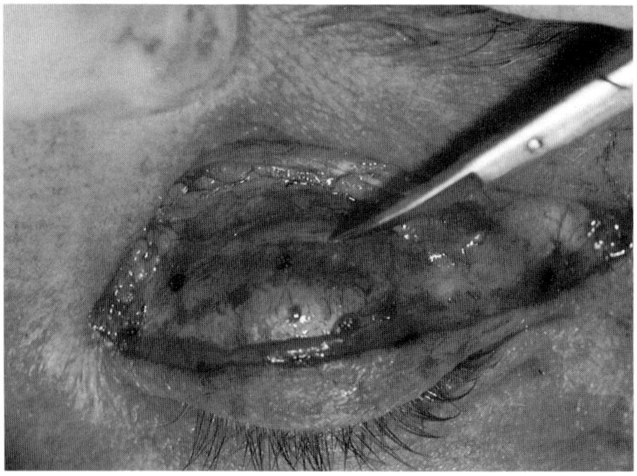

FIG. 5. Aponeurotic surgery. Surgical view showing scissors pointing to separated end of levator aponeurosis; Müller's muscle is underneath.

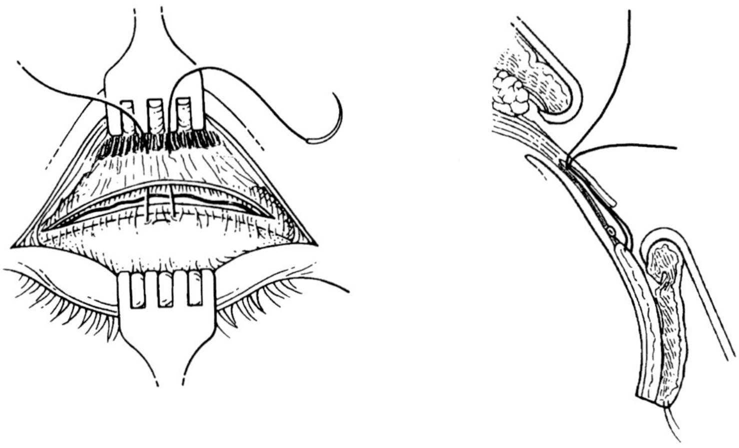

FIG. 6. Aponeurotic surgery. A suture is placed in the superior edge of the tarsal plate in line with the pupil and into the levator at its musculoaponeurotic junction.

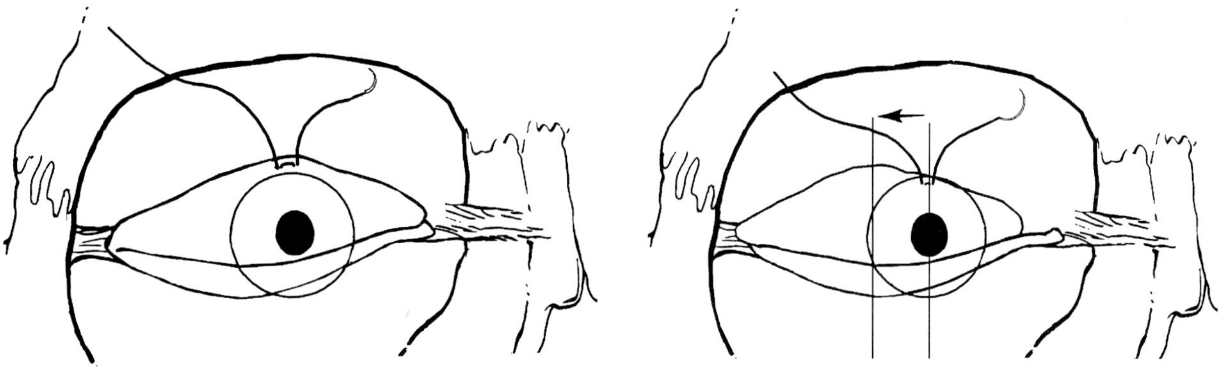

A B

FIG. 7. Aponeurotic surgery. **A:** Positioning of suture at superior tarsal edge in line with the pupil. The patient has no lateral displacement of the tarsus. **B:** Patient with lateral displacement of the tarsus as seen in involutional ptosis and the needed position of the suture in the superior tarsal edge to stay in line with the pupil.

edge of the tarsal plate (Fig. 6). This suture is the central lifting suture and should be placed in the exact vertical line with the pupil. This aspect is important when dealing with involutional patients who have a lateral displacement of the tarsal plate (Fig. 7A, B). A double-armed suture is used, which then can be brought through the levator aponeurosis (Figs. 6 and 8). Insertion of the central lifting suture is made into the levator at the junction of the aponeurosis and the muscular part of the levator (Fig. 6). The central suture is the lifting suture, the "motor" for lifting the lid. The nasal and temporal sutures, if placed, serve more for contour adjustment.

The method of choice to quantitate the ptosis correction is the adjustment of the eyelid height under local anesthesia retaining levator function with the patient cooperating by opening the lid, i.e., *voluntary opening*. After the insertion of the central lifting suture and a temporary tying, the patient is asked to open and close his or her eyes or fixate on a cotton applicator stick in the primary position (Fig. 9) (8). It has not been necessary in the authors' experience to have the patient sit up on the operative table to do this. The central lifting suture is then further tightened or loosened until the lid is 1 mm higher than the desired final result. The additional elevation is needed to compensate for the weakening of closure muscles (orbicularis) by the anesthetic. Additional sutures are then inserted to adjust

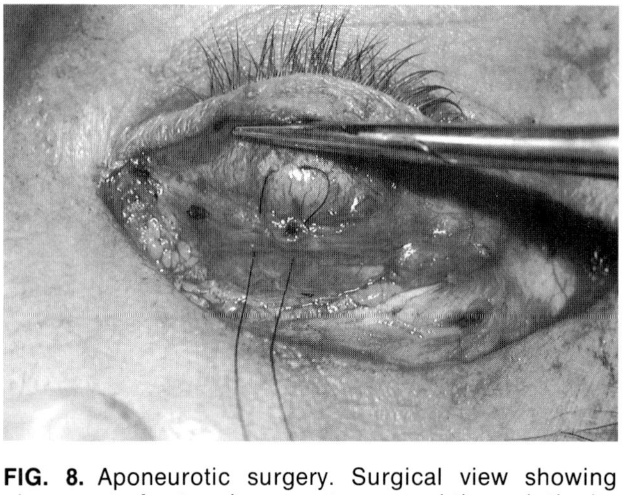

FIG. 8. Aponeurotic surgery. Surgical view showing placement of suture in upper tarsus and through the levator.

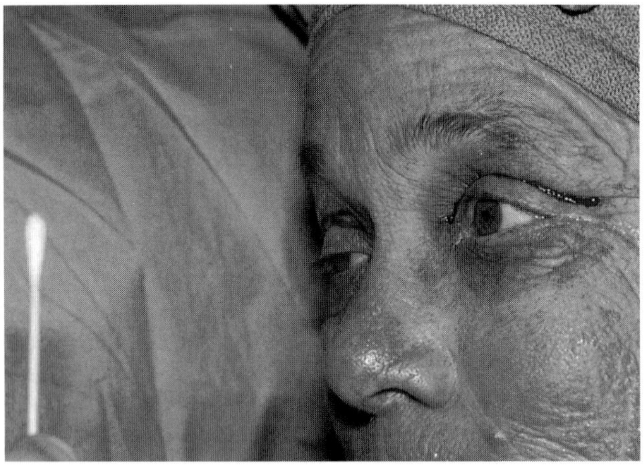

FIG. 9. Intraoperative adjustment of levator with voluntary opening by the patient. The left eye has been adjusted to the desired position slightly higher than the final result.

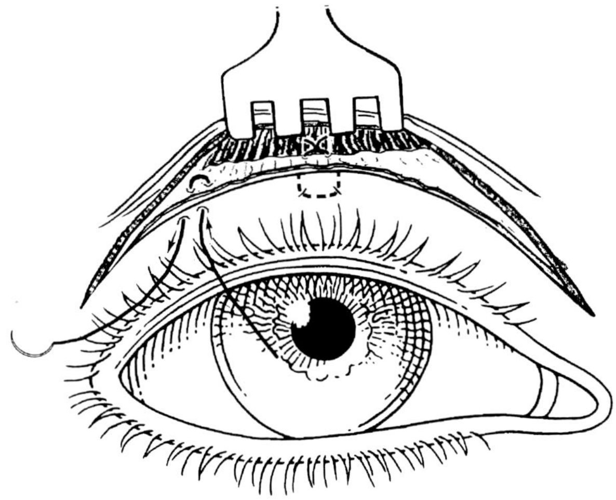

FIG. 10. Central lifting suture has been tightened and a transcutaneous suture has been inserted laterally through the pretarsal skin into the levator aponeurosis.

the contour (Fig. 10). It is important to have cooperation from the patient; therefore heavy intravenous sedation should not be used. The levator should not be akinetic and should be tested by the surgeon 10 min after the initial blocks are given to determine if the levator has been affected due to akinesia of the orbicularis muscle. Poor cooperation of the patient or oversedation can markedly affect this method.

Another pitfall in this method is lid retraction from stimulation of Müller's muscle if epinephrine is used in the anesthetic. This increased elevation of the lid is not consistent and is apparent soon after local takes effect. The amount of elevation caused by this can be taken into consideration with the voluntary opening method of quantitation. Anesthesia without epinephrine can be used but increased bleeding will occur.

If the levator function is affected by the anesthetic it is generally best to convert to another method of quantitation.

Gapping Method

The gapping method has a good degree of predictability. It correlates the gapping of the upper and lower eyelids during surgery with the postoperative position of the eyelids. Figure 11 shows calipers being used to measure the gapping of the eyelid. In general, in patients with acquired ptosis, the eyelids are gapped on the operating table 1 mm more than the amount of ptosis one wishes to correct. In congenital cases, the amount of gapping is 3 mm more than the amount of ptosis one wishes to correct because the amount of permanent lift one gains in congenital ptosis is less. A patient with acquired ptosis of 3 mm will be gapped 4 mm on the operating room table, and a patient with congenital ptosis of 3 mm will be gapped 6 mm on the operating table. It must be emphasized that there are many variables involved in setting the eyelid level. All formulas are simply starting points; each ptosis surgeon must adapt these formulas to his or her own specific techniques. Other variables that exist are variations in location of suture placement on the tarsus, the amount of dissection employed, and the tension in the tying knot.

After the desired gapping has been obtained with the central lifting suture, additional nasal and temporal

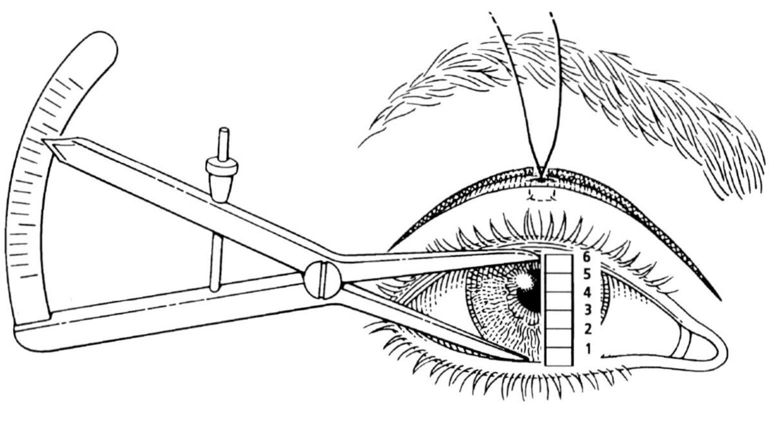

FIG. 11. Aponeurotic surgery. Gapping method of correction when the levator is akinetic. For acquired ptosis the amount of gapping equals the amount of ptosis plus 1 mm. For congenital ptosis gapping equals ptosis plus 3 mm.

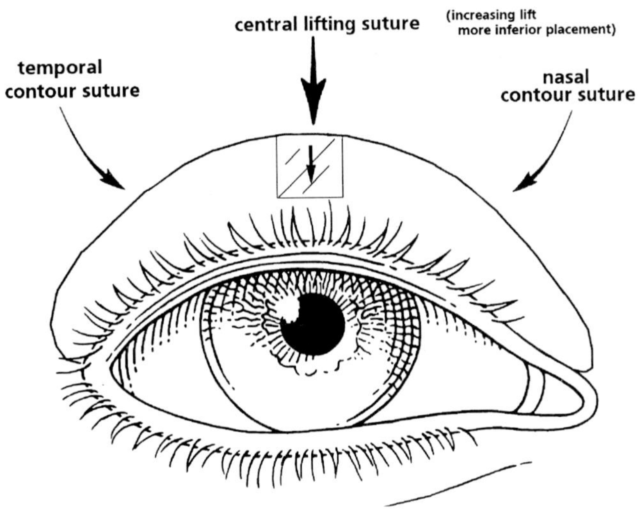

FIG. 12. Diagram of aponeurotic surgery emphasizing the fact that the central suture in ptosis surgery is the lifting suture, in contrast to the nasal and temporal sutures which are used to adjust contour as needed.

sutures between the tarsal plate and the aponeurosis are placed to ensure proper contour. Two sutures are usually required to maintain proper lid contour when orbicularis tone returns. The central lifting suture and a lateral contour suture are the most commonly used. It is usually not necessary to use a nasal contour suture. It has been useful to recognize that the central suture is primarily responsible for the lifting of the eyelid whereas the other sutures are primarily for adjusting contour (see Fig. 12). It is important to place the central lifting suture near the superior edge of the tarsus. It is a more physiologic position when it is then introduced into the musculoaponeurotic junction and postoperative undercorrections are more easily corrected by further downward advancement if needed.

Skin closure sutures are then used to attach the skin-muscle edges of the levator or the superior tarsal border, depending on the desired position of the final crease (Fig. 13). Any unwanted lid contour arching or notching can usually be noted at this time and should be corrected. Contour asymmetry usually results from sutures tied too tightly or placed too far down on the anterior tarsal surface. Overcorrections and undercorrections may occur and adjustments can be made 7 or more days postoperatively by massage or by loosening of sutures or tightening of sutures before firm healing takes place (9–11). Figure 14A and B shows the patient

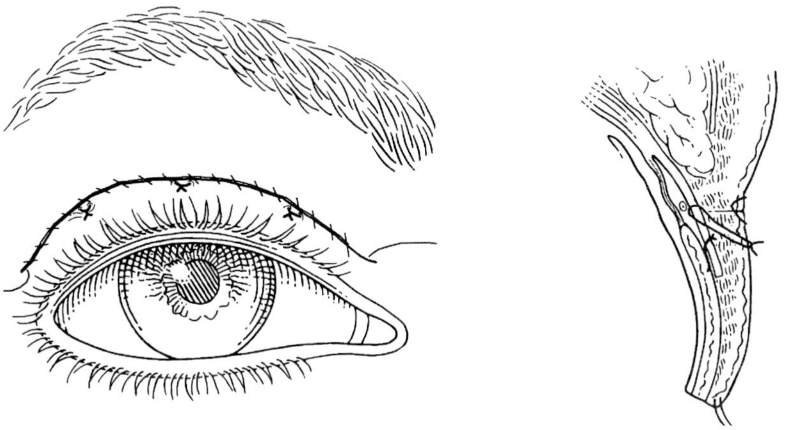

FIG. 13. Frontal and lateral views showing final suture placements of crease sutures plicating the pretarsal skin to the levator and skin closure.

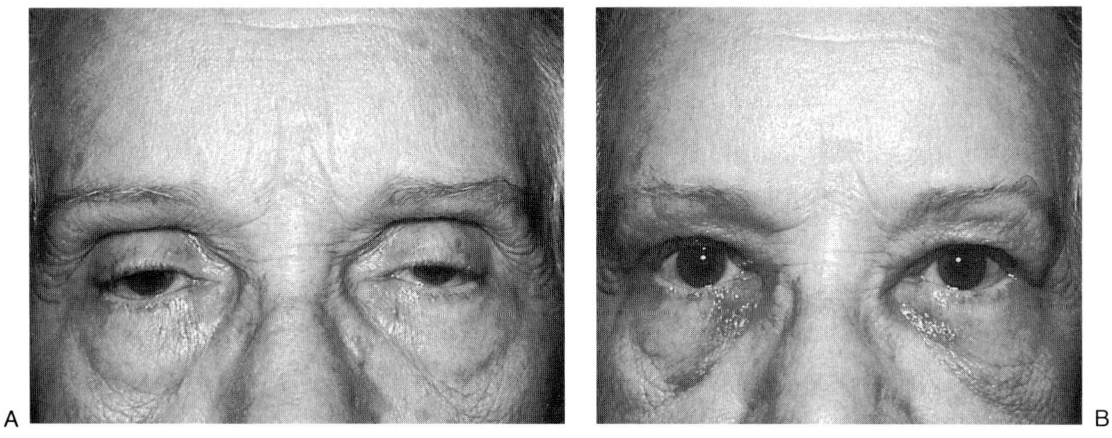

FIG. 14. A: Patient with involutional ptosis and levator aponeurotic defect prior to surgery. **B:** Patient 1 week postoperatively with skin suture removal. If there is any overcorrection or undercorrection, adjustments can be made at this time.

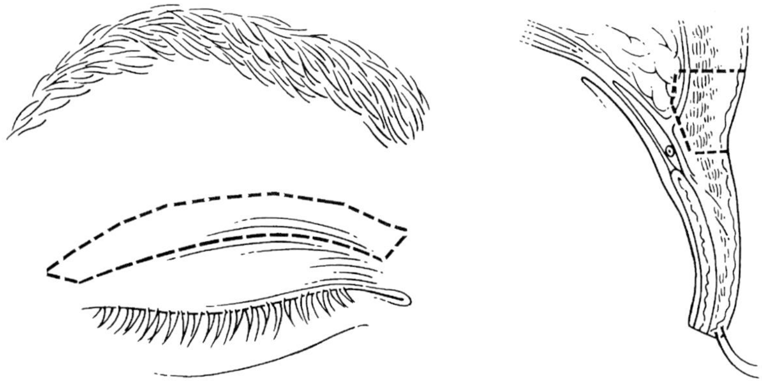

FIG. 15. Levator resection with dissection. Outline of skin incision and initial tissue removal.

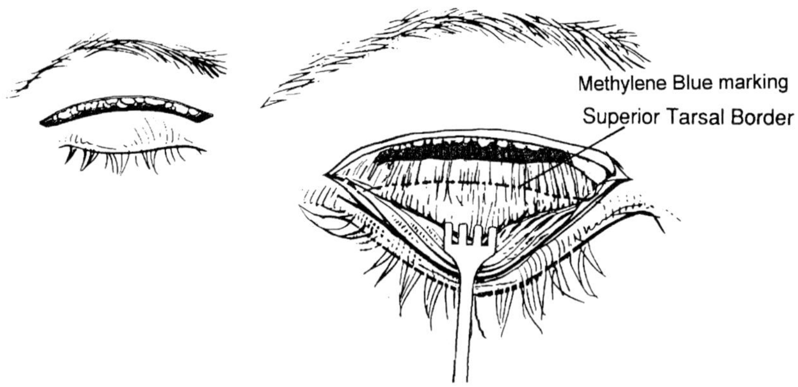

FIG. 16. Levator resection with dissection. Marking of levator aponeurosis at superior tarsal edge.

intraoperatively before surgery and a week postoperatively. No adjustments were necessary.

EXTERNAL LEVATOR RESECTION WITH EXTENSIVE DISSECTION

External levator resection with extensive dissection is the best surgical approach for the correction of ptosis in patients with fair (5–10 mm) levator function. The most common patients in this category are congenital ptosis patients. Certain categories of acquired ptosis such as posttraumatic ptosis may be found in this grouping.

Technique

A lid crease incision is made and dissection carried down to the superior border of the tarsal plate (Fig. 15). A strip of skin and orbicularis muscle is usually needed to produce symmetry with the opposite side. The excision of this tissue can be accompanied with the opening of the orbital septum, which should be in-

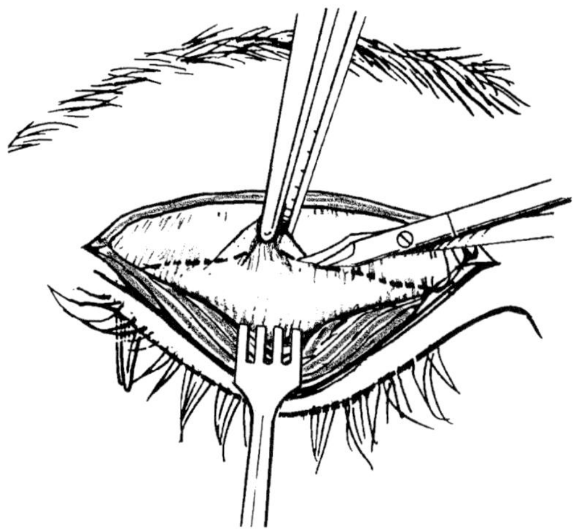

A

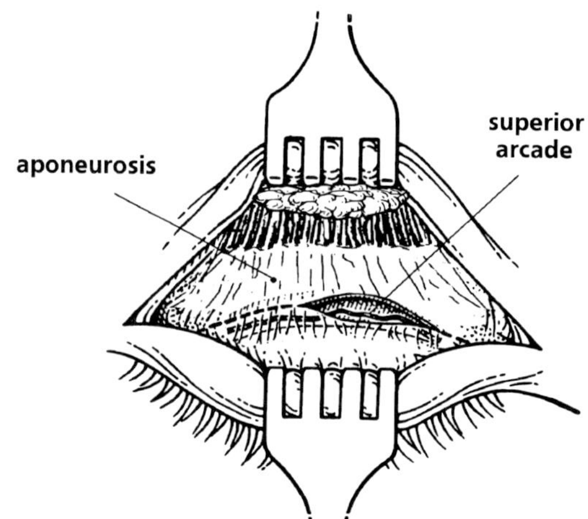

B

FIG. 17. Levator resection with dissection. **A:** Incision of levator aponeurosis at marking by tinting levator over tarsal plate. **B:** Placement of initial incision through levator.

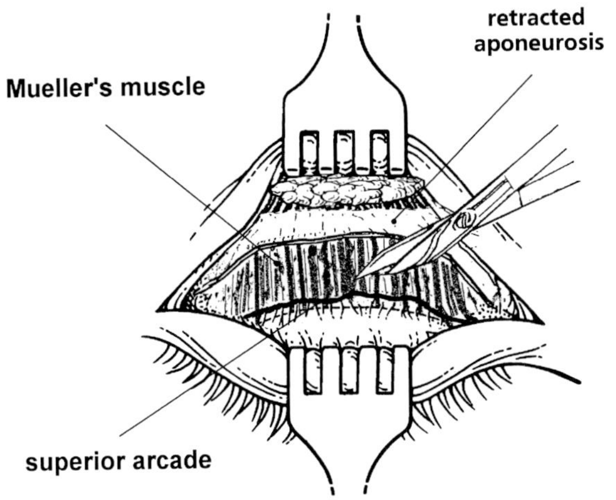

FIG. 18. Levator resection with dissection. Levator has been freed from tarsus and inferior incision and incision through Müller's muscle above the superior arcade is made superficial to the underlying conjunctiva.

cised and opened through its entire width for exposure of the levator and separation from the levator to the prevention of postoperative tethering of the lid and excessive lagophthalmos. Gentle pressure on the orbital contents against the lower lid will cause the preaponeurotic fat to bulge forward behind the orbital septum, ballooning it outward. The septum then can be incised. The most valuable anatomic guideline for the surgeon performing a levator resection is identification of the preaponeurotic fat because just beneath it is the levator muscle and aponeurosis.

Once the aponeurotic and muscular portion of the levator is exposed, the aponeurosis is marked with methylene blue at the level of the superior tarsal edge (Fig. 16). The aponeurosis is incised and dissected from Müller's muscle (Fig. 17A, B). Müller's muscle is then dissected from the underlying conjunctiva starting above the superior arcade to reduce bleeding (Fig. 18). The levator–Müller's complex is then dissected together from the conjunctiva superiorly into the upper fornix area. This dissection is facilitated by tensing the conjunctiva downward with a cotton applicator stick to avoid buttonholes and upward traction on the levator (Fig. 19A, B).

In most cases the check ligaments of the levator must be loosened to increase the elasticity and "stretchiness" of the levator. With traction on the levator with forceps or clamp, the lateral expansion (levator horns) is incised (Fig. 20A, B). In reality, the incision of the levator horns is more of a "nibbling" procedure. The medial check ligament takes the form of a ligamentous strand (interpad septum) that separates the nasal and

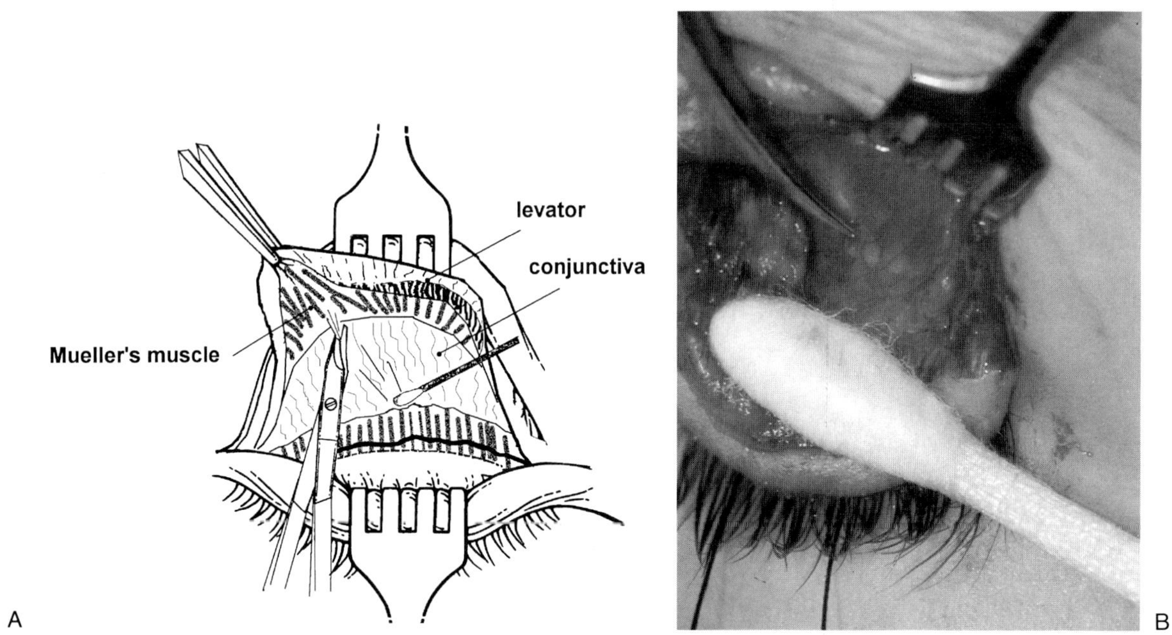

FIG. 19. Levator resection with dissection. **A:** Müller's muscle and the levator complex is tinted upward with dissection of Müller's from its detachment to the underlying conjunctiva. **B:** Surgical slides showing dissection of Müller's from conjunctiva. Accessory lacrimal glands are encountered and should be preserved. Scissors tip is pointing to accessory lacrimal gland.

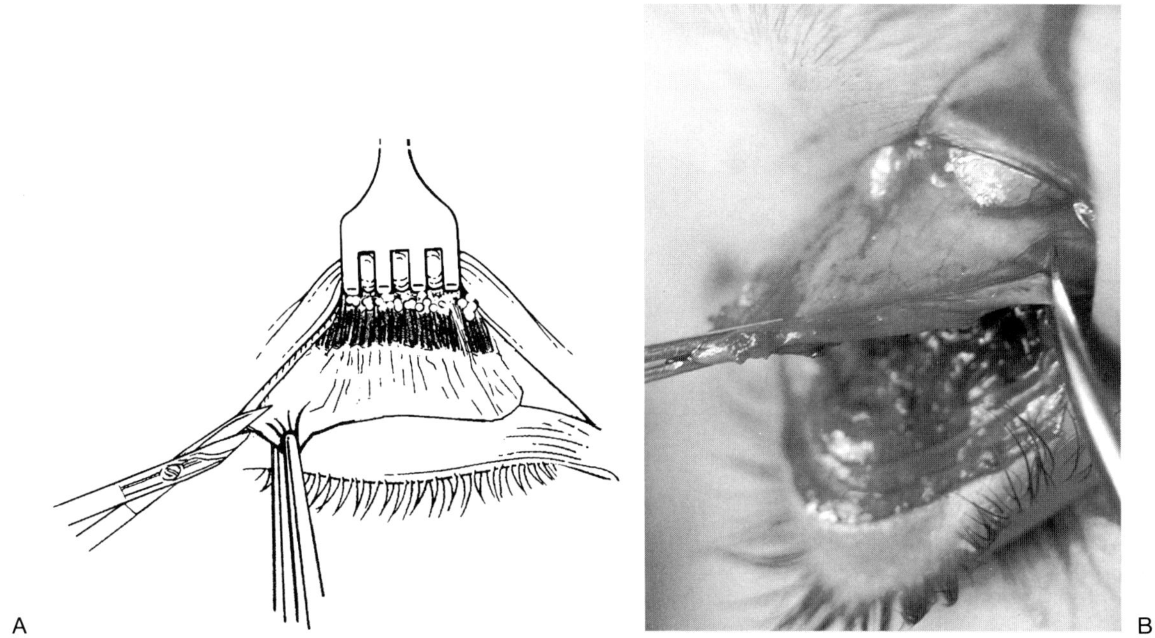

FIG. 20. Levator resection with dissection. **A:** The lateral horn is lysed as conservatively as possible with a nibbling maneuver with traction to feel when there is loosening of the horn. **B:** Surgical slides showing lysing of the lateral horn.

intermediate fat pad (Fig. 21). Just enough of the lateral and nasal check ligaments of the levator are incised to allow the levator to be stretched forward (Fig. 22). Overly aggressive dissection can actually weaken the lifting power of the levator. Once the levator horn and check ligament are loosened by dissection, the surgeon must make sure all additional attachments of the orbital septum are freed from the levator so that the levator becomes "stretchy."

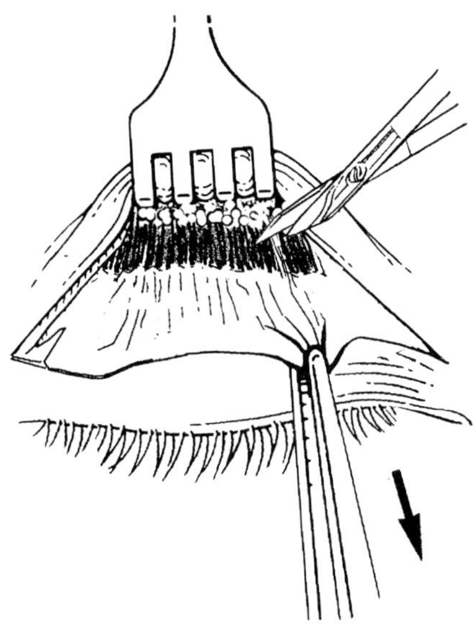

FIG. 21. Levator resection with dissection. **A:** Nasal traction shows the tethering of the nasal levator with the inter pad septum extending from the transitional fat area to the aponeurosis. The nasal horn is not lysed; only the interpad septum to gain stretchability of the levator is lysed.

Quantitating the Effect

There are two basic approaches to quantitating the amount of levator that is resected to produce the desired lift of the lid.

Measured Amount of Levator Excised

A method favored by Beard is to measure the amount of the levator that is excised (Fig. 23). If the method of quantitation to be used is the amount of levator excised, then the sutures are placed in the desired part of the levator to allow the proper amount of resection to be performed and then tightened and the level of the lid noted measuring the amount of levator resected according to Table 1 (12,13).

TABLE 1. *Amount of levator resection according to levator function and ptosis*

Amt. ptosis	Amt. levator resection (mm)	Levator function (mm)
Mild	10–13 (small)	7–10
Moderate	14–17 (moderate)	6–7
Severe	18–22 (large)	4–6

Modified from Beard (12).

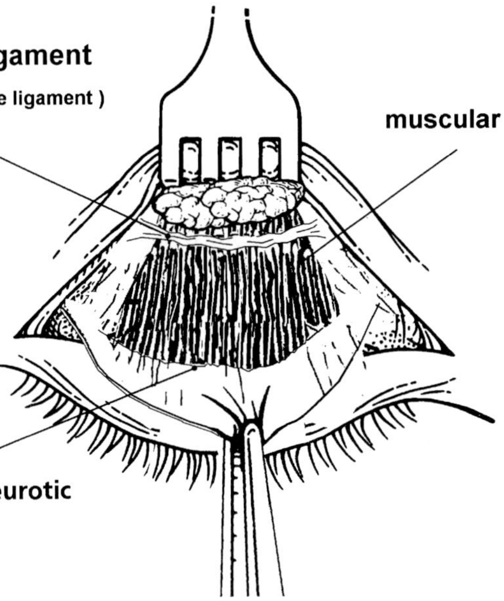

FIG. 22. Following lysis of the lateral horn and lysis of the inner pad septum the levator can be stretched forward and its "springiness" determined.

Gapping Method

An alternative method is described by Berke in which one does not actually measure the amount of levator resected but measures the amount of "gapping" or separation of the upper and lower lids on the operating table (14). Berke was able to correlate the gapping on the operative table with the postoperative position when the patient was awake and unanesthetized, and has developed a table of the expected "lift" or "fall" of the lid postoperatively according to how much levator function is present preoperatively. An advantage of this method is that it neutralizes many surgical variables, such as how much dissection of the levator occurs and how much the levator is stretched when measuring the amount to excise. Table 2 illustrates the amount of gapping of the eyelid or the position of the upper lid in the relationship to the upper limbus with the expected postoperative result.

This lid gapping formula has been adapted for use in patients who have levator functions from 5 to 10 mm (function below 5 mm requires frontalis suspension, above 10 mm are best corrected by aponeurotic repair). It is to be emphasized that no formula is perfect and any formula is just a starting point for the ptosis surgeon to make his or her own judgment as experience is gained. With experience, each individual ptosis surgeon can adjust the basic quantitating technique to his or her surgical bias to gain the predicted result.

Following the decision on the type of quantitation to use, a central double-armed lifting suture (6-0 silk) is placed in the anterior tarsal surface, half-thickness, in the upper one fourth of the tarsal plate with a double

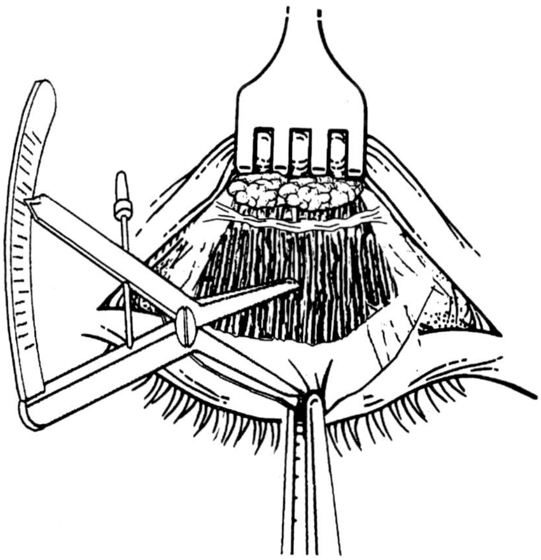

FIG. 23. Levator resection with dissection. Initial measurement of position for suture placement in levator resection. Anatomically there is approximately 11 mm of levator resected at the musculoaponeurotic junction and from the musculoaponeurotic junction to Whitnall's ligament is an additional 20–22 mm.

TABLE 2. *Quantitation of ptosis correction by intraoperative "gapping"*

Placement of the upper lid position intraoperatively in relationship to desired postoperative position	Levator function (mm)
Slightly lower	8–10
Same level	6–8
Slightly higher	4–6

Modified from Berke (14).

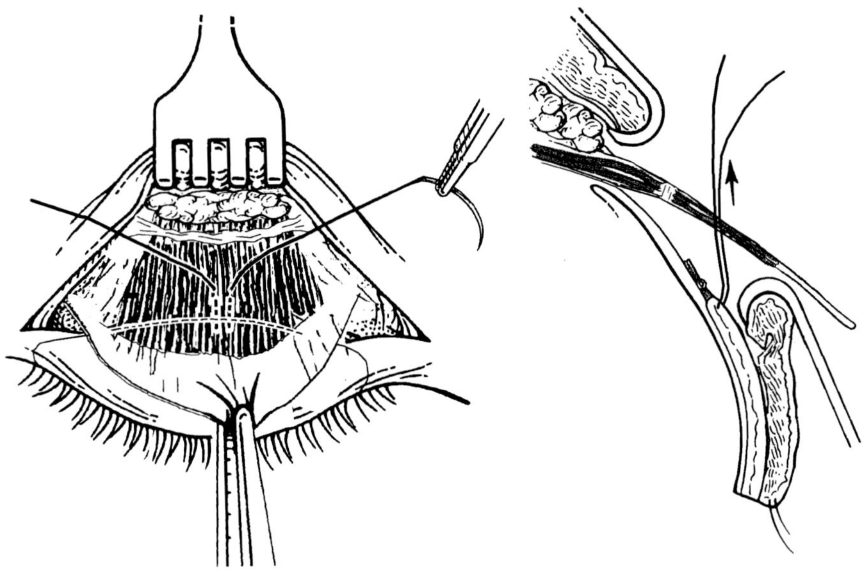

FIG. 24. Levator resection with dissection. Diagram showing positioning of suture and central lifting suture from superior tarsal edge into the muscular levator.

stitch. The sutures are then brought underneath and through the levator–Müller's muscle complex, which had been dissected (Figs. 24 and 25). If the gapping method is to be used, the sutures are tightened until the lid reaches the desired elevation and contour (Fig. 26A, B). An additional suture is placed laterally to ensure a lateral lift. It has been found that it is not necessary to use a nasal suture. Following both of these methods, some redundant levator is resected.

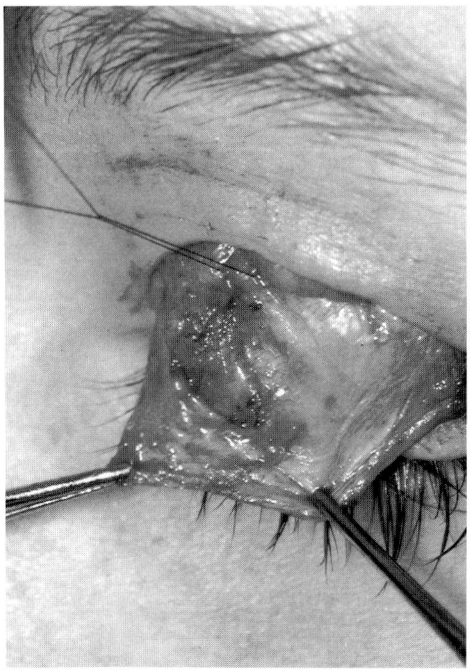

FIG. 25. Surgical slides showing placement of central lifting suture through muscular levator.

It is to be emphasized that this is the "moment of truth" in the ptosis procedure. The surgeon may have performed a superb anatomic dissection with a technically precise suture placement but may still compromise the surgical correction if great care is not given to the last tightening or loosening of the sutures and its effect on the level of the lid.

The last step is the recreation of the lid crease. In most levator resections it is important to have performed a small skin incision to avoid redundant skin in the newly elevated lid. It is important to include in the skin closure sutures that will allow attachment of skin-muscle edges to the levator muscle in a manner that assures a proper lid crease position. Transcutaneous absorbable sutures in the central, lateral, and nasal portions of the pretarsal skin area are used as in the aponeurotic repair.

Frost sutures to close the eye are usually not required postoperatively unless there is an impairment in the eye protective mechanisms. Antibiotic ointment can be used to protect the cornea postoperatively, and it is recommended that ice compresses be used postoperatively. Compression bandages should be avoided because of the possibility of abrading the cornea.

Berke Dissection Technique

The Berke dissection technique is not needed in the usual ptosis cases but is a helpful alternative in reoperated cases and some posttraumatic cases in which the tissue is scarred and the anatomy difficult to identify or dissect. In these cases the standard Berke dissection can be employed to assure identification of the levator.

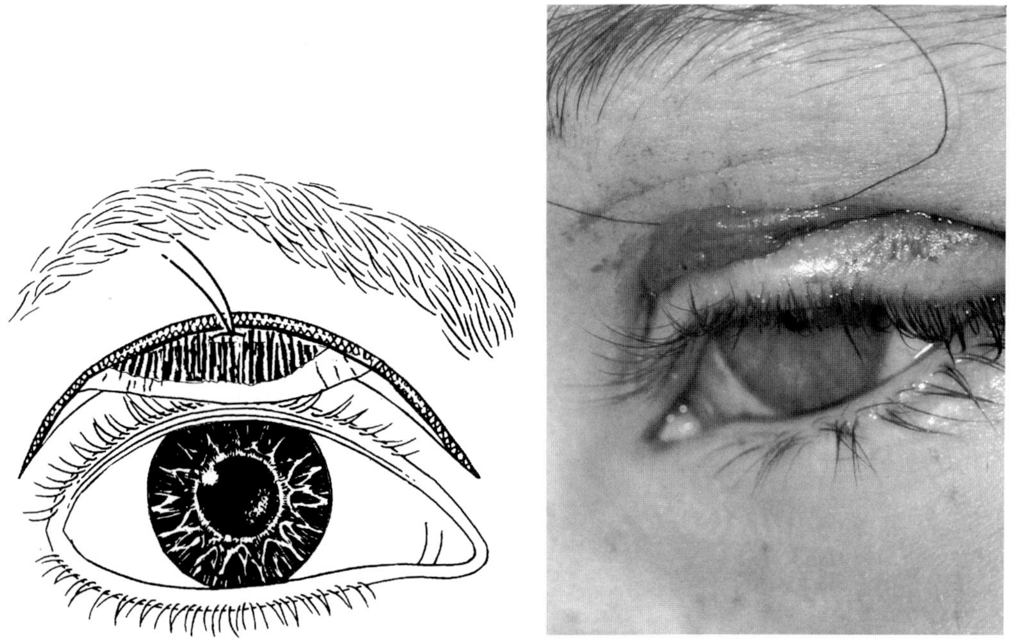

A B

FIG. 26. Levator resection with dissection. **A:** The central lifting suture has been tied and the amount of gapping or separation of the upper and lower lid on the operative table is noted. **B:** Surgical slide showing intraoperative gapping after tying of central lifting suture.

The orbital septum is opened to try to identify the preaponeurotic space and levator. The dissection of the levator–Müller's complex is then undertaken. With downward traction of the lid, buttonholes are made just above the superior tarsal border, 2 cm apart, with a punch-through maneuver (Fig. 27A). The globe should be protected during this maneuver. A ptosis clamp or hemostat is then used to clamp the tissue inserting on the superior tarsal border, which includes levator aponeurosis, Müller's muscle, and conjunctiva (Fig. 27B). The tissue within the contents of the clamp is then separated from the superior tarsal border, avoiding any excision of the superior tarsal edge (Fig. 28). The conjunctiva is then dissected free from the undersurface of Müller's muscle (Fig. 29A). A preliminary maneuver of ballooning the conjunctiva by injection of saline before dissection is helpful. Dissection should avoid the fornix attachment of the conjunctiva to prevent postoperative conjunctival prolapse. The conjunctival edge is then resutured to the superior tarsal border with 6-0 gut, placed so as to avoid irritation of the cornea (Fig. 29B). Following this maneuver, Müller's muscle, levator aponeurosis, and orbital septum are contained within the ptosis clamp. The lateral

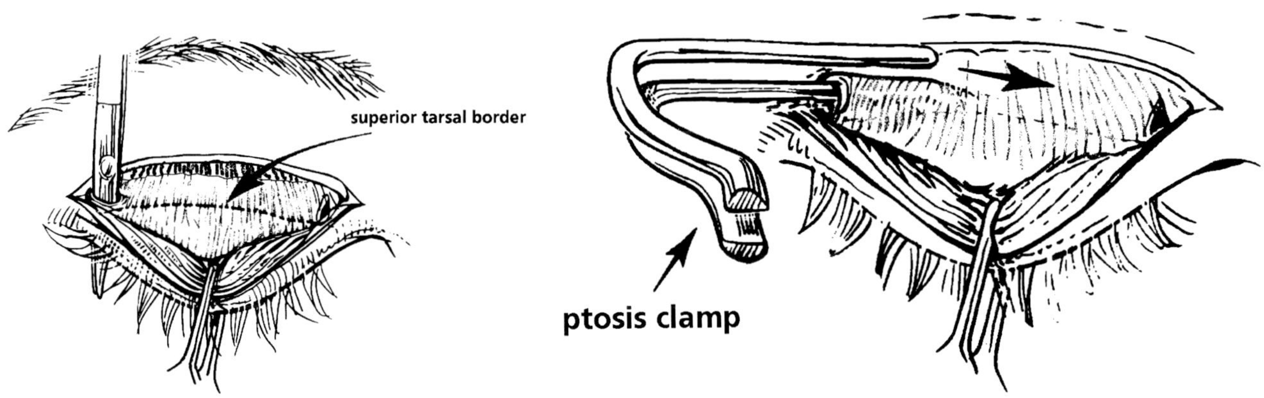

A B

FIG. 27. Classic Berke external levator resection. **A:** After the levator is marked at the superior tarsal edge, buttonholes, full thickness, externally through the conjunctiva are made nasally and temporally approximately 2 cm apart. **B:** The ptosis clamp is inserted between the two buttonholes clamping the full-thickness eyelid including conjunctiva Müller's muscle and levator above the superior edge of the tarsal plate.

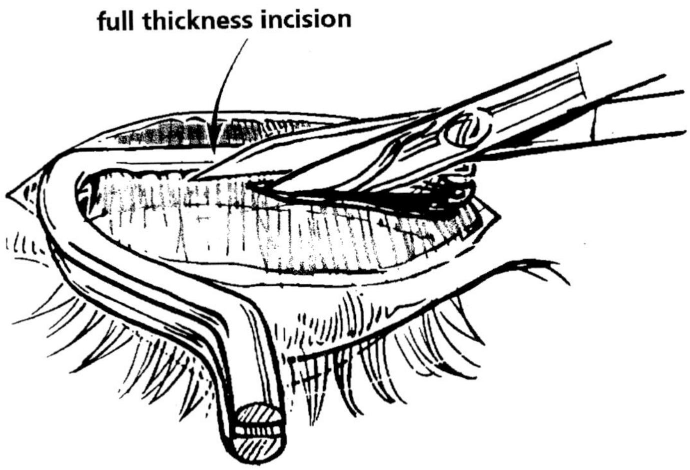

FIG. 28. A full-thickness incision of the clamp tissue between the clamp and the superior edge of the tarsal plate.

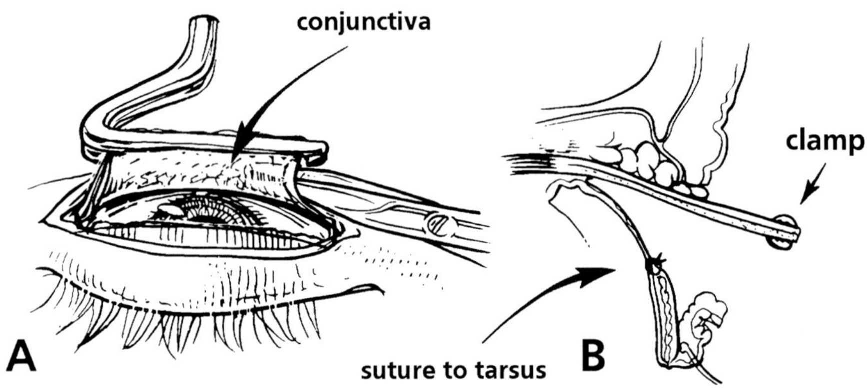

FIG. 29. A: The conjunctiva is dissected free from the clamp tissue. **B:** It is then resutured to the superior edge of the tarsus leaving levator and Müller's muscle within the clamp. The orbital septum has been opened.

horn and check ligament are lysed as described previously (Fig. 30).

Levator Excision

In patients with aberrant eyelid retraction in whom the anomalous movement is a problem either functionally or cosmetically, inactivation of the levator by segmental excision is used to eliminate the movement. This must be followed by a frontalis suspension procedure to elevate the lid back to a normal level. This is most commonly needed in children with the jaw winking syndrome but can occur in other conditions such as aberrant regeneration of a third nerve palsey.

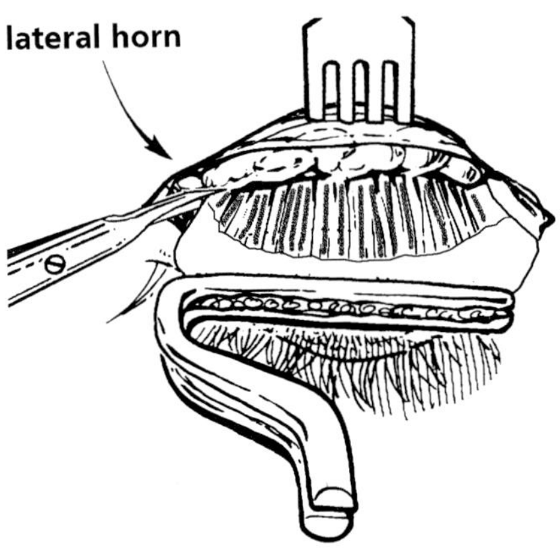

FIG. 30. Classic Berke external levator resection. Lysis of the lateral horn of the levator while grasping the levator Müller's complex and the clamp.

With a frontalis procedure, the patient must use his or her brow for lid elevation. There is a tendency not to use the brow if there is a normal lid on the opposite side, which has led Beard to recommend excision of the levator on the opposite ("normal") side with secondary frontalis suspension which forces the patient to use the brow symmetrically (15). Many surgeons prefer not to excise the levator on the normal side but only place frontalis suspension material there to produce a more symmetric movement with both upper lids. This approach has become known as the "chicken Beard" procedure. The authors generally take the "chicken" approach.

Anterior levator resection to eliminate the anomalous retraction requires extensive anterior dissection of the levator and all existing check ligaments, as well as removal of any strands of tissue that may transmit a pull to the upper lid postoperatively. This type of dissection causes a large loss of support structures for the upper lid and tarsal plate, which makes it very difficult to get a full correction of the ptosis with a frontalis suspension procedure.

A technique of levator excision to produce inactivation of the movement without weakening anterior eyelid support is to excise the levator posterior to Whitnall's ligament, leaving all of the anterior levator and eyelid support structures intact. This can then be followed by a frontalis suspension in the same surgical session.

Technique

The first part of the procedure is to create the standard levator exposure as previously described. The anterior levator is bypassed and a Blair retractor is placed on Whitnall's ligament. The levator is pulled forward exposing the ribbon-like orbital segment of the levator muscle (Fig. 31A). A muscle hook is placed under the levator to isolate and bring a segment of it forward (Fig. 31B). At the same time the globe is rotated to ensure that the superior rectus is not incorporated in the hook. The muscle is clamped in two places with hemostats, a 5-mm segment is excised, and after cauterization of the cut end the muscle is allowed to retract

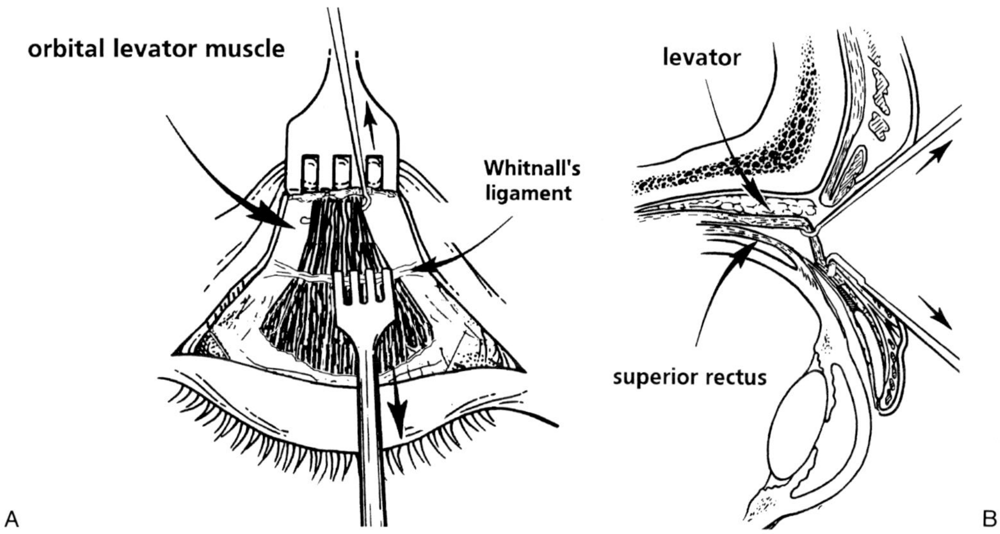

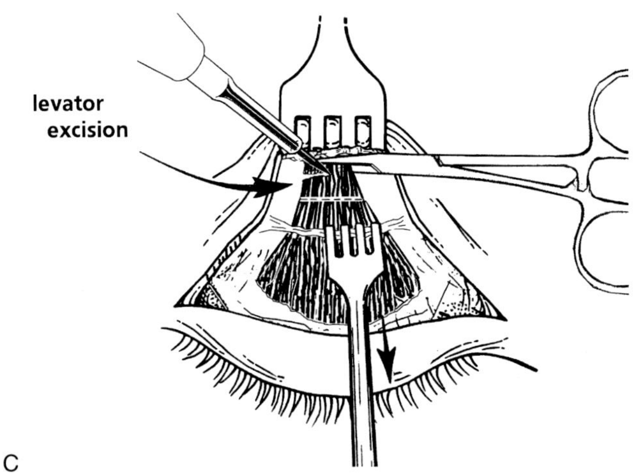

FIG. 31. Levator excision for jaw winking syndrome. **A:** After initial exposure of the levator muscle with opening of the orbital septum and retraction of the orbital fat, a Blair retractor is placed on Whitnall's ligament and the levator complex is brought forward until the thin orbital portion of the levator can be seen. A muscle clamp is then inserted underneath the orbital portion of the levator muscle. **B:** Sagittal view showing placement of the clamp sparing the superior rectus muscle. With the muscle clamp on the orbital segment of the levator, the globe should be rotated to ensure that the superior rectus is not incorporated with the muscle hook. **C:** Hemostats are used to clamp a segment of the orbital portion of the levator and a segment is excised immobilizing levator movement. The proximal cut end of levator can be preserved and sutured to the periosteum in the roof if desired.

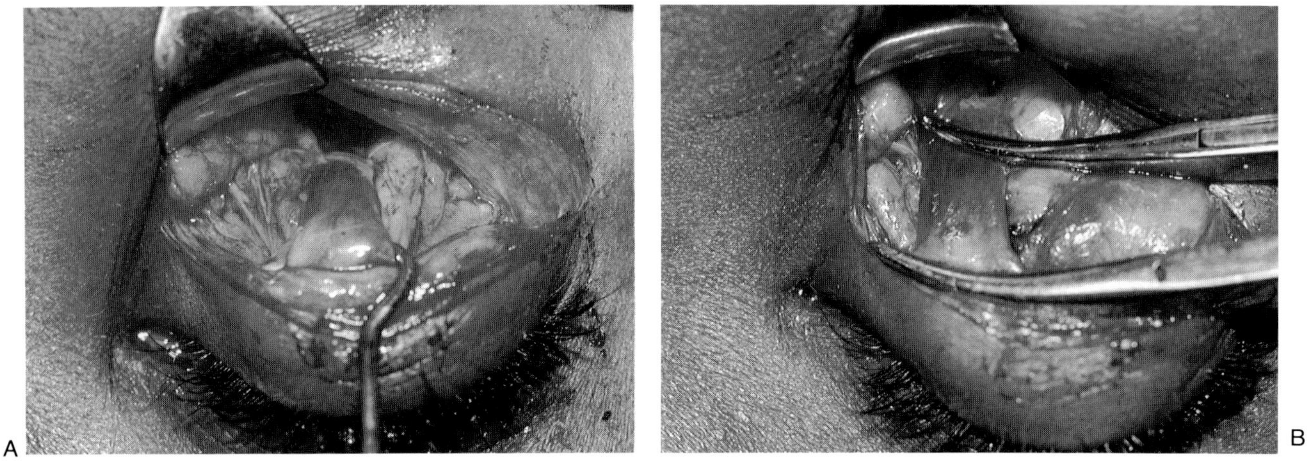

FIG. 32. A: Surgical view of orbital portion of the levator muscle behind Whitnall's ligament. **B:** Portion of orbital levator muscle clamped for excision.

into the orbit (Fig. 31C). The frontalis procedure is then performed. Figure 32A shows a surgical view of the orbital portion of the levator isolated with a muscle hook. Figure 32B shows clamping of the section of levator muscle to be excised.

REFERENCES

1. Epstein GA, Putterman AM. Supermaximum levator resection for severe unilateral congenital blepharoptosis. *Ophth Surg* 1984;15:911–979.
2. Anderson RL, Jordan DR, Dutton JJ. Whitnall's sling for poor function ptosis. *Arch Ophthalmol* 1990;108:1628–1632.
3. Fasanella RM, Servat J. Levator resection for minimal ptosis: Another simplified operation. *Arch Ophthalmol* 1961;65: 493–496.
4. Paris GL, Quickert MH. Disinsertion of the aponeurosis of the levator palpebrae superioris muscle after cataract extraction. *Am J Ophthalmol* 1976;81:337–340.
5. Anderson RL, Gordy DD. Aponeurotic defects in congenital ptosis. *Ophthalmology* 1979;86:1493–1499.
6. Jones LT, Quickert MH, Wobig JL. The cure of ptosis by aponeurotic repair. *Arch Ophthalmol* 1975;93:629.
7. Anderson RL, Dixon RS. Aponeurotic ptosis surgery. *Arch Ophthalmol* 1979;97:1123.
8. Linberg JV, Vasquez RJ, Chao GM. Aponeurotic ptosis repair under local anesthesia. Prediction of results from operative lid height. *Ophthalmology* 1988;95:1046.
9. Shore JW, Bergin DJ, Garrett SN. Results of blepharoptosis surgery with early postoperative adjustment. *Ophthalmology* 1990;97:1502–1511.
10. Dortzbach RK, Kronish JW. Early revision in the office for adults after unsatisfactory blepharoptsis correction. *Am J Ophthalmol* 1993;75:68–75.
11. Jordan DR, Anderson RL. A simplified procedure for adjusting eyelid position after aponeurotic ptosis surgery. *Arch Ophthalmol* 1987;105:1288.
12. Beard C. The surgical treatment of blepharoptosis: a quantitative approach. *Trans Am Ophthalmol Soc* 1966;64:401.
13. Beard C. *Ptosis*. 3rd ed. St Louis: CV Mosby Co; 1981:89–91.
14. Berke RN. Results of resection of the levator muscle through a skin excision in congenital ptosis. *Arch Ophthalmol* 1959;61: 177–201.
15. Beard C. *Ptosis*. 3rd ed. St Louis: CV Mosby Co; 1981:213–217.
16. Baylis HI, Shorr N. Anterior tarsectomy reoperation for upper eyelid blepharoptosis or contour abnormalities. *Am J Ophthalmol* 1977;84:67.
17. Putterman AM, Urist MJ. A simplified levator palpebrae superioris muscle recession to treat overcorrected blepharoptosis. *Am J Ophthalmol* 1974;77:358.
18. Gladstone GJ, Putterman AM. Internal vertical shortening for the correction of diffuse or segmental postoperative blepharoptosis. *Am J Ophthalmol* 1985;99:429.
19. Scott KR, Tse DT, Kronish JW. Vertically oriented upper eyelid nerve fibers. A clinical, anatomical and immunohistochemical study. *Ophthalmology* 1992;99:222.

CHAPTER 9

Frontalis Suspension

The indication to use frontalis suspension for correction of ptosis is generally considered to be levator function of 4–5 mm or less. This amount of function occurs commonly in patients with congenital ptosis, which may be bilateral in many cases. Poor levator function also occurs in patients with acquired ptosis but is not common and is usually the result of trauma or paralysis. In patients with poor levator function (usually children), unilateral frontalis suspension can correct the ptosis but will produce noticeable asymmetry in lid movement and lagophthalmos in downgaze postoperatively. For this reason, bilateral frontalis suspension procedures have been advocated for patients with unilateral ptosis. Better symmetry in movement and lagophthalmos is obtained with bilateral surgery and this approach has become a standard one by many ptosis surgeons (1).

Many substances have been advocated for use as the suspending element, including Gore-tex, suture material (braided and monofilament nylon), preserved eye bank sclera, preserved fascia lata, and silicone (2–7). The best suspensory substance is autogenous fascia lata, which provides the most long-lasting and predictable results (8–13). More recently, temporalis fascia has proven effective in frontalis suspension, although it is somewhat more friable; it is more difficult to obtain longer strips than with fascia lata. The "double-strand" techniques are preferred by the authors because of better contouring and purchase. Silicone is best used as a single strand (14).

FRONTALIS SUSPENSION WITH SKIN-FAT RESECTION AND CREASE FORMATION

The traditional method of frontalis suspension has produced satisfactory results (8–14). As one operates on a large number of ptosis patients, however, one finds that some postoperative problems can occur with this technique. The most common postoperative problem that can occur in patients who have undergone frontalis suspension in the traditional manner is loss of the upper lid crease with lash ptosis and, in some cases, entropion of the upper lid from slippage of skin. These cases require a secondary eyelid crease–entropion procedure for correction. In addition, it is often the case with the traditional technique in young children that, the eyelid may seem overly puffy and bulky postoperatively.

Problems found with the traditional technique may be prevented by a modification. The modification consists of a skin-muscle-fat excision in the area of the desired crease and crease-tensing sutures such as those seen in upper lid entropion procedures. This crease incision also makes the passage of the suspensory material easier and more precise.

Fat removal is ideally done in bilateral cases, but even if done in unilateral cases the inserted suspensory material usually prevents deep asymmetric crease formation when fat is removed.

Standard Technique with Alloplastic Material

Three markings are made above the brow hairs in the brow area with methylene blue (Fig. 1A). In the supralash areas, one marking is made in line with the pupil. The central brow incision should correspond to the pupillary incision. The area is infiltrated with local anesthetic with adrenalin and incisions are made. The crease is marked and the desired amount of skin (muscle-septum) is outlined. The upper marked incision is made first to expose the preaponeurotic space and the yellow, loose-lying fat in the preaponeurotic space (just in front of the levator) is grasped and removed with the cutting bovie. Usually only the amount that presents itself is removed. The skin-muscle-septal flap is then excised (Figs. 1B, 2A, B). Hemostasis is usually obtained with a bipolar cautery. The suspensory material can then be inserted.

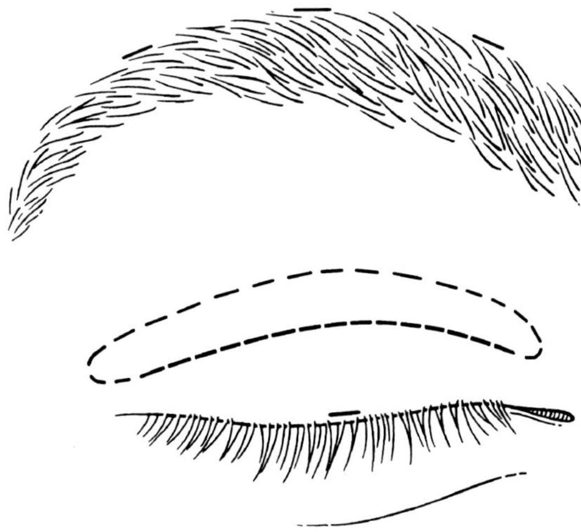

A

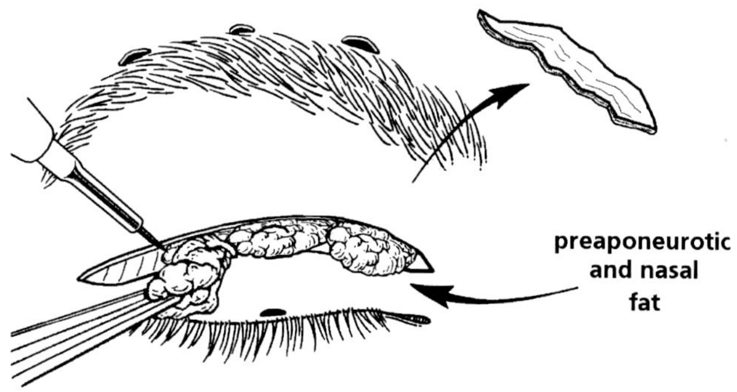

B

FIG. 1. Alloplastic material. **A:** Marking of skin for skin excision and incisions for passage of suspensory material. **B:** Excision of skin muscle layer above crease and removal of preaponeurotic fat.

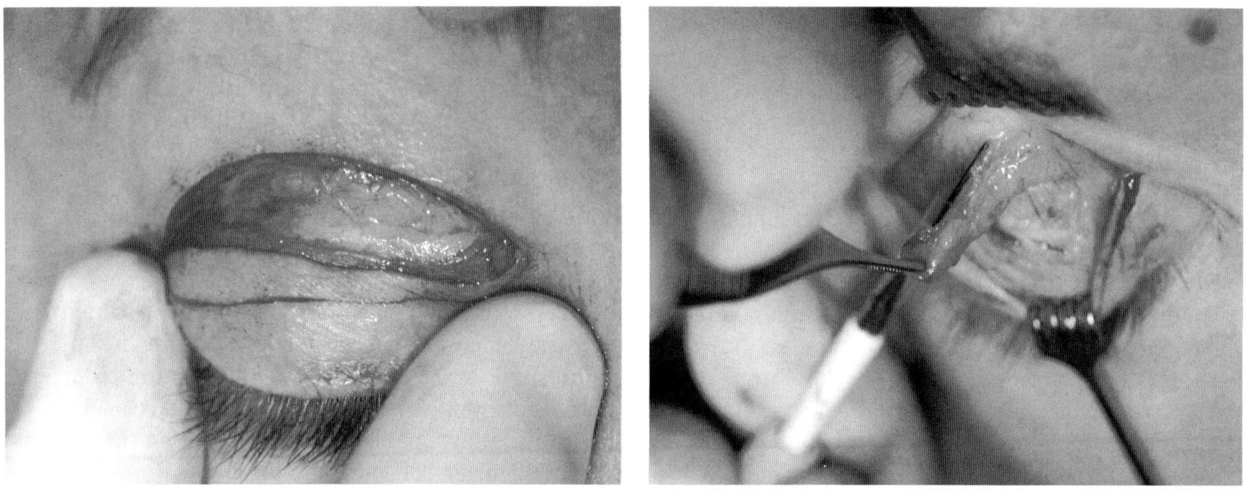

A B

FIG. 2. Alloplastic material. **A:** Surgical view showing opening of orbital septum with marked skin muscle for removal. **B:** Excision of preaponeurotic fat.

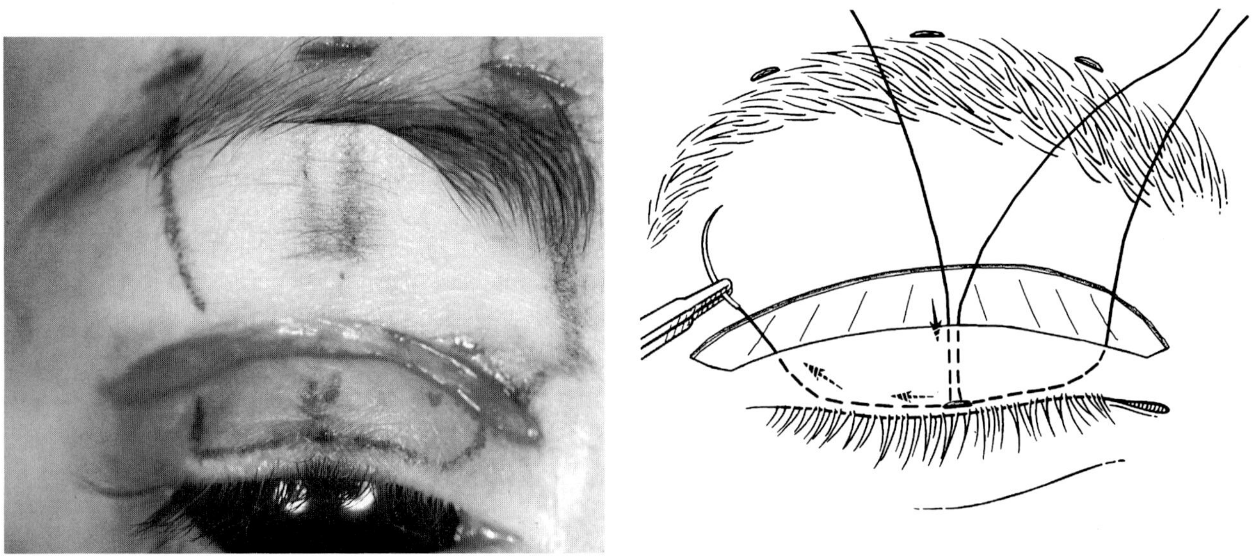

A B

FIG. 3. Alloplastic material. **A:** Marking with methylene blue on the surface of the skin after skin excision and incisions are made. Marking shows the direction of passage of the alloplastic suspensory material. **B:** Passage of alloplastic material through pretarsal area. Material is brought out through lid crease incision after being threaded above the lashes in the pretarsal plane.

It has been found that the use of a cutting general closure needle for the vertical passage and a Keith needle for the horizontal passages is easier and safer than the larger fascia needle. Some suture material will already have a swedged-on needle that is satisfactory for the passage in the tarsal area (Ethicon 4-0 Nurolon, PS-2 cutting needle no. 5654). The suspensory material is threaded from the crease incision into the central incision above the lashes in a double strand. The desired placement of the suspensory material is marked on the lid to serve as a guide for passage (Fig. 3A). Each strand is then threaded horizontally in the supralash area and to the nasally and temporally and back into the crease incision (Fig. 3B). In the horizontal passage between the incisions in the supralash area, care must be taken not to penetrate the tarsal plate, and the

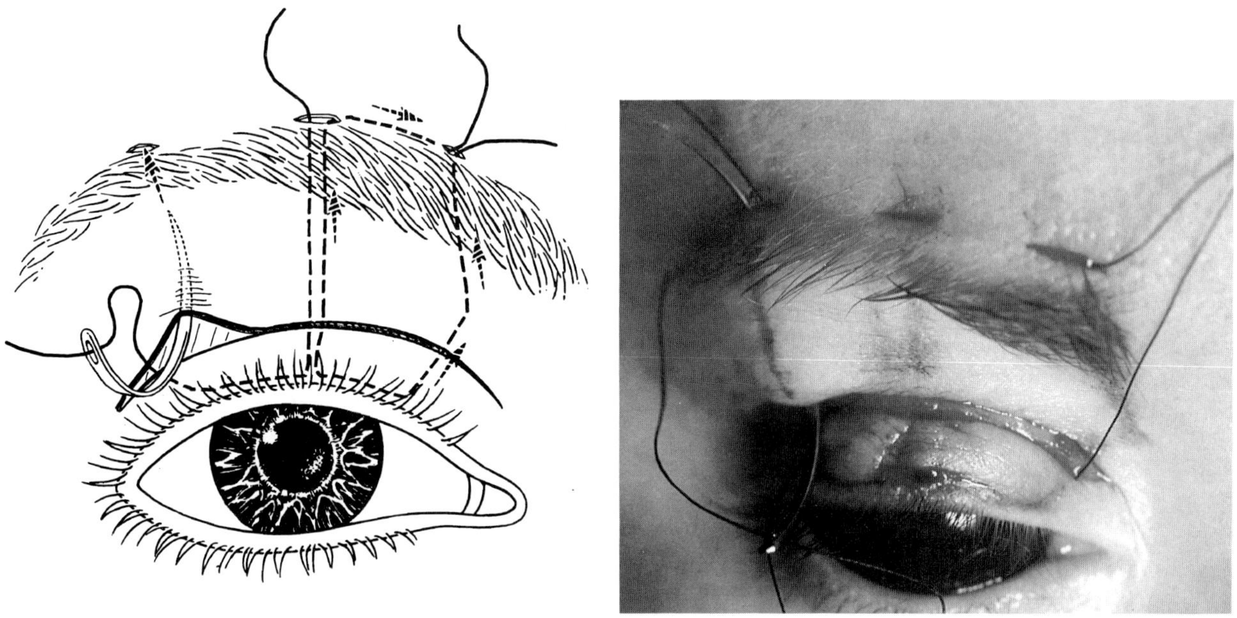

A B

FIG. 4. Alloplastic material. **A:** Passage of the alloplastic material through the crease incision to the brow incisions. **B:** Surgical view showing passage of alloplastic material through the crease incision into the brow incisions with a general closure cutting needle.

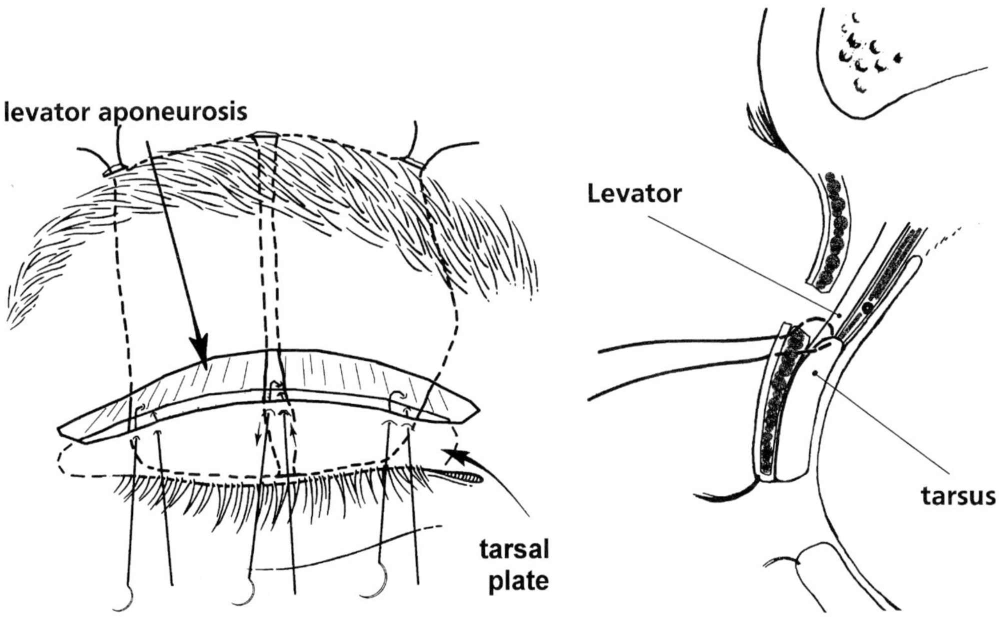

A B

FIG. 5. Alloplastic material. **A:** After the alloplastic material has been threaded through the marked passage ways, the eyelid crease formation is accomplished with tensing of the pretarsal skin to the superior edge of the tarsal plate with transcutaneous crease sutures. **B:** Sagittal view showing placement of crease sutures through pretarsal skin to the superior edge of the tarsal plate tensing the pretarsal skin.

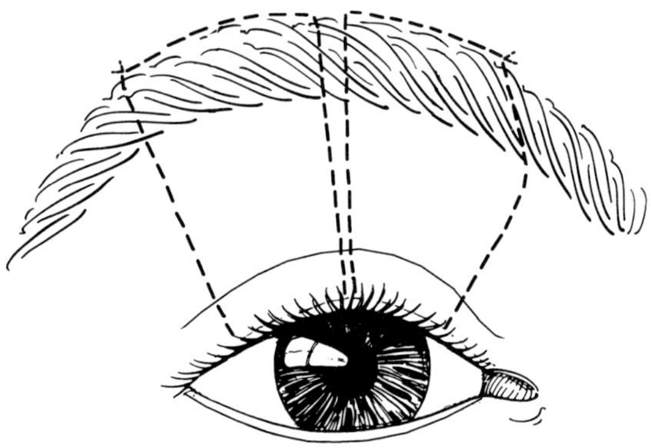

FIG. 6. Alloplastic material. Final configuration of the alloplastic material after it has been tightened showing the lid elevation.

material should be threaded between the musculocutaneous layer and the tarsus. Little dissection should be carried out so that the material will be secured firmly into position with each passage. The strands can be looped at the central incision above the lashes to prevent cheesewiring through the tissue over time with lowering of the lid (15).

The pathway of the strands from the crease incision to the brow should also be made in the submuscular plane and generally should not penetrate the orbital septum to prevent tethering (Fig. 4A, B). In some cases a pulley effect can be created (16). This is best accomplished with a larger needle such as a cutting general closure needle. The passage from the crease to the nasal brow incision seems to cause less notching if it is slightly angulated. In the brow area the strands from the central incision are then threaded to the nasal and temporal brow incisions. The final positioning of the strands takes the form of two rhomboids, as shown in Fig. 5A. The suspensory material is tensed through the brow incisions to test their ability to elevate the lid and produce the desired contour. Modifications can be made at this time if needed.

The crease incision is then closed with transcutaneous sutures tensing the pretarsal skin, forming the crease, and preventing lash rotation. The incision is closed completely with a running suture. The suspensory material in the brow can then be tightened (Fig. 5A, B).

Adequate dissection should be done in the brow incisions to allow a securing of the strands to the frontalis muscle buried beneath the skin–subcutaneous layer of the brow. In the brow area, there is a plane of fatty tissue that is present between the skin and the frontalis muscle, and dissection must be carried through that in order for the strands to find a resting place on the frontalis muscle. It is important that all of the material be buried deep beneath the skin fat to avoid subsequent granuloma formation from irritation in the subcutaneous tissue. Adjustment of the upper lid position before securing the material is then made. The placement of the upper lid margin at the time of surgery should be slightly higher than one wishes it to be postoperatively (Fig. 6). When adjusting the frontalis suspension, care must be taken that all traction on the forehead skin, including drapes, be relieved to eliminate any false elevation of the brow. The eyes should be in the primary position when the surgeon makes the judgment for the proper elevation. Care must be taken with patient cooperation under local anesthesia or the depth of anesthesia under general because the eyes will tend to roll upward if general anesthesia is lightened toward the end of the case. Figure 7A and B shows a child before and after alloplastic frontalis suspension bilaterally.

Autogenous Fascia

Fascia is usually the suspensory material of choice for frontalis suspension unless it cannot be obtained

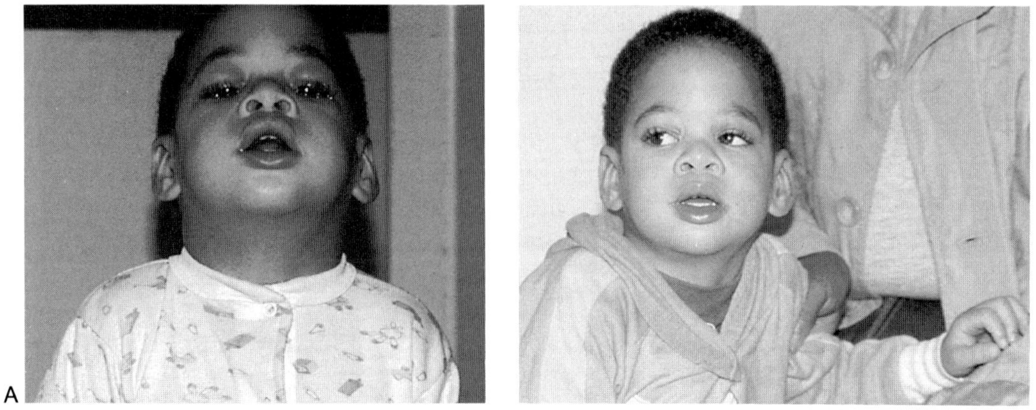

FIG. 7. Alloplastic material. **A:** A young child with a backward head tilt because of congenital ptosis and poor levator function. **B:** Same child following frontalis suspension with alloplastic material.

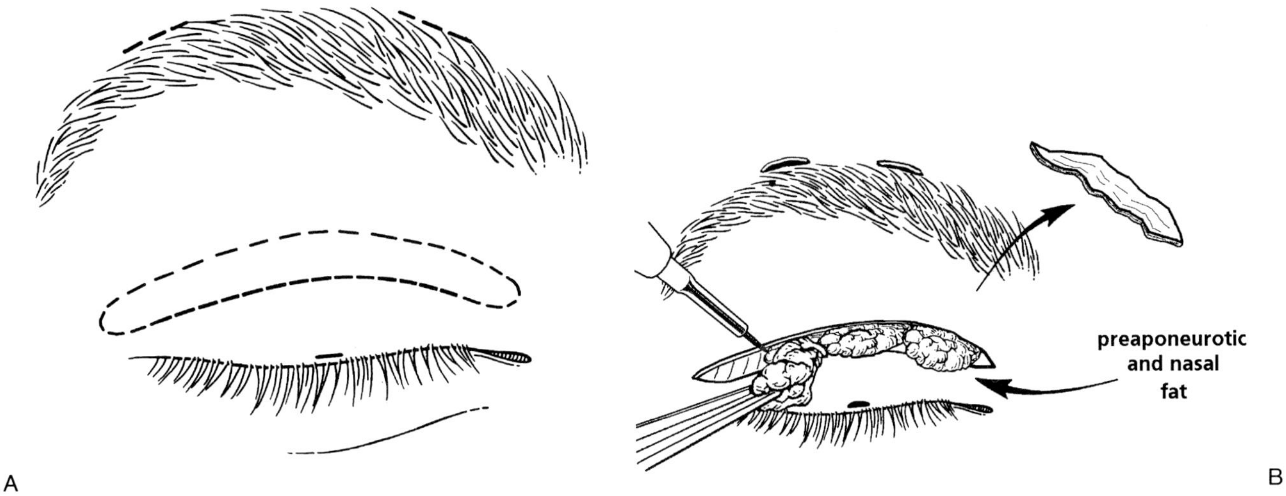

FIG. 8. Fascia. **A:** Marking of the skin for excision and skin incision for placement of fascia strips. **B:** Excision of the skin muscle strip above the crease and preaponeurotic fat.

from the patient. It should not be used in patients who have poor eye protective mechanisms and who may need postoperative loosening. There may be other extenuating circumstances. The difference in technique when fascia is used is that there are only two brow incisions centered above the limbal areas (Fig. 8A). The skin-muscle-septal flap is excised as previously described (Fig. 8B). The fascial strands are passed in the pretarsal area similar to alloplastic material; however, a larger needle with an adequate eyelet for threading the fascia must be used (Fig. 9A). A Keith needle or a small general closure needle can be used. From the crease incision the fascia strands are threaded into the brow incisions, so that the final configuration of the strands is two base-down triangles since there are only two brow incisions (Figs. 9B, 10). In our experience, a third brow incision has not offered any more correction or movement with the fascia and increases the bulkiness of the suspensory material. In some cases, supplemental 6-0 silk sutures can be in-

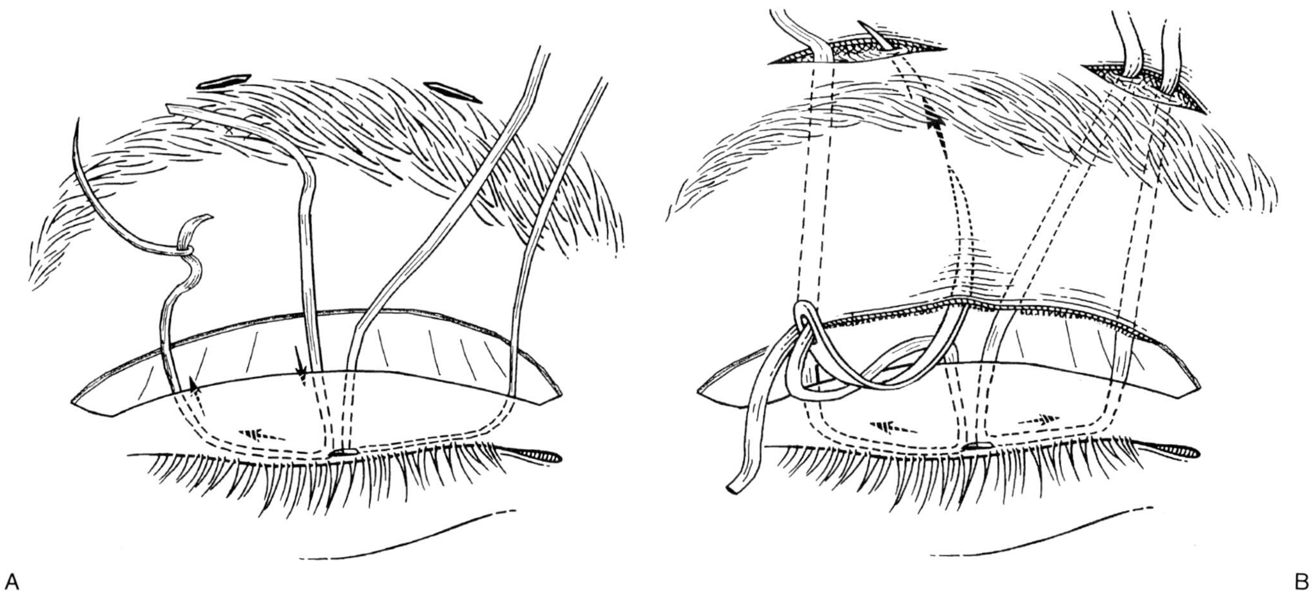

FIG. 9. Fascia. **A:** Threading of the fascia strips in the pretarsal area. The strips are threaded through the central incision, then nasally and temporally in the pretarsal plane above the lashes, and then up into the crease incision nasally and temporally. **B:** Passage of the fascia strips from the crease incision into the brow incisions. The direction of passage is anterior to the orbital septum and periosteum, into the frontalis muscle superiorly. The superior incisions have been undermined so that the fascia can be buried adequately beneath the brow skin.

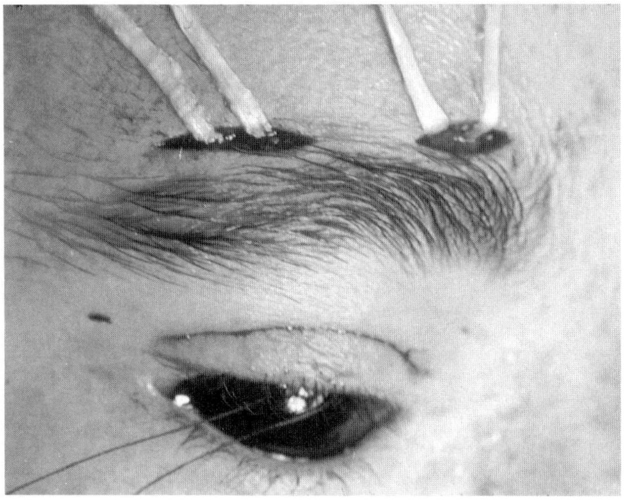

FIG. 10. Fascia. Surgical view showing the fascia strips having been threaded into the brow incisions.

serted through the crease incision to anchor the fascial strands to further adjust the contour if desired. This maneuver is particularly helpful in difficult cases such as the blepharophimosis syndrome.

The crease incision is then closed with transcutaneous sutures tensing the pretarsal skin, forming the crease, and preventing lash rotation. The incision is closed completely with a running suture (Fig. 11A). The suspensory material in the brow can then be tightened. The fixation of fascia in the brow area is accomplished by fixating the two strands together with 4-0 silk with the first half of a surgeon's knot (double throw) and observing the elevation and contour (Fig. 11B). When the desired elevation and contour is obtained the second throw is completed. Additional tightening and elevation can be accomplished, if desired, by reintroducing the 4-0 silk into the strands of fascia at a lower level in the loop and tightening. After the proper elevation and coutour of the lid is obtained, the redundant fascia and suture is trimmed and the knot buried beneath the skin-fat layer beneath the brow skin (Fig. 11C). Failure to bury the material adequately will result in subcutaneous irritation and granuloma formation. Figures 12 and 13 show patients before and after bilateral fascia frontalis suspension with this technique.

Horizontal Tightening with Frontalis Suspension

When there is significant laxity in the upper lid, the tension of the suspensory strands may tend to evert or separate the eyelid from the globe. Contour adjustment

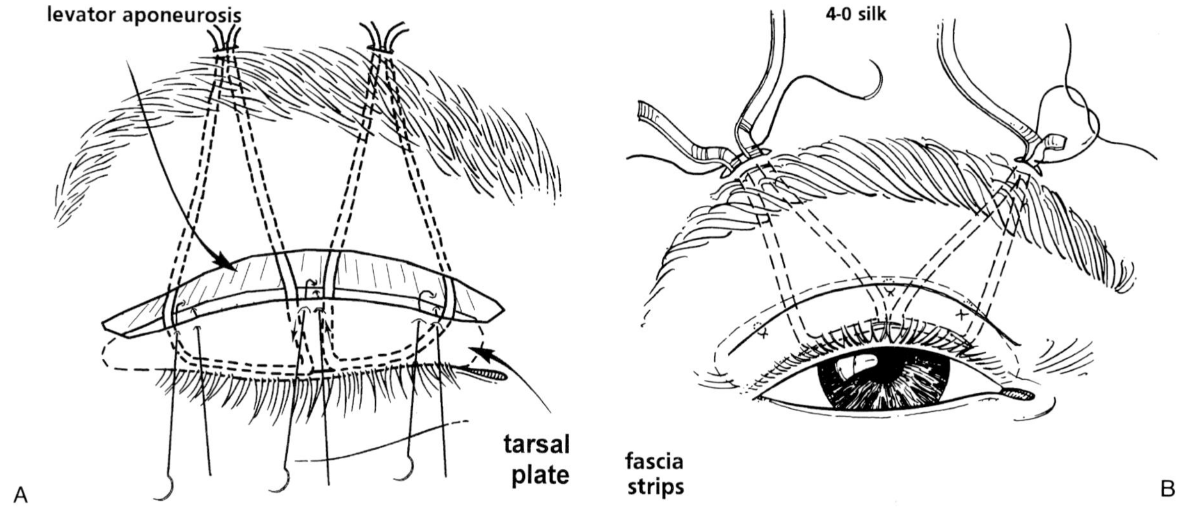

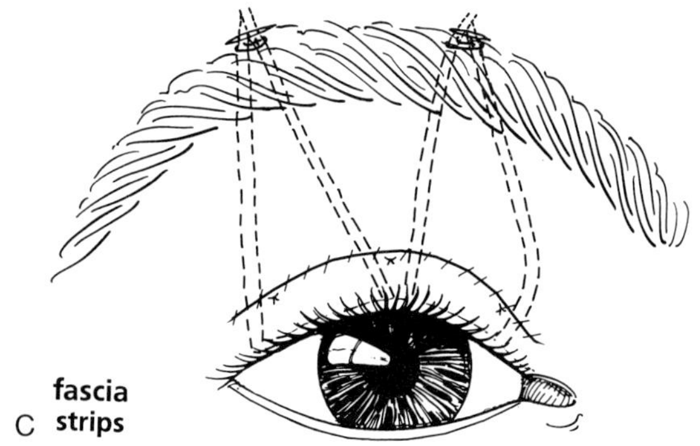

FIG. 11. Fascia. **A:** After the fascia strips have been threaded into the brow incisions, the eyelid crease sutures are placed transcutaneously tensing the superior edge of the pretarsal skin to the superior edge of the tarsus. Care is taken to place the sutures between the strips in the tarsus or supporting tissue, not the strips themselves. **B:** The fascia strips can then be tensed in the brow incisions elevating the lid and the formation of the crease can be observed. Initial anchoring of the strips to observe the effect on contour can be done with 4-0 silk suture. **C:** The fascia strips have been tightened in the brow until the eyelid has reached the desired level and the 4-0 silk suture has been advanced and sutured to the fascia strips beneath the thick eyebrow skin. An additional suture in the frontalis muscle can be taken.

can be very difficult in these cases. Increased laxity can occur commonly in patients following trauma or with prosthetic eyes. An adjunctive procedure of horizontal tightening of the upper lid tenses the lid, allowing the suspensory strands to produce the desired elevation without eversion or notching (Fig. 14A–C). Figure 15A–C shows the use of this adjunctive procedure in a patient.

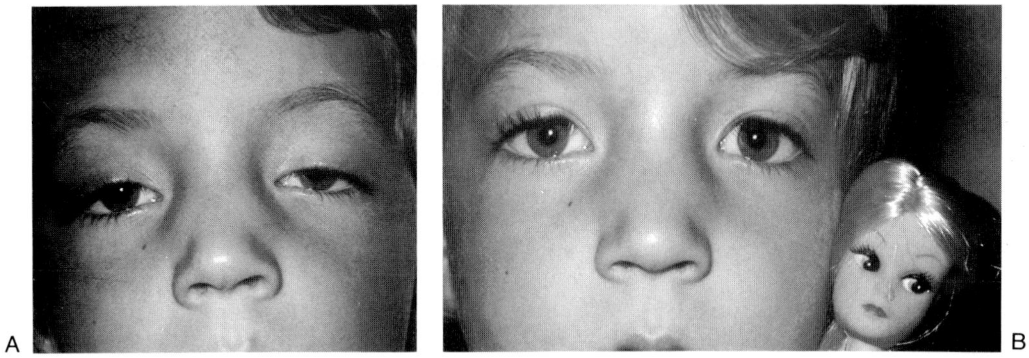

FIG. 12. Fascia. **A:** A young child with congenital ptosis with poor levator function and poor eyelid crease formation. **B:** Same child following frontalis suspension with eyelid crease procedure.

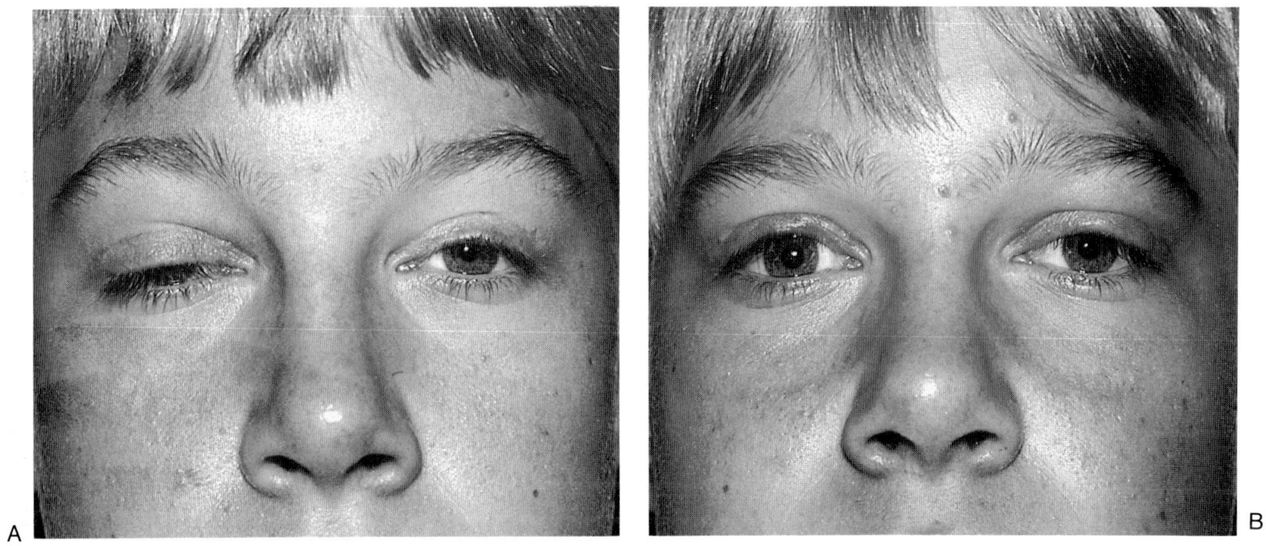

FIG. 13. Fascia. **A:** A young male who has had previous levator resection with poor elevation because of poor levator function. Patient is shown preoperatively before frontalis suspension with fascia. **B:** Same patient 2 weeks postoperatively following frontalis suspension with autogenous fascia lata.

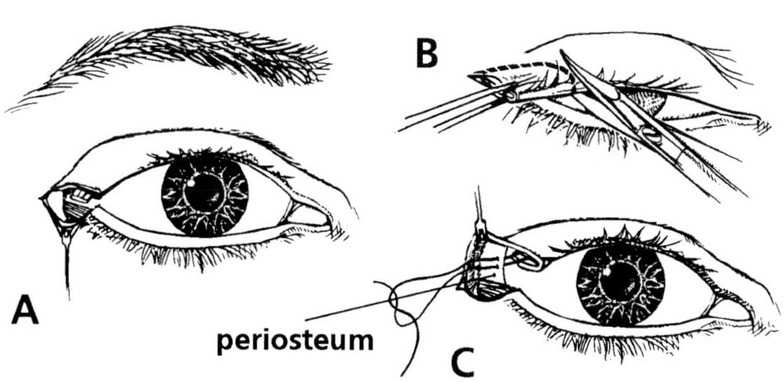

FIG. 14. Horizontal tightening of upper lid for unstable lid prior to frontalis suspension. Contour adjustment is extremely difficult with frontalis suspension when there is significant laxity in the upper lid. This commonly occurs with patients with prosthetic eyes but can also occur in other situations. **A:** A canthotomy and cantholysis of the upper limb of the canthal tendon is performed. **B:** A full-thickness resection of the lid at the outer edge including margin is performed after the lid is tensed to the orbital rim to determine the amount to resect. **C:** A 4-0 prolene suture is used to insert into the edge of the tarsal plate and into the periosteum laterally to tense the upper lid and correct the laxity so that the frontalis suspension will have adequate purchase.

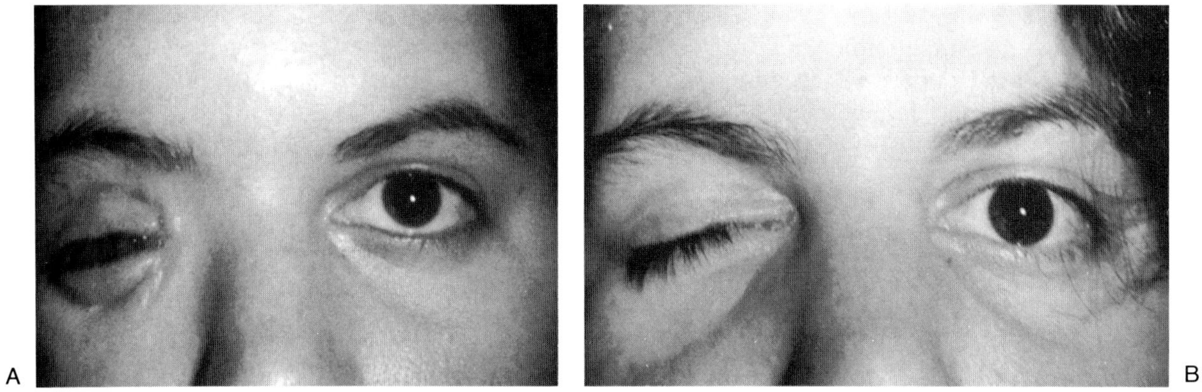

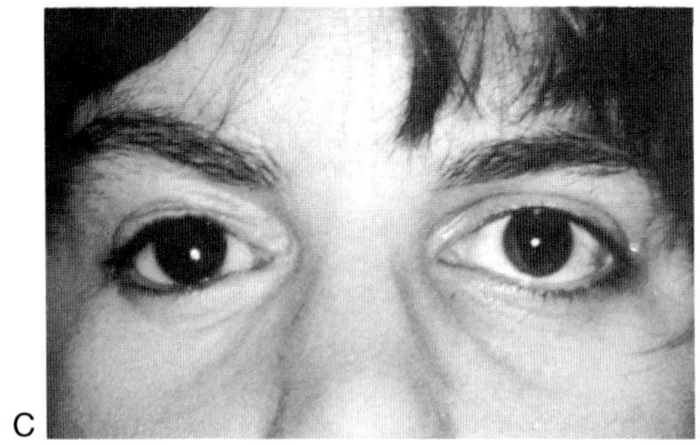

FIG. 15. Horizontal tightening with frontalis suspension. **A:** A young woman who had a severe facial injury with soft tissue and orbital deformities and loss of the right eye. She has dehiscence of the canthal tendons and no levator function. **B:** Patient following transnasal wiring correcting the right medial canthal dehiscence. **C:** Patient following frontalis suspension on the right with reasonable upper lid contour and elevation, which could only be accomplished after tightening of an otherwise lax lid with a lateral resection as well. The patient wears a prosthetic eye on the right.

FRONTALIS SUSPENSION USING THE SILICONE ROD

Silicone rod frontalis suspension is recommended in patients with poor eye protective mechanisms because of its ease of loosening or adjustment postoperatively (14,17,18). Lagophthalmos from any ptosis procedure can produce severe exposure keratopathy in patients with poor eye movement or extremely dry eyes. Patients who have weakness of eyelid closure from denervation or corneal anesthesia are also at risk for exposure keratopathy following ptosis surgery. The chapter on ptosis evaluation reviews the common situations with this risk. The solid silicone rod (1-mm) is ideal for this purpose (Fig. 16). Various retinal bands have been used in the past and cannot be configured to the eyelids successfully. Dow Corning has discontinued marketing the product, probably for medicolegal reasons, but it can be obtained from retail surgical supply houses. At the time of writing, in the state of Georgia, it can be obtained from Technical Products of Georgia (1-800-226-8434; 1-800-969-3366; TPI# 515-1; pack of three unsterile).

Technique

The following materials are needed:

1-mm silicone rod
Cutting general closure needle
Watzke sleeve (hollow polyethelyne tubing)
Braided nylon suture

A frontal block is performed and the brow and upper eyelid are injected with red-labeled xylocaine and Wydase. A 1.5 cm suprabrow incision is made, centered over the pupil. The incision is undermined, the frontalis muscle exposed, and the superior wound edge undermined for 1–2 mm for later fixation of the rod to the

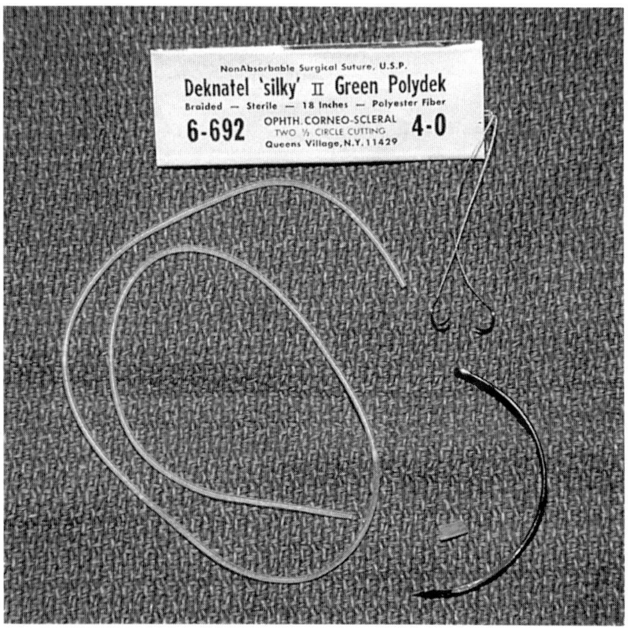

FIG. 16. Silicone. The materials required for frontalis suspension with this technique are shown: a 1-mm silicone rod, a Watzke sleeve, a general closure cutting needle, a soft nonabsorbable suture to secure the Watzke sleeve, in this case, polydek suture.

frontalis muscle. The proposed lid crease is marked, and a skin-muscle incision made to expose the central superior tarsus. If there is excess skin in the upper lid, a small strip of skin and orbicularis may be excised but one should be conservative when excising skin. The silicone rod is sutured to the tarsus centrally in the pupillary line, 4–5 mm below the superior tarsal border with an interrupted suture of 6-0 silk (Fig. 17A).

A general closure needle is then used to pass the rods through the eyelid into the brow incision. The needle is passed in the plane of the levator aponeurosis, through the preaponeurotic fat, exiting the brow in the center of the suprabrow incision, 4–5 mm apart. The arcus marginalis and frontalis muscle should not be engaged because this inhibits postoperative mobility of the eyelid (Fig. 17B). When passing the medial rod, the needle should first be angled toward the glabella for a distance of 1.5 cm before turning cephalad toward the center of the brow. This gives the correct vector forces on the tarsus and prevents bunching, tarsal buckling, and contour deformities from horizontal forces on the tarsus as the rod is tightened, elevating the lid. When the strands are pulled into the brow incision, the lifting force on the upper lid can be tested. If the central lid cannot be satisfactorily elevated, then the central lifting fixation suture should be placed further down on the tarsus for more purchase.

The medial and lateral sutures, which are mainly contour sutures, are placed and centered over the medial and lateral limbus, respectively. The position of these sutures can be changed later if necessary to make fine adjustments in lid contour. The ends of the rod in

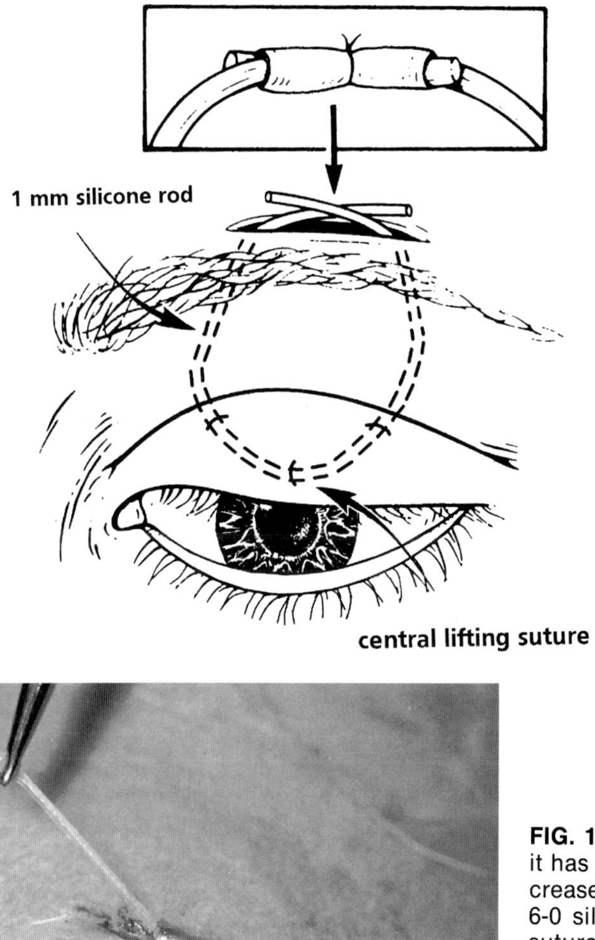

A

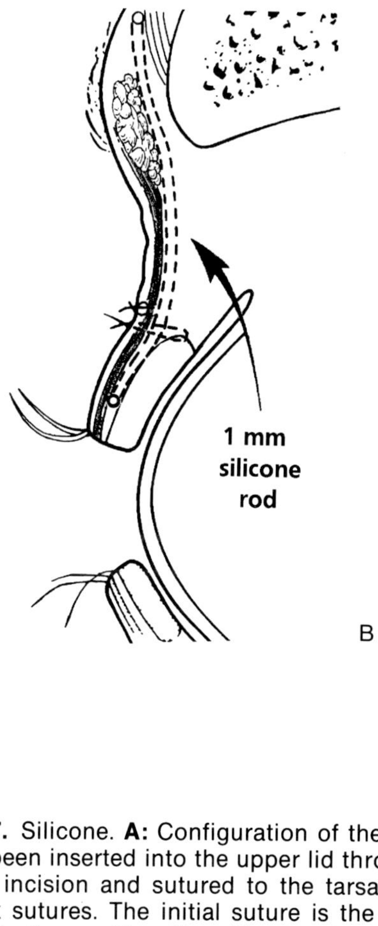

B

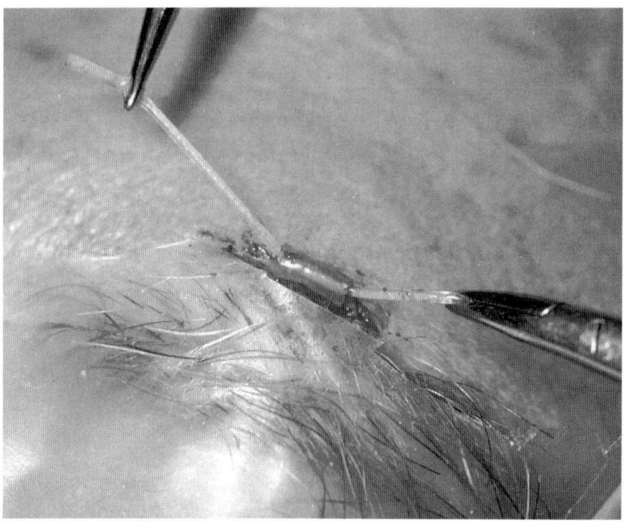

C

FIG. 17. Silicone. **A:** Configuration of the silicone after it has been inserted into the upper lid through an eyelid crease incision and sutured to the tarsal surface with 6-0 silk sutures. The initial suture is the central lifting suture in the pupillary line. The nasal and temporal sutures are adjusted according to the contour desired. The ends are threaded through a Watzke sleeve and secured with a nonabsorbable suture (4-0 braided nylon). **B:** Horizontal view showing the placement of the silicone rod on the anterior tarsal surface and the submuscular plane in its path to the frontalis muscle. Lid crease sutures have been inserted. **C:** Surgical view showing tightening of the silicone rod through the Watzke sleeve to obtain the desired lid elevation.

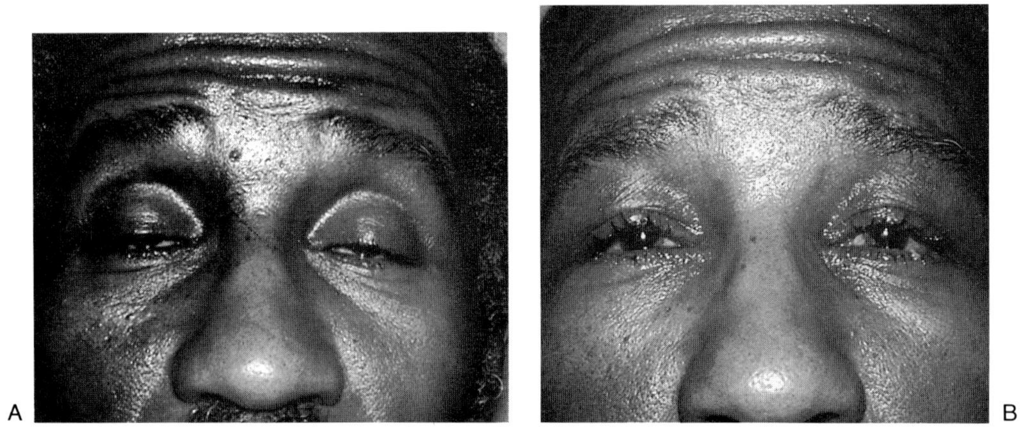

FIG. 18. Silicone. **A:** Patient with ocular myasthenia whose eyelids are unresponsive to Mestinon treatment with continued ptosis and visual obstruction. **B:** Same patient following silicone rod insertion. The patient is able to tolerate the elevation well without exposure despite poor ocular motility.

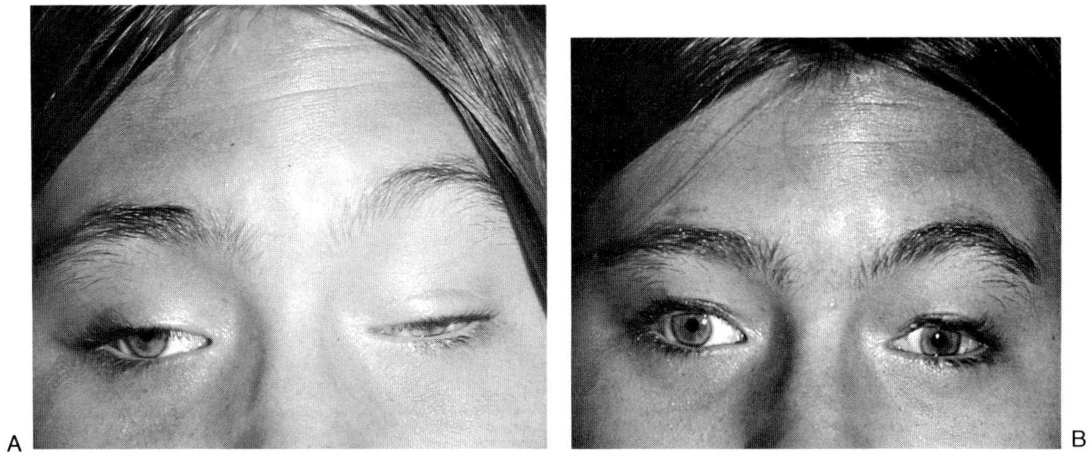

FIG. 19. Silicone. **A:** Young woman with congenital orbital fibrosis syndrome with poor extraocular function and poor eye protective mechanisms with risk of corneal exposure. **B:** Same patient after silicone rod frontalis suspension. There is less lagophthalmos than with other materials and good ability to elevate the eyelids. No corneal exposure was experienced.

the brow incision are now passed through a Watzke sleeve and pulled tight to adjust the eyelid to its upper height (Fig. 17C). The ends of the rod are trimmed long for later loosening if necessary. Do not overcorrect lid height by more than 1 mm. One braided nylon suture (4-0 Polydek) is tied around the Watzke sleeve, which in turn is sutured to the frontalis muscle. Bites deep in the galea should be avoided except in patients with facial nerve paresis who have no frontalis motility. The suprabrow incision is closed in layers. It is important to avoid superficial placement of the silicone to avoid granuloma formation. The eyelid wound is closed with a 5-0 subcuticular suture. The eyelid crease is formed with three double-armed 6-0 silk sutures. A Frost suture is usually not required. Ocular lubricants and ice provide comfort and decrease postoperative lid edema. Figures 18 and 19 show patients before and after frontalis suspension with a silicone rod bilaterally.

POSTOPERATIVE OFFICE ADJUSTMENT

One can adjust the eyelid position in the office if necessary. Infiltrate the brow with red-labeled xylocaine. A 1.5-cm incision is made through the previous scar in the brow and the Watzke sleeve is exposed. The Polydek suture is removed and the rods tightened or loosened to adjust the lid to the desired position. The sleeve is again secured to the frontalis muscle as previously described and the wound closed in layers.

REFERENCES

1. Beard C. *Ptosis*. 2nd ed. St Louis: CV Mosby; 1976.
2. Steinkogler FJ, Kuchar A, Huber E, Arocker-Mettinger E. Gore-tex soft-tissue patch frontalis suspension technique in congenital ptosisi and in the blepharophimosisptosis syndrome. *Plast Reconstr Surg* 1993;92:1057–1060.

3. Dickson JB. The use of a pedal extensor tendon in frontalis suspension surgery. *Ophth Surg* 1986;17:581–583.
4. Billet E. Bovine fascia lata in ptosis surgery. *Am J Ophthalmol* 1968;65:561–571.
5. Katowitz JA. Frontalis suspension in congenital ptosis using a polyfilament, cable-type suture. *Arch Ophthalmol* 1979;97: 1659–1663.
6. Beyer CK, Albert DM. The use and fate of fascia lata and sclera in ophthalmic plastic and reconstructive surgery. *Ophthalmology* 1981;88:869–886.
7. Bodian M. Repair of ptosis using human sclera. *Am J Ophthalmol* 1968;65:352–358.
8. Wright WW. The use of living sutures in the treatment of ptosis. *Arch Ophthalmol* 1922;51:99–102.
9. Crawford JS. Repair of ptosis using frontalis muscle and fascia-lata. *Trans Am Acad Ophthalmol Otolaryngol* 1956;60:672–678.
10. Berke RN. Discussion of repair of ptosis. *Trans Am Acad Ophthalmol Otolaryngol* 1956;60:678.
11. Crawford JS. Fascia lata: its nature and fate after implantation and its use in ophthalmic surgery. *Trans Am Ophthalmol Soc* 1968;66:673–745.
12. Crawford JS. Repair of ptosis using frontalis muscle and fascia lata. *Trans Am Acad Ophthalmol Otolaryngol* 1956;60:672–678.
13. Crawford JS. Frontalis sling operation. *J Pediatr Ophthalmol Strabismus* 1982;19:253–255.
14. Waller RR, McCord CD, Tanenbaum M. Evaluation and management of the ptosis patient. In: McCord CD, Tanenbaum M, eds. *Oculoplastic surgery*. New York: Raven Press; 1987: 365–371.
15. Antosyzyk JH, Tucker N, Ling C, Codere F. Interlocking Crawford triangles in frontalis suspension. *Arch Ophthalmol* 1993; 111:875–878.
16 Patrinely JR, Anderson RL. The septal pulley in frontalis suspension. *Arch Ophthalmol* 1986;Z104:1707–1710.
17. Tillett CW, Tillett GM. Silicone sling in the correction of ptosis. *Am J Ophthalmol* 1966;62:521–523.
18. Leone CR, Rylander G. A modified silicone frontalis sling for the correction of blepharoptosis. *Am J Ophthalmol* 1978;85: 802–805.

CHAPTER 10

Decision Making in Ptosis Surgery

Ptosis surgical technique requires skill and precision in handling of tissue and a thorough knowledge of anatomy. After acquiring these skills it is important for the surgeon to know how to apply each technique to a specific case. A system of decision making in ptosis surgery is as important as a knowledge of anatomy or surgical skills, and this section of the book is devoted to it.

The first step in the surgeon's system of logic is to decide which ptosis procedure to use (Fig. 1). After the selection of the procedure for a particular case, the success of ptosis surgery depends on intraoperative decision making (Figs. 2 and 3). Although many decisions are made preoperatively as to the application of a specific procedure, decision making that affects the grading of effect often occurs intraoperatively and depends on existing conditions that the surgeon observes during surgery. A logical series of responses to these observations intraoperatively can lead the surgeon to more predictable results.

PREOPERATIVE DECISION MAKING

The factor with which the surgeon must be concerned in choosing of procedures for postoperative safety and patient tolerance is the presence of adequate eye protective mechanisms. The factor that determines the type of procedure from the standpoint of surgical technique is the amount of levator function. Almost all ptosis surgery, except very conservative aponeurotic repair, will produce some lagophthalmos. Patients with deficient eye protective mechanisms may be tipped over into corneal exposure by ptosis surgery. It is well known that the most common postoperative problem in ptosis surgery leading to a medical-legal situation is corneal exposure following the ptosis surgical procedure. The presence of deficient eye protective mechanisms should lead to a more conservative approach to the surgery, a possible choice of an alternative procedure that is more reversible, and an explicit description of the possible consequences of surgery to the patient, which would include the potential necessity for reversing the surgical effect (see Fig. 1).

If eye protective mechanisms are determined to be normal in the preoperative exam, then the surgeon can proceed in the preoperative evaluation to the assessment of levator function. The preoperative decision with regard to choice of surgical technique depends on the amount of levator function.

In patients with good levator function of approximately 10 mm or more, there is most commonly an anatomic defect in the levator aponeurosis that is the basis of the ptosis, with the muscular portion of the levator usually being unaffected. The surgery in most of these cases should address the defect, and aponeurotic repair or advancement is the procedure of choice.

Patients with less than 4 mm of levator function are usually congenital or posttrauma ptosis patients with a "stiff" levator. The "supermaximal levator resection" or the "suspension of the lid on Whitnall's ligament" type of resection techniques can in many cases elevate the lid, but in most of these cases the amount of postoperative lagophthalmos may be severe and in some cases extreme and unacceptable. It has been the authors' experience that frontalis suspension offers a good elevation, good cosmesis, and a smaller amount of lagophthalmos because of brow motility in patients with extremely poor levator function. The arbitrary cutoff point of 5 mm is not rigid but in general terms it is felt that below 4 mm of levator function, resection is the less desired procedure.

The patients who have levator function between these two extremes are candidates for the classical levator resection, in which dissection of the horns and resection of Müller's muscle is carried out. These patients are usually not responsive to purely aponeurotic surgery, which would produce an undercorrection. Patients in this levator function range can get good elevation with mild lagophthalmos and should not be sub-

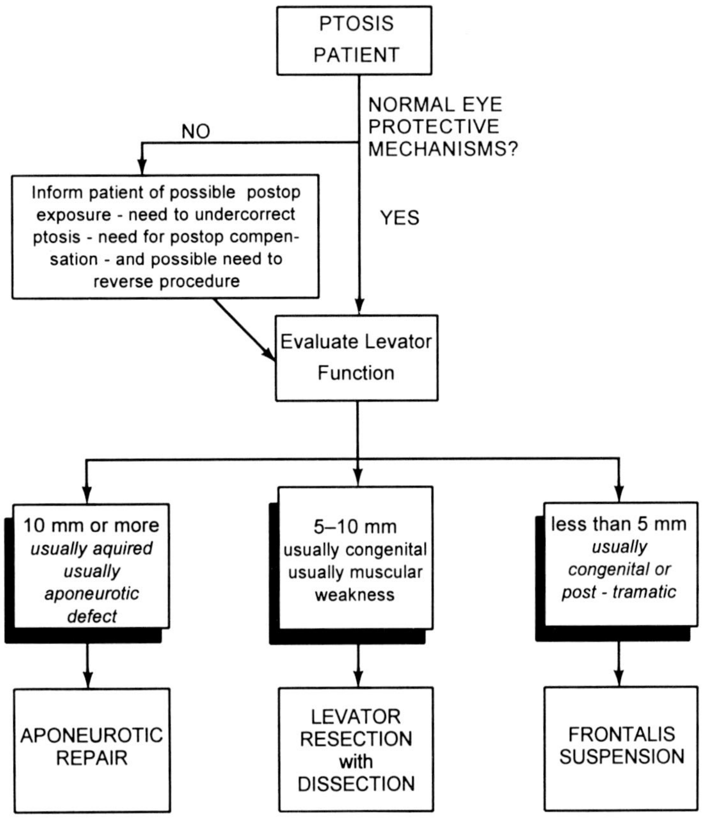

FIG. 1. Preoperative decision making.

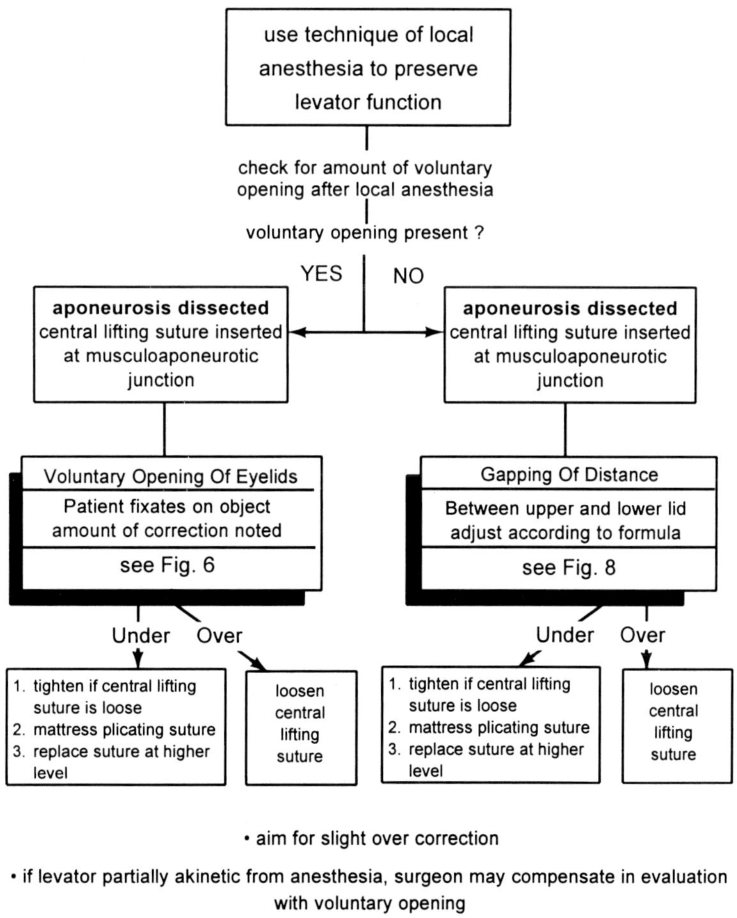

FIG. 2. Aponeurotic levator surgery (levator function 10± mm).

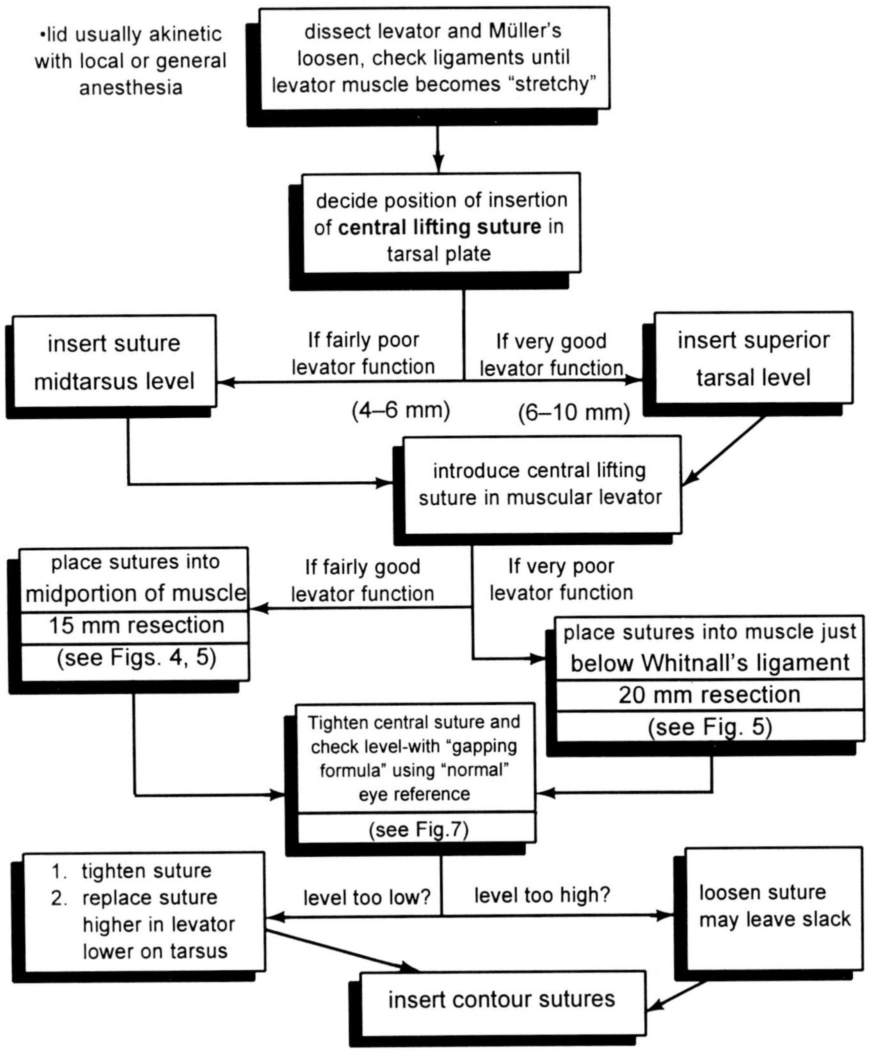

FIG. 3. Levator resection with dissection (levator function 4–10 mm).

jected to frontalis suspension. It is this "in-between" category of 5–10 mm of levator function that the patients get the best results with the classic levator resection with dissection (Berke).

INTRAOPERATIVE DECISION MAKING

Frontalis Suspension

Intraoperative decision making in frontalis suspension is not an issue since the lid is simply "set" on the operating table while the surgeon ensures good contour. There is usually little change postoperatively. This is simply a matter of observing good surgical technique. The placement of the upper lid intraoperatively is slightly higher than the desired postoperative position because of postoperative droppage. Care must be taken to loosen head drapes before adjusting the level. Traction by surgical drapes may produce artifactual elevation in the forehead area and cause postoperative undercorrection.

Levator Surgery

The patients who undergo levator surgery (aponeurotic surgery or levator muscle surgery with dissection) require that much more intraoperative judgment be applied. There are probably more intraoperative decisions to be made in aponeurotic surgery than in levator muscle surgery. Because of the greater leverage of effect one has with the levator in aponeurotic patients and the fact that aponeurotic patients can be adjusted via their own voluntary eyelid opening, there are more opportunities for "fine tuning" in these patients. Many of the patients undergoing levator resection with dissection are under general anesthesia and do not lend themselves to voluntary opening judgment. If local anesthesia is used the levator muscle usually becomes

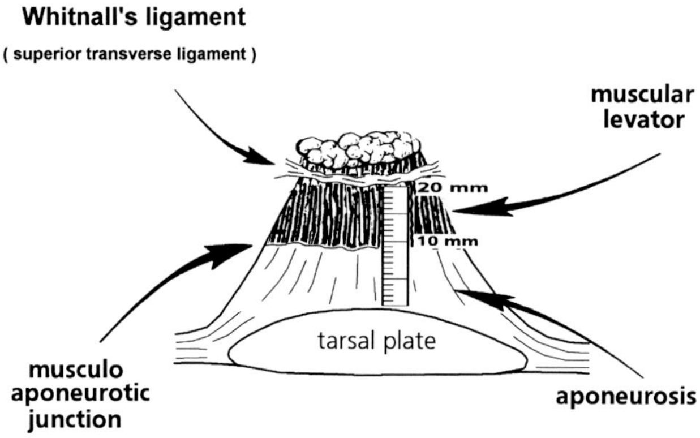

FIG. 4. Anatomic landmarks in the tarsolevator complex and approximate dimensions.

anesthetized and akinetic, also precluding use of the voluntary opening method.

Anatomic Starting Point

In all levator surgery the initial judgment that is made in order to place the central lifting suture is an anatomic one. In all cases the sutures that are brought from the tarsus are introduced in the levator at a predetermined position. This should be considered as the starting point for the two levator procedures and the secondary fine tuning of the lid level involves either intraoperative voluntary opening in aponeurotic surgery or intraoperative gapping of the lid in levator surgery with dissection.

Aponeurotic Repair

The musculoaponeurotic junction is the starting place for the insertion of the central lifting suture (Fig. 4).

Levator Resection with Extensive Dissection

The central lifting suture is placed in the muscular portion of the levator at a place determined by the amount of levator function with a method described by Beard (see previous chapter and Fig. 5 of this chapter).

In the aponeurotic patients, the surgeon may need to resort to an intraoperative gapping technique because of an inability to use the voluntary opening technique (because of anesthesia causing akinetic levator or because of the patient being uncooperative due to oversedation). Figure 2 shows the decision making involved in patients undergoing aponeurotic surgery. Figure 3 shows the decision making and intraoperative decision making involved in patients undergoing levator resection with dissection.

Voluntary Intraoperative Opening

Voluntary opening requires a kinetic (unanesthetized) levator and patient cooperation (light sedation) and is most commonly used with aponeurotic repair.

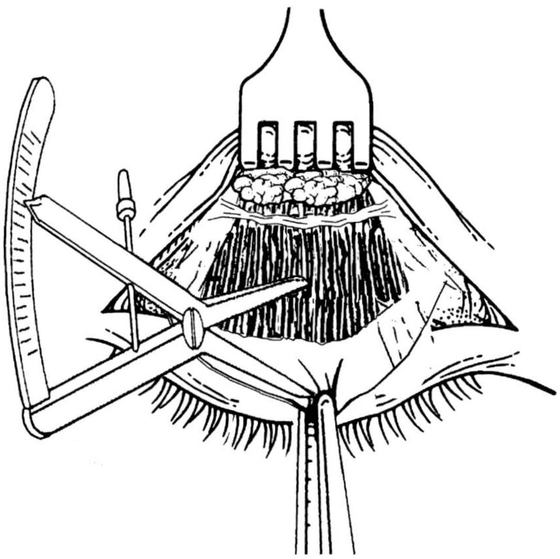

FIG. 5. Patient undergoing levator resection with extensive dissection measuring the location for placement of the central lifting suture, which would equate with the amount of resection performed.

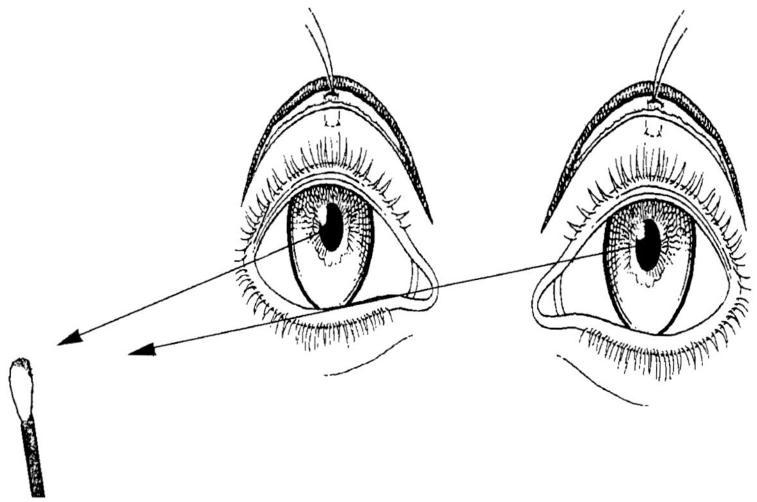

FIG. 6. Quantitation of eyelid elevation with voluntary opening during surgery. A kinetic (unanesthetized) levator is necessary as is light sedation to allow patient cooperation. If surgery is unilateral, the eyelid is set 1 mm above the desired level to compensate for loss of orbicularis tone. If surgery is bilateral, then adjust for elevation and symmetry.

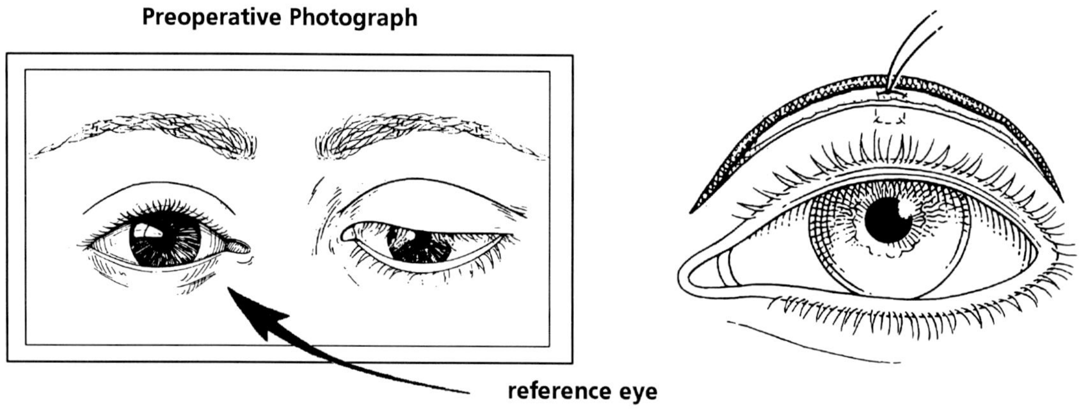

FIG. 7. Method of quantitating ptosis correction in patients undergoing levator resection with extensive dissection with general anesthesia or an akinetic (anesthetized) levator. A photograph of the patient must be used to determine the level of the normal eyelid, which is the point of reference for positioning the level of the operated eyelid during unilateral surgery. If the case is bilateral, then level and symmetry must be observed.

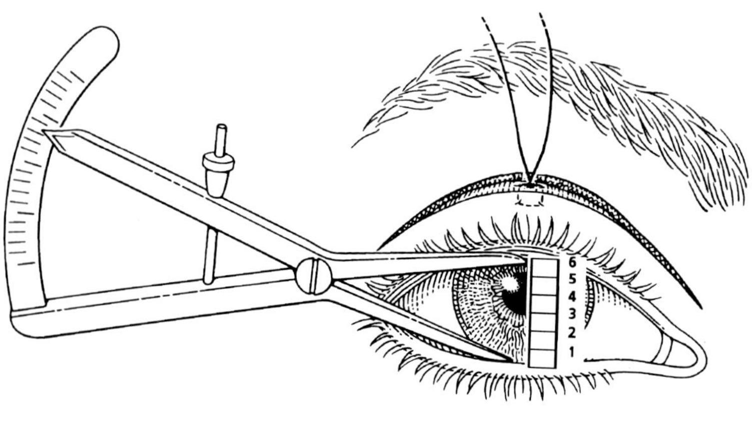

FIG. 8. Method of adjusting patients undergoing aponeurotic surgery if the levator becomes akinetic. The gapping method can be used to confirm other methods of quantitation. This is the least precise method but can be used if needed. The formula is included in the text. Spring-back symmetry can be helpful for confirmation.

The surgeon can adjust eyelid level and symmetry bilaterally. The surgeon can have the patient focus on a cotton applicator stick for this judgment (Fig. 6). If the surgery is for unilateral ptosis, then the operated lid must be placed slightly higher than the unoperated side to compensate for loss of tone of the orbicularis muscle from anesthesia. It is unusual to be able to use voluntary opening to quantitate patients undergoing levator resection with dissection because the amount of anesthesia needed to allow dissection usually causes akinesia.

Intraoperative Gapping

Intraoperative gapping is used in patients with an akinetic levator (general anesthesia or akinesia from local anesthesia) which is most commonly the patient undergoing levator resection with dissection. A modified gapping technique is used in patients undergoing aponeurotic surgery in whom the voluntary opening technique cannot be used because of an akinetic levator or poor cooperation.

Levator Resection with Extensive Dissection

The upper lid is set against the pupil or upper limbus. The position or point of reference is the level of the contralateral or normal eye (Fig. 7). The eyes must be straight ahead in the primary position for this judgment to be made. Light anesthesia must be avoided because it causes the eyes to roll upward from the primary position.

Aponeurotic Repair

The preoperative amount of ptosis is noted and a gapping of the upper and lower lids (distance in mm of the upper lid from the lower lid) is produced by tightening of the central lifting suture. It is quantitated for correction with the formulas:

Congenital ptosis = amount ptosis in mm + 4 mm

Acquired ptosis = amount of ptosis in mm + 2 mm

These formulas are used only in patients with good (>10 mm) levator function. This evaluation may be double-checked with the pupil–margin relationship for confirmation as one would do in patients undergoing levator resection with dissection. The amount of gapping corresponds in most cases.

"Spring-back" Evaluation with Gapping Methods

The confirming technique of spring-back evaluation with gapping methods is used in bilateral cases in which symmetry is needed (Fig. 8). After performing levator surgery according to the formula, the operative levels may seem equal but there still can be postoperative asymmetry due to other variables. This inequality can be discovered intraoperatively with the spring-back test. Because of asymmetries in suture placement between the two sides (further down on the tarsus or higher up on the levator, which the surgeon may use as compensation to get equal gapping by adjusting suture tension), postoperative asymmetric results can occur because of unequal leverage of the pull of the levator. This problem can in most cases be compensated for by ensuring that the passive tensions of the eyelids on the operating table are the same. In eyelids that appear to be gapped properly but have different tensions as shown by the spring-back test, in the looser lid the suture should be tightened with a plicating suture or replaced with a new suture until the spring-back is the same with equal gapping.

CHAPTER 11

Complications of Ptosis Surgery and Their Management

Correction of ptosis in many cases does not produce an entirely physiologic result and one should differentiate between expected side effects of the ptosis procedure and their effect on the patient, and true complications, i.e., unexpected results resulting from the ptosis operation.

In most ptosis operations, particularly in the congenital patient or those in whom frontalis suspension is performed, there is always stiffness of the eyelid postoperatively, which may cause stiffness in downgaze or lagophthalmos and some separation of the eyelids at night. The ptotic eyelid, although corrected for primary straight ahead gaze, will not move as quickly or have as wide an excursion as the normal side. The patient should be informed of this before surgery.

Another side effect that can take place in the presence of a surgically "perfect" ptosis procedure is that of corneal exposure and dry eye symptoms. Even if the person has a perfectly positioned lid postoperatively in the primary position and the expected amount of lagophthalmos or separation of the lids at night, the patient can still have severe symptoms of corneal exposure and pain if he or she does not have good eye protective mechanisms. It is to be emphasized that patients who demonstrate a deficiency in one of the protective mechanisms preoperatively should be approached with caution. They should be informed of the possibility of these symptoms postoperatively and told that if the eye does not tolerate being open the procedure will have to be reversed. This will save the patent from a prolonged course of postoperative pain and potential corneal damage, and shield the surgeon from medicolegal risk.

Complications are unexpected or unintended results that are not side effects of the surgery that may occur despite the surgeon's best intentions. They are often the result of deficiency in patient selection, improper judgment in surgical technique, or uncontrollable circumstances. Table 1 lists some of the more common complications.

OVERCORRECTION OF PTOSIS

Possible causes of postoperative overcorrection of ptosis are inaccurate measurement of levator function preoperatively, failure to identify the appropriate ptosis patient (acquired vs. congenital), and application of an inappropriate procedure in levator resection such as the use of a levator resection with extensive resection when an aponeurotic surgery would be proper. Overcorrection is a much more common problem following levator resection surgery than frontalis suspension surgery. A common situation is a localized temporal overcorrection in involutional patients with a lateral shift of the tarsal plate. It is obvious, however, that poor judgment and tightening of the suspensory material in frontalis suspension can result in overcorrection in some cases. For the large part, a discussion of overcorrection will be appropriate for patients who have undergone levator resection.

If areas of overcorrection are present postoperatively in patients who have undergone frontalis suspension, lysis of the offending strands can be performed.

Early Overcorrection

The treatment of overcorrection in most cases involves early postoperative adjustment. If the patient is severely overcorrected at 1 week; then with local infiltration office loosening of the central lifting suture can be performed. If mildly overcorrected at 1 week, the patient can be instructed to massage the lid downward.

TABLE 1. *Complications of ptosis surgery*

Undercorrection
Overcorrection
Excessive lagophthalmos
Corneal exposure or keratitis
Eyelid contour abnormality; temporal overcorrection
Eyelid crease asymmetry or abnormality
Eyelash ptosis or lash abnormalities
Entropion of the upper lid, ectropion of the upper lid or lid eversion
Extraocular muscle imbalance
Brow granuloma
Conjunctival prolapse
Hemorrhage and/or infection
Lacrimal gland cysts, damage, or dry eye syndrome

Technique of Massage

The patient is instructed to grasp the lashes of the upper eyelid with two fingers, hold the lid downward, and look upward while pulling the lid downward. The patient is told to do this for 40 times with sets of four per day. The eyelid margin position will be the highest at the end of the day when overnight swelling is gone, so the patient should look into the mirror at the end of the day and notice if the lid is still overcorrected. If it is, then a repeat set of massage should be performed the following day. At the end of that day, if the lid position is normal when the patient looks in the mirror, then the patient should omit the next day's exercises and rejudge the position the following afternoon.

Clipping the Central Lifting Suture

If the overcorrection is more than the patient will be able to correct by massage or if early attempted massage has produced no improvement in the overcorrection, then lysis of the central lifting suture and stretching of the upper lid in the office can correct most overcorrections. This must be done within the first 5–10 days before firm healing takes place (1–5).

A small amount of local anesthetic is placed in the crease incision. The incision can be grasped with forceps and separated by pulling, exposing the central lifting suture. The suture is then cut and the lid stretched downward, observing the margin position after each tug, until the desired position is reached. If the correction is done very early, topical anesthetic can be used (Fig. 1A,B). A patient undergoing early adjustment can be seen in Fig. 2A and B.

Spacer Material Implant

Either massage or clipping sutures and massage will almost always remedy the overcorrection if treated early. In patients with overcorrections that are "old"—either patients referred by other doctors or those who have returned with poor follow-up—it is difficult to lower the lid by dissection without insertion of spacer material and have the lid stay down. Healing will contract and reelevate the lid. In these patients, the lid crease incision is made over the area of overcor-

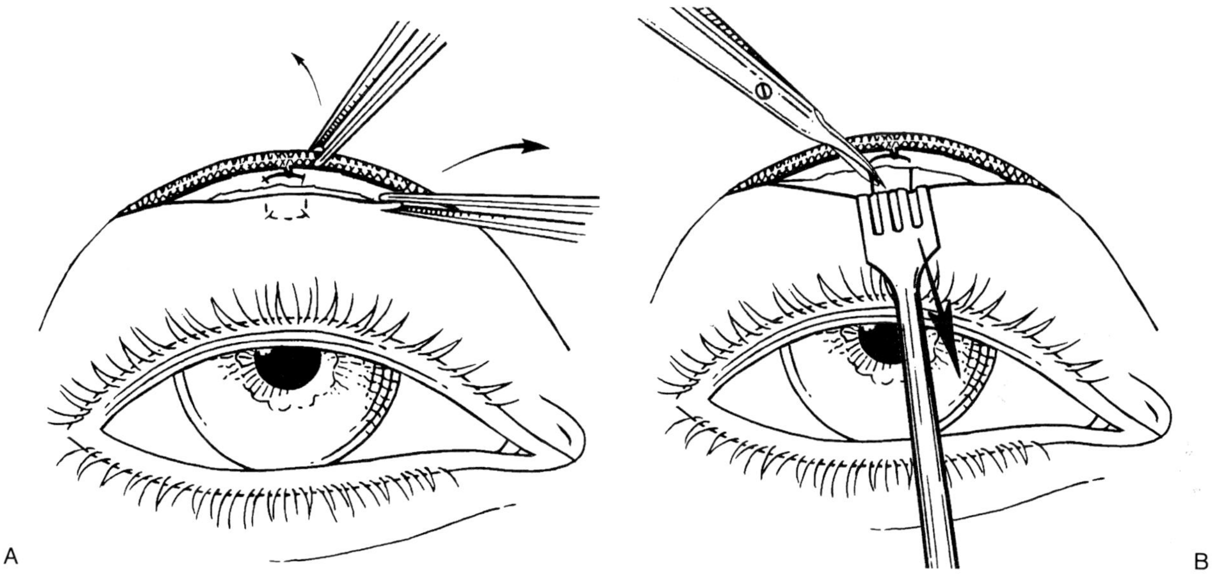

FIG. 1. Early overcorrection. **A:** If within 5–10 days the patient is overcorrected; a loosening of the central lifting suture can be performed with superficial local anesthesia in the office. The wound can usually be separated giving access to the central lifting suture. **B:** Lysis of the central lifting suture will allow the lid to be lengthened with downward retraction. The "tissue glue" at this point will maintain the lid position at the loosened position even though the suture has been partially or completely lysed.

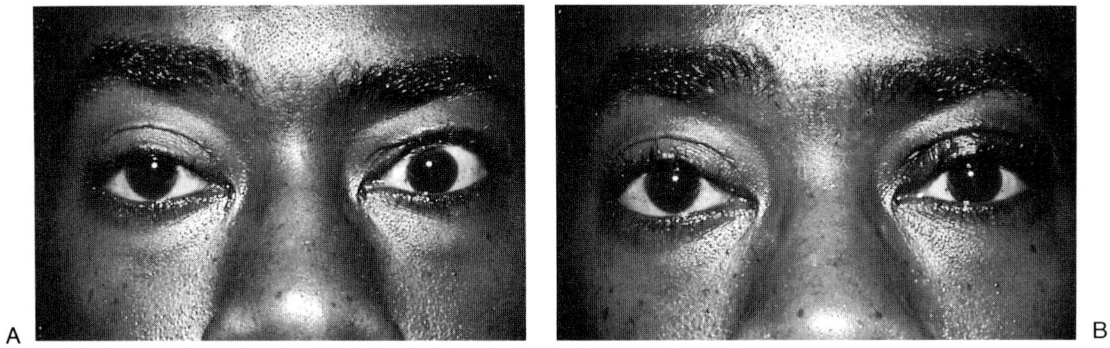

FIG. 2. Early overcorrection. **A:** Patient on first postoperative visit following levator resection in the left upper lid with overcorrection. **B:** Following loosening of the central lifting and lateral suture under superficial anesthesia in the office.

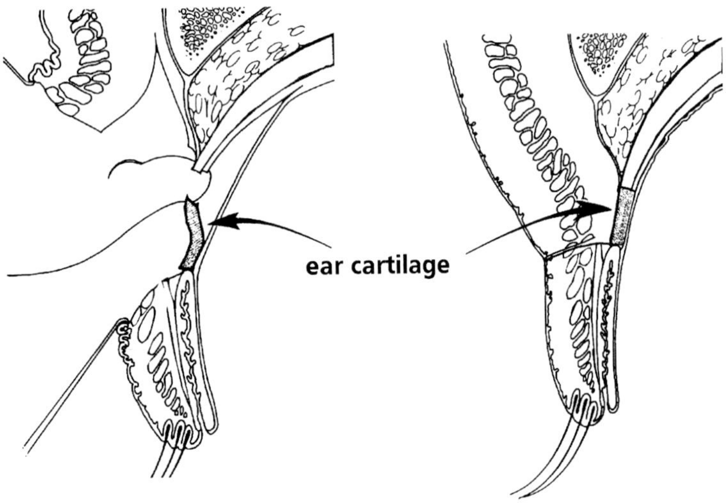

FIG. 3. Late overcorrection. Once the tissue has firmly healed, the eyelid cannot be loosened by relaxation of the lifting suture because the tissue adhesions are too strong. Simple recession of the levator will generally result in only a temporary correction since during the healing, the lid will tend to retract back upward. To prevent this, spacer material must be inserted to lower the lid or lengthen the lid the desired amount to overcome the retraction during healing.

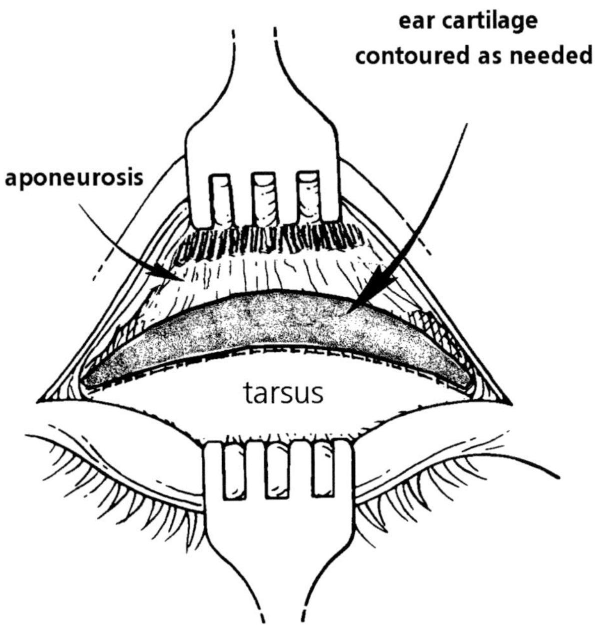

FIG. 4. Late overcorrection. This shows the levator aponeurosis (and Müller's muscle) recessed with spacer material interposed between the superior edge of the tarsal plate and the retractors. If dissection is carried out only at the superior edge of the tarsus, a one-for-one vertical amount of tissue can be used.

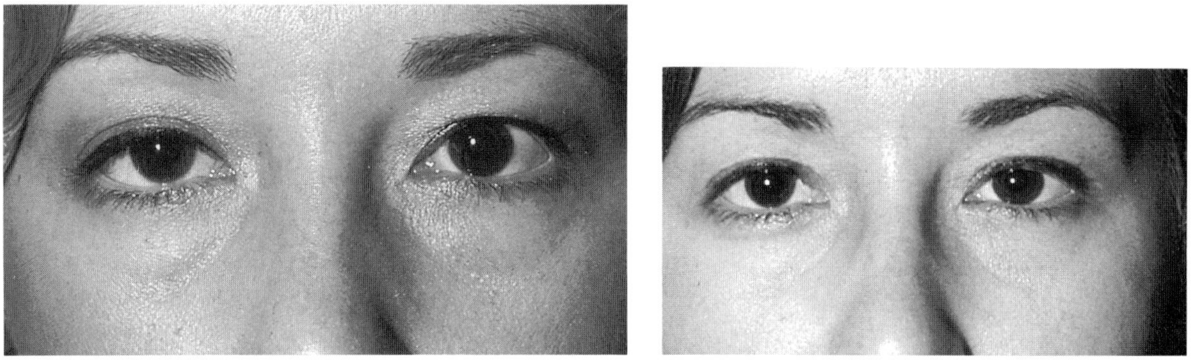

FIG. 5. Late overcorrection. **A:** A patient who had a symmetric overcorrection of the left upper lid following levator resection that had taken place approximately 5 months prior. **B:** Same patient following recession of the levator complex with a spacer material implant.

rection and lysis of the levator from the superior edge of the tarsal plate is performed. Ear cartilage in one-to-one ratio to the overcorrection is then placed between the superior edge of the tarsal plate and the recessed levator (and Müller's muscle). Care is taken to reform the crease in the desired position with transcutaneous sutures (Figs. 3 and 4). Figure 5A and B shows a patient corrected by this technique.

UNDERCORRECTION OF PTOSIS

Often mild undercorrection of ptosis is not confirmed until 3–4 weeks following surgery because postoperative swelling of the lid may mask where the final position of the lid margin will be. In general, cases of acquired ptosis with good levator function will elevate postoperatively with time whereas congenital cases with poorer levator function will tend to fall as edema subsides. Cases that are moderate to severely undercorrected will usually be obvious at the outset.

In most cases undercorrection of ptosis occurs in the patient undergoing levator resection because the surgeon overestimated the levator function. Many times this happens because in measuring levator function the brow is not adequately splinted or there is poor patient cooperation. Failure to recognize a congenital ptosis case that may first present in an adult will also cause the surgeon to underestimate the amount of levator resection needed and the incorrect procedure may be chosen for correction. In most cases patients with poor levator function do not respond well to Fasanella-type procedures or aponeurotic surgery alone.

Undercorrection can also occur with frontalis suspension because of failure to secure the suspensory material adequately in the soft tissue or because of inadequate intraoperative adjustment. Tight surgical drapes in the forehead area can cause the surgeon to overestimate the surgical correction intraoperatively.

In some cases, such as in children with blepharophimosis syndrome, it is extremely difficult to elevate the lid enough to get a full correction because of the tissue anomalies and this must be accepted.

If the undercorrection is mild and the patient has gotten a good lid crease formation that was lacking before surgery, the patient may be pleased enough to accept the mild undercorrection. Undercorrections that are not acceptable require surgical modification.

The treatment of undercorrection is more involved than that of overcorrection because in most cases it involves surgical intervention. In patients who have had aponeurotic surgery alone, often tightening of the central lifting suture can be done under local anesthesia in the office over a 5- to 10-day interval. For patients with congenital ptosis who have had extensive dissection or who will not accept office surgery, or in cases of frontalis suspension, a formal reoperation is usually necessary.

Technique of Advancing the Central Lifting Suture

The lid crease and pretarsal area is infiltrated with a small amount of local anesthetic. A crease incision is made and an adequate area of the pretarsal area exposed. The edge of the aponeurosis is exposed and dissected free. A new double-armed suture is advanced further downward on the tarsal plate from its previous position on the tarsus, reinserted higher in the aponeurosis, and tightened to observe the effect with voluntary opening of the eyelid by the patient. If the suture placement in the initial operation was near the upper edge of the tarsus, the surgeon may need only to advance the suture downward. To avoid multiple insertions it is better that the surgeon overestimate and slightly exaggerate the suture placements initially. Slack can always be left in the suture to obtain the proper level (Fig. 6A, B).

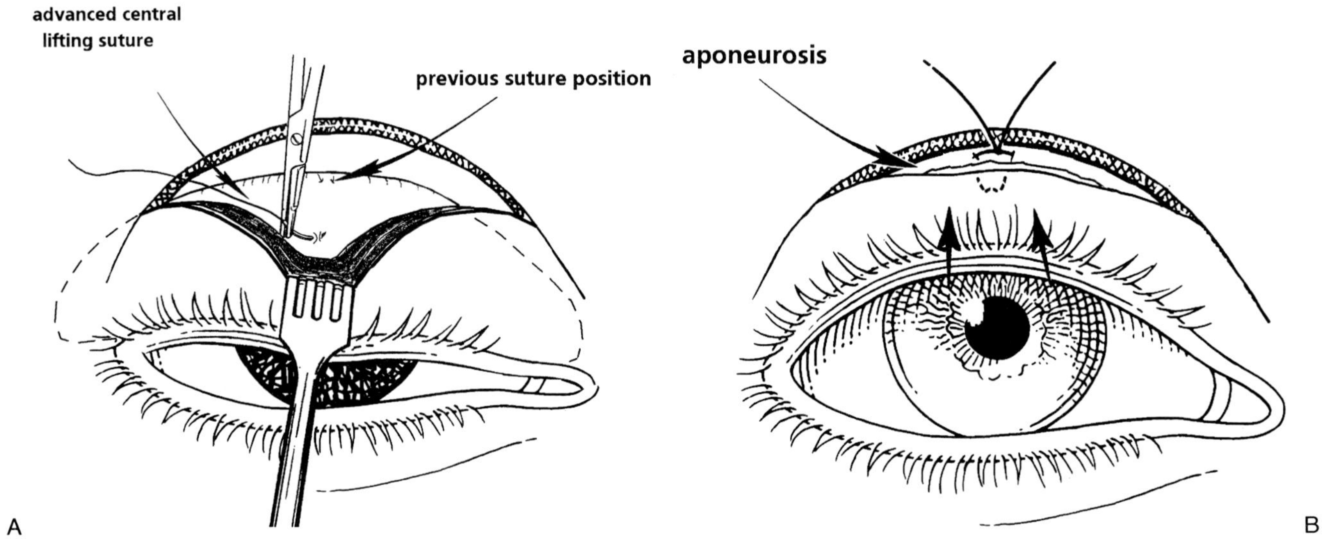

FIG. 6. Mild to moderate undercorrection. **A:** With superficial crease anesthesia the superior edge of the tarsal plate can be exposed and an additional central lifting suture can be inserted further down into the tarsus, advancing the tissue onto the tarsal plate with a plicating lifting suture. **B:** Tightening the suture shows the desired elevation of the undercorrected lid being obtained. More elevation can be obtained by also placing the suture higher in the aponeurosis.

EXCESSIVE LAGOPHTHALMOS WITH CORNEAL EXPOSURE

As previously mentioned, some lagophthalmos is inherent in most ptosis surgery. However, excessive lagophthalmos to the point of being cosmetically unacceptable or producing symptoms can occur from imprecise application of surgical techniques. In patients with poor eye protective mechanisms this presents a more acute and distressing situation. In levator resection surgery, overestimation of the amount of levator to be resected, particularly if a Whitnall's ligament sling is used or the levator is stiff and inelastic, can produce excessive lagophthalmos. More commonly, incorporation of the orbital septum into the skin or wound, or failure to open the septum adequately, will result in severe lagophthalmos.

Severe levator fibrosis from intrinsic causes or postoperative fibrosis can also result in lagophthalmos. If the lagophthalmos is associated with lid retraction, then recession of the lid with spacer material can help. It is usually difficult or impossible, without finding a specific strand that plays a role in lagophthalmos, to restore elasticity to the eyelid.

With patients who have levator resection with extensive dissection, care must be taken to completely separate the levator–Müller's complex from the underlying conjunctiva and fornix. Incorporation of the fornix into the levator resection will cause eyelid retraction when the eye moves upward, extreme separation of the eyes at night, and severe lagophthalmos with corneal exposure. This can be avoided with careful anatomic surgical dissection. At the end of the procedure, the globe should be grasped by the rectus muscles and passively rotated to ensure that the globe moves independently of the eyelid.

CONTOUR ABNORMALITY

A very common cause of eyelid contour abnormality is the result of failure to recognize a "lax" lid or diplaced tarsus. This can occur in patients with floppy upper lid syndrome, patients who have lateral tarsal shift from involutional changes, and patients who have prosthetic eyes.

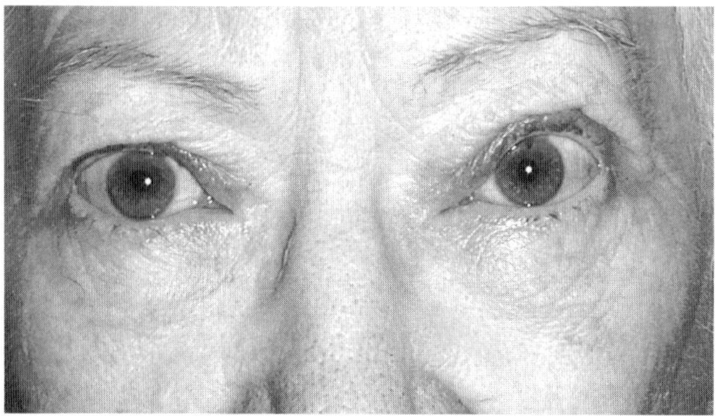

FIG. 7. Contour abnormality. In this patient, who had involutional ptosis and a "lateral tarsal shift," the postoperative temporal flare seen is the result of placing the central lifting suture in the apex of the tarsal plate that had been shifted laterally.

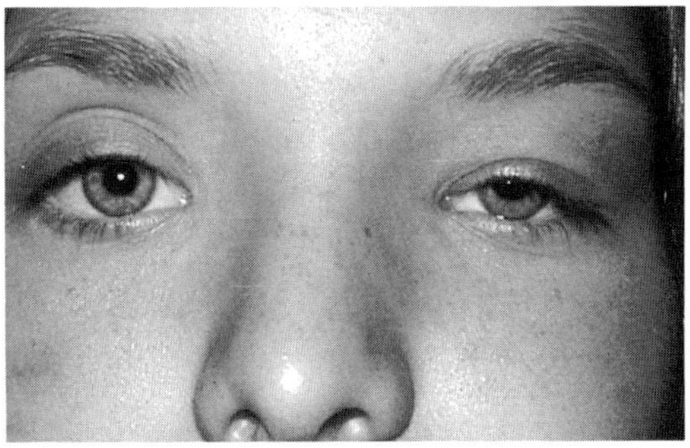

FIG. 8. Eyelid crease asymmetry. This patient was reported to have had different amounts of levator resection in both eyes and some fat removal from the right side. The resulting failure to attach the crease and asymmetric fat removal resulted in eyelid crease asymmetry.

Figure 7 shows a contour abnormality from failure to recognize a lateral tarsal shift. Faulty placement of the central lifting suture in patients who have lateral tarsal shift will cause a temporal overcorrection commonly noted in these patients in the past. In patients undergoing frontalis suspension (or levator resection), if the upper lid is extremely lax and does not lend itself to the contouring with the purchase points of the sutures or suspensory material, then a horizontal tightening procedure should be done in the upper lid laterally to tense the lid so that it will conform to the globe. Purchase points of the suspensory material or lifting sutures can then be placed more successfully to produce a pleasing contour.

Postoperatively, contour adjustments can be made with focal plications of the levator-tarsus in the office. Lysis or plication of the suspensory material in frontalis suspensions may require return to the operating room because many of the patients are children.

Postoperative contouring can be performed by localized resections of the tarsal plate; however, it is probably best to avoid tarsal resection when possible to avoid tarsal instability (6,7).

EYELID CREASE ABNORMALITY

Asymmetry of the eyelid crease can occur particularly if there is a levator resection in a unilateral case (Fig. 8). In the unilateral case of levator resection, a small strip of skin can be excised to compensate for some redundancy but no fatty tissue should be removed. There is a tendency to place the lid crease too high if it is sutured to the levator muscle, so the lid crease should be formed with transcutaneous crease sutures fixing it directly to the tarsal plate at a position symmetric to the opposite side. Crease problems are also a problem with frontalis suspension procedures (8).

Another reason for asymmetric crease positioning is continued asymmetric eyebrow arching by patients with congenital ptosis. Despite the postoperative elevation of the lid the patient will out of habit continue to arch the brow, which will pull the eyelid skin up and cause an asymmetric-appearing crease. Asymmetric eyebrow arching should be noted preoperatively and pointed out to the patient. A trans-lid eyebrow pexy (see Chapter 14) can be performed in many cases to stabilize the brow if needed.

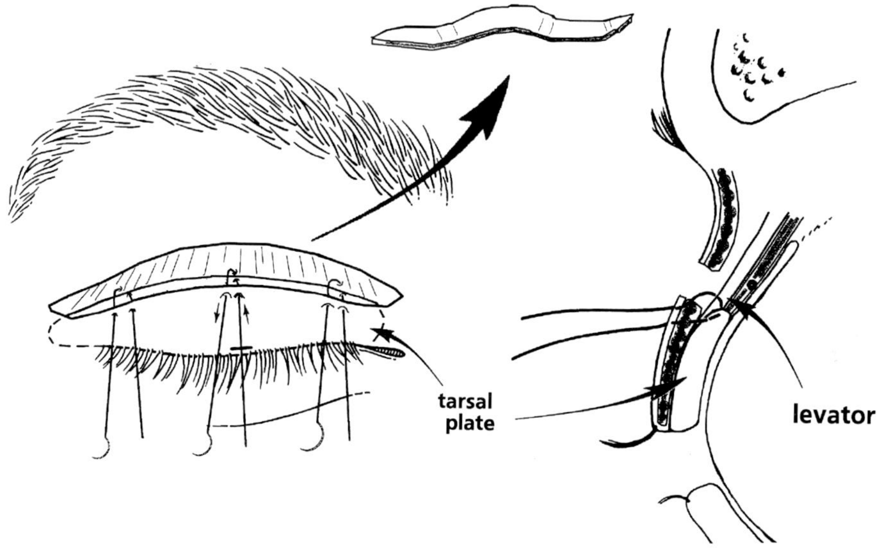

FIG. 9. Diagrammatic representation of the eyelid crease procedure that involves excision of skin-muscle strip above the desired position of the crease and plication of the pretarsal skin to the superior edge of the tarsus incorporating some of the levator aponeurosis to reform the crease. This can also have a rotational effect on the eyelashes depending on how far down in the pretarsal skin the plicating sutures are introduced.

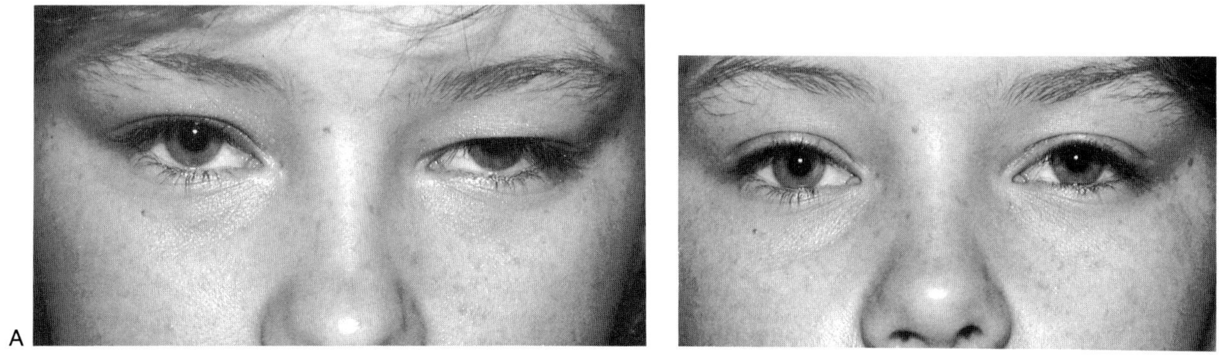

FIG. 10. Loss of eyelid crease in left upper lid following levator resection. **A:** Patient preoperatively. **B:** Patient following eyelid crease procedure with skin excision and plication of pretarsal skin.

The failure of stimulus to arch the brows can occur postoperatively when the lid reaches a more normal level causing the person to relax the brow, and then redundant skin will appear. This should be considered in the preoperative planning and an appropriate amount of skin removed to ensure the formation of the desired position of the lid crease without excessive folding.

In patients who have had previous surgery or trauma, the pretarsal skin will often contract postoperatively and the lid crease will be lost. This can also occur in patients who have had frontalis suspension in which the pretarsal skin is plicated to the suspensory material itself, such as fascia, as opposed to the superior edge of the tarsal plate. Chronic pulling of the suspensory material will pull the lid crease loose.

Patients who have had prior surgery or trauma have great difficulty in maintaining the position of a lid crease despite revisional surgery. For such patients it is recommended that when the new lid crease is formed, crease sutures be inserted and additional transcutaneous sutures used to further create adhesions of the pretarsal skin to the tarsal plate (9–11) (Fig. 9). A patient requiring a reformation of the crease is shown in Fig. 10 A and B.

EYELASH PTOSIS AND ENTROPION OF THE UPPER LID

If the pretarsal skin is not adequately tensed and a strong eyelid crease formation is created at the time of the initial ptosis procedure, whether it be levator resection or frontalis suspension, a postoperative laxity and downward migration of the lashes can occur. This is a particularly severe problem when operating on patients who have had previous ptosis surgery in whom the pretarsal skin may contract or the tarsus is unstable. Prolonged swelling of the pretarsal skin can also aggravate this problem. If the tarsal plate is other-

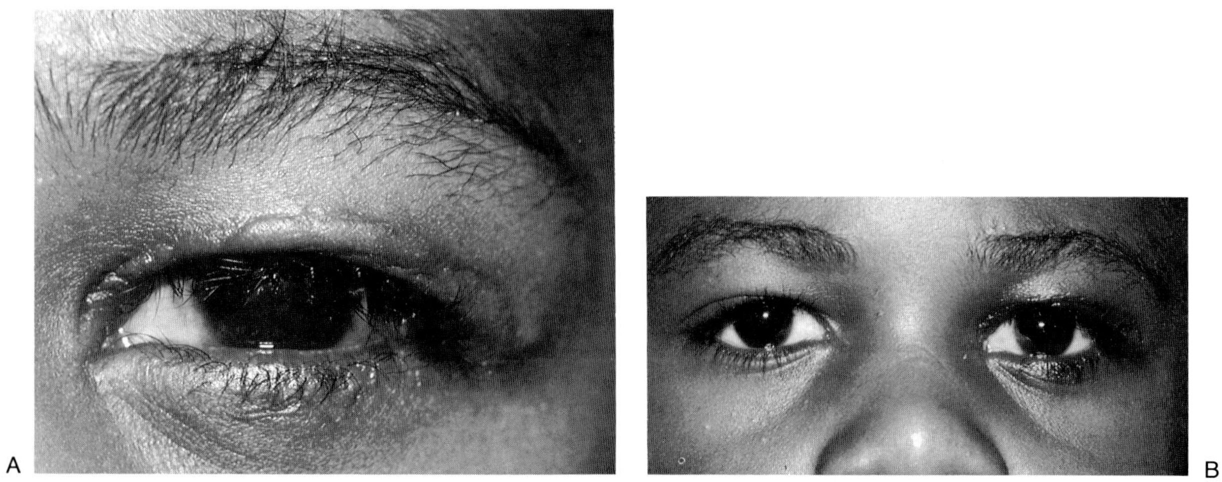

FIG. 11. Loss of eyelid crease and entropion of left upper lid with corneal abrasions. **A:** Patient who had had three previous levator procedures with loss of crease and inverting of the eyelid margin and lashes causing multiple corneal abrasions. **B:** Same patient postoperatively after resection of scar tissue and plication of pretarsal skin with the eyelid crease procedure.

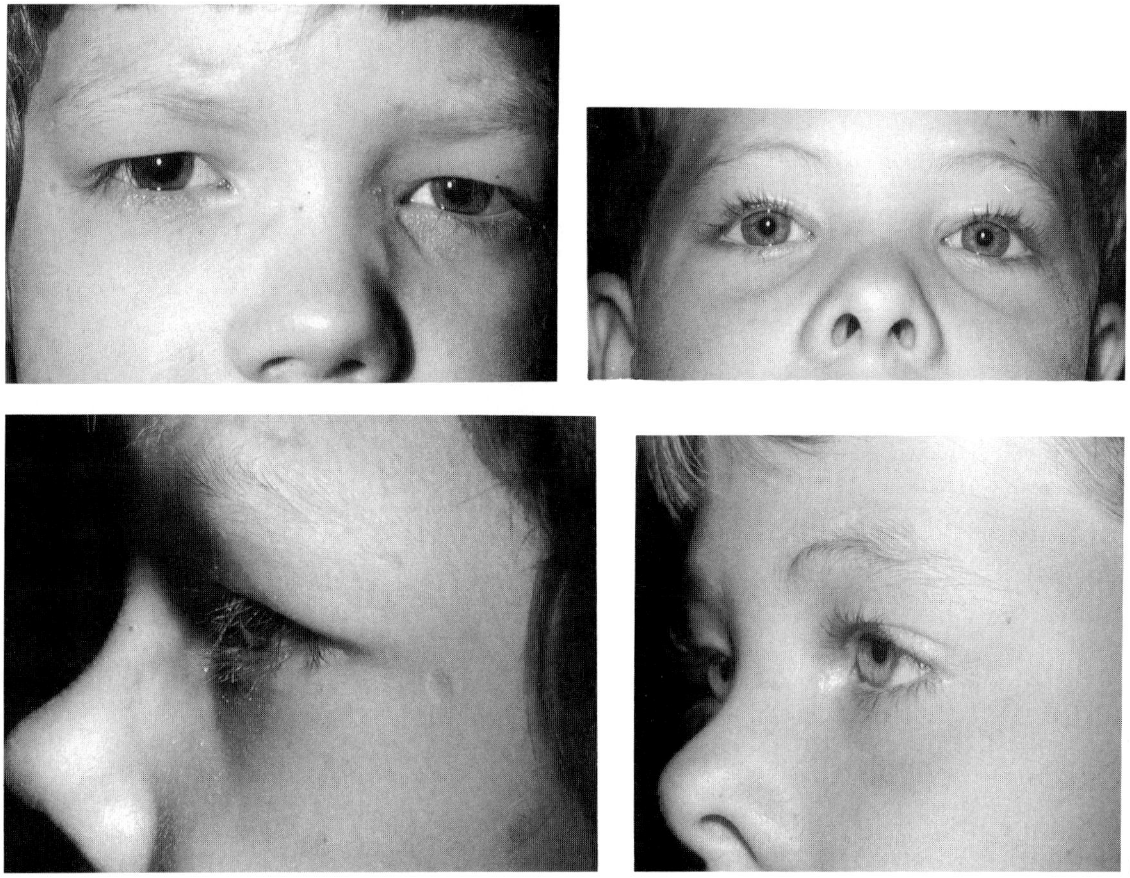

FIG. 12. Entropion and loss of eyelid crease following frontalis suspension. **A:** Young boy who had had a frontalis suspension shows entropion with lashes touching cornea, loss of crease, and a bulkiness and redundancy of tissue in upper lids. **B:** Same patient following resection of skin and fatty tissue plication of pretarsal skin to reform eyelid crease with rotation of lashes. **C:** Same patient preoperatively showing side view. **D:** Same patient postoperatively showing rotation of lashes and reformation of crease.

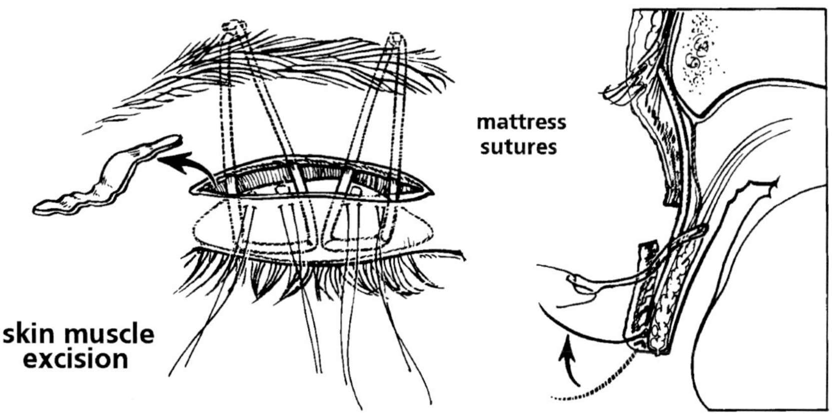

FIG. 13. Diagram of procedure for the correction of entropion and lash ptosis following frontalis suspension. A skin-muscle strip is removed exposing the superior edge of the tarsal plate. Transcutaneous pretarsal skin sutures can be used to plicate the skin to the superior edge of the tarsus. This will correct entropion and eyelid crease abnormalities in these patients. Patients who also have an undercorrection from the frontalis suspension can gain elevation with attachment of sutures to the strands of the suspensory material and with plication, elevating the lid.

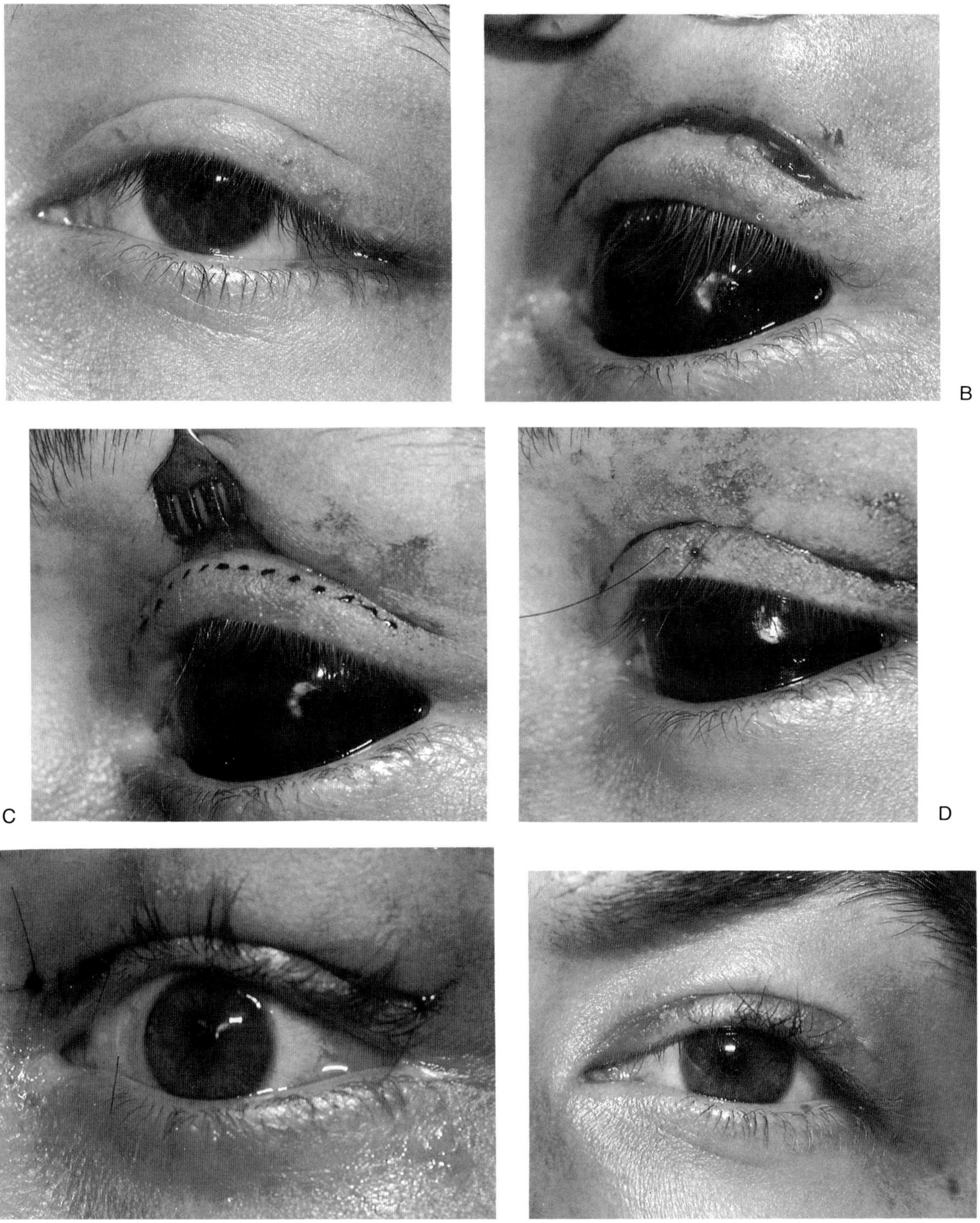

A B C D E F

FIG. 14. Undercorrection and rotation of the lashes following frontalis suspension. **A:** Patient eyelid shown preoperatively with undercorrection, lash ptosis, and entropion. **B:** A skin eyelid crease incision is made exposing the suspensory strands in the superior edge of the tarsal plate. **C:** After testing the desired tension required in the pretarsal skin, a strip of skin is removed at the superior edge. **D:** Transcutaneous sutures are placed in the pretarsal skin to tense the skin for lash rotation and are also placed in the suspensory elements for elevation of the lid. **E:** The transcutaneous pretarsal sutures have been tightened rotating the lid and elevating the lid, and the skin has been closed. **F:** The view of the same eyelid following suture removal at 1 week.

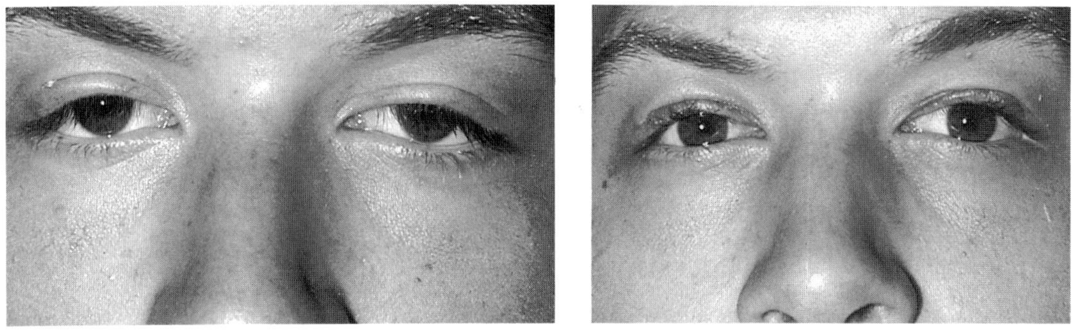
A B

FIG. 15. Undercorrection and lash ptosis following frontalis suspension. Same patient whose eyelid was seen in Fig. 14. **A:** Patient preoperatively. **B:** Same patient postoperatively at 10 days following suture removal.

wise stable and undistorted, then a surgical crease procedure and tensing of the pretarsal skin to the superior edge of the tarsus can be performed (12,13). One can use additional quilting sutures in the pretarsal area to further form the crease. An actual entropion of the upper lid can occur from a buckling outward of the superior edge of the tarsal plate or folding of the tarsal plate if either suspensory material has caused buckling of the tarsus over a period of time (14).

This can also occur after levator resection if the levator is plicated to the tarsal plate too far down in front of the lashes and is a very distressing problem. In patients who have had levator resection, a revision of the wound with respositioning of the levator attachments, plication of the pretarsal skin, and straightening of the tarsal plate with quilting sutures will in most cases correct this problem (Fig. 11A and B).

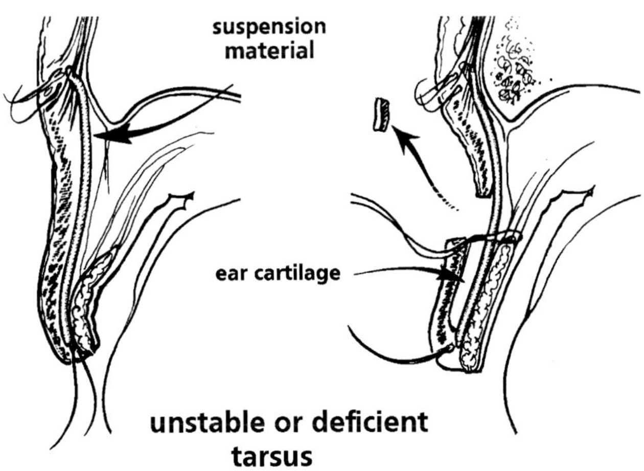

FIG. 16. Entropion of the upper lid following frontalis suspension in patients who have deficient tarsus or unstable tarsal plate. The diagram shows the necessary placement of a stabilizing ear cartilage graft in the pretarsal area. The pretarsal skin is then tensed over the graft to the superior edge of the existing tarsus to stabilize the area and to rotate the lashes.

Entropion of the upper lid is more common and more commonly seen following frontalis suspension procedures. Revision of the lid crease, usually with excision of a strip of skin and tensing of the pretarsal skin with mattress sutures, can correct most cases (Figs. 12–15).

In some of these cases, after frontalis suspension the tarsal plate becomes completely folded with time. Even if the tissue is rearranged with revisional surgery at a revisional procedure, it will tend to recontract during the healing process because of fibrous strands and the entropion will recur. In a number of these very difficult cases the author has used supplementation of ear cartilage to stabilize the tarsal plate area to provide a full correction for this procedure. This has corrected this problem in severe postfrontalis suspension entropion procedures that have failed with other procedures (Fig. 16).

ECTROPION OR MARGIN ROTATION OF THE UPPER LID

Ectropion or margin rotation of the upper lid is more common in patients who have had frontalis suspension but may occur following levator surgery if the levator fixation sutures are placed too low or the pretarsal skin is overtensed. Excessive traction of suspensory material, particularly if the purchase points are just in front of the lashes, often can produce an outward turning of the lower lid margin. Children who are used to arching their brows many times will continue to arch the brows and with excessive brow arching can separate the lid from the globe. If the lid position is normal when the eyebrow position is relaxed, the parent should be reassured and the children should be retrained to not arch their brow as often. In patients who have some outturning of the margin, even when resting, the levator or suspensory material is attached too far inferiorly or is too tight, and revisional surgery is needed to relax or recess the suspensory material or the levator muscle attachments (8).

EXTRAOCULAR MUSCLE IMBALANCE

Superior oblique paresis following ptosis surgery or, in some cases, superior rectus paresis can occur. This is not a common complication but most likely occurs with overly aggressive dissection of the nasal horn of the levator muscle (which in most cases is unnecessary) with injury to the superior oblique, or failure to identify the levator muscle itself and the confusing of it with the superior rectus muscle.

LOSS OF EYELASHES

Eyelash loss is most likely to occur in patients who have frontalis suspension because the purchase points of the suspensory material is often in the vicinity of the lash follicle roots. Care should be taken when dissecting in this area to avoid damage of follicles with loss of lashes or misdirection of lashes.

CONJUNCTIVAL PROLAPSE

Conjunctival prolapse is an unusual complication but has been seen in some children who have undergone extensive levator resections with dissection. It may be the result of the complete separation of the forniceal attachments of the conjunctiva from the undersurface of the levator combined with postoperative swelling. For refractory cases that don't improve with patching or intermarginal sutures, mattress sutures can be brought through the prolapsed conjunctiva and repositioned into the upper fornix with sutures brought out transcutaneously and tied (15–17). In certain cases, some of the redundant conjunctiva can be resected (Fig. 17A, B).

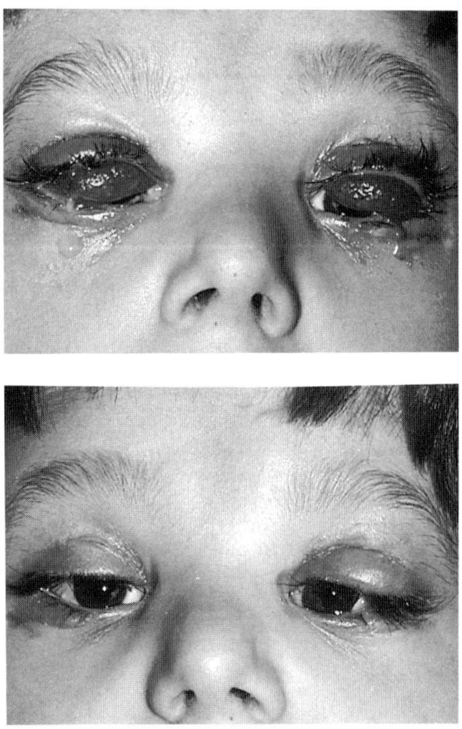

A

B

FIG. 17. Conjunctival prolapse following levator resection with extensive dissection. **A:** Patient 2 weeks preoperatively. **B:** Following partial resection of conjunctiva and suture reforming the superior fornix.

GRANULOMA FORMATION

Granuloma formation occurs in the suprabrow area following frontalis suspension procedures when the suspensory material is close enough to the undersurface of the skin to cause irritation (Fig. 18). It is important to undermine the brow incisions in the plane of the frontalis muscle so that the material can rest beneath the subbrow fat pad. Closure of deep tissue also prevents migration of buried material.

LACRIMAL GLAND DAMAGE; DRY EYE SYNDROME

Dry eye syndrome is a very unusual complication but can occur in patients who have levator resection with extensive dissection. Overaggressive dissection of the lateral horn of the levator in the area of the lacrimal gland can cause severance of the lacrimal ductules. Lacrimal cysts can form postoperatively if ductules are occluded (18).

HEMORRHAGE AND INFECTION

Hemorrhage and infection complications are generally seen early postoperatively. The surgeon should observe the usual preoperative evaluation of the patient for risk factors. Blood coagulating problems, hyperten-

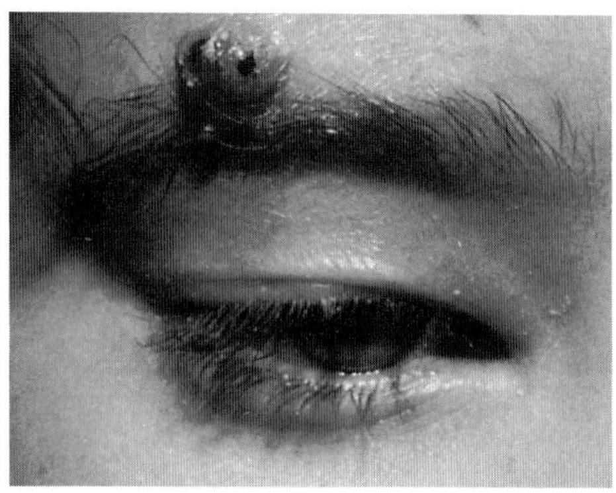

FIG. 18. Granuloma formation in the eyebrow at the site of skin incision following frontalis suspension. This is the result of the suspensory material being too close to the skin surface and with chronic irritation subcutaneously causing a granuloma formation.

sion, or the use of blood-thinning medication should be detected. Instruction to the patient to avoid postoperative Valsalva maneuvers should be considered. Infection is extremely uncommon following ptosis surgery but can occur if non-absorbable or slow absorbing sutures are left in the lid communicating with the skin for a significant period of time.

REFERENCES

1. Shore JW, Bergin DJ, Garrett SN. Results of blepharoptosis surgery with early postoperative adjustment. *Ophthalmology* 1990;97:1502–1511.
2. Dortzbach RK, Kronish JW. Early revision in the office for adults after unsatisfactory blepharoptosis correction. *Am J Ophthalmol* 1993;75:68–75.
3. Jordan DR, Anderson RL. A simplified procedure for adjusting eyelid position after aponeurotic ptosis surgery. *Arch Ophthalmol* 1987;105:1288.
4. Linberg JV, Vasquez RJ, Gung-Mei C. Aponeurotic ptosis repair under local anesthesia. *Ophthalmology* 1988;95:1046–1052.
5. Berlin AJ, Vestal KP. Levator aponeurosis surgery: a retrospective review. *Ophthalmology* 1989;96:1033–1037.
6. McCord CD. An external minimal ptosis procedure: external tarsoaponeurectomy. *Am Acad Ophthalmol Otolaryngol* 1975; 79:683–686.
7. Baylis HI, Shorr N. Anterior tarsectomy reoperation for upper eyelid blepharoptosis or contour abnormalities. *Am J Ophthalmol* 1977;84:67–71.
8. Smith B, Bosniak SL. Frontalis sling complications. *Ophth Surg* 1980;11:614–616.
9. Pang HB. Surgical formation of upper lid fold. *Arch Ophthalmol* 1961;65:783–784.
10. Cies WA, Baylis HI. Surgical revision of the upper eyelid fold. *Am J Ophthalmol* 1975;80:1019–1023.
11. Putterman AM, Urist MJ. Reconstruction of the upper eyelid crease and fold. *Arch Ophthalmol* 1976;94:1941–1954.
12. Dortzbach RK, Callahan A. Repair of cicatricial entropion of upper eyelids. *Arch Ophthalmol* 1971;85:82–89.
13. McCord CD, Tanenbaum M, Dryden RM, Doxanas MT. Eyelid malpositions: entropion, eyelid margin deformity and trichiasis, ectropion and facial nerve palsy. In: McCord CD Jr, Tanenbaum M, eds. *Oculoplastic surgery*. 2nd ed. New York: Raven Press; 1987:279–324.59.
14. Patipa M, Wilkins RB. Vertical tarsal buckling as a complication of levator aponeurosis repair for acquired blepharoptosis. *Am J Ophthalmol* 1984;97:93–99.
15. Wolfley DE. Preventing conjunctival prolapse and tarsal eversion following large excisions of levator muscle and aponeurosis for correction of congenital ptosis. *Ophth Surg* 1987;18;491–494.
16. Biglan AW, Chang A, Hiles DA. Prolapse of conjunctiva following external levator resection. *Ophth Surg* 1980;11:581–583.
17. Buckman G, Levine MR. Treatment of prolapsed conjunctiva. *Ophth Plast Reconstr Surg* 1986;2(1):33–39.
18. Gonnering RS, Carroll RP. Cystic lesions of the eyelid following ptosis repair. *Ophth Plast Reconstr Surg* 1986;2(2):89–93.

CHAPTER 12

Blepharoplasty: Preoperative Evaluation

SURGICAL GOALS

If planned and performed well, blepharoplasty can be a pleasing experience for both the patient and the surgeon. Before surgery is undertaken, careful evaluation of the patient as to his or her specific anatomic problems and attitude toward expected results from surgery must be carried out. Each patient must be aware of what the surgeon can and cannot do with surgical techniques, and the surgeon must be aware of what the patient expects from the surgery. Realistic goals must be met in order to produce a happy patient and a satisfied surgeon.

PATIENT EDUCATION

It is very important to point out to the patient the specific anatomic problems that can be improved by surgery. This can be done very easily with a "mirror" discussion with the patient or with a detailed examination of Polaroid photographs taken during the interview session. It should be emphasized to the patient that the only thing that will take place as the result of surgery is a change in the anatomic features discussed. Blepharoplasty may give the patient an emotional lift but it will not by itself make the patient younger, improve his or her love life, solve marital problems or other life situations. The surgeon should beware of the demanding and/or impatient individual, the patient who brings photographs of movie stars, the highly labile or emotional individuals, and the patient who seems to be a "doctor hopper." In general, if the patient exhibits unrealistic expectations in what he or she wishes to obtain from a blepharoplasty surgical procedure, then the surgeon should very courteously refrain from pursuing any surgery with that individual.

SAFETY IN BLEPHAROPLASTY: EYE PROTECTIVE MECHANISMS

It should be explained to the patient that the eyelids are not "decorations" but are eye protective devices that are basically designed to protect the cornea and preserve the function of the eye. An adequate evaluation of other eye protective mechanisms should be done before planning blepharoplasty surgery. Table 1 contains a list of mechanisms that are needed for protection to compensate for stiffness of the lids that may occur following blepharoplasty surgery.

Ocular Motility

Normal ocular rotations, particularly Bell's phenomenon, are important for eye protection following blepharoplasty. The patient may, for a period of time, suffer some stiffness of closure and "gapping" of the eyelids at night. This is particularly true if the surgeon becomes overzealous with skin removal. Corneal drying and keratitis can occur.

Tear Film

The precorneal tear film is needed to moisten and protect the cornea. Patients with a history of "dry eyes" requiring ocular lubricant should be approached with caution. Tests for tearing that are appropriate in the preoperative blepharoplasty patient are the Schirmer test with anesthesia, evaluation of the precorneal tear meniscus with slit-lamp examination, and the tear film break-up time. Patients should be asked, "Has anyone told you that you have dry eyes?" because there is a correlation with postop discomfort and a preoperative history of dryness.

TABLE 1. *Eye protective mechanisms*

Ocular motility and Bell's phenomenon
Adequate tear film
Orbicularis and eyelid closure strength
Corneal sensation
Lower lid position and movement

Eyelid Closure

Orbicularis function and tone is important for the eyelid to have its normal "windshield wiper" effect in protecting the cornea. Any preexisting weakness of orbicularis strength or the inability of the orbicularis muscle to close the eye from nerve paresis or unusual stiffness of the lid, skin stiffness, or other should be noted. Such patients should also be approached with caution.

Corneal Sensation

The eye protective mechanisms can only work to compensate for a corneal dry spot if the cornea tells them to do so, and a decrease in corneal sensation from corneal disease or a fifth nerve paresis can also place the patient at risk for postoperative corneal exposure.

Lower Lid Position

Postoperative gapping of the eyelid and exposure can be aggravated by preexisting lower lid retraction or scleral show, amplifying any postoperative lagophthalmos and gapping of the eyelids. Laxity of the lid may predispose the patient to have ectropion or scleral show postoperatively.

ANATOMIC EVALUATION OF THE UPPER LID

The potential blepharoplasty patient may present to the surgeon with nonspecific general complaints of fullness and a "droopy" look in the upper lid, but very specific anatomic problems causing the laxity and fullness may be present and should be recognized. It is important for the surgeon to analyze each patient's anatomic changes and help the patient to understand how these specific changes cause the unwanted appearance (Fig. 1).

Brow Position and Laxity

When evaluating patients who are potential candidates for upper lid blepharoplasty, an extremely important determination is eyebrow laxity and position. The

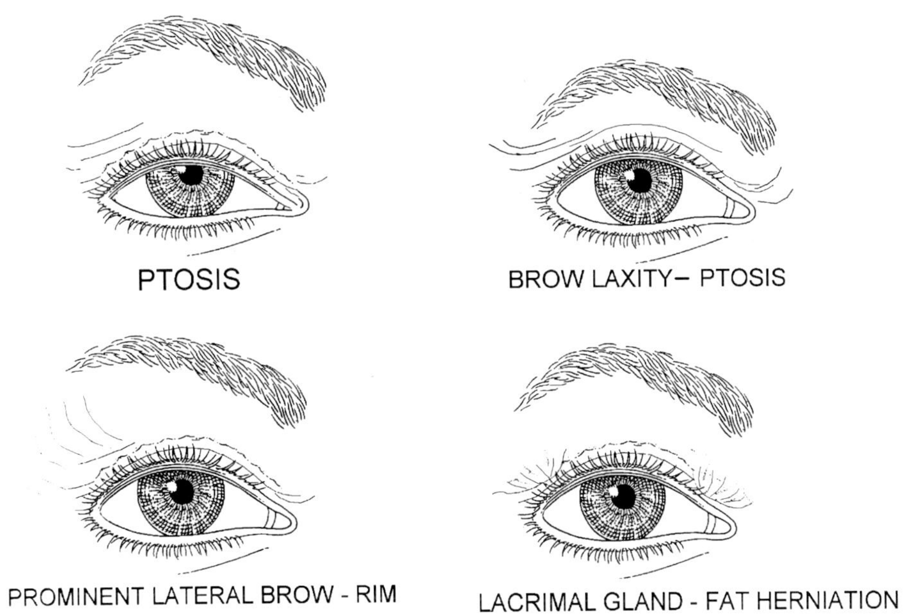

FIG. 1. Important anatomic situations to recognize in the preoperative blepharoplasty patient. True ptosis with downward movement of the eyelid margin should be noted. Any abnormalities in the brow should be noted, specifically eyebrow laxity and the positioning of the brow with the brow–lash distance. Many patients' main complaint when presenting for blepharoplasty will be of the lateral fullness of the orbital rim and lateral brow skin as opposed to the lid fullness. This should be noted preoperatively since it will not be corrected with standard eyelid skin-fat removal. Subcutaneous protuberances in the upper lid producing fullness can be caused not only by herniated fat but also by lacrimal gland prolapse laterally and should be noted.

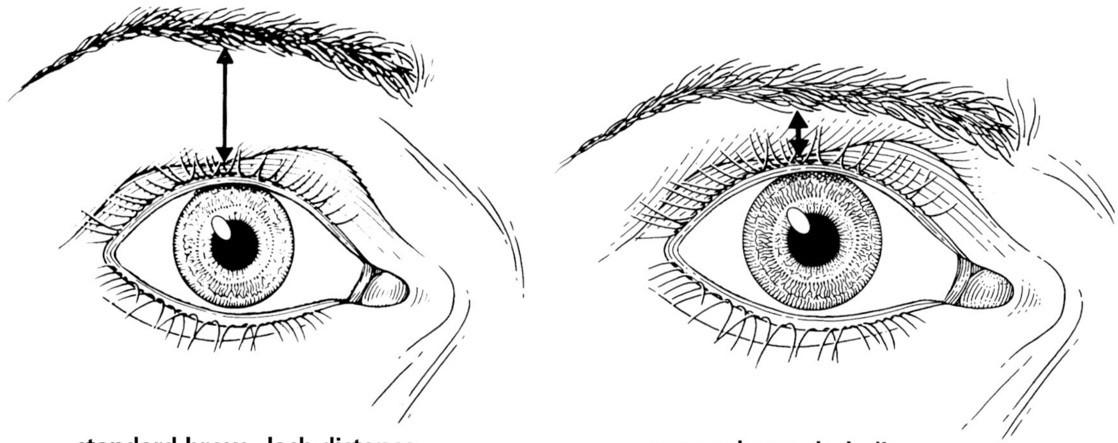

FIG. 2. A: Normal or standard eyebrow–eyelash distance. **B:** Diagrammatic representation of narrowing of the eyebrow–eyelash distance from droppage of the brow.

eyebrow and eyelid skin are basically a unit with the eyebrow. The eyebrow is the "curtain rod" of the eyelid and the eyelid skin the curtain. A problem that can occur with upper lid blepharoplasty in the presence of a lax brow is *eyebrow drop* and *narrowing of the brow–lash distance*. It is important to remember that some brow drop will normally occur following a standard upper lid blepharoplasty. In patients who have a fairly firm and stable brow the drop is usually minimal and not noticed by the patient. If the eyebrow is lax, when significant amounts of skin are removed from the upper lid the brow is pulled down to some degree. This can produce a reduced effect from upper lid blepharoplasty that can take the form of recurrent temporal folds laterally from a lateral lax brow, decrease in the brow–lash distance centrally from downward migration, and failure to correct nasal folding and laxity from looseness of the medial portion of the brow (Fig. 2A, B). A nasal lowering of the brow accentuates glabellar folds and produces a "worried" or "mean" look. A lateral lowering of the brow results in a "sad" look with residual folds. If a person has these changes at the time of the evaluation for upper lid blepharoplasty, it is quite clear that a brow procedure is needed as an adjunct to the upper lid blepharoplasty. Sometimes the brow changes are subtle but the surgeon must carefully evaluate the brow stability and position preoperatively to avoid the postoperative sequela. Figure 3A and B shows a patient with brow droppage following upper lid blepharoplasty requiring correction with a coronal forehead-eyebrow lift.

Lateral brow laxity can be corrected by either a coronal forehead lift, direct brow pexy with an extended incision line laterally, or, to a lesser degree, internal brow pexy. If skin folds extend lateral from the brow toward the hairline, then the smoothing must be accomplished with the coronal forehead brow lift with attention to pull in the lateral area.

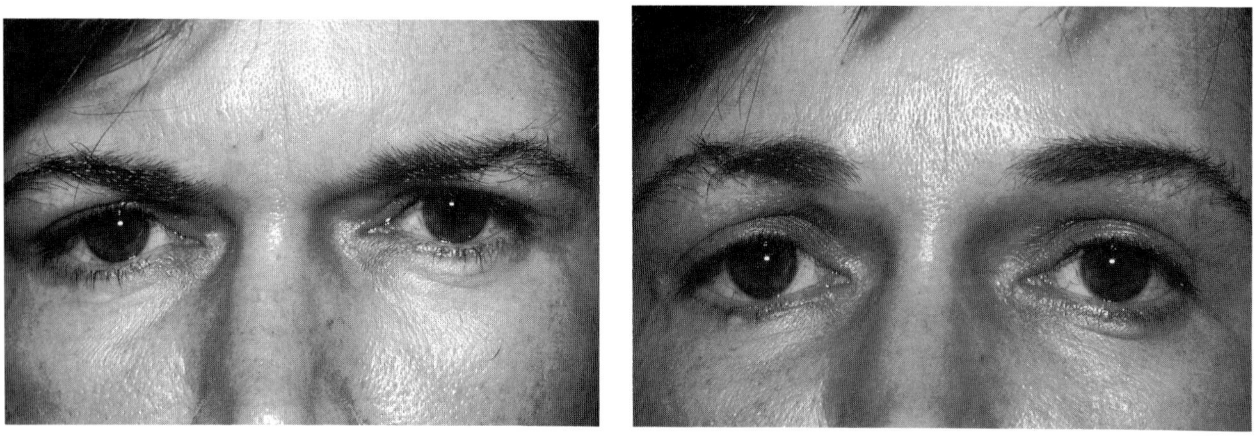

FIG. 3. A: Patient following upper lid blepharoplasty who developed narrowing of the eyebrow distance and brow drop postoperatively. **B:** Same patient with a more normal eyebrow–eyelash distance following coronal forehead lift that restored the distance to normal.

Laxity of the brow in the nasal or glabellar area is very difficult to correct with a direct brow pexy. Internal brow pexy, which has a lateral effect, offers no correction for nasal laxity and can actually accentuate it. The only procedure that offers a good improvement in the glabellar-nasal area is the coronal forehead brow lift, which produces an "opening-up" look to the nasal area, brow, and eyelids with smoothing of the glabellar area.

Laxity in the central portion of the brow can be corrected by a coronal forehead brow lift or a direct eyebrow pexy in males or in indicated females.

Preexisting Ptosis of the Upper Lid

The upper lid may appear droopy not because of the overfolding of skin and weighing down of the eyelid with the eyelid and brow tissue but because of a downward position of the margin of the lid that occludes the pupil. True ptosis of the lid may be present with dermatochalasis and brow ptosis, and if not specifically addressed it will still be present postoperatively. An adequate assessment of the level of the edge of the lid with respect to the pupil should be made and ptosis can be corrected, if necessary, with blepharoplasty combined with aponeurotic repair.

Prominent Supraorbital Rim

An exaggerated lateral superior orbital rim can be caused by either a bony prominence or a thickening of the brow fat pad laterally. In many cases patients who have been specifically asked to point to the area that bothers them point to the fullness in the temporal aspect of the orbital rim area or brow. Brow plasty techniques for reducing the prominence of the lateral brow involve bone sculpting with ostectomy of the edge of the superior orbital rim. Sculpting of the subbrow fat pad in this area through the blepharoplasty incision is also a very effective way to thin the fullness in this area.

Fatty Pad Location

The upper lid contains one long preaponeurotic fatty pad resting on the surface of the levator, a nasal fatty pad, and a small junctional fat pad between those two. A subbrow fat pad may extend from beneath the orbicularis muscle in the brow area into the preseptal area, also causing a fullness of the lid (Figs. 4 and 5) (1–3). A preoperative attempt should be made to assess the contribution of each of these to the fullness.

Herniated Lacrimal Gland

Fullness in the lateral portion of the lid may be due to a prolapse of the lacrimal gland, which can add fullness to the lid and, if not repositioned, can reduce the desired crease effect laterally. The orbital portion of the lacrimal gland should not be excised because of the danger of reducing tear flow to the eye. The lacrimal gland can be enlarged in patients who have had thyroid disease or sarcoidosis.

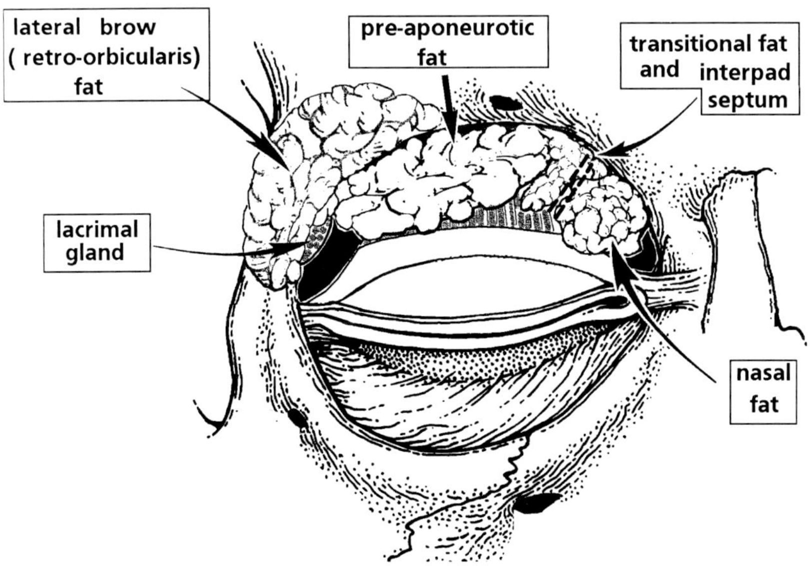

FIG. 4. Diagrammatic representation of the fatty areas and compartments in the upper lid and brow area.

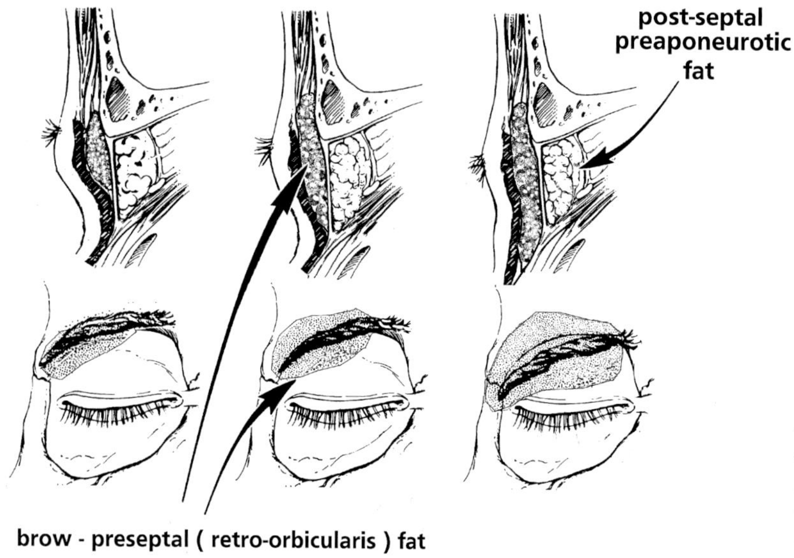

FIG. 5. Variations in positioning and extent of the subbrow or fat pad, which is contiguous with the preseptal fat. Age and other factors can cause a widening of area of the subbrow fatty tissue and thickening of this tissue producing fullness. After McCord and Doxanas (1).

PREEXISTING OCULAR DISEASE

Close examination should be made of the cornea to note any preexisting corneal scars, pterygia, or pingueculae formation, which may be a sign of an incipient corneal problem. If these findings are not noted and recorded preoperatively, they may be assumed to have been caused by the surgery if noticed postoperatively by someone else (Table 2).

Conjunctivochalasis

In some patients a redundancy of conjunctiva, particularly at the lateral canthus, can swell postoperatively and cause a tendency to postop chemosis. This may cause a prolonged course of chronic corneal dry spots for the patient; consequently, some resection of the redundant conjunctiva may be indicated at the time of blepharoplasty.

Eyelid Disease

The eyelid margin should be examined for signs of chronic staph blepharoconjunctivitis, recurrent chalazia scars, or a cicatrizing disease such as ocular pemphigoid. If present, such condition should be diagnosed and recorded preoperatively. If these conditions do exacerbate postoperatively, it may be assumed by the patient that they were caused by the surgery. Rosacea can be a particular nuisance in some patients.

OTHER PREEXISTING DISEASE

There are other peripheral ocular conditions that should be recognized preoperatively (Table 3).

Blepharospasm

Benign essential blepharospasm, which is a progressive involuntary contracture of the eyelids, will in its early stages have only subtle signs in many patients. These patients may present to a plastic surgeon because their eyelids are "droopy." If active orbicularis contracture is seen around the eyes and a history of light insensitivity or involuntary eyelid closure is obtained, then one must entertain this diagnosis as a possibility and advise the patient to have further evaluation. Eyelid surgery can be performed on blepharospasm patients to ameliorate some of the laxity problems, but will have no effect on the spasms themselves which may well progress. Other treatment such as botulinum toxin injections may be indicated.

TABLE 2. *Preexisting eye–eyelid disease*

Chronic blepharoconjunctivitis (staph, seborrhea, and rosacea)
Conjunctivochalasis
Cicatrizing eyelid disease (e.g., pemphigoid)
Corneal disease

TABLE 3. *Preexisting systemic disease*

Benign essential blepharospasm
Hypothyroidism
Underlying orbital disease, tumor
Active Graves' disease
Obstructive sinus disease
Chronic recurrent fluid retention or allergies
Systemic infiltrative disease, lymphoproliferative

Thyroid Disease

Hypothyroidism can cause puffiness of the eyes. If the patient demonstrates any other signs or symptoms, such as hair loss or cold intolerance, further tests should be performed. Graves' disease, with or without hyperthyroidism, can of course cause severe eyelid changes. These permanent anatomic changes can be helped by blepharoplasty and related procedures; however, caution should be observed with regard to timing. The patient should have surgery only when the active inflammatory stage has subsided. Surgery in the active phase of the disease can aggravate the tissue changes and the patient may feel that the surgery has actually worsened the problems.

Underlying Orbital disease

Lacrimal gland enlargement (resulting from lymphoid tumors and other problems) and orbital tumors can present with fullness of the brow and eyelid. The authors have seen a patient with a sphenoid wing meningioma who had undergone a blepharoplasty before being diagnosed.

Underlying Sinus Disease

Chronic sinusitis, particularly obstructive sinus disease, can cause eyelid puffiness. The obstructive component should be remedied before any surgery is undertaken. Any inflammatory processes should be suppressed before blepharoplasty.

Blood Dyscrasias

Local infiltrates can present as eyelid fullness although this is unusual as a presenting sign. The authors have seen a patient referred for blepharoplasty who had fullness of the eyelids from the infiltrates of chronic lymphocytic leukemia (Fig. 6).

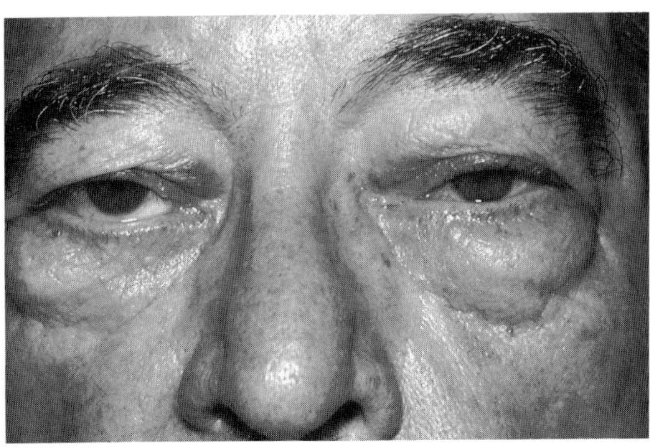

FIG. 6. Patient with chronic lymphocytic leukemia referred for a lower lid blepharoplasty. The protuberances in the lower lid were not herniated fat but lymphocytic infiltrates in the lower lid.

Severe Allergies and Fluid Retention

The fullness and puffiness of the eyelids caused by this problem can be ameliorated by surgery. Surgery will not alter the underlying tendency and some changes may recur, so that the patient should be informed as such.

ANATOMIC CHANGES IN THE LOWER LID

The patients who complain of puffy lower lids may have a wide variety of anatomic changes and conditions that must be recognized preoperatively. The specific changes must be recognized and pointed out to the patient (Fig. 7).

Location of Herniated Fat Pads in the Lower Lids

It has been traditional to describe three fat prominences in the lower lid—central, medial, and lateral—although some of the fatty tissue actually may be contiguous at a deeper level in the orbit. The specific locations of these prominences vary from patient to patient and should be noted preoperatively and recorded with photographs (Fig. 8).

Lower Lid Laxity or Malposition

Skin resection with the lower lid blepharoplasty in the presence of preexisting lower lid retraction or scleral show may aggravate the situation postoperatively, particularly if the eyelid is loose. Further scleral show, corneal exposure, and, in some cases, an actual ectropion will usually be the result. The lower lid can be evaluated by inspection to note any preexisting scleral show and the laxity can be noted by pulling on the lashes and determining if the lid elasticity is strong enough to immediately reposition it against the globe. This is the so-called spring-back test and can be helpful in evaluating this situation. Horizontal tightening procedures with lateral canthoplasty should be used in these patients to prevent this complication and probably should be incorporated as part of the routine procedure.

Cheek Bone Prominence

Very high cheek bones, particularly if prominent laterally or nasally, are important to note because exces-

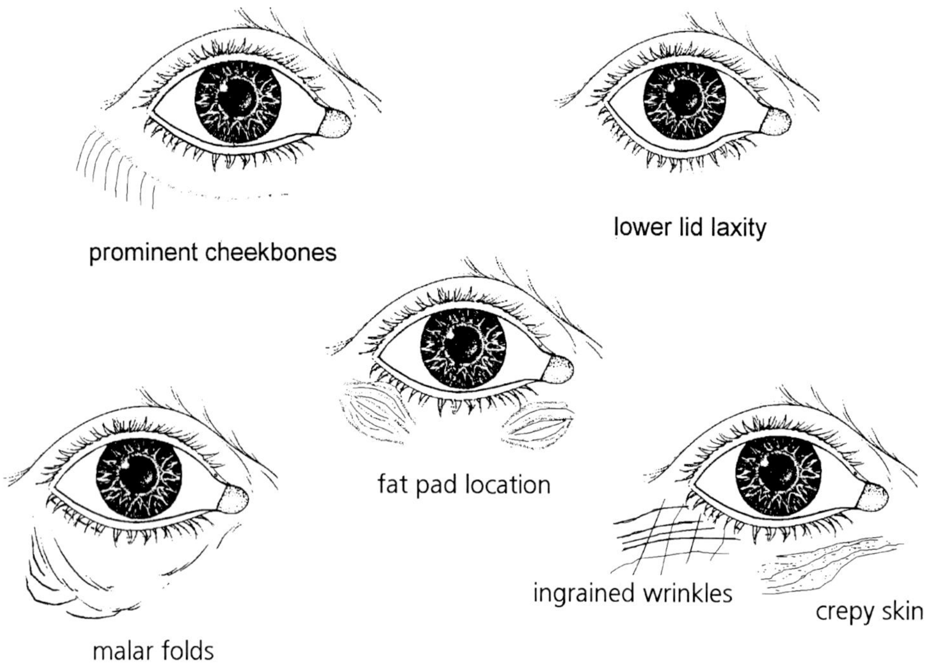

FIG. 7. Diagrammatic representation of important anatomic aspects of the lower lid that should be recognized prior to blepharoplasty.

sive fat removal in these areas will further accentuate them and produce a sunken look. In some patients, an overly prominent malar bone, more commonly nasally, can be sculpted at the time of lower lid blepharoplasty if needed.

Orbicularis Hypertrophy

The fullness or puffiness in the lower lids in many patients is due not to herniated fat but to hypertrophy and thickening of the orbicularis muscle. This is most commonly seen when the patient is squinting slightly. This thickening will not go away with simple fat removal and skin stretching, and specific resection of portions of the orbicularis are necessary to remedy this problem (Fig. 9).

Prominent Eyes

Patients who have prominent eyes from familial tendency or Graves' disease have a tendency to downward migration of the eyelid margin and scleral show. This problem in some patients can be remedied by a lateral tightening, but in patients with more prominent

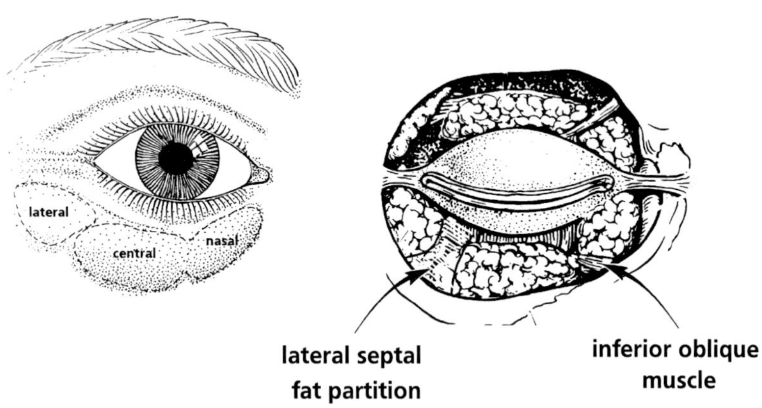

FIG. 8. Diagrammatic representation of the fat pad components in the lower lid area.

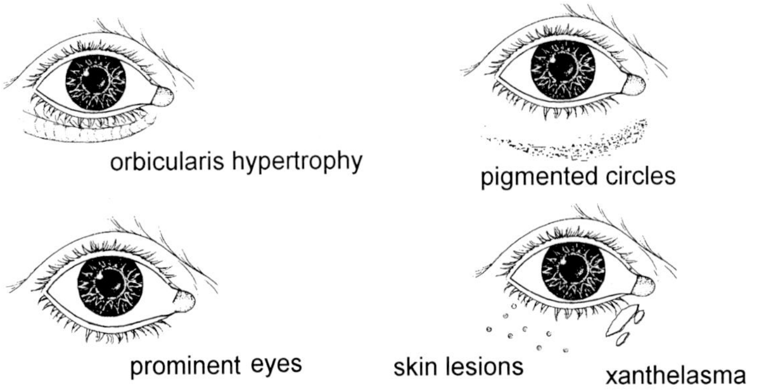

FIG. 9. Diagrammatic representation of important anatomic characteristics of the lower lid that should be considered before doing lower lid blepharoplasty.

eyes the lateral tightening of the eyelid will simply "clothesline" the margin of the lid further downward. A specific technique for loosening the lid and supraplacement of the tendon will be presented to deal with this problem.

Ingrained Wrinkles—Crepy Skin

Many patients who have prolonged sun exposure, very commonly seen in women golfers, will acquire a leathery quality to the skin with wrinkles that cannot be smoothed by tensing the skin. In this parched skin, some wrinkles that can be smoothed by tensing will actually form new wrinkles 90° to the original direction.

Crepy skin has a peculiar elasticity and the small lines and wrinkles cannot be removed completely by usual skin excision. This should be noted preoperatively and the patient should be warned that an incomplete smoothing of the skin will be obtained because of the crepy nature.

Pigmented Circles Under the Eye

Many patients complain of dark circles under the eye and want to know if they will be gone after lower lid blepharoplasty. The circles that are due to shadows, i.e., the shadow produced by the convexity of the herniated fat and downlighting, will indeed be improved or corrected with removal of the fat and tensing of the skin. Many patients will have pigmentation of the skin in this area, however, and this will remain following surgery. It should be explained to the patient that the pigmentation will not be removed by skin stretching and excision.

Coexisting Skin Lesions and Xanthelasma

Many times during the course of a lower lid blepharoplasty, some of the existing skin lesions and xanthelasma can be excised, if they happen to lie in the surgical area that will normally be excised. Even if they don't, small excisions can be performed, but not if it will produce an overstretching of the skin and a tendency for lower lid malposition. The patient should be informed that this is a limiting factor and that some of the lesions will have to be excised at a later date. Nasally occurring xanthelasma can often be excised with a specially designed skin excision for lower lid blepharoplasty with a nasal flap as opposed to a temporal flap, which will be described.

Malar Festoons

Many patients will have, in addition to the puffiness and folding of skin in their lids, a folding of skin and puffiness further down on the lateral aspect of the cheek bone. In the past this was called "malar festoons" or "bags on bags." There has been some difficulty in correcting this problem adequately in the past; therefore, the patient should be informed that the condition probably will not be fully corrected in that it will take a special technique to get much effect in this area. The options for correcting this are an extended incision and undermining with lower lid blepharoplasty, or in many cases a direct excision of the more severe folds. A definitive correction can be obtained with a cheek lift (see Chapter 16).

DOCUMENTATION OF VISUAL DEFECT—ANATOMIC CHANGES EFFECT ON VISUAL FIELD—PREOPERATIVE PHOTOGRAPHS

Photographs are particularly helpful in the preoperative discussion with the patient and as a record of the effects of surgery. They also serve as a guide during the surgical procedure to remind the surgeon of specific anatomic aspects. They also serve the purpose of providing information to the insurance company for a prior approval in patients who may have a functional deficit from upper lid problems. Larger format photographs with blown-up black-and-white glossies are quite excellent. However, black-and-white polaroid or color photographs taken with a CU-5 medical–dental polaroid camera with the full-face frame are quite satisfactory and in many cases can be suitable for reproduction in scientific articles. The standard views taken are a straightahead facial view, a nose-down view to highlight the lower lid puffiness and malar folds, and a lateral view to show the overlying hooding and shelf effect of the brow and redundant upper lid skin.

Visual Acuity Check

A visual acuity taken with the glasses or pinhole should be documented to determine any preexisting reduction in vision. If this is not done, any postoperative reduction in vision that is noted may be automatically assumed to be the result of the surgery.

Visual Fields

Visual fields are performed with the patient gazing straight ahead with the eyelid and brow relaxed, and then with the eyelid and brow elevated to a normal position. The difference in visual field between the two positions can be considered to be the deficit produced by the deformity. The percentage of deficit has varied in the past, but usually 30% of the upper field of vision is considered a functional deficit. The visual field can be performed by a tangent screen, perimeter, or automated perimeter. As of this writing, there is no standard technique for determination of visual fields. It should be mentioned that there is an excellent correlation between the visual field deficit and the distance between light reflex in the cornea and the upper lid fold or upper lid margin. Numerous articles have referred to correlations in the reduction in visual field with the narrowing distance between these two (4–7). In many cases this is more precise than the actual visual field measurement, which is purely subjective. However, it has not yet been accepted as a criterion by the existing carriers.

PREOPERATIVE COMMUNICATION AND PSYCHOLOGICAL MANAGEMENT OF THE PATIENT

This chapter has emphasized that care should be taken in determining the patient's expectations and in adequately describing to the patient what can be accomplished with a blepharoplasty procedure and cannot be done. Many patients who are excellent candidates, not only from the anatomic standpoint but psychologically as well (i.e., with realistic expectations), may have certain apprehensions about the surgery. If it is felt by the surgeon that the patient is a good candidate, then an attempt should be made to encourage the patient to consider the surgery.

When talking with potential blepharoplasty patients, it is important to understand that what you say—and the exact words that you use—in discussion of the surgery are very important. The words that are used should reassure patients, not frighten them. Some of the following words should be worked into the conversation.

Safe. Probably the biggest fear on the part of the patient is of having a loss of vision or one of the extreme results that are sometimes discussed as gossip. The patient should understand that a good outcome is your priority and that your first concern as a surgeon is that he or she come through the surgery in a healthy way. It should be emphasized to the patient that the surgeon understands that the eyelids are not decorations, that they exist to protect the eyes and vision, and that the planned surgery will always take that into consideration first.

Natural. The purpose of blepharoplasty for patients is to make them look more attractive, but in a natural way. All patients (or most of them) want to avoid a stark and stretched look, and they do not want to look like "someone else." They want to have an improved appearance but do not want anyone to come up to them following surgery and say, "Gosh! You must have had plastic surgery!" The preferred comment is, "Gee, you look better, rested, you must have lost weight." In these sophisticated times if someone looks a lot better very rapidly, then many people will guess that some surgical procedure must have taken place. But a natural look is the preferred improvement.

Friendly. This word is particularly helpful with male patients. It is used in conjunction with the idea that conservatism will be used, that some of the anatomic changes that are desired will take place, but that the surgeon will not become too aggressive. This is a corollary of the word "natural." This implies that following surgery the patient will look better but will maintain a personal, friendly look. This term can also be used as a hedge against undercorrection or residual postoperative folds or laugh lines after surgery.

Sculpt. In spite of the modern education of patients, many have a morbid fear of scalpels and blood. When describing to the patient what will be done anatomically, the surgeon in many cases would best avoid using terms like "cut," "excision," "hemorrhage," "resection."

Thin. This is another good word to use in describing how one will treat the anatomic changes. This word does not frighten patients and it gives a lot of latitude to the surgeon. It implies that there is room for judgment in the mind of the surgeon as to how much the surgeon wants to change or "thin" the lid.

Enhance; clean up. These are nonspecific words that imply improvement in certain areas while giving the surgeon a hedge against implied results.

INFORMED CONSENT

It seems ironic that after reassuring a candidate for blepharoplasty the surgeon must then turn around and describe a series of problems that may occur. Although in most cases the odds are small that the patient will have problems, it is considered legally necessary, and probably considerate to the patient, to describe to them problems that can occur. The risks that are mentioned to the patient by these authors on a routine basis are as follows: unusual bruising and swelling, dryness of the eye or dry spots of the eye following surgery that may require lubricants on a long-term basis, the need for secondary surgery (either office touch-up or revisional surgery at a surgical facility), and recurrence of folds in the upper lid if the brow loosens with time. Each state has its own set of laws with regard to required disclosure of "material risks." These can be more severe in nature, such as death, blindness, and paralysis. Routinely in our office a specific "general informed consent" videotape is shown to patients that describes the material risks. Following that, a very detailed consent form is signed by the patient.

MEDICAL EVALUATION OF THE PATIENT

All patients, particularly those in an older age group who may take medication or have hypertension, should have clearance from their primary care doctor. Even though most blepharoplasty surgery can be performed with local anesthesia and sedation, severe medical conditions should be evaluated and accounted for preoperatively.

The most common surgical concern is excessive bleeding, which may produce swelling and hematoma formation that can threaten vision and compromise the surgical result. The most common problems causing this are uncontrolled high blood pressure and medications that decrease blood clotting. Every attempt should be made to eliminate aspirin or aspirin-like medications for a week prior to surgery. Vasodilating medications such as Persantin or Cyclospasmol can be discontinued under the guidance of the patient's personal physician. True anticoagulants such as coumadin can also be discontinued and the protime monitored preoperatively by the patient's internist.

After a thorough examination and evaluation of the patient's anatomic changes, expectations, and general medical condition, the surgeon may feel that the indications are good for surgery and proceed to schedule the patient for blepharoplasty surgery. However, in certain situations the surgeon may feel that it is not in the patient's or the surgeon's best interest to proceed with surgery, and in such a case should tactfully discourage surgery (Table 4).

TABLE 4. *Identifying the problem patient*

Psychological—"won't be happy"
Technical—difficult to correct with surgery
Medical—risky for eye health

REFERENCES

1. McCord CD, Doxanas MT. Browplasty and browpexy: an adjunct to blepharoplasty. *Plast Reconstr Surg* 1990;86:248–254.
2. Lemke BN, Stasior OG. The anatomy of eyebrow ptosis. *Arch Ophthalmol* 1982;100–981.
3. Weiss R. Thesis for membership in the American Society of Ophthalmic Plastic and Reconstructive Surgery, 1987.
4. Cahill KV, Burns JA, Weber PA. The effect of blepharoptosis on the field of vision. *Ophth Plast Reconstr Surg* 1987;3:121–125.
5. Meyer DR, Linberg JV, Powell SR, Odom JV, Quantitating the superior visual field loss associated with ptosis. *Arch Ophthalmol* 1989;107:840–843.
6. Patipa M. Visual field loss in primary gaze and reading gaze due to acquired blepharoptosis and visual field improvement following ptosis surgery. *Arch Ophthalmol* 1992;110:63–67.
7. Meyer DR, Stern JH, et al. Evaluating the visual field effects of blepharoptosis using automated static perimetry. *Ophthalmology* 1993;100:651–659.

CHAPTER 13

Brow Surgery

EVALUATION OF THE EYEBROW

Eyebrows are normally positioned above the level of the superior orbital rim but may migrate below the superior rim causing a magnification of the redundancy of the upper eyelid skin (Fig. 1). A common error in upper lid blepharoplasty is failure to diagnose brow laxity preoperatively causing an undercorrection of effect of the surgery. The residual upper lid folding and narrowing of the brow–lash distance may produce a "mean" or "sad" look in the patient postoperatively causing patient dissatisfaction.

ANATOMY

There are differences in bony anatomy in the forehead and eyebrow between males and females (1–3). The supraorbital ridges form the upper boundary of the orbit and males tend to have a more flat contour and females a more arched contour. The protrusion of the supraorbital rim is more prominent in its lateral third in males. This area is followed by a flatter area of the midforehead before the convexity of the upper forehead. Pneumatization of the frontal sinus can cause prominent frontal bossing and protrusion of the frontal bone. This occurs more characteristically in males. The female has a smoother, gentler, continuous curve from the supraorbital rim to the upper forehead. This is due to the lack of frontal bossing and less prominent supraorbital rim.

The soft tissue of the eyebrow is normally fixed to the superior orbital rim through fibrofatty connective tissue. The muscular component of the eyebrow is composed primarily of the frontalis muscles. Nasally, the frontalis muscle interdigitates with the orbital orbicularis muscle and the obliquely oriented corrugator superciliaris muscle, and the nasal-most portion of the frontalis muscle is attached to the nasal bones to form the procerus muscle. The remaining frontalis muscle does not have periosteal attachments and does not extend to the orbital rim laterally. The frontalis muscle is encapsulated by a split in the galea aponeurotica that forms its anterior and posterior muscular sheaths and the posterior sheath extends to the periosteum at the superior orbital rim. This inferior extension of the frontalis posterior muscular sheath contributes to the orbital septum of the eyelid. The eyebrow fat pad occurs anterior to the posterior fascial sheath. The eyebrow fat pad enhances eyebrow mobility, especially in the lateral brow, where it is most pronounced and has been referred to by some surgeons as "lateral fat." In many individuals, the brow fat pad may extend inferiorly into the suborbicularis-preseptal plane in the eyelid to become the "preseptal fat" that has been recognized previously by blepharoplasty surgeons (4–6).

BROW SURGICAL TECHNIQUES

The *internal brow pexy* is a valuable adjunct to upper lid blepharoplasty but has limited ability for much elevation of the brow (6). It is useful in milder cases for elevation in the lateral brow area. In patients with borderline laxity of the eyebrow in the lateral-central area, it can prevent a postoperative brow drop. In patients who have obvious brow ptosis or in those in whom elevation of the brow is critical to satisfying the patient postoperatively, a direct suprabrow pexy or coronal forehead–brow lift must be performed. In patients who have significant nasal brow ptosis, lateral internal brow pexy can cause an accentuation of the nasal brow ptosis. The surgical technique of internal brow pexy is described in the chapter on upper lid blepharoplasty because it is adjunctive to that procedure.

The *direct brow lift,* in which a strip of skin is removed just above the brow hairs, is most commonly done in males (7–11). This is because there is a better opportunity to hide the scar just above the thicker, bushier brow found in males and because of males'

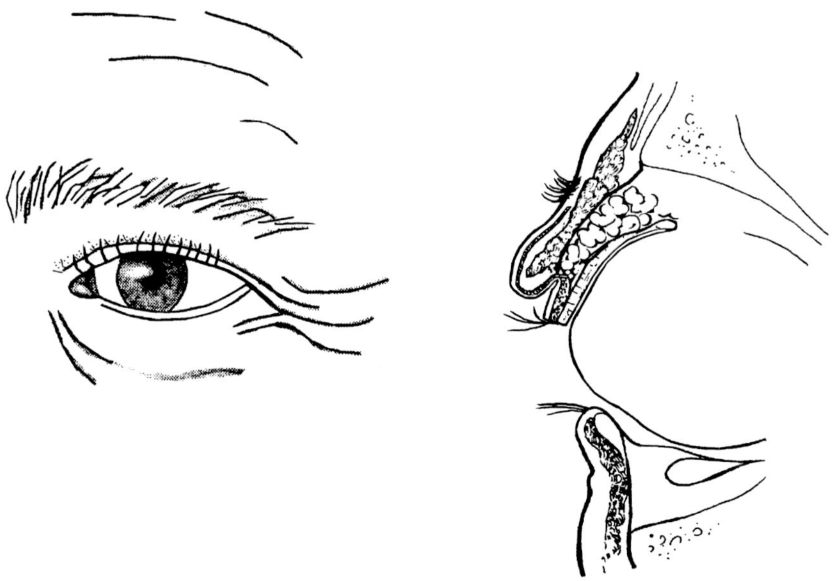

FIG. 1 Diagrammatic representation of a common situation in the lax male eyebrow. The brow migrates down below the edge of the superior orbital rim, resting on the upper lid with the fold of skin obscuring the pretarsal skin area.

adverse feelings about recession of the hairline. The coronal forehead lift is rarely used in males because with the usual incision it pulls the hairline back a small amount. There are occasionally male patients with deep transverse forehead furrows in which coronal flap incisions can be placed without causing recession of the hairline. In fact, it will lower the hairline a small amount.

The *coronal forehead eyebrow lift* is the most effective way of correcting laxity in the eyebrow forehead area (12,13). Its disadvantages are that it can alter hairline position and that it has been perceived by most patients as "extensive surgery." There are three general anatomic problems that the coronal forehead eyebrow lift will correct (see Fig. 9). The main goal in most cases is correction of the brow position in a *narrow brow–lash distance*. A common problem that sometimes goes unrecognized by the patient is *wrinkling in the glabellar area* due to corrugator muscle contracture and laxity in the nasal glabellar area, which causes folding about the nose and nasal upper lid. The coronal lift not only tenses and elevates the lax tissue in this area but allows trimming of the corrugator muscles to prevent future furrowing. Many patients who have severe brow laxity will have developed *transverse furrows in the forehead area* from constant arching of the brow that can be improved with the procedure, although in most cases it is not the primary reason for performing the coronal forehead lift. The coronal forehead lift allows smoothing of the furrows with incisions in the galea under the forehead flap in the course of performing the coronal forehead lift. As mentioned before, these deep transverse furrows in male patients often present an opportunity for the incision placement for the coronal forehead flap. A pretrichial incision at the edge of the hairline can be used as an alternative but also has the disadvantage of producing a visible scar. A pretrichial incision can be used in patients who want no recession of the hairline and can tolerate the visible incision line or cover it with hair arrangement.

Direct Brow Lift or Supra Brow Pexy

The most common placement of the skin excision ellipse is centrally. The incision lines do not usually extend the full length of the brow (Fig. 2A). The skin design must be customized from patient to patient, however, and if a temporal laxity is more evident, then the skin excision can be extended or placed more temporally as shown in Fig. 2B. A more aggressive brow lift can be obtained by extending the skin excision throughout the entire width of the brow and this is most commonly used in patients who have had a facial paralysis with a paralytic brow (Fig. 2C). The skin excision by itself does not elevate the brow the full amount and underlying fixation of the brow to the frontalis muscle is needed. The width of the skin excision can be determined preoperatively by facing the patient, elevating the brow the desired amount, and measuring the width of skin movement with a ruler.

Surgical Technique

The brow is stretched with two-finger traction after the ellipse of skin is marked. The skin is incised down to the subbrow fat pad with the Bard–Parker blade and at the upper edge of the brow is slanted in the direction of the hair follicles so as to avoid significant hair loss, although this is not as important in the male patient (Fig. 3A). After the skin has been incised, a small skin hook is placed in the nasal end of the wound for greater

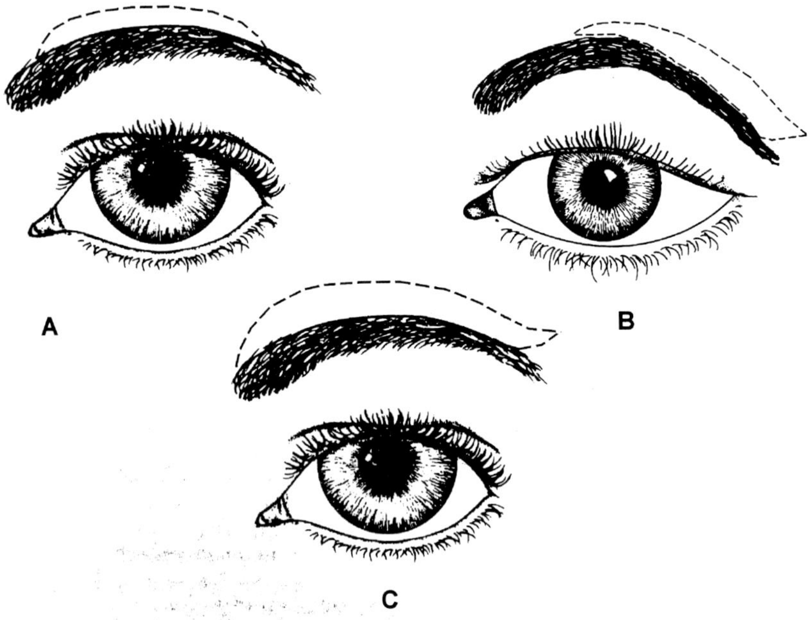

FIG. 2. Direct eyebrow lift. **A:** The area of skin to be removed is marked. In most cases the marked ellipse does not extend to the nasal or temporal end of the brow to avoid scarring. The amount of skin can be estimated by movement of the brow with the patient upright in determining the millimeters of movement required to reposition the brow to the desired location. **B:** Modification of placement of the brow with patient with a marked temporal laxity. **C:** Placement of direct brow fixation in the patient with a paralytic brow, which requires a larger area of skin excision and direct fixation to the galea.

traction, and with additional traction, the segment of incised skin can be tensed. Sharp scissors can then be used at the upper edge of the incision to incise through the subbrow fat pad until the plane of the frontalis muscle is reached (Fig. 3B). With additional traction the sharp scissors are then introduced beneath the subbrow fat pad in the plane between it and the frontalis muscle; then the ellipse of skin-fat is undermined from the underlying frontalis muscle and excised (Fig. 4A). Efforts are made to "square off" the excision of the skin and fat. However, invariably the depths of the incision are not squared off and fatty tissue slopes into the bed of the wound, interfering with good skin closure and good approximation of the wound. The deep fatty edges of the wound are then squared off with the use of the coagulating Bovie tip, which allows the surgeon to sculpt the fat from the frontalis muscle (Fig. 4B). Following this, the liquified fat is irrigated with cold water. The Bovie tip is then also used for hemostasis in the area of the frontalis muscle and other areas. Care is taken not to cauterize hair follicles. Figure 5A shows a surgical view of the area of brow skin-fat excision with vertical wound edges. Figure 5B shows the ellipse of skin-fat removed.

The lifting part of the procedure, the fixation of the subbrow fat pad to the frontalis muscle, is then undertaken. The upper edge of the wound is undermined to allow better exposure to the frontalis muscle and allow for better wound eversion. 4-0 Prolene sutures are introduced first into the subbrow fat pad underneath the brow and then into the frontalis muscle under the undermined superior edge of the wound, and then brought out through the fat pad of the superior wound edge at a level that approximates the entry into the subbrow fat pad underneath the brow (Fig. 6A). This is done in two or three areas, in the desired area of lift. When the

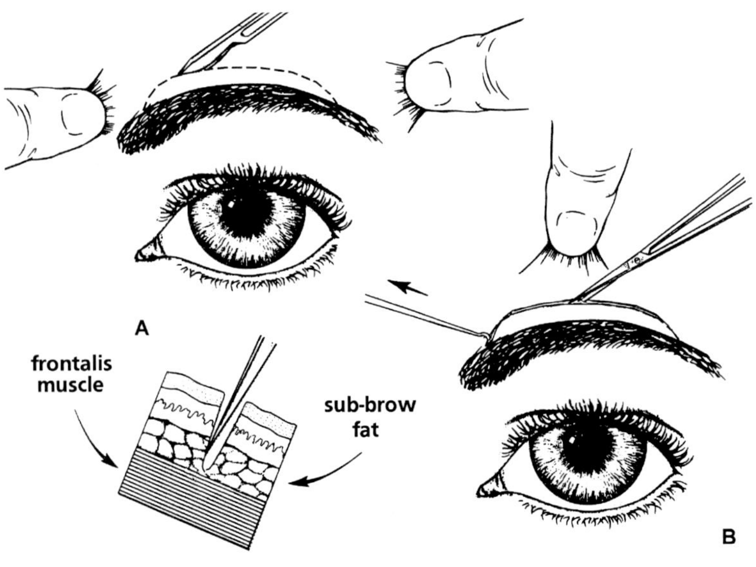

FIG. 3. **A:** Direct brow lift. With traction, the marked area is incised with the Bard–Parker through the thick skin and into the subbrow fat. **B:** With finger traction with skin hooks in two directions, sharp scissors can incise into the brow fat down to the level of the frontalis muscle.

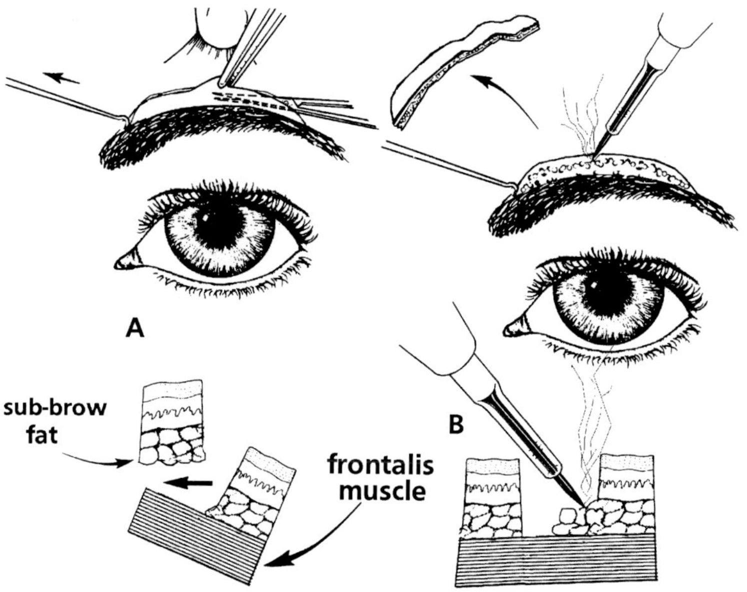

FIG. 4. Direct brow lift. **A:** With traction on the wound and the flap, the scissors can be used to dissect the thick skin and subbrow fat away from the frontalis muscle. The skin-fat ellipse is then excised. **B:** The wound can be "squared off" for more even closure. The residual fat at the base of the incision can be sculpted with the coagulating Bovie needle to ensure a rectangular-sided wound.

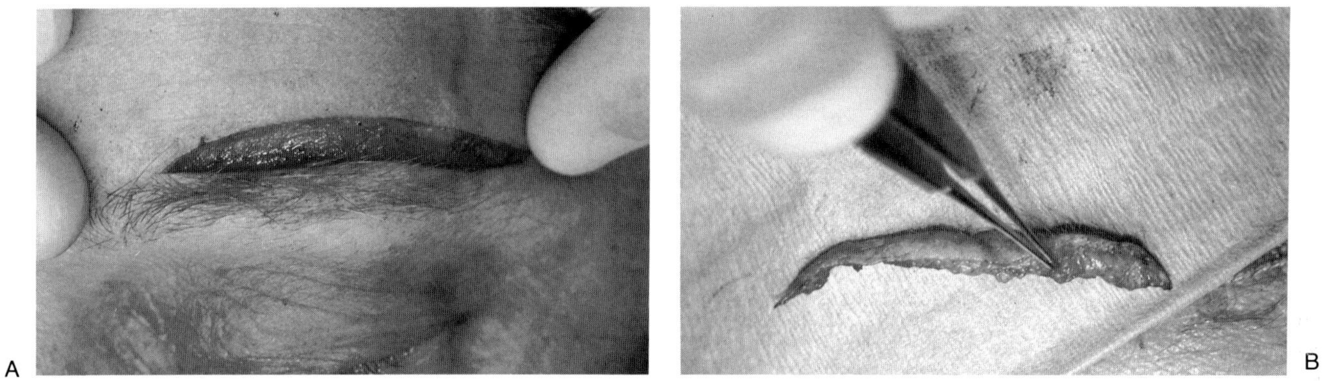

FIG. 5. Direct brow lift. **A:** Surgical view after skin and subbrow and subskin fat has been removed showing the frontalis muscle. **B:** The segment of skin and fat that has been removed.

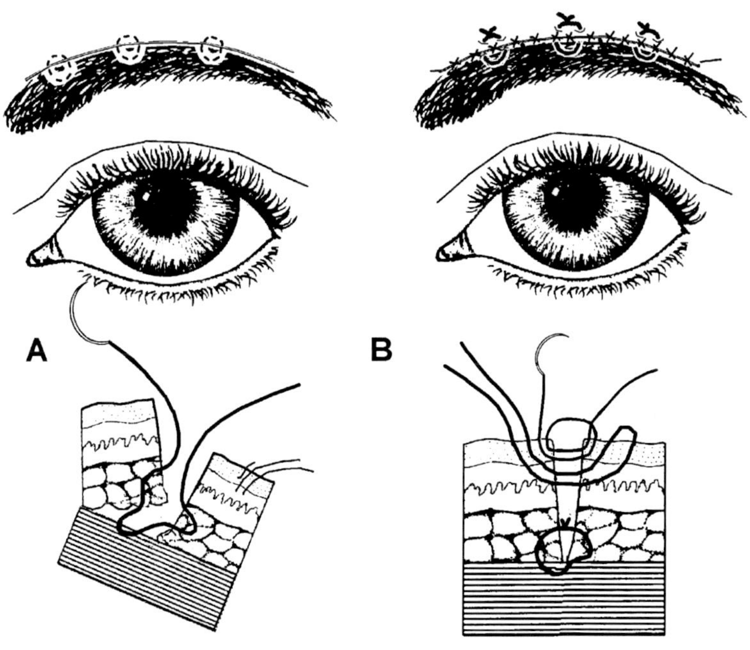

FIG. 6. Direct brow lift. **A:** The subbrow fat pad is sutured to the frontalis muscle and then to the inside superior edge of the incision. The superior edge of the incision has been undermined. **B:** Closure of the skin is accomplished with mattress everting sutures followed by continuous vertical mattress sutures to minimize scar formation in this conspicuous area of thick skin.

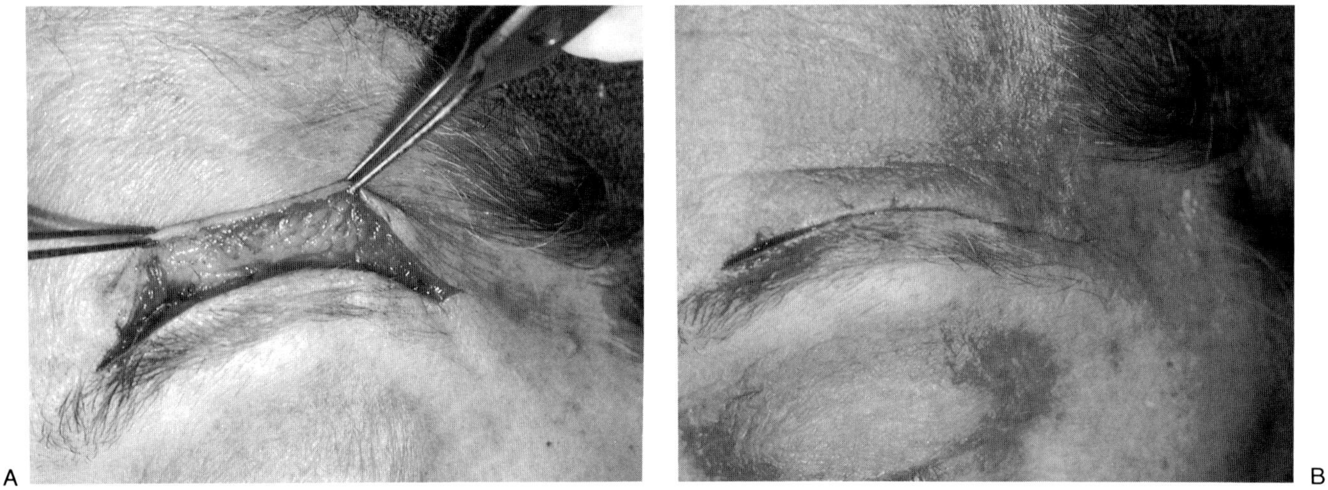

FIG. 7. Direct brow lift. **A:** The subbrow fat underneath the brow has been fixated to the frontalis muscle. The upper edge of the incision has been undermined and is being everted. **B:** With proper placement of the deep fixating sutures, the skin edges will approximate with closing the deep sutures alone. This ensures minimal tension on skin sutures and reduces scar formation.

sutures are tightened, the skin above the brow should approximate well to allow good closure and reduce scar formation in this conspicuous area. Figure 7A and B shows good deep approximation for closure of the brow incision. Further closure is accomplished with mattress everting sutures of 4-0 prolene to assure that the skin wound edges are everted before final closure. Final closure is then accomplished with continuous suture vertical mattress sutures of 6-0 nylon. The 6-0 nylon sutures are placed to encompass full-thickness wound edge (Fig. 6B). The sutures are removed in 1 week. Figure 8A and B shows a patient before and after direct brow lift.

Coronal Forehead Eyebrow Lift

The three anatomic deformities that are corrected by the coronal brow forehead lift are narrowing of the brow–lash distance, glabellar furrowing, and transverse forehead furrows. The coronal flap surgical procedure may be tailored to emphasize the correction of one of the problems or all three (Fig. 9).

Surgical Technique

Anesthesia

The coronal forehead lift can be performed under general or local anesthetics. It is generally combined with upper and lower lid blepharoplasty and, because of the duration of the procedure, is usually performed under a general anesthetic. If one chooses to perform the coronal lift under local anesthesia with sedation, then adequate anesthesic blocks can be obtained by bilateral frontal nerve blocks and infiltration of the zygomatic or temporal nerve branches just in front of the ear.

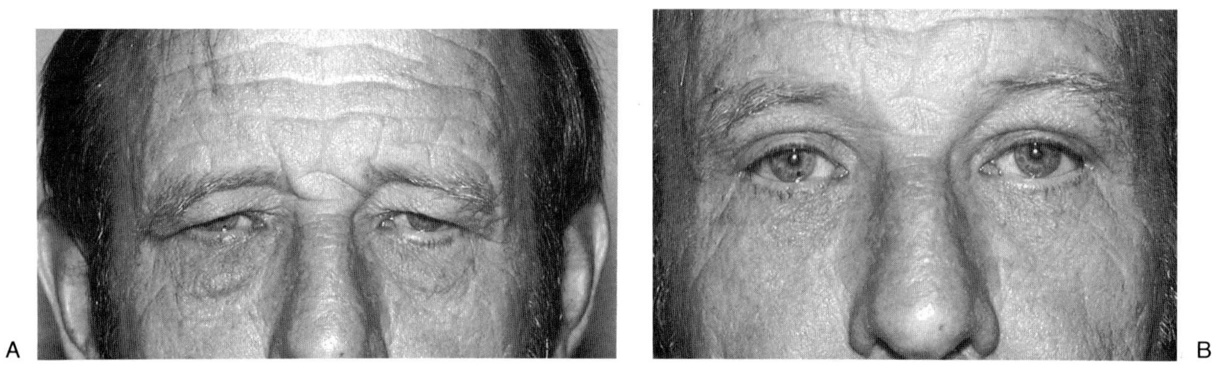

FIG. 8. Direct brow lift. **A:** A patient preoperatively with brow laxity and brow ptosis and a narrowed brow–lash distance. **B:** Same patient postoperatively with good brow elevation and fixation. In addition to a direct brow lift the patient also had an upper and lower blepharoplasty.

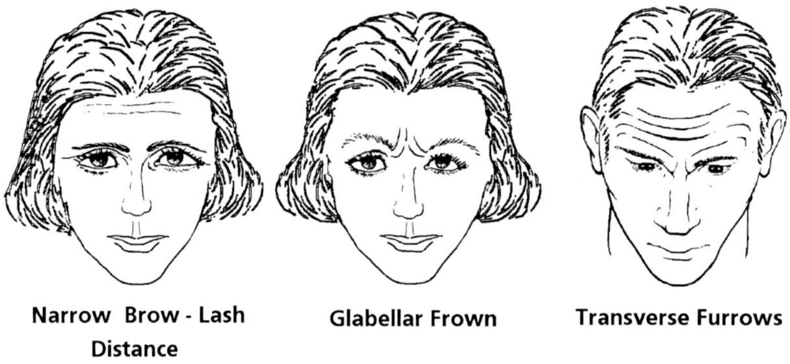

FIG. 9. Diagrammatic representation of the three deformities that can be corrected by a coronal forehead lift.

Technique

After anesthesia is obtained, the patient is positioned in the slightly head-up tilted position. The face and hair are scrubbed with Betadine sponge, and protective contact lenses are put into position. The incision line in most cases is placed behind the hairline, as shown in Fig. 10A(a) and B. This occurs most commonly in females who do not have a receding hairline or who wear their hair in the forward position. In women or in patients who have a receding hairline, the incision can be placed at the edge of the hairline, as in Fig. 10A(b); in some males who have deep transverse furrows, the incision can be placed in the midforehead area, as in Fig. 10A(c). In the usual situation, the placement is behind the hairline and the hair is parted with a comb at the desired position of the incision. The tract of scalp to be excised is then shaved and the incision line placed at the posterior edge of the shaved area. Usually it forms a slightly arcuate or bilobed incision that extends toward the root of the ear. A modification of the incision has been proposed by authors that extends behind the ear to allow greater mobility of the flap downward to expose the superior orbit (14).

The glabellar area, superior orbital rim area, and scalp area to be incised are infiltrated with red label

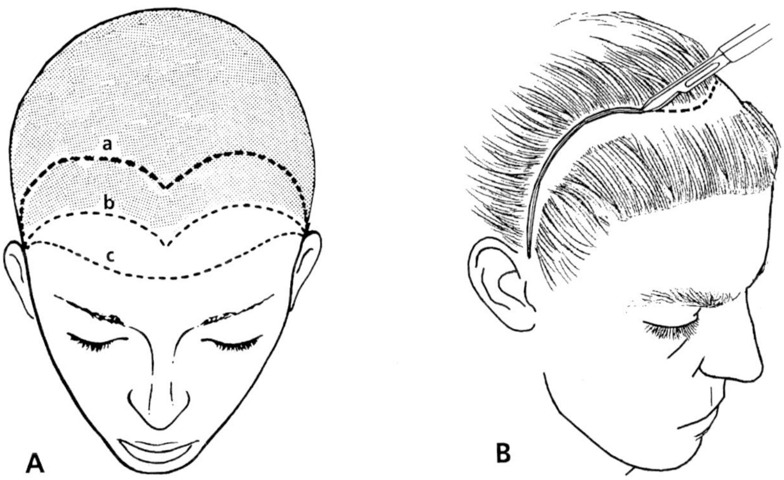

FIG. 10. Coronal forehead lift. **A:** Variations in incision placement with coronal forehead lift. (a) Standard placement of incision in females behind the hair line. (b) Pretrichial placement of the incision at the edge of the hairs in patients with receding hair line who wish the hair line to be brought downward. (c) Midforehead incision in patients who have deep transverse furrows in the forehead area, usually males. **B:** Initial incision is being made in the standard placement of the coronal incision. Over the temporalis muscle area, the incision is initially made only half-thickness through the scalp to avoid cutting the fascia and muscle.

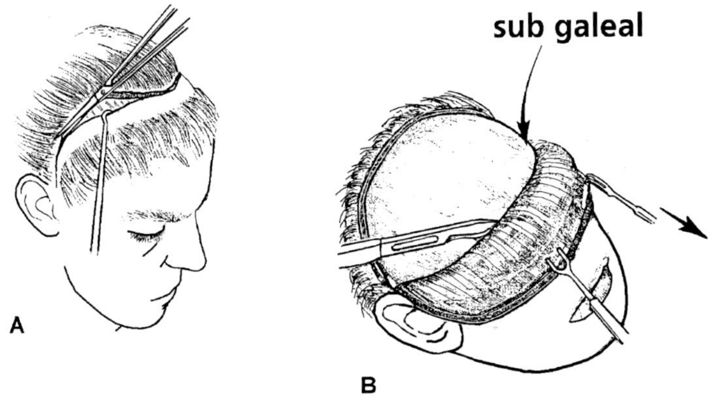

FIG. 11. Coronal forehead lift. **A:** Following the full-thickness incision in the central cranial area, the flap is retracted and scissors are used to complete the half-thickness incision that had been made over the temporalis muscle. The one arm of the scissors can be introduced in the plane between the scalp flap and the temporalis fascia and the incision completed without damage to the fascia or muscle. **B:** With downward traction on the flap, the flap can be everted and separated easily with a Bard–Parker blade dissecting in the subgaleal plane.

xylocaine and allowed 10 min for vasoconstriction. An incision with a Bard–Parker no. 12 blade is then made half scalp thickness starting at the ear portion of the incision over the temporalis muscle and carried to the central dome (Fig. 10B). Over the cranium, the incision is then full thickness to the periosteum. Skin hooks are then inserted to separate the anterior edge of the incision. Large Metzenbaum scissors are then introduced into the wound and the one tip subgaleal, and the other in the half-incised skin incision. The scissors are then used to complete the excision down toward the base of the ear (Fig. 11A). This allows completion of incision in an easier manner, and avoids inadvertent nicks into the temporalis muscle or fascia. The similar technique is used to incise the opposite side of the coronal incision.

Raney clips may be used in very vascular areas along the wound edges. In most cases they are not used because it has been found that adequate vasoconstriction and familiarity with the points of bleeding make them unnecessary. The most common sites of bleeding are in the superior temporal area of the flap and these are adequately cauterized with a bipolar cautery. Many times the middle branch of the superficial temporal artery is incised just above the ear, and this must also be cauterized with a bipolar cautery. Eliminating the use of the Raney clips has also in this author's experience reduced the incidence of hair loss from compression and damage to the hair follicles.

Using traction with large, double-pronged skin hooks, the coronal flap is then dissected in the subgaleal plane with the Bard–Parker blade as shown in Fig. 11B. As one reaches the superior orbital rim, the hooks should not be advanced down on the flap for fear of injury to the superficial temporal branch of the facial nerve. At this point the flap can be grasped with 4 × 4 gauze and fingers for downward traction. As one reaches the glabellar area and superior orbital rim area, the sharp dissection with the Bard–Parker blade is discontinued and further dissection is carried with the "peanut" gauze dissector and a hemostat, as shown in Fig. 12A. The dissection can be carried down laterally over the superior temporal portion of the lateral rim, if some sculpting of the bony lateral rim is desired (15,16). It can be carried down further centrally in a subperiosteal plane into the superior orbit if the removal of superior orbital fat from the eyelid is desired.

The outline of the corrugator muscles can be seen and a mosquito hemostat used to dissect out each corrugator muscle (Figs. 12B and 13A). When the muscles themselves are isolated, they are severed in a piecemeal manner with sharp scissor dissection in such a way as to spare sensory branches of the supratrochlear nerve, which will reduce the amount of postoperative numbness in the forehead. In most cases a fairly large branch of the supratrochlear nerve can be seen and saved. No portion of the corrugator muscle is actually removed but is simply lysed as completely as possible. In the author's experience, extensive removal of the soft tissue in the glabellar area can produce an unwanted flattening postoperatively. Following the lysis of the two corrugator muscles, the procerus muscle in

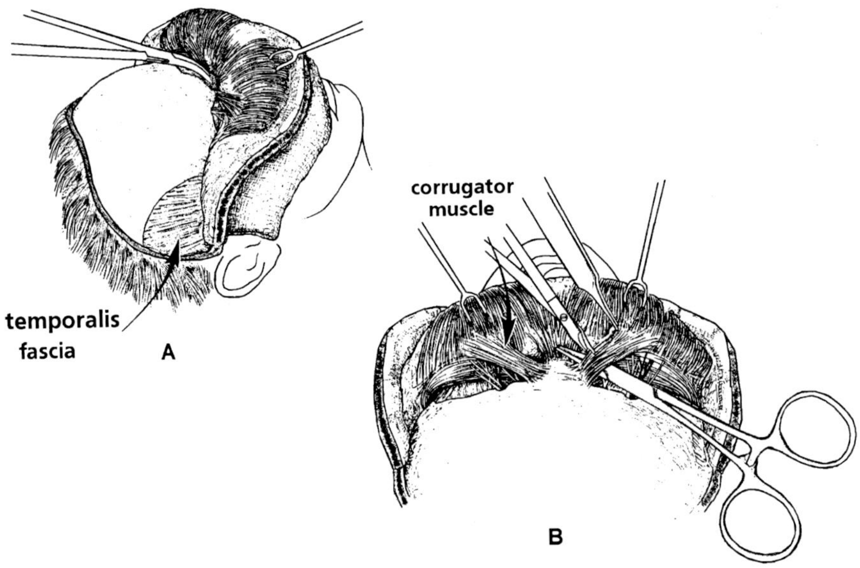

FIG. 12. Coronal forehead lift. **A:** When the flap has been reflected downward to the superior orbital rim, the "peanut" dissectors are used to further dissect the glabellar portion of the flap for isolation of the corrugator muscle. **B:** Mosquito hemostats are then to be used to dissect through the fascial planes and underneath the corrugator muscles isolating the muscles. With sharp dissection and direct visualization, the muscle can be lysed sparing the sensory nerves that run through the muscle, reducing numbness in the forehead area.

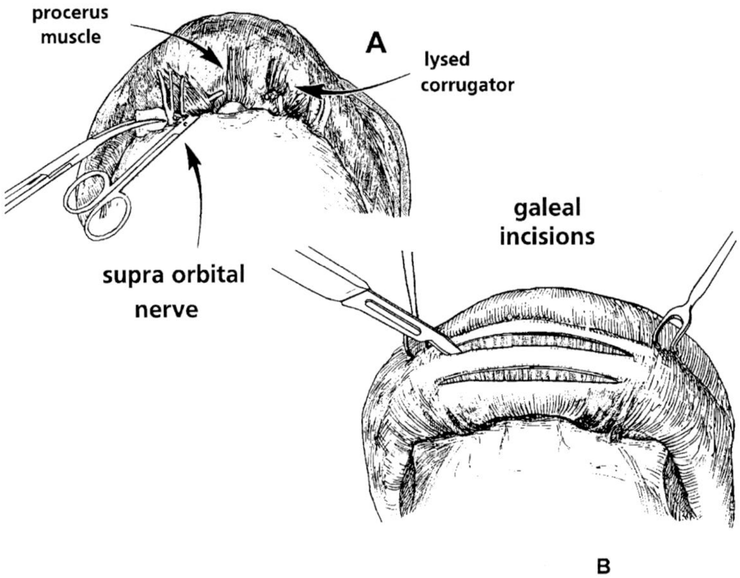

FIG. 13. Coronal forehead lift. **A:** The corrugator muscle has been lysed on the right side and isolated on the left for dissection. The supraorbital nerves can be identified and retracted from the dissection area. The thin procerus muscle in the midline can also be lysed. **B:** Following the lysis of the corrugator and procerus muscles conservative incisions in the galea can be made, if desired, to allow more stretchability of the flap for smoothing of transverse furrows. The frontalis muscle is left intact.

the central area can be lysed in a similar manner, although many times simple incision of the galea and lysis of a few strands with a Bovie cautery is sufficient. Some undermining can be carried down into the nasal dorsum if desired. After hemostasis is obtained with the bipolar cautery, the area is irrigated with cold water to facilitate identification of any potential bleeders.

Before replacement of the flap, if there are visible transverse furrows that are unsightly, some smoothing of these can be obtained by incisions in the galea at the approximate location of the furrows (Fig. 13B). This author has found this to be satisfactory in smoothing the transverse furrows. Actual excision of frontalis muscle in strips can be performed and is recommended by other authors, but unfortunately in some cases it can produce an "overstretched" and shiny look to the forehead. Consequently, it is not used by this author.

The flap is then replaced. Relaxing incision and cardinal sutures are placed in the advanced flap in the areas that require the greatest lifting. In patients who have an exaggerated glabellar frown, two relaxing incisions are made in a vertical line beginning at the nasal third of the brow area to gain the greatest lift in this area (Fig. 14B). Additional relaxing incisions are made temporally. In the standard situation of generalized brow laxity or in patients who have more of a temporal laxity, a single relaxing incision is made in the central

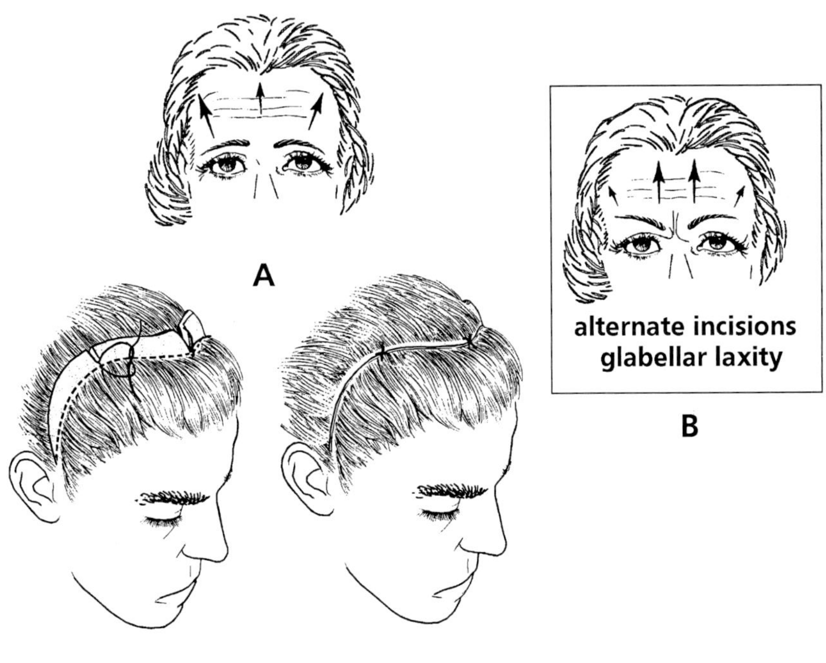

FIG. 14. Coronal forehead lift. The incisions for placement of the cardinal sutures in advancement of the flap can be varied according to the maximum areas of laxity. **A:** If the maximum area of laxity is temporal, then usually one central relaxing incision is made and two temporal incisions are made. **B:** If the laxity is greater in the glabellar area, two incisions are made over each eyebrow area for greater purchase of the cardinal sutures in the nasal brow area. With either set of incisions, the flap is advanced, cardinal sutures are placed advancing the flap, and the redundant rectangles and triangles of scalp are excised before closure. The galea is closed meticulously with 3-0 vicryl sutures, which ensures hemostasis and prevents later spreading of the incision line.

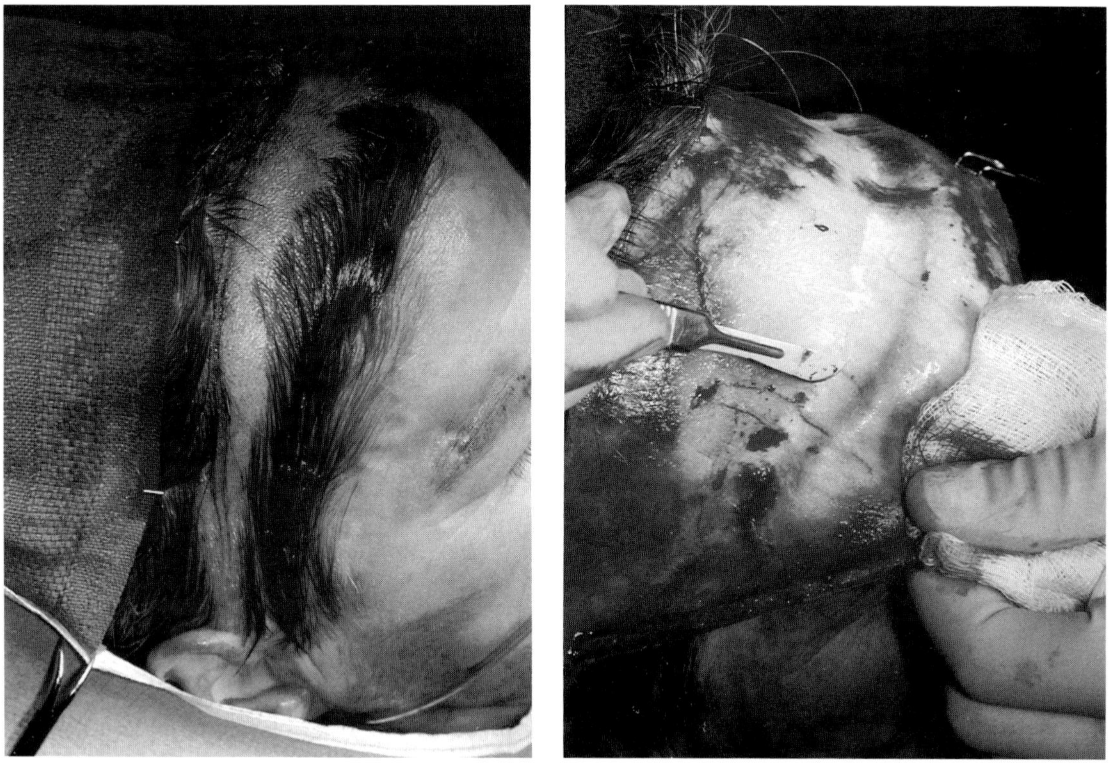

A B

FIG. 15. Coronal forehead lift. **A:** Surgical view showing shaved area with incision line marked at the posterior edge of the shaved area. **B:** The coronal flap has been dissected downward in the subgaleal plane with sharp dissection. Digital retraction with a gauze pad is preferred to hooks to avoid possible injury to the temporal branch of the facial nerve.

portion of the flap in line with the dorsum of the nose and then relaxing incisions temporally, as shown in Fig. 14A. The widths of the relaxing incisions generally correspond to the width of the shaved scalp if the incision is behind the hairline. However, one should judge intraoperatively the positioning of the brow and further adjustments in the length of the incision should be made. Cardinal sutures of 3-0 prolene are then used in

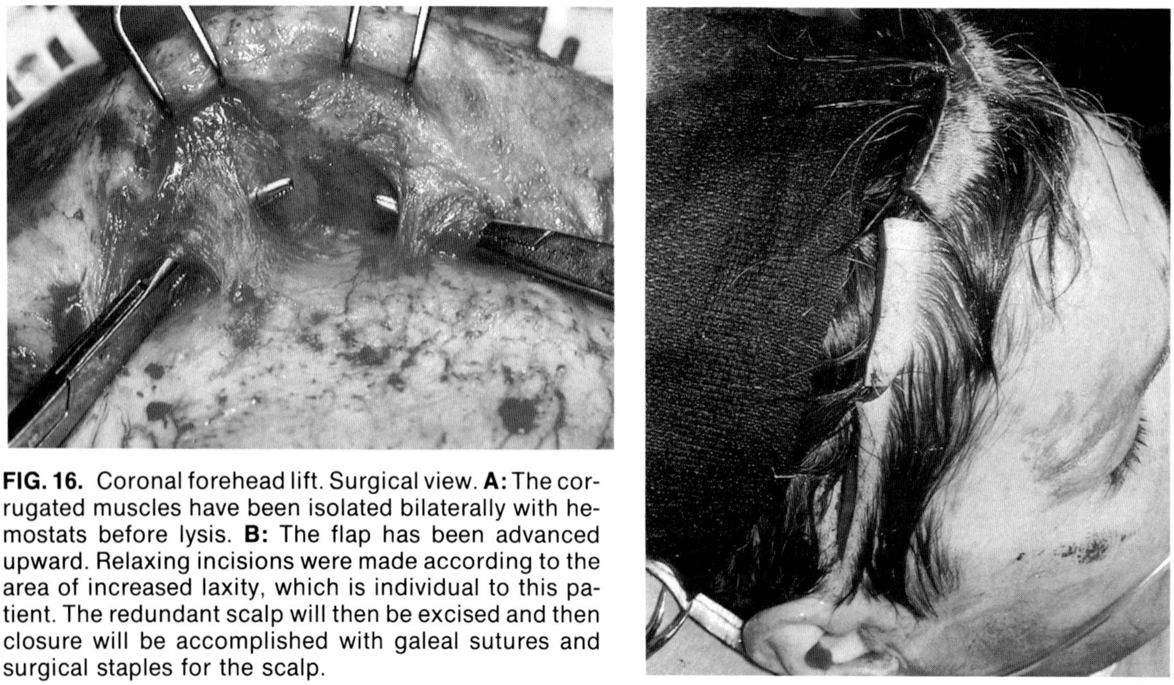

A B

FIG. 16. Coronal forehead lift. Surgical view. **A:** The corrugated muscles have been isolated bilaterally with hemostats before lysis. **B:** The flap has been advanced upward. Relaxing incisions were made according to the area of increased laxity, which is individual to this patient. The redundant scalp will then be excised and then closure will be accomplished with galeal sutures and surgical staples for the scalp.

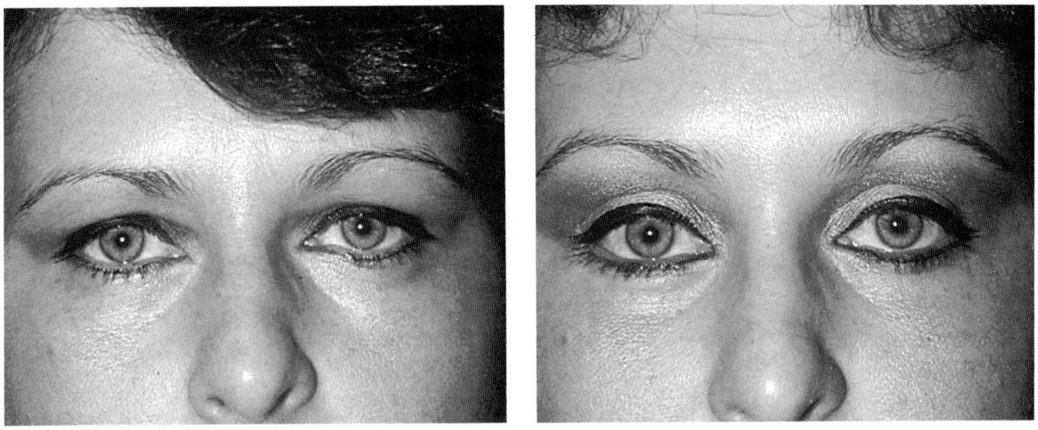

A B

FIG. 17. Coronal forehead lift. **A:** Patient preoperatively before conservative coronal forehead lift and upper and lower lid blepharoplasty. **B:** Same patient postoperatively.

the areas of the relaxing incisions to advance the flap and elevate the brow glabellar area. Occasionally, multiple adjustments are needed to gain symmetry or the desired effect.

Once the flap has been advanced to the desired position, the rectangular areas of scalp that are redundant are then excised as is the triangular temporal flap that is most adjacent to the ear. If new bleeding occurs at this time, the flap edges can be injected with saline to reduce the bleeding and the bipolar cautery can be used.

Sutures are then placed in multiple areas in the galea for closure, particularly across the dome of the head. These galea sutures are important for hemostasis and also reduce any "spreading" of the scar postoperatively. (It is always annoying to have a patient return with complaints from a hairdresser about the width of the scar a year or so later.) 3-0 Vicryl on a half-circle needle seems to be the easiest suture to use for this closure. Final closure of the incision if placed behind the hairline is performed with surgical staples, which give excellent closure and reduce damage to the hair follicles.

Figure 15A and B shows surgical views of the coronal incision and dissection of the scalp flap. Figure 16A shows a surgical view of isolation of the corrugator muscles with hemostats and Fig. 16B the advancement of the scalp flap with relaxing incisions.

It has been found that proper attention to hemostasis during the procedure will eliminate the need for any postoperative drain in most patients. If the incision is placed at the hairline edge or in the midforehead area, staples should not be used to close the visible skin incision. Closure in this area is accomplished with 4-0 prolene everting mattress sutures and skin sutures of 6-0 nylon. The galea should also be closed meticulously in this area.

Figures 17–19 show pre- and postoperative views of patients following coronal forehead lift with varying techniques.

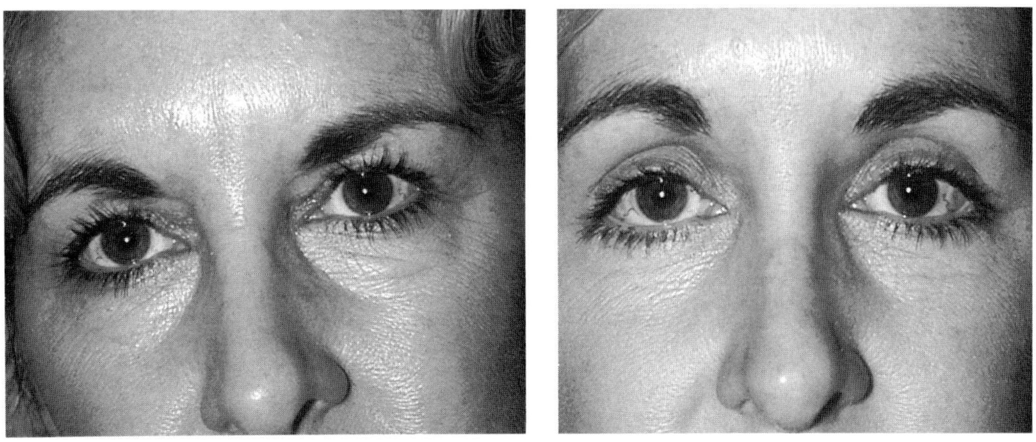

A B

FIG. 18. Coronal forehead lift. **A:** Patient before coronal forehead lift and upper and lower lid blepharoplasty. **B:** Because of the patient's wishes, more arching of the brow and a higher lid crease was created.

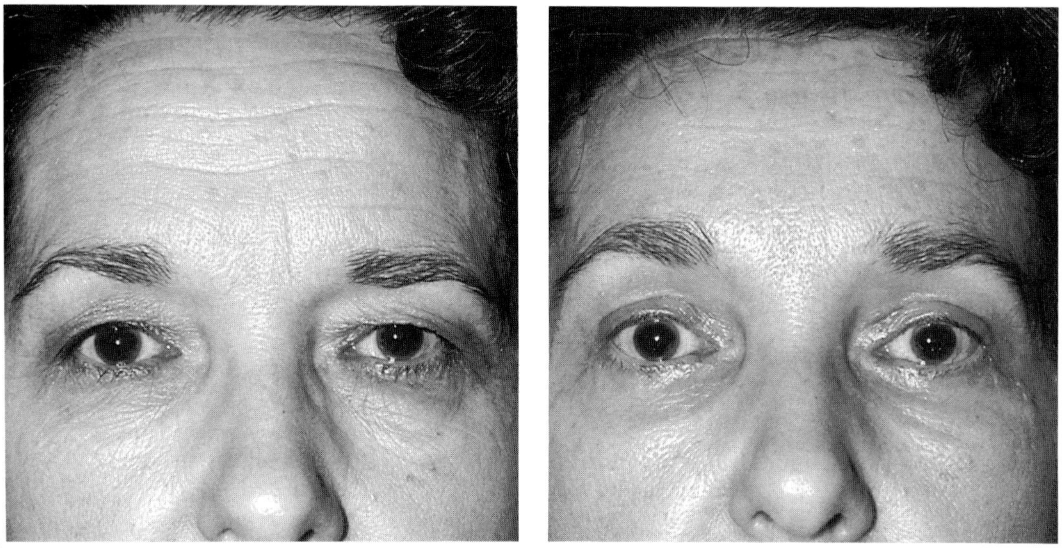

A B

FIG. 19. Coronal forehead lift with pretrichial incision. **A:** Patient with receding hair line preoperatively. **B:** Same patient at 4 weeks following coronal forehead lift with pretrichial incision and upper and lower lid blepharoplasty. The hair has been brushed backward to show the placement of the healing incision.

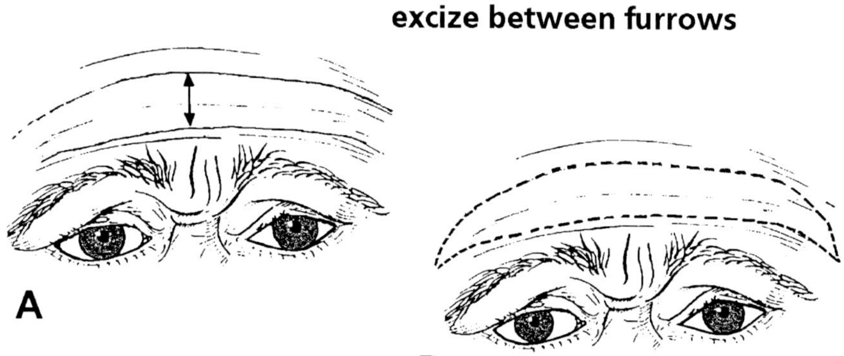

A B

FIG. 20. Coronal forehead lift, midforehead incision. **A:** Area of skin to excise between the two deepest furrows should be marked for excision. **B:** Marking of the area to be excised.

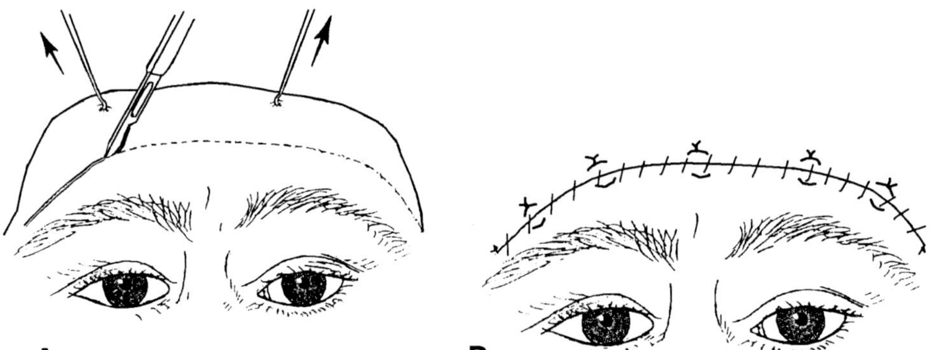

A B

FIG. 21. Coronal forehead lift, midforehead incision. **A:** The flap in the forehead area has been developed with an incision through the upper marking and the segment of skin is then completely excised with a Bard–Parker blade. **B:** Closure in the galea has been performed before final closure with mattress sutures everting the skin and continuous sutures.

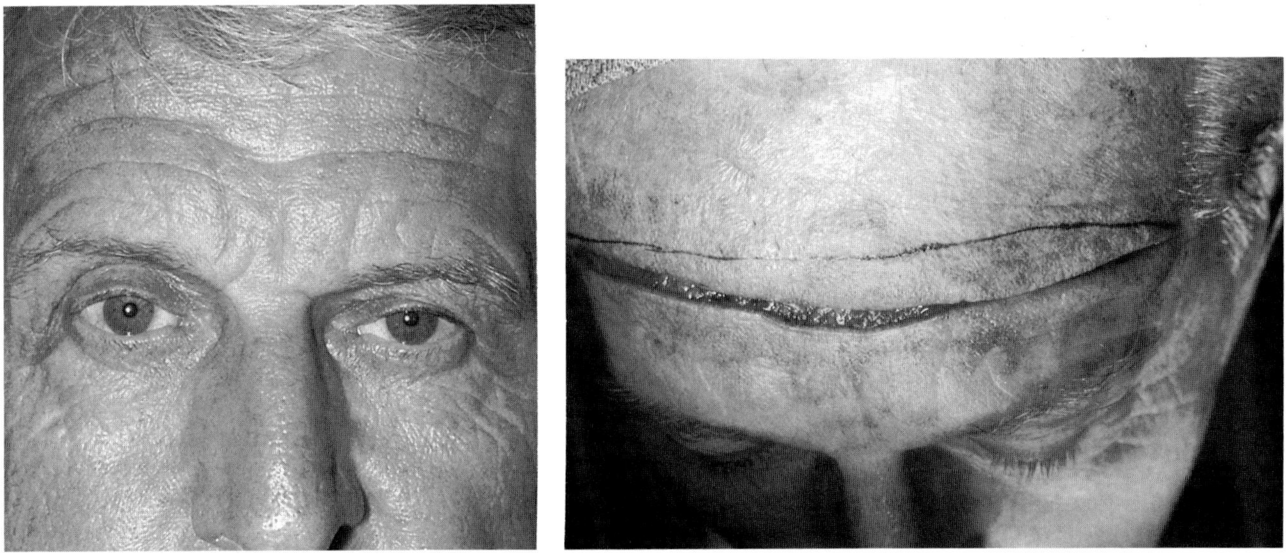

A B

FIG. 22. Coronal forehead lift, midforehead incision. **A:** Patient preoperatively. **B:** Surgical view showing the area of skin and forehead tissue to be excised in this patient.

Coronal Forehead Lift Through a Midforehead Transverse Incision

Coronal forehead lift through a midforehead transverse incision is done almost exclusively in males and in patients who would benefit from forward advancement of the hairline. The most common anesthesia used is frontal nerve block and local infiltration of the forehead area. When placing the skin incision, the surgeon should try to find two furrows and plan to make the initial incision in the upper one and develop the flap for advancement inferiorly, although the opposite direction has been used successfully. If the amount of forehead skin to be resected coincides with a lower furrow, then a much better scar and smoothing effect in the forehead can be obtained (Fig. 20A, B).

The resection of skin and flap development can be subgaleal or subcutaneous. The subgaleal flap is easier to elevate and easier to close with less of a scar but transects the sensory nerves with marked forehead numbness postoperatively. The subcutaneous flap does not cause quite as much sensory loss but closure is more difficult with tension on the skin edges of the wound. When the wound is closed, separate galeal closure is needed if it is incised. The forehead skin is then closed with exaggerated everting vertical mattress sutures (4-0 prolene) and vertical mattress sutures (6-0 nylon) (Fig. 21A, B).

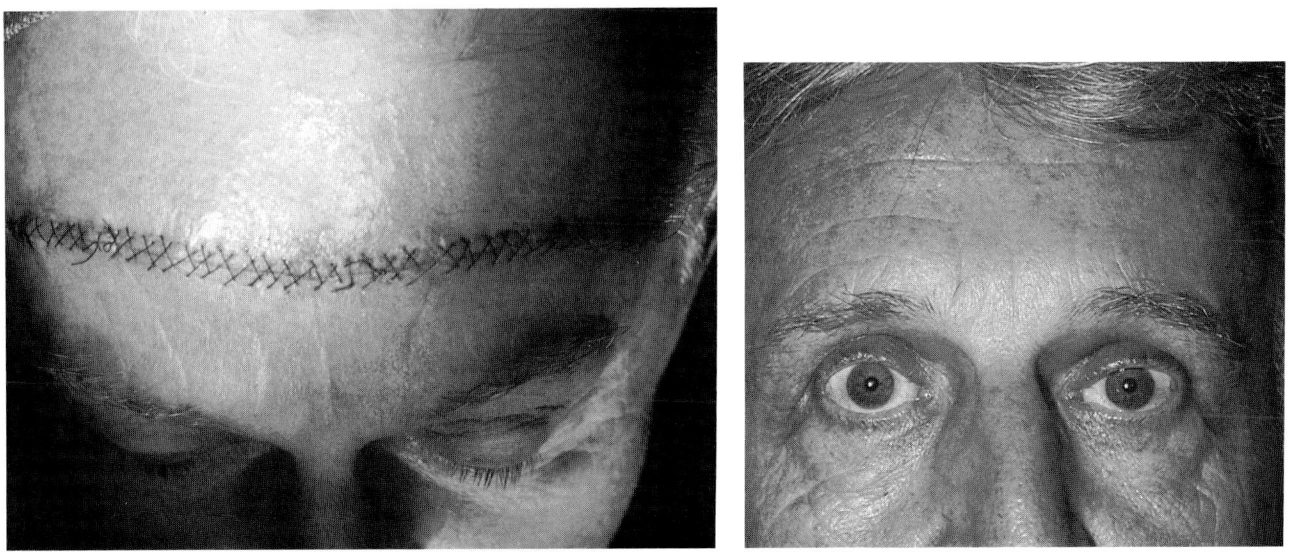

A B

FIG. 23. Coronal forehead lift, midforehead incision. **A:** The skin segment has been excised in this patient with closure of the galea and vertical mattress skin closure. **B:** Same patient as seen in the previous views 6 weeks postoperatively.

Figure 22A and B shows a patient for a midforehead coronal incision preoperatively and a surgical view of the developed scalp flap. Figure 23 A and B shows closure of the incision and a 6-week postoperative result.

For cosmetic brow surgery, see Chapter 29, "Endoscopic Forehead Lift."

SIDE EFFECTS AND COMPLICATIONS

Numbness behind the incision line is always present postoperatively and should be thoroughly described to the patient preoperatively. Sensation will return over a period of 8–10 weeks but may not completely return for several months.

Hairline displacement will always occur to some degree and the specific technique that is acceptable to the patient should be used.

Incisions placed within the hairline have the potential of causing *hair loss* by damage to the follicles. Strangulating mattress sutures should not be used to close the scalp incision in these areas because of the production of follicle ischemia. Surgical staples seem to avoid this problem.

Hematoma formation can occur in patients with specific problems such as elevated blood pressure, blood thinning medication, or other factors. Suction drains are not used routinely by the authors but should be used if there is a question of a problem.

Overflattening and *thinning in the glabellar area* can occur if the corrugator and procerus muscles are overly excised. Some subcutaneous atrophy of fat may occur.

Overcorrection and the "surprised" look are responsible for causing the greatest fear in patients considering the coronal procedure. The surgeon should maintain good intraoperative attention and control with this problem in mind when adjusting the brows.

REFERENCES

1. Giles E, Elliot O. Sex determination by discriminant function analysis of crania. *Am J Phys Anthropol* 1963;21:53.
2. Snow CC, Gatliff BP, McWilliams KR. Reconstruction of facial features from the skull: an evaluation of its usefulness in forensic anthropology. *Am J Phys Anthropol* 1970;33:221.
3. Stewart TD. Sex determination of the skeleton by guess and by measurement. *Am J Phys Anthropol* 1954;12:385.
4. Doxanas MT, Anderson RL. *Clinical orbital anatomy*. Baltimore: Williams and Wilkins, 1984.
5. Zide BM, Jelks GW. *Surgical anatomy of the orbit*. New York: Raven Press; 1985.
6. McCord CD, Doxanas MT Browplasty and browpexy: an adjunct to blepharoplasty. *Plast Reconstr Surg* 1990;86:248–254.
7. Wilkins RB, Hunter GJ, McCord CD, Tanenbaum MN. Blepharoplasty: cosmetic and functional. *Oculoplastic surgery*. 2nd ed. New York: Raven Press; 1987:451–457.
8. Hinderer UT. Blepharocanthoplasty with eyebrow lift. *Plast Reconstr Surg* 1972;56:402.
9. Connell BF. Eyebrow, face, and neck lifts for males. *Clin Plast Surg* 1978;5:15–28.
10. Castanares S. Forehead wrinkles, glabellar frown and ptosis of the eybrows. *Plast Reconstr Surg* 1964;34:406.
11. Vinas JC, Caviglia C, Cortinis JL. Forehead rhytidectomy and browlifting. *Plast Reconstr Surg* 1976;57:445.
12. Rees TD, Wood-Smith D. *Cosmetic facial surgery*. Philadelphia: WB Saunders; 1973.
13. Shore JW. Essential blepharospasm. *Oculoplastic surgery*. 2nd ed. New York: Raven Press; 1987:479–487.
14. Cartwright MJ, Elner V, Polley, et al. A modification of the transcoronal flap that enhances orbital exploration and cosmesis. *Ophth Plast Reconstr Surg* 1993;9:139–142.
15. Lassus C. Ostectomy of superior orbital rim in cosmetic blepharoplasty. *Plast Reconstr Surg* 1979;63:481.
16. Whitaker LA, Morales L Jr, Farkas LG. Aesthetic surgery of the supraorbital ridge and forehead structures. *Plast Reconstr Surg* 1986;78:23.

CHAPTER 14

Upper Lid Blepharoplasty

SURGICAL CONSIDERATIONS

Preoperative plans for upper lid blepharoplasty should have specific anatomic goals in mind for the patient's postoperative appearance. The past perceptions that if the surgeon has excised some upper lid skin and a little fat a satisfactory upper lid blepharoplasty has been performed should be abandoned. In most cases, by today's standards, this would be considered a token or incomplete blepharoplasty, likely to result in dissatisfaction.

The usual goal in upper lid blepharoplasty is to expose (or reexpose) a clear strip of skin between the lashes and the upper lid crease (the pretarsal skin or "eyeshadow space" in females) so that it is not covered by the upper lid fold. The degree of this effect may vary from exposing a large area with production of a high lid crease and a "deep-set" look in females (Fig. 1) to a smaller amount in males (Fig. 4). This effect is accomplished by removal and debulking of the overhanging fold of skin-muscle layer, removal of orbital septum and orbicularis, adequate removal of fatty tissue, and crease fixation. Figure 2A–D shows the desired effect in an older female. Figure 3A–D shows the desired effect in a younger female.

TREATMENT OF ORBITAL SEPTUM AND MUSCLE

The surgeon must utilize more than skin excision and minimal fat removal through little holes in the septum.

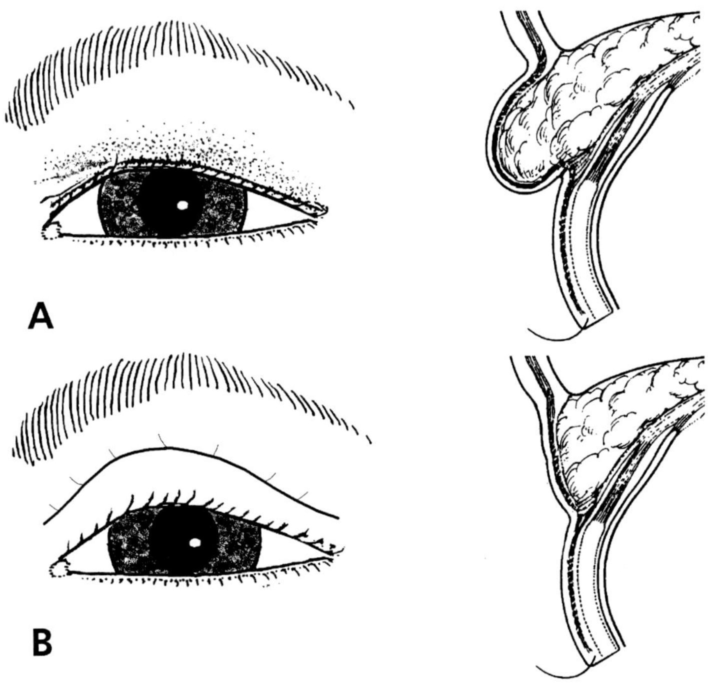

FIG. 1. Goal of blepharoplasty in female upper lid. **A:** Diagrammatic representation of an upper lid fold in the female patient obscuring the pretarsal area. **B:** Postremoval of skin-muscle-septum and preaponeurotic fat and crease fixation to produce more exposed pretarsal area.

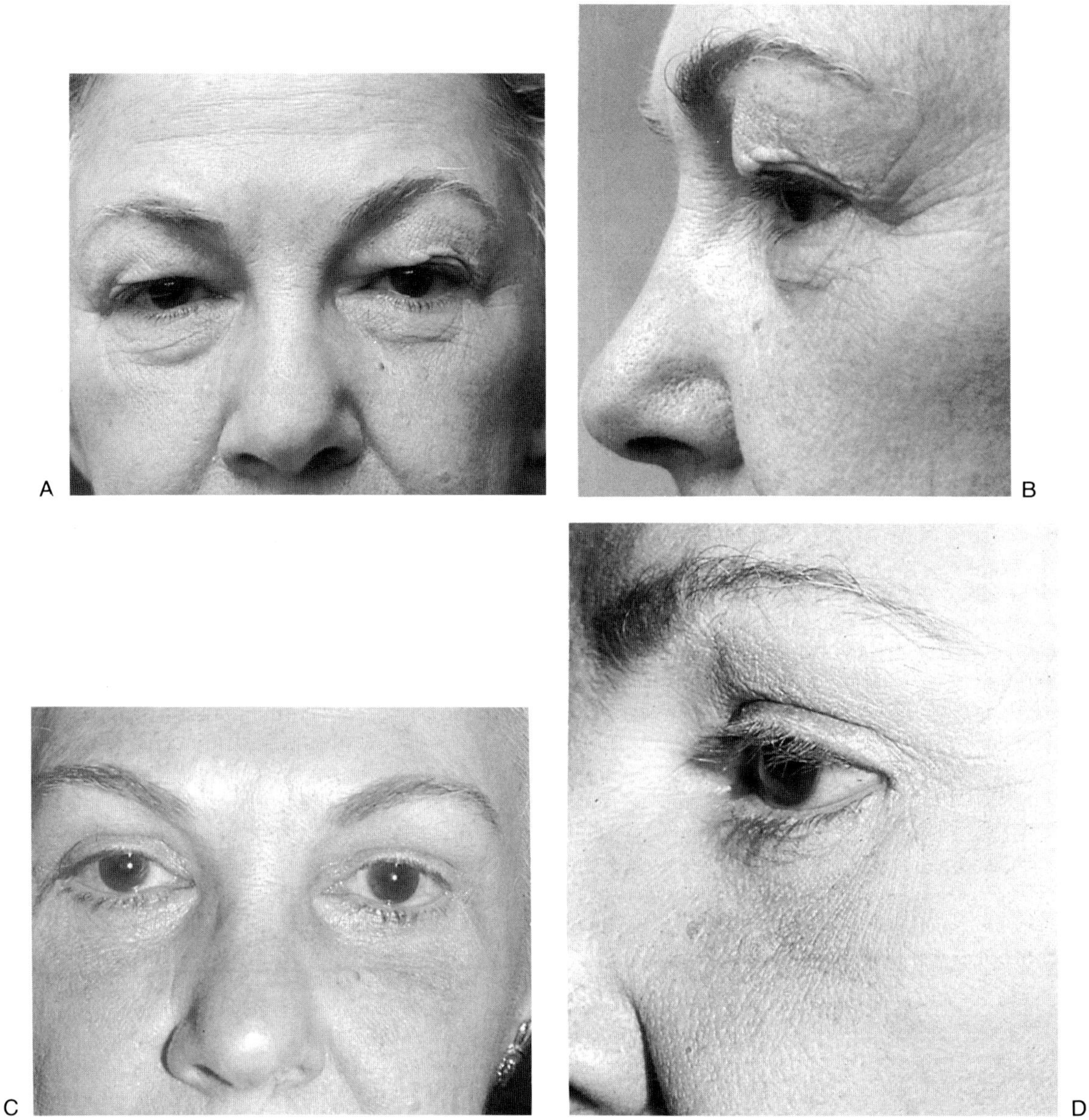

FIG. 2. A: Patient with pronounced folding of skin and fatty tissue obscuring the pretarsal space (eye shadow space). **B:** Side view of the same patient preoperatively. **C:** Same patient following an upper lid blepharoplasty with formation of a lid crease and exposure of the pretarsal "eye shadow" space. The patient has also had a lower lid blepharoplasty. **D:** Same patient postoperatively from side view.

Complete removal of the underlying orbital septum and orbicularis reduces some of the lagophthalmos that may be seen postoperatively if they are left intact (1). Septal scarring can produce unwanted stiffness in the lid postoperatively. Closure of skin over unexcised orbicularis, besides decreasing the thinning effect in the lid, will stiffen eyelid closure.

SKIN EXCISION DESIGN

The desired surgical approach should have the effect of forming a well-defined lid crease, clearing the pretarsal space and producing a pleasing amount of upper lid concavity with conservative skin excision. This results in less lagophthalmos and less chance of making the patient have exposure or dry eye symptoms postoperatively.

In general, the surgeon has much more latitude in excising skin in the lateral portion of the upper lid. The lateral brow area is much more forgiving and even if unwanted stiffness occurs laterally it seems to produce fewer symptoms in the patient. This is not true nasally and even small amounts of stiffness and lagophthalmos can produce severe symptoms in a patient, particularly

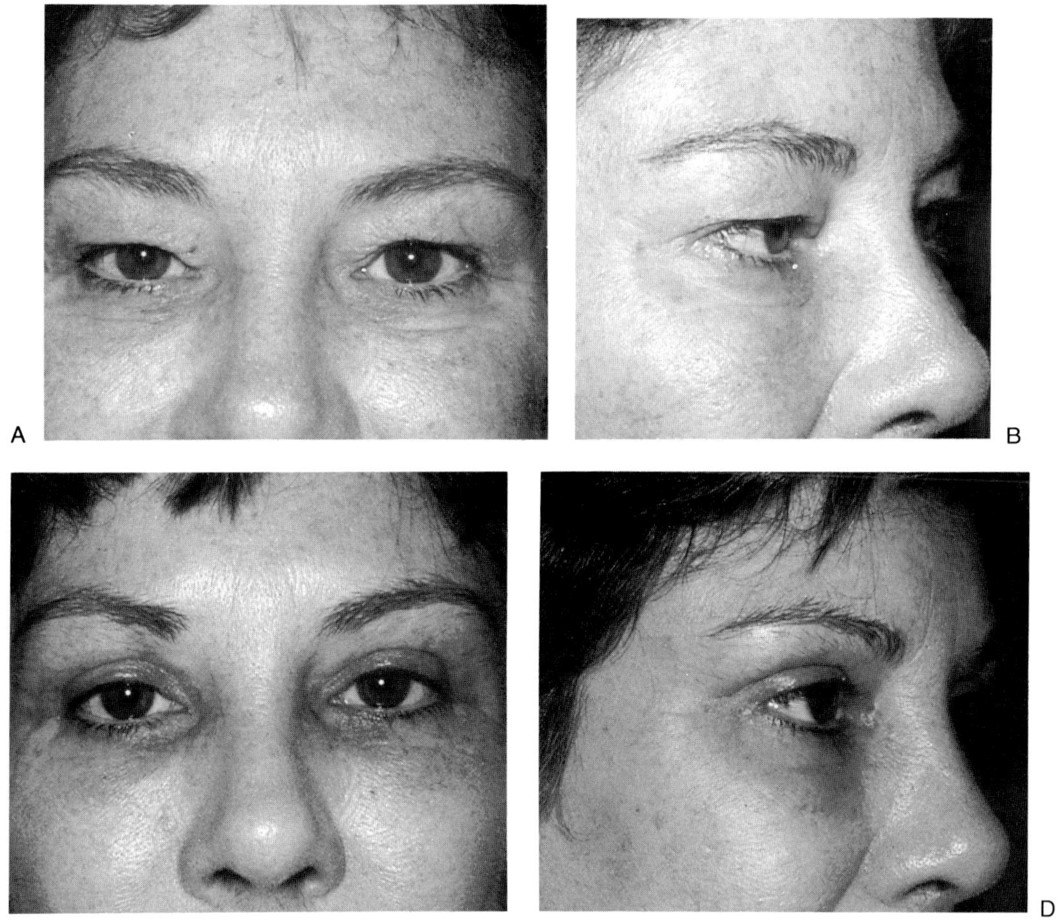

FIG. 3. Younger patient with hooding of the upper lids and loss of visibility of the pretarsal skin and eyelid crease. **A:** Patient before surgery. **B:** Side view of the same patient. **C:** Patient following upper lid blepharoplasty with good visibility of the pretarsal eye shadow space and formation of eyelid crease. The patient has also had a lower lid blepharoplasty. **D:** Same patient from the side view.

if he or she has a reduced tear film. The position of the upper lid crease is placed in females 9–10 mm and in males 8 mm above the lash line but can vary according to the desired effect.

BROW

As previously discussed, a lax brow requires some brow treatment or the surgeon will never be able to "clear" the pretarsal area of the skin fold even with large amounts of skin excision, because the brow will simply migrate downward postoperatively, producing a new fold of skin on the eyelid.

SPECIAL CONSIDERATIONS IN MALE BLEPHAROPLASTY

As indicated above, the surgeon usually takes a different approach to upper lid blepharoplasty in males patients than females. The percentage of males who undergo blepharoplasty has been increasing. Probably the most important reason for this is the fact that males, busy executives or professional people, have become aware that surgery is available, can be performed safely, and is usually not time consuming. In addition, the new trend toward "fitness" and being "in shape" body-wise is now being applied to the face. It seems incongruous to many males or females to be in shape physically but have baggy eyelids. The competitiveness in today's job market hinges on one's appearance and ability to project youthful energy.

The range of men undergoing this procedure is increasing, from young males with puffy eyelids of a familial nature to older males who are undergoing changes due to the passage of time and other factors.

Most males do not want as much change in appearance as their female counterparts, wanting to retain a "natural" look. In the upper lids this usually is reflected by a removal of a portion of the lid fold that comes out over the lid, obscuring the lid skin above the lashes, and a slight elevation of the brow or simple restoration of the brow to its normal position on the superior orbital rim. The male brow is flat and rests just above the level of the rim. Most males do not want a deep-set upper lid crease, so a more conservative amount of skin-muscle and fat is removed with less clearing of the pretarsal skin.

In many cases eyebrow ptosis is the main problem in the male patient. A very common combination of procedures in the male is eyebrow fixation with a direct of internal approach with a conservative upper lid blepharoplasty. A lower lid procedure that may commonly enhance the above is a conservative lower lid blepharoplasty externally or fornix fat removal as described in the next chapter.

UPPER LID BLEPHAROPLASTY SURGICAL TECHNIQUE

Anesthesia is performed by frontal block, pretarsal infiltration, and nasal fat infiltration. Wydase is used to reduce tissue distortion and a 10-min wait before surgery is customary to allow vasoconstriction to occur (Fig. 4).

Skin Marking

Patient should have a soap (Betadine) prep blotted dry instead of scrubbed with water so methylene blue will adhere to skin. The central position of the upper lid crease is marked at 9–10 mm in females and 8 mm in males, with the tissue on a stretch. The lid crease incision marking is drawn freehand but placing it above the lashes approximately 6 mm at lateral canthus and 5 mm nasally (Fig. 5A–C). At the lateral end of the crease it is angled upward pointing toward the end of the brow. Medially it is angled upward just beyond the punctum. Symmetry should be checked from side to side.

A general idea of skin removal can be gained with the ''bunching technique'' but it should only be used at the lateral canthus area. This is in keeping with the idea that the postoperative result doesn't depend on exactly how much skin is removed, but the treatment and recontouring of the subcutaneous structures for rearranging of the eyelid skin. If the bunching technique is used, it is to be used only at the lateral canthus. The proper amount of bunching should show some slight eversion of lashes. Bunching should not be used in the central lid or nasally because the amount of skin excision in these areas should be conservative and less than that obtained with the bunching technique. In general terms, the surgeon should maximize the skin excision laterally and minimize the skin excision centrally and nasally. It is to be emphasized that the desired effect in the upper lid, the creation of a crease and a smooth exposed pretarsal skin area, is obtained not by skin stretching but by rearrangement of tissue, adequate fat removal, septal muscle excision, and fixation of the pretarsal skin.

One way of ensuring symmetry in skin excision from both upper lids is to measure the distance of the superior edge of the marked ellipse from the brow hairs above (Fig. 5C). The superior ellipse edge should be measured from the inferior edge of the brow hairs and generally is located at the juncture of the thick and thin skin of the upper lid. Symmetric distances will give symmetric creases postoperatively if the brows are symmetric.

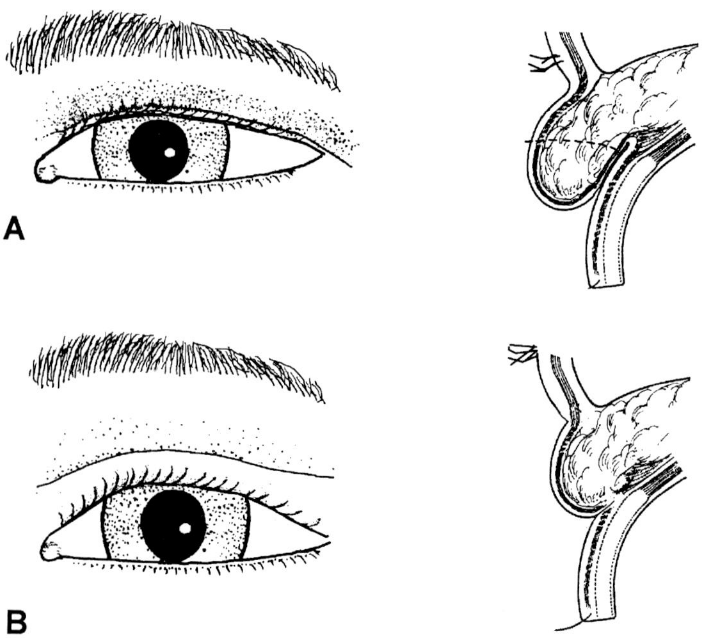

FIG. 4. Goal in male upper lid blepharoplasty. Diagrammatic representation of a more conservative amount of skin-muscle and fat removal in the male to avoid the higher crease. In most males the desired result is a lower lid crease than in the female and not as much skin exposed in the pretarsal area above the lashes. **A:** Preoperatively. **B:** Postoperatively.

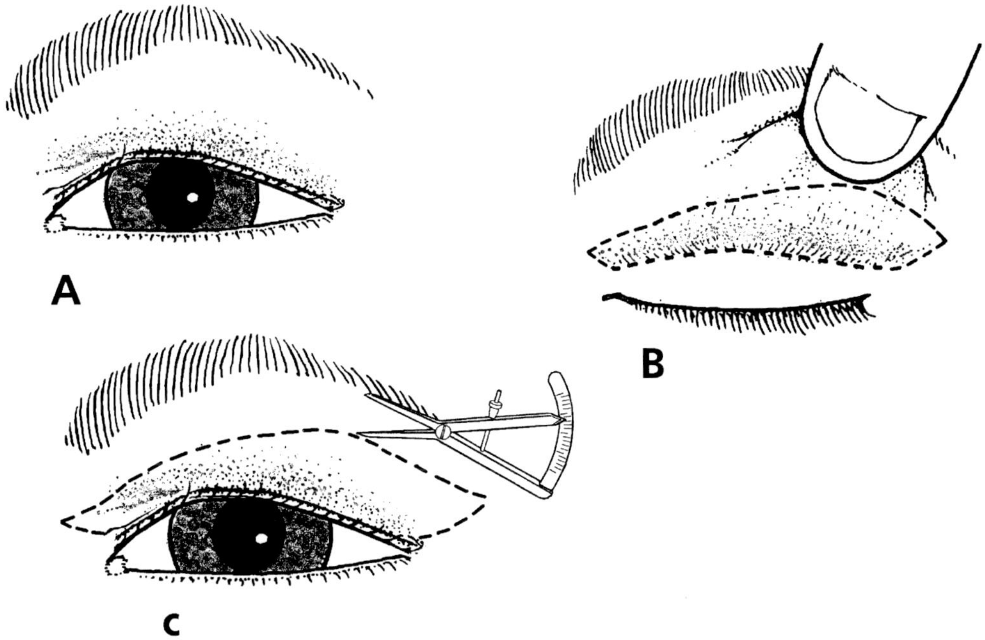

FIG. 5. Upper lid blepharoplasty surgical technique. **A:** Before skin marking. **B:** The skin has been retracted upward and the lid crease has been marked at the desired position above the lash line. The width of the ellipse is determined initially by a bunching technique that gently outturns the lashes. It is safe to remove larger amounts of skin from the lateral portion of the lid. The nasal portion of the lid should have very conservative amounts of skin removed and that shortage in this area produces more severe lagophthalmos. **C:** In order to ensure postoperative symmetry in brow crease positioning, the upper edge of the ellipse distance should be measured from the brow and should be equal from side to side.

Skin Incision; Tissue Removal

For ease of skin incision, the surgeon must tense the skin for incision and incise only through skin in the marked ellipse (Fig. 6A). The next incision is through the orbicularis muscle in the upper edge of the ellipse. Use the Bovie on cutting and incise some through the subbrow fat or preseptal fat pad temporally (Fig. 6B).

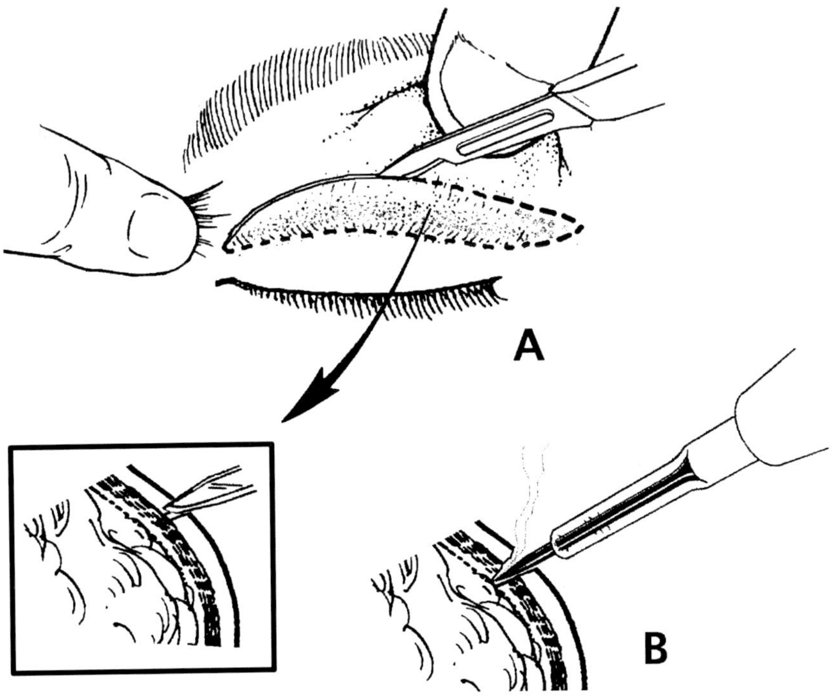

FIG. 6. Upper lid blepharoplasty surgical technique. **A:** An incision is made initially through the skin only on the marked area of the ellipse. Two- or three-point traction is needed to tense the skin for ease of excision. **B:** Following the skin incision the muscle is incised with a cutting Bovie needle along the upper edge of the ellipse only.

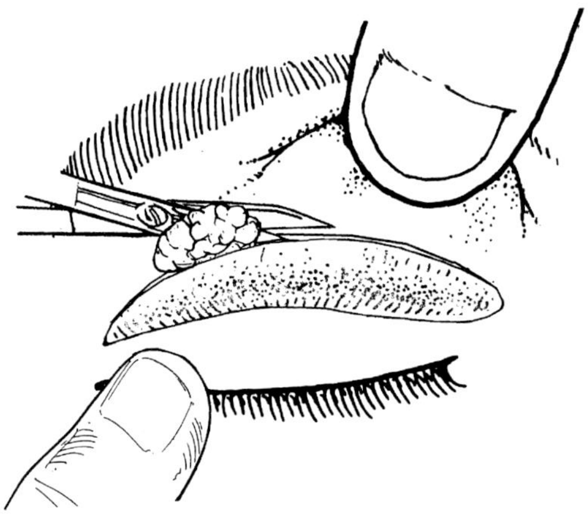

FIG. 7. With pressure on the globe, sharp scissors can then be introduced into the upper edge of the incision through the orbital septum, opening the septum throughout its entire width to allow prolapse of fat with an "open sky" technique.

With pressure on the globe and sharp Wescott scissors, an incision is then made through the orbital septum across its entire width allowing the fat to balloon through ("open sky incision") (Fig. 7). One should avoid incising the lacrimal gland, which may present laterally (it is grey-brown and firm) (Fig. 8). Figure 9A shows a surgical view of incision of orbicularis muscle with the Bovie needle and Fig. 9B the open sky removal of fat.

With a Blair retractor, the skin-muscle septal flap is pulled down, exposing the preaponeurotic fat, junctional fat, and nasal fat pads. With forceps traction, the loose preaponeurotic fat is excised with a bovie on coagulation. Some traction on the preaponeurotic pad in a nasal direction will allow removal of the "tail" extension of the pad. The edge is cauterized (Fig. 10A).

With an additional rake retractor placed in the inner canthus and pressure on the globe, incision is made

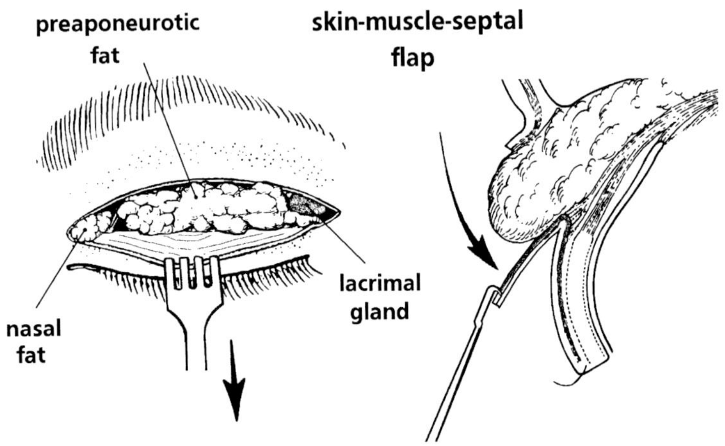

FIG. 8. The complete incision through the upper edge of the orbital septum has been performed with retraction of the skin-muscle septal flap downward exposing the preaponeurotic and nasal fat.

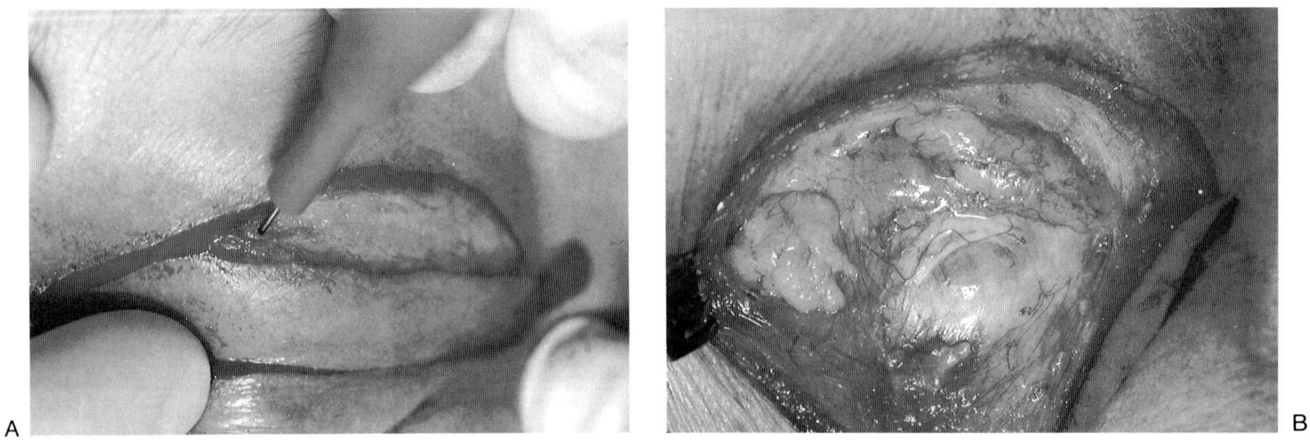

FIG. 9. Upper lid blepharoplasty surgical view. **A:** Incision of the orbicularis in the upper edge of the incision with the cutting Bovie needle. **B:** Open sky exposure of the fat in the right upper lid following complete incision of the septum in the upper incision and retraction of the skin-muscle septal flap downward. The whitish rounded nasal fat and the horizontally oriented preaponeurotic fat can be seen centrally. The superior transverse ligament can be seen just beneath the preaponeurotic fat and some portion of the muscular and aponeurotic parts of the levator.

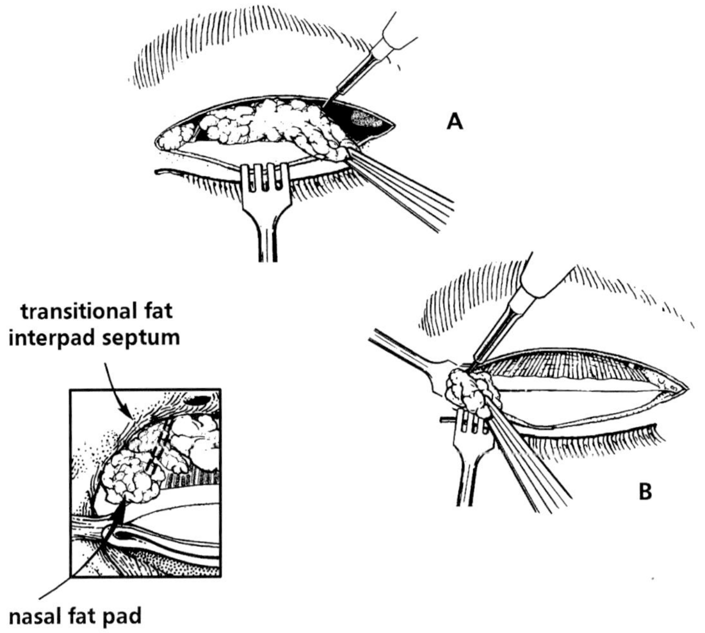

FIG. 10. Fat removal in upper lid blepharoplasty. **A:** The preaponeurotic fat is grasped and retracted away from the levator and the lacrimal gland laterally and excised with the Bovie needle coagulating current. **B:** The nasal and inferior edge of the blepharoplasty incision is retracted and, with pressure on the globe and incision in the capsule, the nasal fat pad can be made to prolapse and also is excised with the coagulating Bovie needle. Following this, the residual fat is in the transitional zone over the septum and is conservatively removed if needed. Excessive removal of the transitional fat can cause an unwanted sunken look to the eye and excessive dissection in this area can damage the superior oblique tendon.

with a cutting Bovie through the capsule covering the white nasal fat. The nasal fat pad is teased out with the forceps and the cotton applicator stick, avoiding vessels. With forceps traction on the nasal fat the coagulation bovie is used to excise the nasal fat pad (Fig. 10B). Vessels can be selectively cauterized. Touch-up cautery along the edges is used on all the fat to sculpt the fat and to cauterize the vessels. The saponified, or liquid, fat should then be dabbed away with the gauze

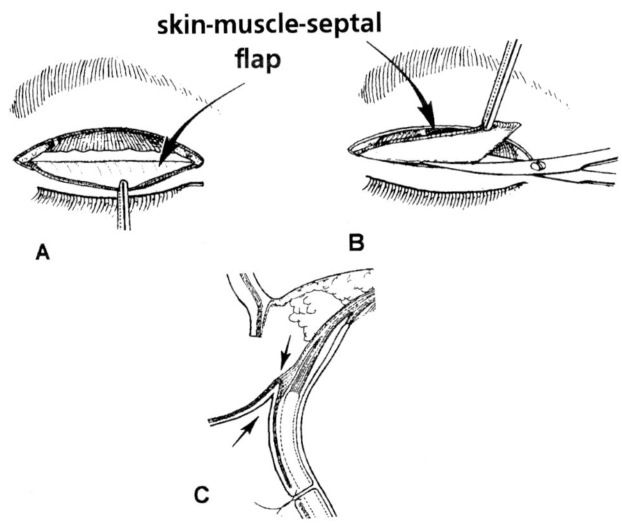

FIG. 11. Excision of the skin-muscle septal flap in upper lid blepharoplasty. **A:** The skin-muscle septal flap is retracted downward. **B:** Straight scissors are used and are slanted to excise the flap at the lower marked skin incision. **C:** Arrows emphasize the fact that slanting of the scissors minimizes disruption of any strands of the levator aponeurosis to the pretarsal skin.

pad to remove it from the wound and the wound irrigated with icy water. The fat is reinspected to cauterize any potential bleeding vessels.

The skin-muscle septal flap is then excised through the lower incision of the marked ellipse. The flap is elevated with gentle traction, separating the edges of the skin incision. The skin-muscle septal flap is then excised. Straight scissors are slanted away from the insertions of the levator aponeurosis so as not to disrupt the insertions of the aponeurosis (Fig. 11A–C). Crease sutures will repair any dehiscences but it is wise to avoid too much disruption in the levator attachments. Figure 12A is a surgical view showing the usual fat excised and 12B the excision of the skin-muscle flap.

Potential bleeding areas are in the orbicularis and subcutaneous layer of the lower crease incision. The pretarsal skin is retracted with cotton applicator sticks and the bipolar cautery used to cauterize the vessels in this area. The lacrimal gland is examined. If prolapsed, it can be reposited by surface cautery with a coagulation Bovie sealing it in position or sutured inside the orbital rim with 4-0 chromic to the periosteum inside the rim (2).

Crease Formation

Proper positioning and symmetry of the upper lid crease is very important and must be specifically surgically addressed (3–6). This allows the surgeon to ensure its postoperative position. Direct suture fixation of the crease (pretarsal skin) to the levator ensures its position and also compensates for any weakening or

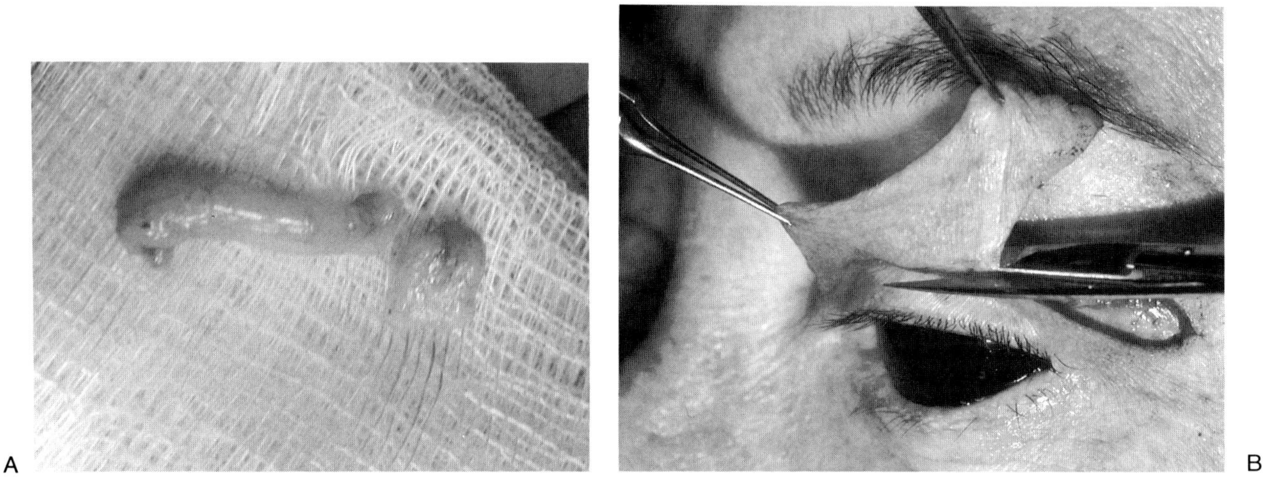

FIG. 12. Upper lid blepharoplasty surgical view. **A:** Rounded nasal fat pad and horizontal preaponeurotic fat that have been removed from a patient in an upper lid blepharoplasty. **B:** Excision of the skin-muscle septal flap at the edge of the lower crease incision in the skin. The scissors are slanted away from the levator aponeurosis.

dehiscence of the levator that may occur when the skin-muscle septal flap is excised. 6-0 Absorbable sutures (usually vicryl) are used to attach the pretarsal skin-muscle layer to the levator aponeurosis in three areas. Sutures are taken with 6-0 vicryl, near the upper edge of the crease incision transcutaneously, a bite through the aponeurosis, and then back out through the skin and tied loosely (Fig. 13A and B). The lid is stretched until there is no gaping of the lid on the operative table. This may cause some slack in the 6-0 vicryl suture, but that is the tension that is appropriate to avoid overelevating the lid. The sutures are then tied permanently. This is done centrally, at the lateral canthus, and nasally to form the crease. The position of the sutures in the skin will determine the height and contour of the crease. Symmetry can be obtained in this manner. Figure 14A is a surgical view of the upper lid after the excisional part of the blepharoplasty has been completed. Figure 14B shows the crease sutures in position.

Skin Closure

The lateral portion of the incision is closed first by stretching the skin laterally to create even incision sides and placing the first suture at the lateral canthus through the skin-muscle layer with 6-0 nylon. The skin edge must be everted and tied loosely. Sutures of 6-0 nylon are then placed laterally, equally spaced in the lateral portion of the wound. Usually a small dog ear forms at the most lateral edge, which is excised with

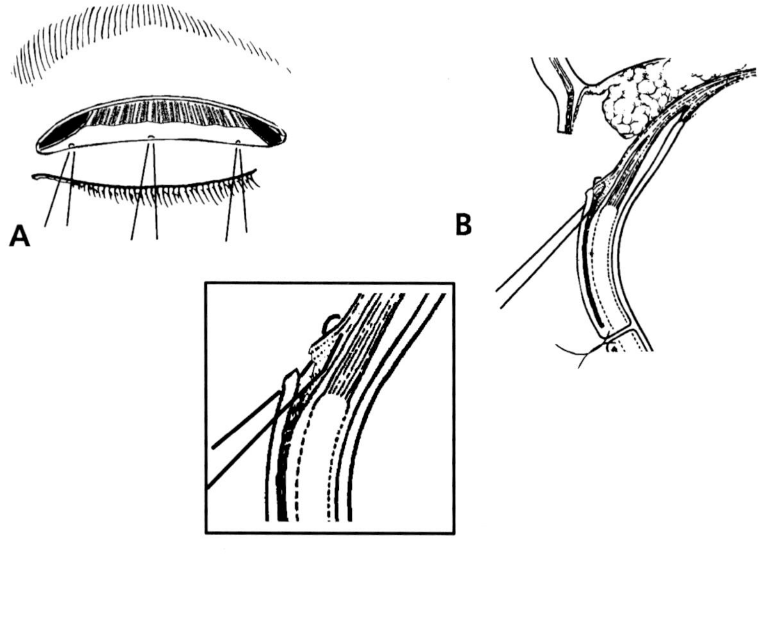

FIG. 13. Upper lid blepharoplasty crease formation. **A:** Transcutaneous sutures (usually 6-0 vicryl) are used to plicate the upper edge of the pretarsal skin-muscle to the levator aponeurosis with the desired tension. **B:** Side view showing placement of the sutures. This not only fixates the eyelid crease in a very precise manner at the desired position but also repairs any inadvertent levator dehiscence that has occurred during excision of the skin-muscle septal flap. These sutures can actually be advanced higher on the levator aponeurosis to create some lifting effect of the lid in patients with mild ptosis.

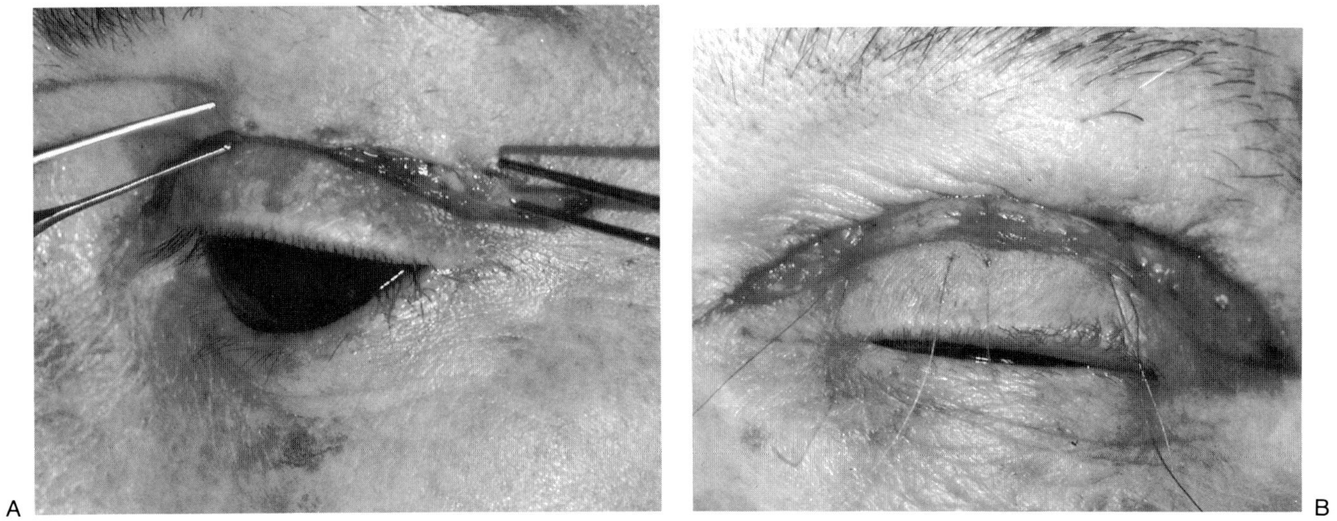

FIG. 14. Upper lid blepharoplasty surgical view of crease formation. **A:** If the skin excision has been designed properly, the skin edges can be brought together with good approximation in an even manner. **B:** The transcutaneous sutures are placed at the upper edge of the pretarsal skin plicating the edge to the levator to reform the crease at the desired position.

a (Burow) triangle before complete closure (Fig. 15A and B). The sutures should be tied loosely. With traction on the temporal and nasal side of the wound, a continuous suture of 6-0 nylon is then started, first introduced at the lateral canthus from the inferior edge, and a continuous slanted suture of 6-0 nylon, including skin and orbicularis muscle, is brought across the eyelid into the inner canthus (Fig. 16). The inner canthus is then stretched nasally, and some deep sutures in the aponeurosis or connective tissue are taken to form crease concavity in that area. A small (Burow) triangle is usually excised to equalize the wound edges. Care must be taken to avoid extending the upper lid incision onto the thicker skin of the nose to avoid postoperative epicanthal fold formation. If a lower blepharoplasty is to be performed, the lateral end of the 6-0 nylon suture

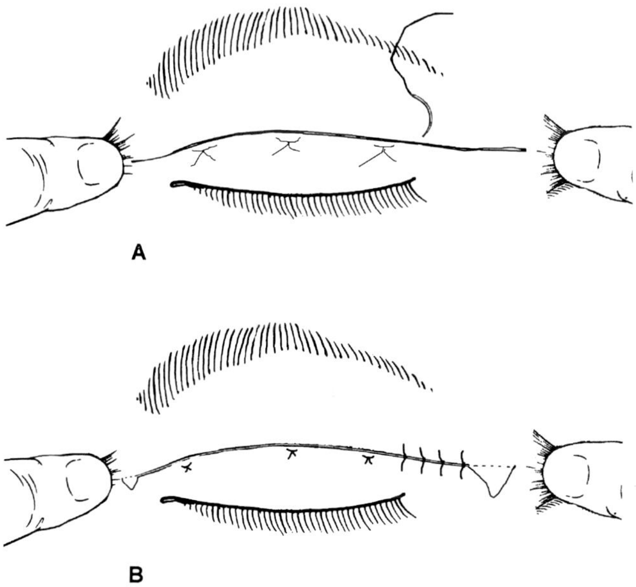

FIG. 15. Skin closure and upper lid blepharoplasty. **A:** Following placement of the crease sutures with the skin on stretch, interrupted sutures are used to close the wound laterally. **B:** In many cases a small dog ear formation at the ends of the incision can be corrected with a Burow triangle excision.

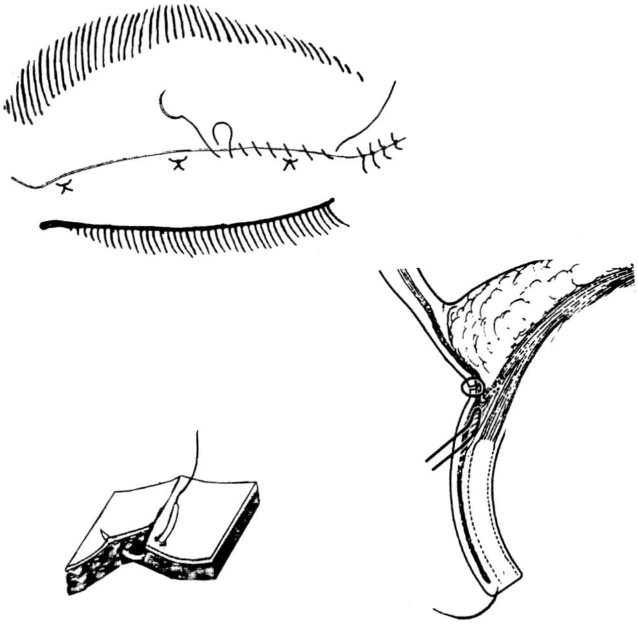

FIG. 16. Skin closure and upper lid blepharoplasty. Final closure of the central portion of the incision is made with a continuous 6-0 nylon suture. It is important to close the skin and muscle layer with skin eversion to reduce visible scar formation.

is left long enough that it can be retracted and clamped to the superior drap or brow hairs to avoid interfering with the lower lid surgery. The symmetry of the crease position and skin folding is then checked and late adjustments can be made as necessary with trimming of the pretarsal skin and reinsertion of sutures if needed.

ADJUNCTIVE PROCEDURES FOR UPPER LID BLEPHAROPLASTY

Browplasty

Lateral brow fullness is sometimes a major complaint of the patient presenting for an upper lid blepharoplasty. This anatomic change is not corrected by the standard upper lid blepharoplasty technique. This fullness can be caused by prominent bony superior rim but is most commonly caused by super abundance of the subbrow fat.

When the subbrow fat layer extends down onto the surface of the lid it becomes preseptal fat, which can commonly be seen. In these patients the usual adjunct to the standard upper lid blepharoplasty is surgical excision and sculpting of the brow fat in the overly prominent area and is defined for present purposes as browplasty (7).

Technique

After marking of the redundant upper eyelid skin to be removed with blepharoplasty, the supraorbital notch is palpated and marked to identify the location of the supraorbital nerve and vessels. In addition, the area of brow fullness should be marked, followed by infiltration of the eyelids and brow with the local anesthetic. After the skin and orbicularis muscle have been excised during a standard blepharoplasty, the dissection is extended in the submuscular plane (postorbicularis fascia) toward the eyebrow. Upward traction on the superior edge of the skin-muscle flap exposes this area. Once the dissection extends approximately 1–1.5 cm above the superior and lateral orbital rim, the brow fat pad should be clearly identified overlying the lateral orbital margin. Dissection should not extend nasally to the previously marked superior orbital notch to avoid damaging the nerves and vessels in that area. The extent of the fat pad to be removed is marked with methylene blue on the skin surface and two Blair rake retractors are inserted to pull the skin-muscle edge back, exposing the superior orbital rim and fatty tissue (Fig. 17A and B). The area of fat on the rim to be removed is marked with methylene blue and is then excised by grasping of the fat with Adson forceps and use of the Bovie coagulating needle. An elliptical segment of brow fat pad is removed measuring approximately 1–1.5 cm in vertical dimension and then tapering nasally and temporally, and should extend laterally to the frontozygomatic suture (Fig. 17C). The fat pad should be removed to the level of the periosteum; however, the periosteum should be left intact to prevent the occurrence of postoperative adhesions in an undesirable area. Care must be taken to avoid the supraorbital nerve and some of the vessels that occur in the area. The liquified fat is then sponged from the area with the 4 × 4 gauze pad and the area irrigated with ice-cold water. Additional tissue or strip of subcutaneous orbicularis fibers from underneath the superior skin edge

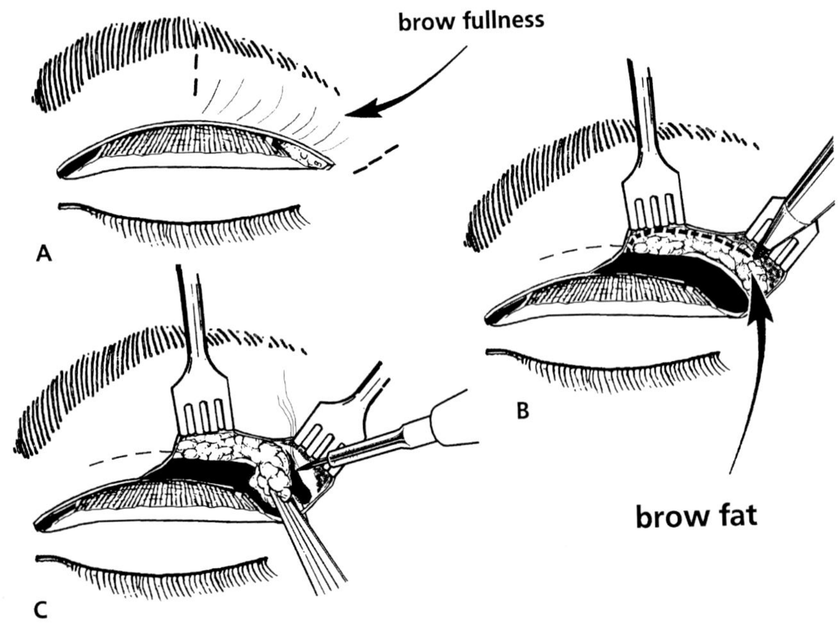

FIG. 17. Browplasty with upper lid blepharoplasty. **A:** The excisional part of the upper lid blepharoplasty has been completed and the area of fullness in the brow marked with methylene blue. **B:** The upper edge of the skin-muscle flap is retracted exposing the superior orbital rim, its central and lateral portion, and the proliferative fat covering the rim. The desired amount of fat removal is marked with methylene blue. **C:** With the coagulating Bovie needle, the marked fat is then excised down to the periosteum of the superior orbital rim. Some sculpting can also be done with cautery and lipolysis.

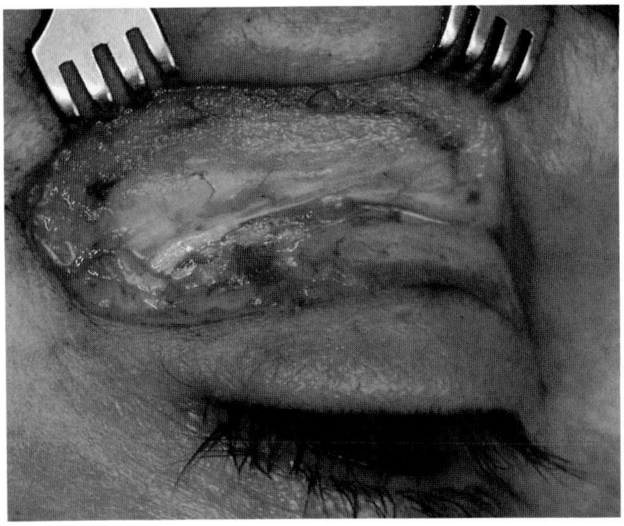
A

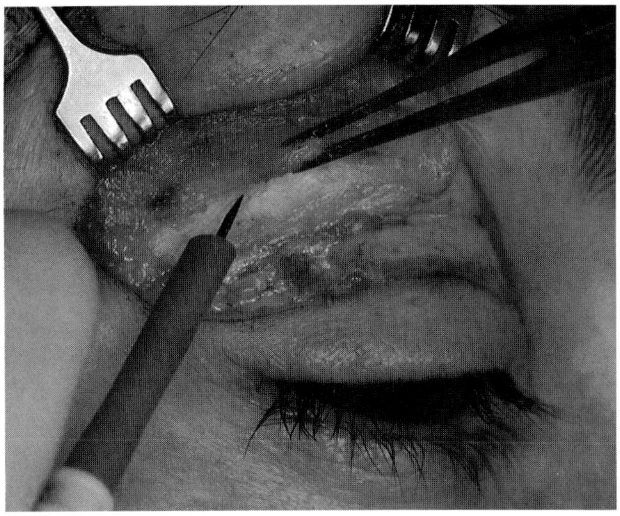
B

FIG. 18. Surgical view of browplasty. **A:** The desired area of brow fat to be removed has been marked with methylene blue. **B:** The fat is being excised down to the periosteum from the brow area with the Bovie needle.

can also be trimmed to accentuate the lid crease if needed. Figure 18A and B shows surgical views of the browplasty technique.

If no brow elevation or fixation is desired at this point, the blepharoplasty is then completed. Figure 19A and B shows a patient preoperatively and postoperatively following the browplasty technique.

Internal Brow Pexy

If brow laxity exists or a degree of brow ptosis needs correction, brow fixation to the superior orbital rim should be performed if a direct brow pexy or coronal brow lift cannot be performed.

In this adjunctive procedure, the surgeon performs a brow fixation to the superior orbital rim periosteum through the blepharoplasty incision, internally, underneath the brow with nonabsorbable sutures (7). The translid brow pexy is performed after the excisional part of the standard upper lid blepharoplasty has been done (Fig. 20A–C). The internal brow fixation should not be used if the person is a willing candidate for a more formal brow procedure, either direct suprabrow pexy or coronal forehead lift. It is a good adjunctive procedure in patients with mild lateral or central brow laxity. It has little or no effect on nasal brow position and can actually accentuate a nasal glabellar laxity. It is commonly used ''prophylactically'' in cases of mild brow laxity to prevent postoperative brow droppage.

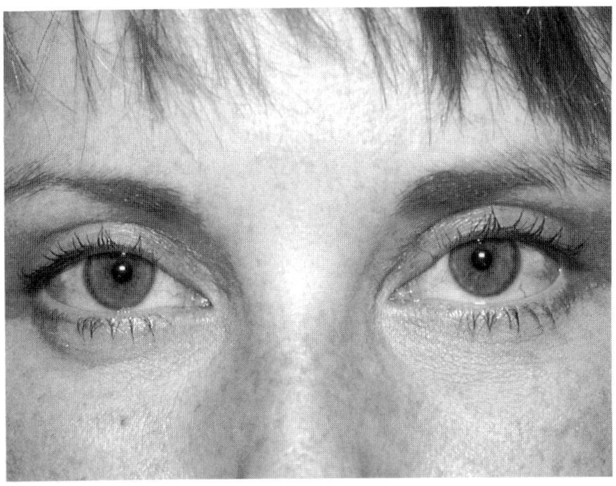
A

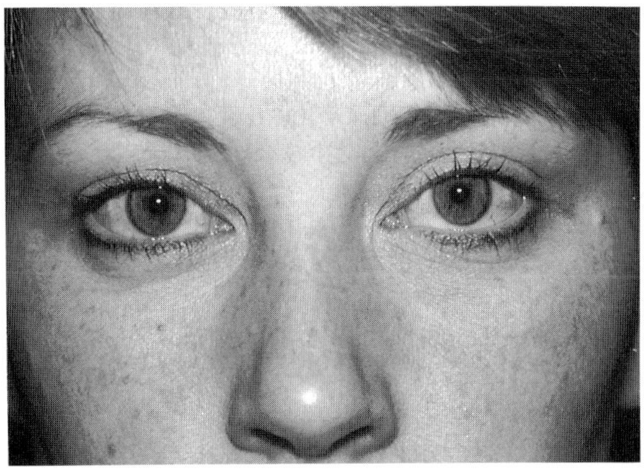
B

FIG. 19. Browplasty. **A:** Young woman who has had a blepharoplasty but was displeased because of the residual fullness in the brow areas laterally—before browplasty. **B:** Same patient following excision of brow fat through a transcutaneous incision with good thinning of the lateral brows.

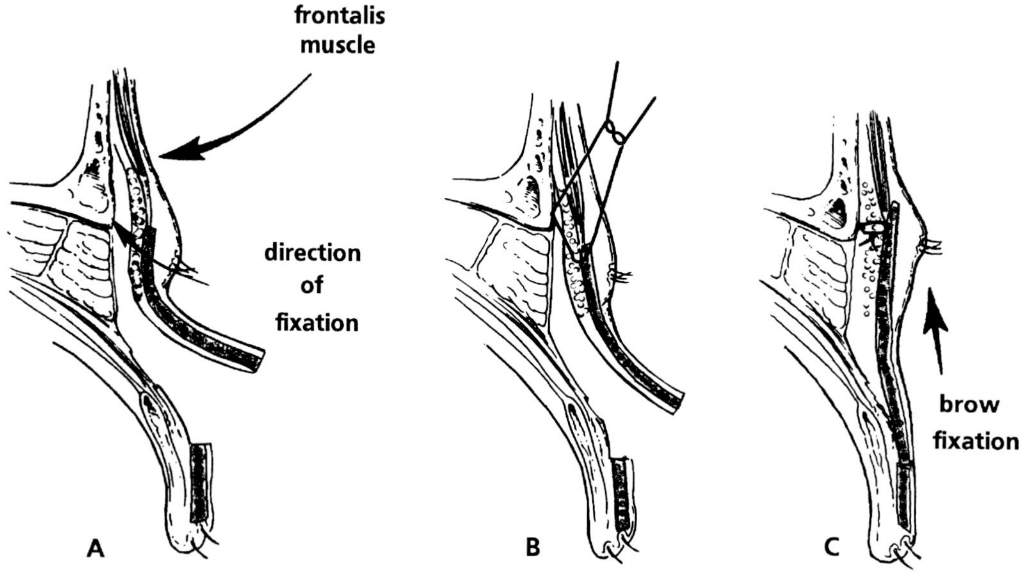

FIG. 20. Internal brow pexy, cross-sectional view. **A:** Following the excisional portion of the upper lid blepharoplasty, dissection is carried out beneath the subbrow fat pad to the orbital rim. **B:** A 4-0 prolene suture is used to plicate the subbrow fat pad and orbicularis beneath the brow hairs to the superior orbital rim. **C:** After tightening of the internal suture, the brow is fixated to the rim.

Internal Brow Pexy Technique

After examining the photographs, vertical marks are made at the lax areas in the brow with methylene blue, where the fixation sutures are to go. There are usually two fixation points, one laterally and one toward the central area. One cannot dissect or place brow fixation sutures in the nasal portion of the brow because the multiple nerves and vessels in that area make dissection difficult. If there is significant nasal brow laxity or ptosis then one should be conservative with lateral lifting because it will accentuate nasal laxity.

The upper lid skin-muscle flap is retracted with the rake retractors and with the needle Bovie coagulating tip dissection laterally. Then the subbrow fat pad is made to separate the brow and its fat pad from the superior orbital rim. This can be done nasally to some degree, but care must be taken to avoid the frontal and supraorbital branches of the frontal nerve in the supraorbital area. Additional dissection may be needed laterally in the fatty plane to allow mobility of the brow.

A suture is then placed transcutaneously at the inferior edge of the brow hairs through one of the marks full thickness to the dissected space underneath. This allows the surgeon to mark the position of the brow hairs while working underneath the dissected flap. This transcutaneous suture serves as a marker so that the surgeon working under the flap of skin in the brow area will know the location of the brow hairs when looking from the undersurface of the flap (Fig. 21A). The suture is then placed through the superior rim periosteum; some overlying fat can be thinned down with the cutting Bovie before this is done (Fig. 21B). The most bites are placed approximately 1 cm from the rim, but the positioning can be done according to the patient's needs. A second bite is taken with the suture (4-0 proline with a PS-5 needle) in the subbrow fat and orbicularis in the area where the transcutaneous markings suture enters the space. This enters the space at the level of the inferior edge of the brow hairs and is the proper position for the fixation suture of the brow (Fig. 21C, D).

The marking suture is then pulled through the skin so that all of the suture is now underneath the brow flap (Fig. 21E). The suture is then tied with a double throw snugly to observe the position of the brow (Fig. 21F). Tugging on the upper lid skin is done to make sure that no inadvertent inclusion of orbital septum or excessive lagophthalmos is reduced by the fixating suture. Once the stretchability of the brow and upper lid skin is confirmed, then the suture is tied permanently (Fig. 21G).

A second suture may be placed nasally or temporally, as the case may be, and again the brow fixation should be firm but stretchable. Two to three mattress sutures of 4-0 prolene are generally used to elevate the brow position. The desired level of fixation of the lateral third of the eyebrow is above the lateral orbital rim. As many as three mattress sutures have been placed to adequately fixate the brow at the desired po-

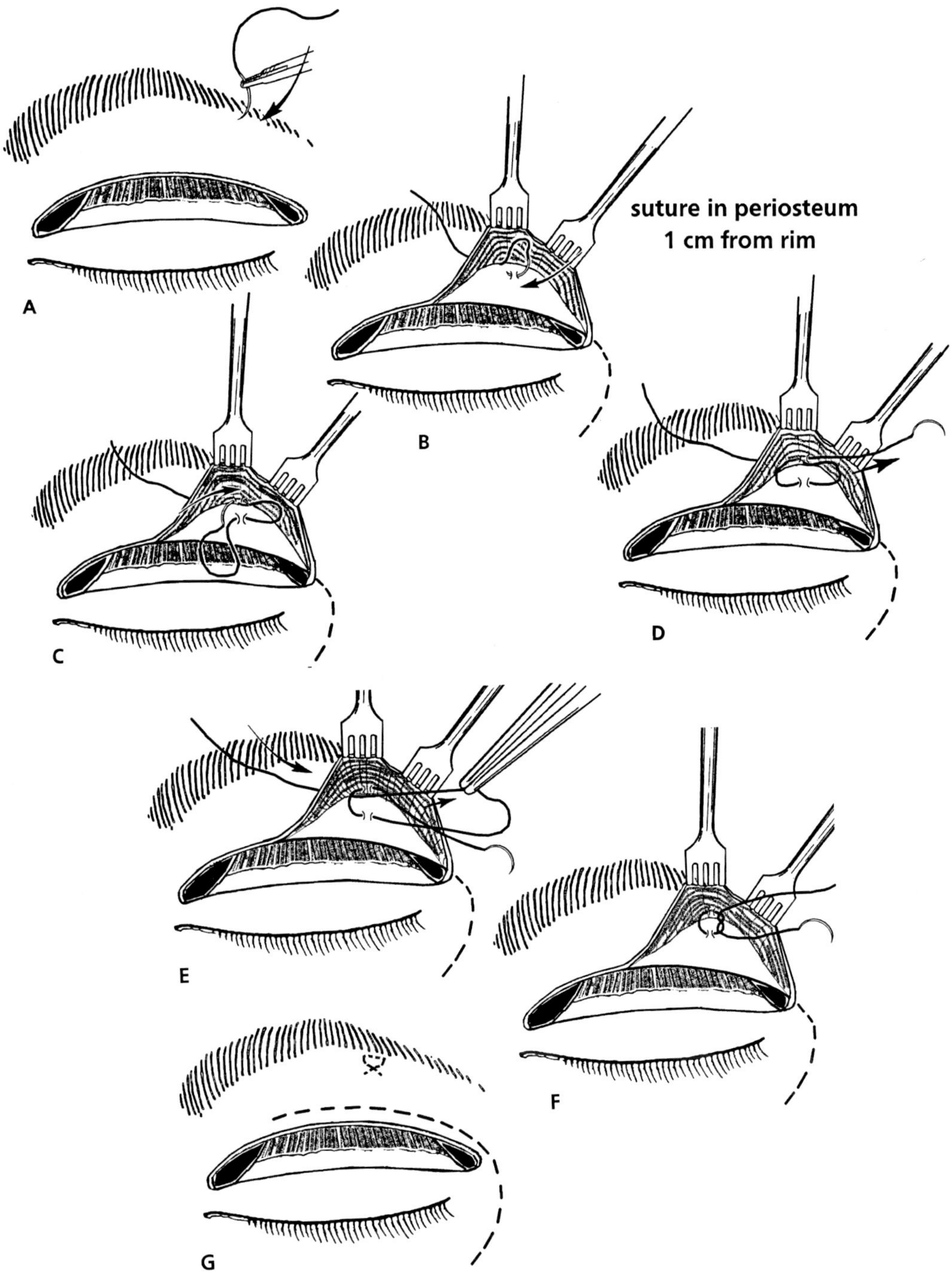

FIG. 21. Internal brow pexy surgical technique. **A:** A suture is introduced transcutaneously at the inferior edge of the brow hairs laterally as a marking device when the flap is everted. **B:** The upper edge of the blepharoplasty flap is everted and the suture introduced into the periosteum of the superior rim at the desired position. **C:** With the transcutaneous marking suture as a guide, the needle can then be introduced on the undersurface of the flap at the level of the inferior edge of the brow hairs. **D:** The suture is taken through the subbrow fat and orbicularis fibers. **E:** The transcutaneous marking suture that was used to identify the inferior edge of the brow hairs can then be pulled through from the undersurface of the flap. **F:** The suture can then be tied and firmed fixating the brow to the periosteum at the desired location. **G:** Following tying of the suture, the brow is tested to ensure that there is still flexibility and stretchability of the brow, so that excessive lagophthalmos will not be produced.

sition. After the brow is fixated, the blepharoplasty procedure is completed. Figure 22A–D shows surgical views of the procedure.

This brow fixation technique is most commonly used to prevent postoperative droppage or to gain a small elevation in brow position. It also has the effect in many patients of correcting brow asymmetry resulting from unequal animation of the brow and in some cases can prevent a person from arching the brow as much when done inadvertently. Figure 23A and B shows a patient before and after upper lid blepharoplasty with internal brow pexy.

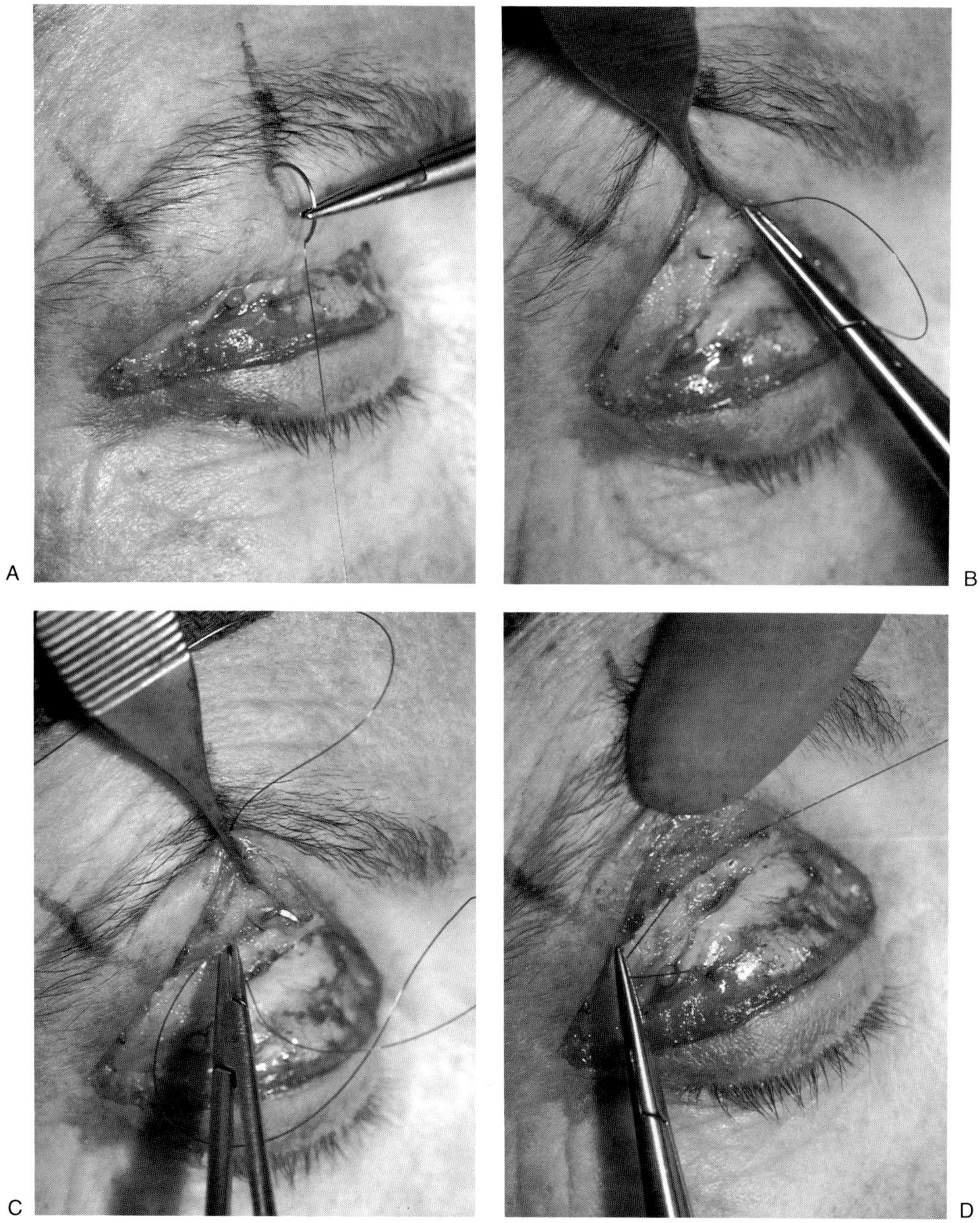

FIG. 22. Internal brow pexy, surgical views. **A:** Introduction of the transcutaneous marking suture at the inferior edge of the brow hairs. **B:** The needle is then introduced in the periosteum at the superior orbital rim at the desired location of brow fixation (usually a centimeter above the edge of the rim). **C:** With the flap everted, the position of the marking suture can be seen and the needle introduced into the subbrow fat and orbicularis at its location. **D:** The marking suture has been pulled through and the suture looped and tied fixating the brow to the periosteum at the desired location.

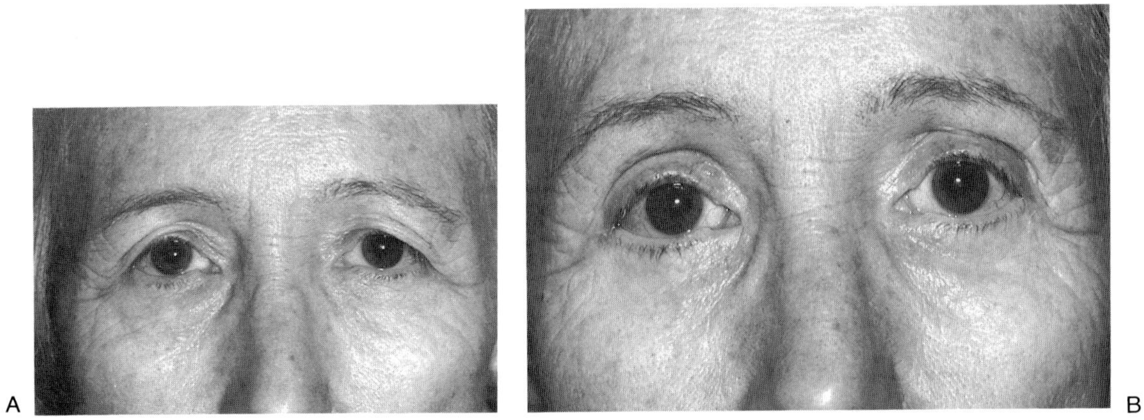

FIG. 23. Patient undergoing upper lid blepharoplasty with internal brow fixation. **A:** Patient preoperatively. **B:** Patient postoperatively following upper lid blepharoplasty and internal brow fixation.

SPECIAL SITUATIONS: UPPER LID BLEPHAROPLASTY

Uncorrected Nasal Brow Ptosis

There will be blepharoplasty candidates with nasal eyebrow laxity or ptosis who have nasal folding in the medial portion of the eyelid. A narrow brow–lash distance and folding of skin in the nasal and glabellar area may also be present. These changes can only be satisfactorily corrected by a coronal forehead lift, which may be refused by the patient or not elected by the surgeon. The upper lid blepharoplasty can be modified in the nasal aspect to try to compensate for the changes in this situation. In the nasal part of the blepharoplasty, a more aggressive removal of the nasal and transitional fat pads, removal of redundant subcutaneous tissue, orbicularis debulking, and aggressive imbricating of the crease sutures (two sutures through upper and lower wound edge) can somewhat compensate for this situation.

Lateral Bony Brow Prominence

Patients with severe lateral brow prominence in whom brow fat pad removal (browplasty) is not adequate to solve the problem may require bony contouring of the lateral rim. In these patients, after the fat is excised from the lateral rim, an incision is made in the lateral rim edge and periosteum flaps are created. In the area of prominence and after reflection of flaps, burring of the bony rim to the desired shape with a rotary osteotome can be performed. Closure of the periosteal flaps is necessary to prevent excessive adhesions in the area.

Upper Lid Ptosis

The most common situation in which upper lid ptosis occurs is in the middle-aged or involutional patient in whom some levator dehiscence has occurred, producing a true ptosis of the upper lid. Aponeurotic repair can be performed after the excisional part of the upper lid blepharoplasty has taken place. In most cases this involves dissection of the aponeurotic edge and direct reattachment to the tarsal plate. In some milder cases the crease sutures can be used to advance the levator as previously described.

Lid Retraction (Dysthyroid)

Many patients who have the eye changes of Graves' disease will request removal of the puffiness and folding of the eyelids. If retraction of the upper lid is present, then recession of the levator can be carried out in the manner described in Chapter 19. This can be done following the excisional part of the upper lid blepharoplasty.

In patients who have residual exophthalmos, conservativism is needed in removal of upper lid tissue and crease formation. Upper blepharoplasty can accentuate the exophthalmos if a high lid crease is produced. Conservative tissue removal, lower crease positioning, and sometimes omission of crease sutures is the proper approach in these patients.

Upper Lid Blepharoplasty in the Asian Eyelid

There are basic anatomic differences between Asian and Western eyelids (8–10). In most Asian eyelids, there is a low insertion of the orbital septum on the

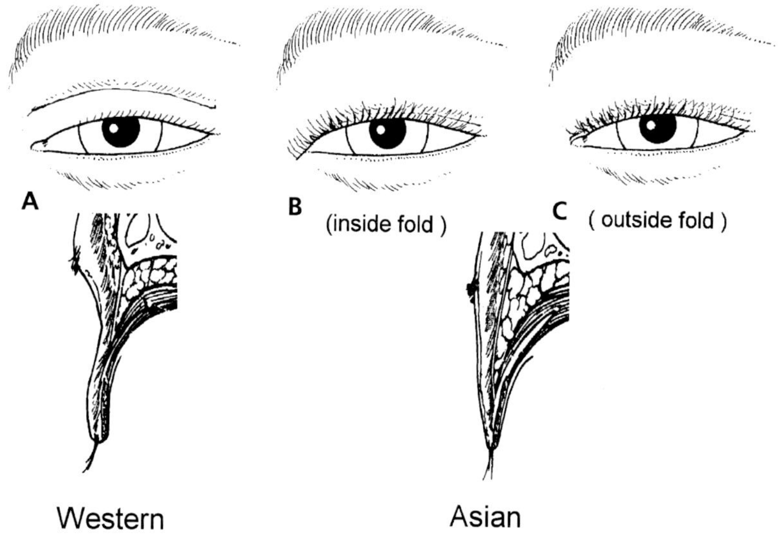

FIG. 24. Comparison of the eyelid crease formation in the Western and Asian eyelids. **A:** In the Western eyelid, the orbital septum inserts above the superior edge of the tarsal plate, retracting the preaponeurotic fat backward and forming a higher lid crease in the visible pretarsal space. **B:** In the Asian eyelid the orbital septum inserts much further down on the lower edge of the tarsal plate allowing the preaponeurotic fat to balloon forward underneath the skin in the pretarsal space. There may be very little, if any, pretarsal space or lid crease in the Asian eyelid. In this diagrammatic representation, there is extension of the fold of skin in the upper lid over the canthus obscuring the inner canthal angle (epicanthal fold). In Asian terminology this represents an inside fold that is inside the angle. **C:** Diagrammatic representation of an Asian eyelid in which the fold does not cover the internal canthal angle and is thereby termed an "outside fold."

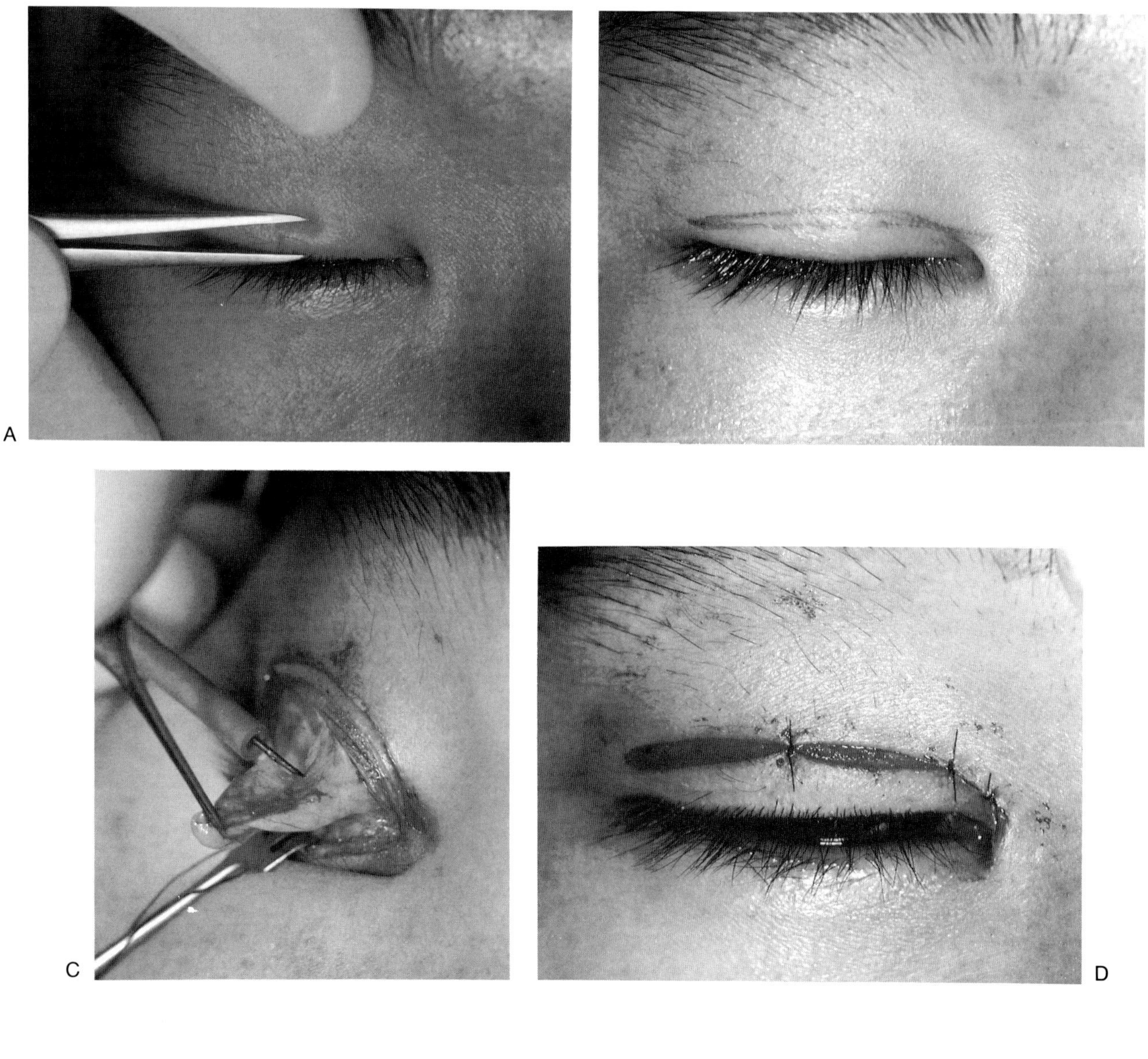

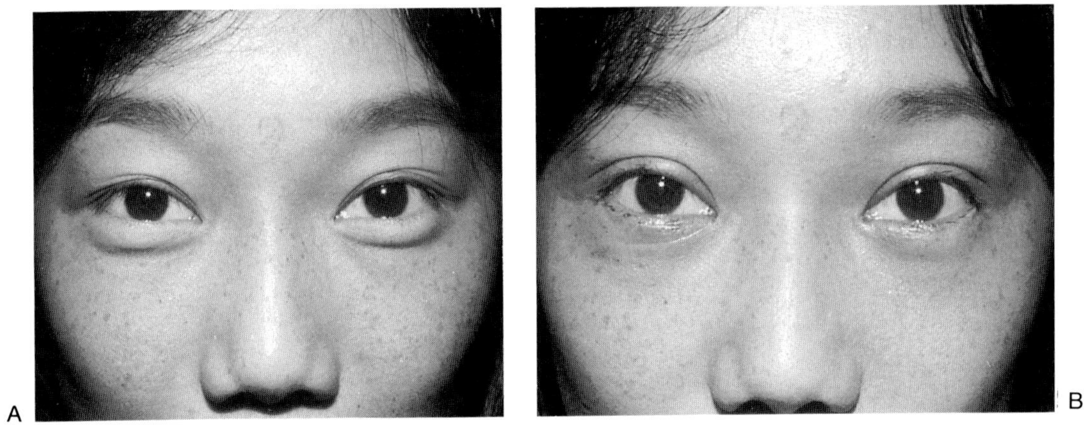

FIG. 26. Surgery in the Asian eyelid. **A:** Preoperative view of Asian patient with puffy folding in the upper lids and orbicularis hypertrophy in the lower lids. **B:** Early postoperative view following upper lid surgery as shown above and excision of hypertrophied orbicularis in the lower lids.

tarsal plate with extension of the preaponeurotic fat into that area. This produces an upper lid with or without a reduced visible crease and with a skin fold protruding over the lashes. There is usually the presence of a medial epicanthal fold extending below the canthus. The upper lid fold and epicanthal fold may in some cases push the upper lid lashes down. The absence of the upper lid crease has been called a "single eyelid" whereas the eyelid with a crease is called a "double eyelid." If a crease is present but the epicanthal fold prevents it from extending to the canthus, it is called an "inside crease." If there is not much epicanthal fold present and the crease extends to above the canthus, it is called an "outside crease" (Fig. 24A–C). The majority of the preoperative evaluation and planning of upper lid blepharoplasty in Asian patients centers around on how much a crease is wanted, how high it should be placed, and whether or not an "inside crease" (epicanthal fold) should be surgically altered. It should be determined preoperatively where the patient wants the crease to be. This can be done with a mirror evaluation. When the desired level has been determined by the patient, a Polaroid photo can be taken with the patient holding the fold up and the desired crease position marked with a felt-tip pen. The photo can be a guide for crease placement intraoperatively and is useful to confirm to the patient postoperatively that the desired result has been obtained. In general, Asians do not want a high crease and do not want much done to the epicanthal fold unless it is producing lash problems. If some correction of the epicanthal fold in needed, then a skin flap procedure as described in Chapter 22.

Asian Eyelid Surgical Technique

A low crease incision 4–5 mm above lashes (individual in each patient) is marked. A conservative amount of skin is excised and the orbital septum is opened in this area (Fig. 25A and B). Fat can be made to protrude through the septum at this location because of its low insertion in these patients. A conservative amount of fat is removed and closure performed. In general, the more skin and fat is removed, the higher the upper lid crease will form (Fig. 25C, D). Figure 26A and B shows a patient pre- and postoperatively who was corrected with this approach.

REFERENCES

1. McCord CD. Techniques in blepharoplasty. *Ophth Surg* 1979; 10:40–55.
2. Horton CT, Carraway TA, Podenzg AO. Treatment of a lacrimal bulge in blepharoplasty by repositioning the gland. *Plast Reconstr Surg* 1978;61:701.
3. Wilkins RB, Hunter GJ, McCord CD, Tanenbaum M. Blepharoplasty: cosmetic and functional. *Oculoplastic surgery*. 2nd ed. New York: Raven Press; 1987:451–454.
4. Baker TJ, Gordon HL, Posrenko P. Upper lid blepharoplasty. *Plast Reconstr Surg* 1977;60:692.
5. Flowers RS. Anchor blepharoplasty. In: *Trans Sixth Int Cong Plast Surg*. Paris: Masson et Cie; 1976:471–472.
6. Sheen JH. Supratarsal fixation in upper blepharoplasty. *Plast Reconstr Surg* 1974;54:424.
7. McCord CD, Doxanas MT. Browplasty and browpexy: an adjunct to blepharoplasty. *Plast Reconstr Surg* 1990;86:248–254.
8. Boo Chai K. Surgery for Oriental eyelids: some refinements in technique. *Aesthet Plast Surg* 1976;1:57.
9. Fernandez L. Double eyelid operation in the Oriental in Hawaii. *Plast Reconstr Surg* 1960;25:257.
10. Sayoc B. Surgery of the Oriental eyelid. *Clin Plast Surg* 1974; 1:157.

FIG. 25. Surgery in the Asian eyelid. **A:** Measurement for placement of the upper crease in a lower position than the Western eyelid. **B:** Marking for conservative or minimal skin excision. **C:** Excision of preaponeurotic fat that extends downward into the pretarsal space in the asian lid. **D:** Initial closure.

CHAPTER 15

Lower Lid Blepharoplasty

Surgical candidates for lower lid blepharoplasty will usually present with complaints of puffy lower lids, a tired look, or the statement that "people say I look like I've been out all night."

It is certainly important to remedy these subjective concerns but, as in upper lid blepharoplasty, the surgeon must preoperatively translate these described problems into anatomic terms. This allows the patient to understand what can and cannot be done surgically and enables the surgeon to plan the operation that best suits the patients needs.

IN FEMALES

The usual anatomic goal for the lower lid in females is the restoration of the visibility of the cheekbone contour (Table 1). This generally requires elimination of loose skin folds over the cheekbone area and a removal of the convexity produced by the fat pads. Special attention must be given to folds that appear only when the person is smiling in that they may represent underlying hypertrophy of orbicularis fibers, which may require excision (1–4).

Most of the dark circles about which patients complain are the result of shadows from downlighting over the convexity of the protuberant fat and skin. In most cases, removal of the skin folds and herniated fat beneath the skin that is producing the puffiness will eliminate "dark circles." Dark circles caused by skin pigmentation are not removed with lower lid blepharoplasty.

Fornix fat removal can be an excellent way to improve the lower lid appearance in some women. The technique does make the assumption that the skin is taut or elastic enough to tighten and reform over the cheekbone and to give more definition. Women who have a specific desire for cheekbone definition but with questionable skin tension should have an external blepharoplasty with skin resections (5–7).

Some women may want improvement of the shape of the eyelid fissure and correction of a downward sloping of the lateral portion of the lid giving a sad look. This can in most cases be improved by a lateral canthoplasty procedure in conjunction with a lower lid blepharoplasty (8–10).

IN MALES

The goal in lower lid blepharoplasty in males is generally much more conservative than in females in that most males do not want tight skin over the cheekbones but rather an improvement in the puffiness and fullness of the lower lids, retaining a more natural look. Males do not usually mind mild residual skin folds because they maintain a "friendly look," which is important to them in their personal interactions. In most cases the male will be satisfied with fat removal and a very conservative skin excision. Usually no orbicularis fibers are excised in the male to preserve the "animated" natural look. In many cases, the male lower lid changes will lend themselves well to fornix fat removal without any skin removal if there is not excessive skin folding present. Lateral canthoplasty with horizontal tightening is also important in the male and should be performed if preoperatively a tendency for ectropion or downward sagging of the eyelid is noted.

SPECIAL CONSIDERATIONS IN LOWER LID BLEPHAROPLASTY SURGICAL TECHNIQUE

The strategy in lower lid blepharoplasty is to obtain the surgical results described without adversely altering the shape of the eyelid fissure (Table 1).

Excision of skin in the vertical direction always has the potential for making the eyelid fissure vertically wider by pulling downward on the lower lid margin causing scleral show or ectropion. Significant horizontal excision laterally can cause an inward pull of the

TABLE 1. *Goals of lower lid blepharoplasty*

Correction of puffiness in eyelid
Avoidance of ectropion or round eye syndrome (scleral show and horizontal narrowing of fissure)
Production of smooth (tight) cheek bones in females

lateral canthus making the fissure horizontally narrow and phimotic.

There are specific surgical techniques to prevent these problems of lower lid eyelid and fissure distortion.

No Skin Resection But Fornix Fat Removal

This approach will work if the patient has taut and elastic skin with minimal folds and is not concerned about absolute smoothness of the skin postoperatively as described above. This avoids any abnormal skin pull on the lower lid margin.

Lateral Canthoplasty

Lateral canthoplasty involves a plication of the tarsoligamentous sling to the periosteum laterally (horizontal tightening of the lid at the lateral canthus) combined with the standard external blepharoplasty (4,11–13). The canthoplasty technique stabilizes the lower lid margin position and fissure width. It has the effect of preventing a downward pulling of the lid preventing lid malposition and also has the positive effect of shaping the fissure. In addition, it produces a smoothing effect on the lid skin just as tightening a loose clothesline has a smoothing effect on sheets that are draped across it. Lateral canthoplasty should be the only technique used for tensing the lower lid. Lower lid shortening techniques, with midlid resections of the tarsal plate, should be avoided because they may pull in the lateral canthus causing phimosis as well as scarring in the eyelid margin.

Periosteal Fixation of Skin-Muscle Flap

Additional stabilization of the eyelid can be obtained by lateral periosteal fixation of the skin-muscle flap. The edge of the flap is attached to the anterior surface of the periosteum laterally in the area of the lateral canthoplasty fixation. This has both a stabilizing and a smoothing effect on the skin in the malar area.

SPECIAL CONCERNS IN LOWER LID BLEPHAROPLASTY

The chapter dealing with blepharoplasty evaluation discusses some special problems. However, it is important to emphasize such problems here. Each patient must be evaluated individually. Many patients will have experienced lower lid anatomic changes requiring special surgical techniques to correct or may have conditions that are difficult or impossible to correct by surgery. This situation must be evaluated ahead of time and the patient informed specifically about what can and cannot be done as well as what procedures will be used. Table 2 provides a list of important things to consider in lower lid blepharoplasty.

TABLE 2. *Lower lid blepharoplasty: special considerations*

Pattern of fat herniation
Skin pigmentation
Malar folds (bag on bag)
Orbicularis hypertrophy
Inferior orbital rim prominence
Crepy skin
Ingrained wrinkles; leathery inelastic skin
Prominent eyes; scleral show
Horizontal laxity
Taut skin
Conjunctivochalasis
Coexistent eyelid disease

The specific *pattern of fat herniation* must be noted and marked in the preoperative plan. It is sometimes difficult on the operating table to note which pads herniate the most; many times the pictures are not as good as they should be, so that proper notes should be made. The most commonly overlooked pad in lower lid blepharoplasty is the temporal fat pad. *Dark circles* under the eye may be due to skin pigmentation, not shadows from puffiness, and it is important to inform the patient that this will not be helped to any degree with lower lid skin smoothing. It is important for the patient to understand that because *skin lesions* do not fall in the usual incision lines it is very difficult to excise them at the same time a lower lid blepharoplasty is performed. Commonly xanthelasma forms in the nasal portion of the lower lid and the skin-muscle flap incisions can be reversed to encompass excision of skin including the xanthelasma.

The folds that occur beneath the edge of the malar bone or *malar folds* (bags on bags) do not lend themselves to the standard incisions of blepharoplasty. It should be explained to the patient that these are difficult to correct and the best chance for achieving some correction is by an extended incision with undermining of the skin in that area and a longer stitch line (14,15). Some of the puffiness that the patient complains about is not herniated fat but *orbicularis hypertrophy*. In particular, when the patient squints or smiles there may be excessive bunching beneath the lashes. This can be helped by excision of the orbicularis fibers, but it is important to note this preoperative complaint so that it may be addressed surgically. Some patients complain of fullness in the lower lid and on examination it becomes apparent to the surgeon that it is a bony *prominence of the inferior orbital rim* as opposed to fatty tissue. When this is the case and the surgeon is willing, some sculpting of the offending bone can be performed with the cutting burr to thin the prominence down. It is important in these patients to recognize this because removal of fatty tissue will only accentuate the problem. Many patients have skin problems in the lower lid that do not respond well to tensing or tightening procedures. *Crepy skin,* despite stretching, can retain a crinkly appearance; it is almost impossible to completely tense crepy skin. This can be noted ahead of time with the inelastic-looking crinkles and should be mentioned to the patient ahead of time.

Ingrained skin wrinkles are usually the product of sun-damaged skin in which the dry and leathery skin has fine lines and wrinkles. Stretching this type of skin generally will not smooth the wrinkles but simply produces another set of wrinkles at 90° to the previous wrinkles. The *prominent eye* condition may occur as a normal or familial characteristic or be the result of a thyroid problem. The pulling down of the lower lid following lower lid blepharoplasty is a greater risk in these patients and the standard horizontal tightening procedure sometimes can aggravate the problem by "clotheslining" the lid margin underneath the prominent eye. A special technique for superplacing the lateral canthal tendon and loosening the lid so the lid will ride up on the globe is needed. In patients who have relatively prominent eyes with known Graves' disease, additional techniques should be used as noted in the chapter on Graves' disease. Laxity of the eyelid was mentioned previously and a standard horizontal tightening procedure is used in these patients who have skin removal. A patient who already has *taut skin* in the lower lid, either because of extreme youth with good skin elasticity, previous blepharoplasty with residual fat, or a similar situation, may be an excellent candidate for a fornix fat removal without any skin surgery. Postoperative chemosis or conjunctival edema can be a temporary problem following some eyelid surgery and patients who have very loose conjunctiva before surgery are at risk for this. The loose conjunctiva or *conjunctivochalasis* should be noted and if it is excessive some resection of the conjunctiva should be performed to prevent this problem. Any *coexistent eyelid disease* such as blepharitis or inflammatory disease, particular that which produces eyelash loss, can be aggravated by a surgical procedure and it very important to point this out to the patient before surgery. If the process is acute, then one should certainly wait until it subsides before proceeding with surgery.

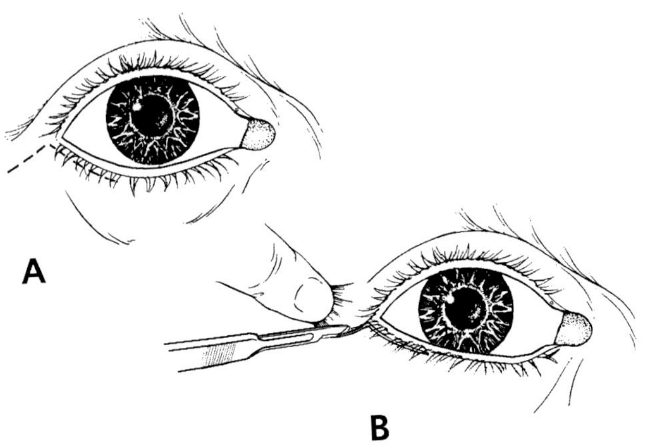

FIG. 1. A: Outline of incision at lateral canthus. The incision should be as high as possible underneath the lashes and extend to the exact canthal angle. **B:** Incision through the skin at the marked incision.

EXTERNAL LOWER LID BLEPHAROPLASTY

In the past external lower lid blepharoplasty was called, simply, lower lid blepharoplasty (16). However, with the popularity of fornix fat removal (internal blepharoplasty) it may be clearer to use the newer terminology. An external skin incision is used and some skin or skin-muscle is resected. The lateral canthoplasty procedure may not necessarily be performed but will be included in a description of the steps because it is commonly used. Lateral periosteal fixation of the skin-muscle flap will also be described in the description of the procedure.

Anesthesia

An infraorbital block is first performed. The lower lid is then infiltrated with with red label xylocaine. Direct injections into the nasal fat pad, central fat pad, and lateral fat pad are made.

Skin Marking

Methylene blue is used to outline the lower lid blepharoplasty incision as high as possible beneath the lashes, extending exactly to the canthal angle and then sloping approximately 45° (Fig. 1A). This exposure makes the lateral canthoplasty procedure easier when performed in conjunction with lower lid blepharoplasty.

Skin–Muscle Incision

With the lower lid on a stretch, the skin is incised beneath the lashes from the temporal third of the lid to the exact corner and then a downsloping incision is made (Fig. 1B). A skin hook is inserted under the upper

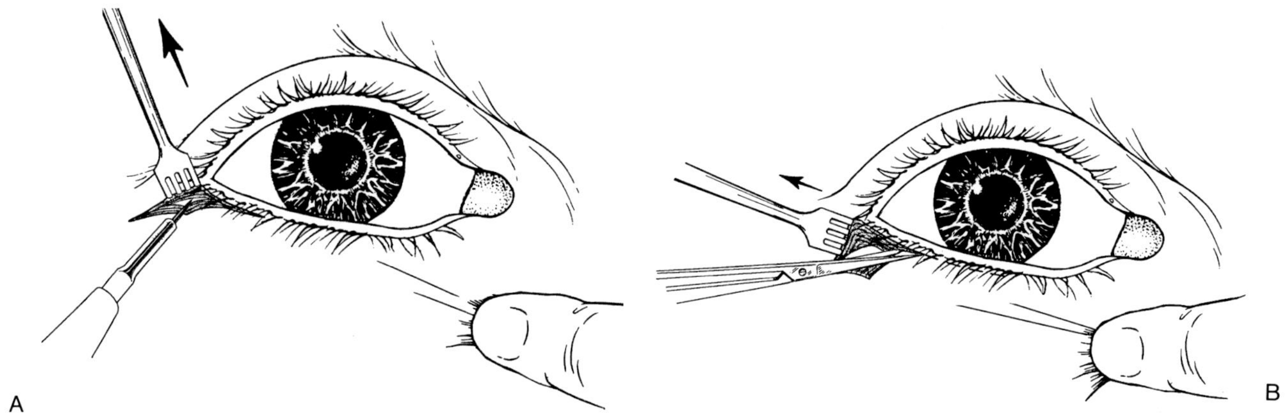

FIG. 2. A: With skin retraction the Bovie needle is used to incise through the orbicularis layer to begin development of the skin-muscle flap. **B:** Scissors are introduced at the skin level and dissection is carried across the lower lid.

edge of the skin incision and the cutting bovie needle is then used to incise through the orbicularis layer beneath the lashes and laterally, developing the skin-muscle flap. Once a small space is created, a small rake retractor (Blair) is inserted. With traction on the flap, the cutting Bovie is used to dissect over the lateral fat pocket area (Fig. 2A). The retractor is turned laterally so that traction is lateral, and the straight-sharp scissors are inserted beneath the skin in the subciliary area, undermining the skin beneath the lashes (Fig. 2B). The skin incision beneath the lashes is made with the straight scissors. The orbicularis muscle is then undermined and incised approximately 3–4 mm below the undersurface of the tarsal plate below the vascular inferior arcade (Fig. 3A). The lower lid skin-muscle flap is retracted downward with the rake retractors as the lower lid is pulled upward. Pressure on the globe then causes protrusion of the fat pockets behind the septum.

Fat Removal

It is helpful to pull the lower lid upward and use a 4 × 4 gauze pad to press on the lower lid to make the fat pockets protrude. When performing this step, the

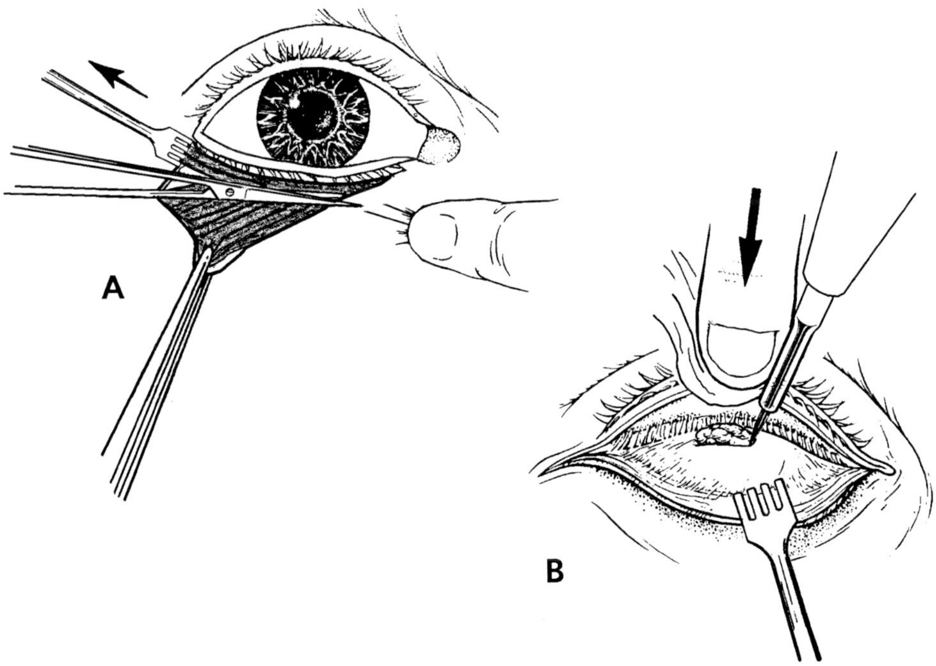

FIG. 3. A: The scissors have undermined the lower lid skin and the skin is incised from the pretarsal orbicularis. Then the muscle is incised to free the skin-muscle flap. Orbicularis muscle over the tarsal plate is not excised. **B:** The lower lid has been retracted upward with a gauze pad and finger pressure on the globe to cause the orbital fat to protrude beneath the septum. The cutting Bovie needle is then used to incise the septum.

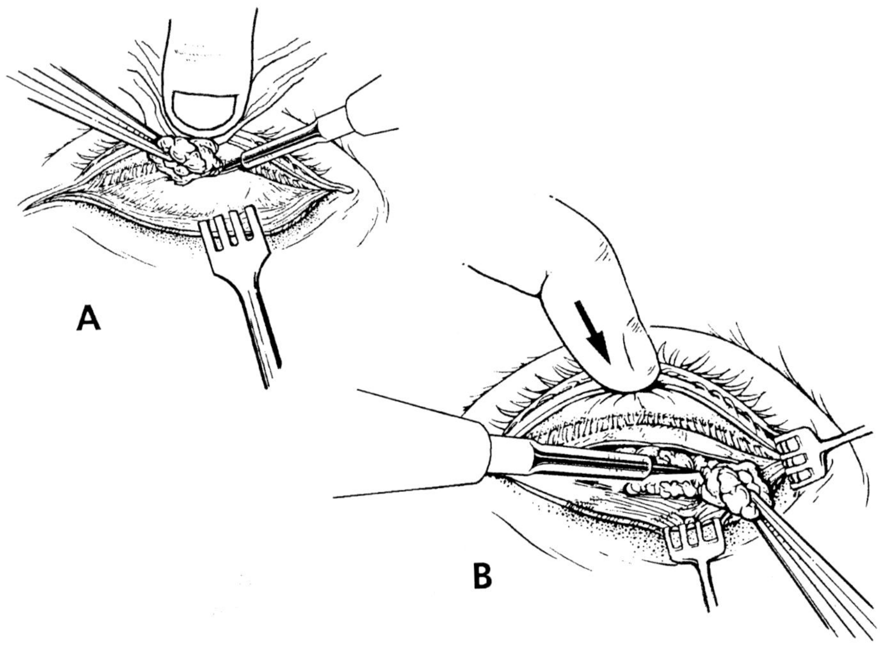

FIG. 4. A: With the same maneuver, the fat is teased from the central pocket and excised with the coagulating Bovie needle. **B:** The rake retractors are used to pull the skin nasally and downward in the nasal edge of the incision. With pressure on the globe the nasal fat is teased outward and excised with the Bovie needle on cutting current.

protective contact lens should be in place, the surgeon should have the assistant retract the skin-muscle flap downward, and a gauze pad should be placed on the pretarsal area of the lower lid. With one hand holding the Adson forceps and the other hand the Bovie cutting needle, a spare finger is placed on the gauze on the eyelid and pressure is applied to cause the fat to protrude. Incisions are then made into the septum overlying the fat pads (Fig. 3B). Incision into the central pocket is done first. Then the fatty pad is grasped with the forceps as it herniates and is excised with the Bovie needle on coagulation (Fig. 4A). A second retractor is inserted nasally, retracting the corner of the eyelid incision over toward the canthus, and with downward pressure the nasal fat pocket is made to protrude. The capsule is incised allowing the whitish fat to herniate. The fat is grasped with forceps, brought outward, and then excised with the Bovie coagulation needle (Fig. 4B). Visible vessels are specifically cauterized. In this area, care is taken to avoid damaging the inferior oblique muscle, which can be seen between the central and nasal fat pockets. Figure 5 is a surgical view showing the nasal and central fat pockets retracted. The fat may be further shrunk and cauterized with the Bovie coagulation needle. Any liquified fat is dabbed with the 4 × 4 gauze pad and the area flushed with cold water. The lateral fat pocket is removed (if needed) after the lateral canthoplasty procedure is performed.

Surgical Technique of Lateral Canthoplasty

This addition to the external lower lid blepharoplasty allows the surgeon to stabilize the eyelid fissure, correct laxity in the lower lid, adjust for the prominent-eye patient, e.g., Graves' disease. It also has the effect of smoothing the skin and allows the surgeon to supraplace the lateral canthal tendon to produce a more exotic look if desired. The lateral canthoplasty procedure is performed before the lateral fat pocket excision because it can affect the prominence of the lateral fat pocket. A canthotomy and lysis of the lower limbus canthal tendon with scissors is performed (Fig. 6A). The lid is then stretched laterally until it is tightened against the lateral orbital rim. When tensing against the orbital rim, if there is redundant overlap of the lid, it is trimmed so that the proper tension is produced.

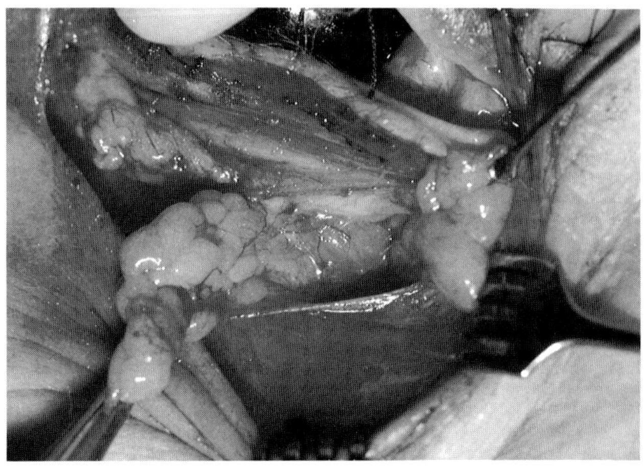

FIG. 5. Surgical view showing the skin-muscle flap retracted during a lower lid blepharoplasty with the nasal fat pad retracted nasally and the central fat pad retracted downward laterally exposing the inferior oblique muscle between the two pads. The lateral fat pocket can also be seen toward the lateral portion of the incision.

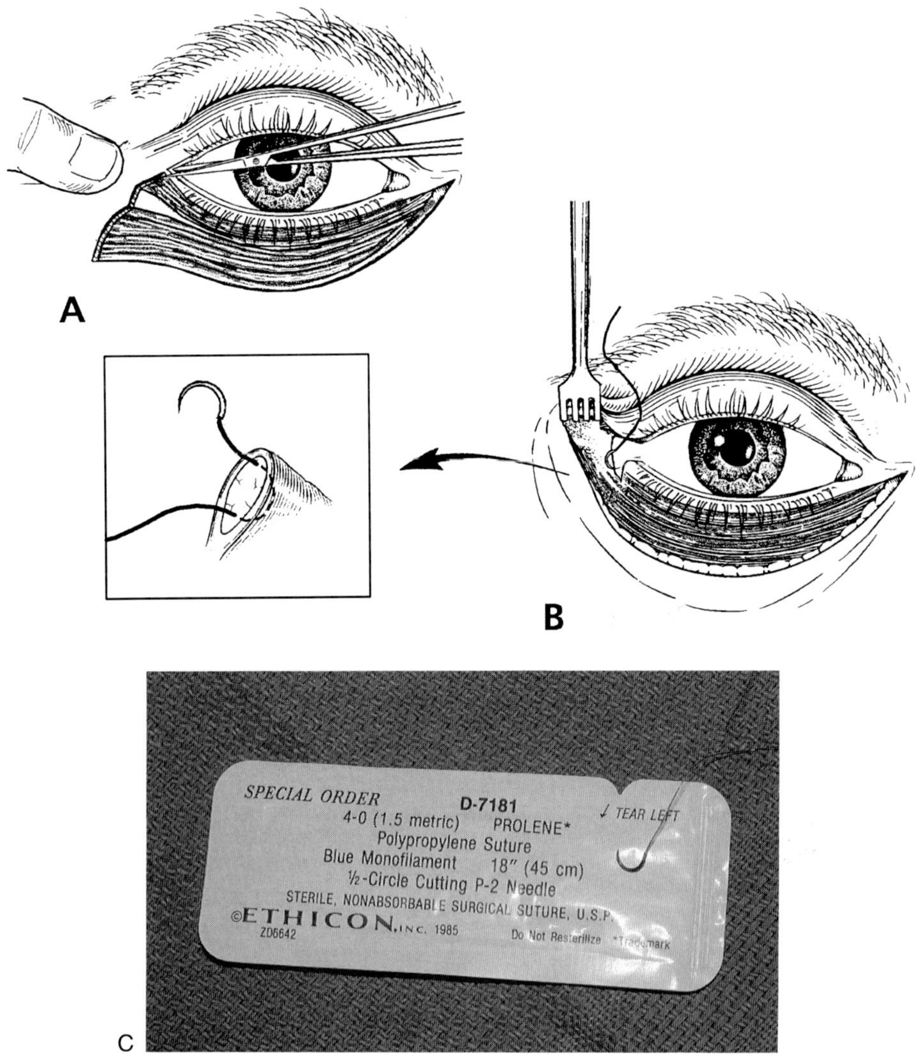

FIG. 6. Lateral Canthoplasty. **A:** Canthotomy and cantholysis is performed. **B:** A 4-0 prolene suture is introduced into the edge of the tarsal plate. **C:** A half-circle needle on a 4-0 prolene suture acquired as a special order which is used for plicating the edge of the lid to the periosteum with the lateral canthoplasty procedure.

The 4-0 prolene suture on P-2 needle (special order, Ethicon) is then inserted through the edge of the lid starting from the inferior tarsus upward and brought out in the tarsal plate, near the edge of the lid (Fig. 6B, C). This is then inserted into the inner edge of the periosteum inside the orbital rim at the level of the midpupillary area and brought from inside the rim outward. A second bite is then taken from outside the rim inward and tightened with a double throw until the lower lid position is in the desired location at the lower limbus with the desired tension (Fig. 7A). If the lid is short and tight, then no tissue is trimmed and the mattress suture that will be inserted can contain slack.

When the suture is tied, care is taken to keep the ends of the suture knot flat so that they will not protrude outward irritating the undersurface of the skin.

Undermining the Skin–Muscle Flap

It is important to undermine the skin-muscle flap over the malar area separating the septal strands and periosteum from the flap. This allows more smoothing of the malar area. Failure to do this will cause anterior distortion of the lateral fat pocket requiring more resection. Once the flap is dissected free the lateral fat pocket is resected if necessary.

Lateral Fat Pad Excision

The lateral fat is grasped with the Adson forceps and then it is trimmed with a cutting Bovie needle and the edges cauterized (Fig. 7B). The area is irrigated with

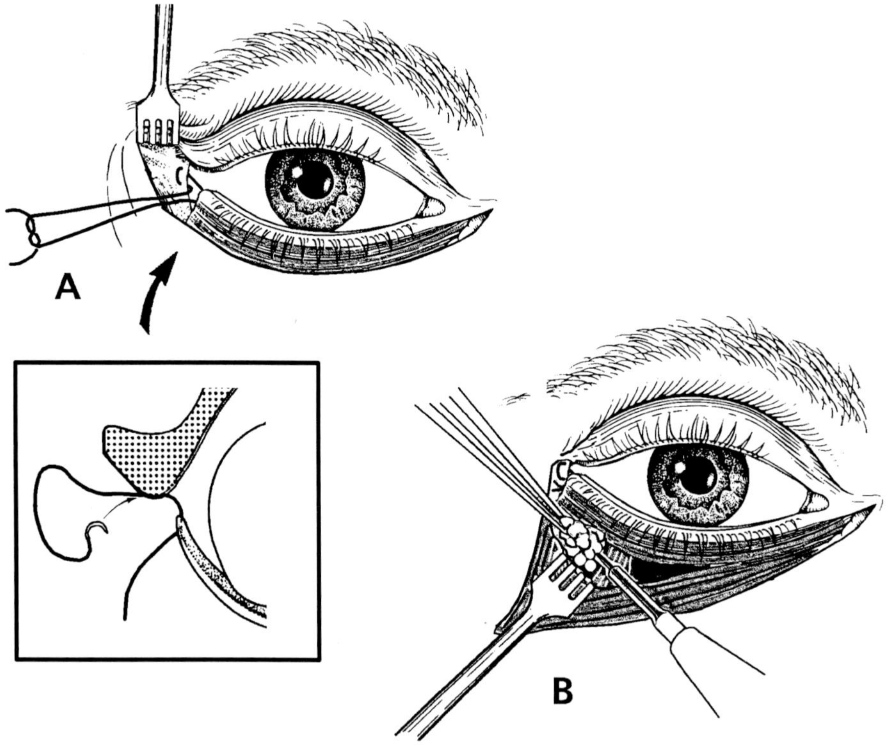

FIG. 7. Lateral canthoplasty. **A:** The 4-0 prolene suture is introduced into the edge of the lateral orbital rim at the pupillary level and in a mattress-like manner tightened with the lower lid to tense the lower lid and complete the canthoplasty. **B:** Following the horizontal tightening and canthoplasty and undermining of the skin-muscle flap, the lateral fat pocket is excised if it is protuberant at this time.

cold water. It is important to preserve the arcuate portion of the orbital septum laterally to prevent recurrence of the lateral pad prolapse postoperatively. The lateral fat and central fat are connected and can be "teased" from behind this portion of the septum without severing it.

Resection of the Skin-Muscle Flap

In order to determine the desired amount of skin-muscle to resect to produce the desired tension over the cheekbone, the lateral slanting incision is held tense with one finger and the tip of the triangular flap is stretched toward the superior tip of the ear until the desired tension is obtained (Fig. 8A). When it is noted how much the lateral triangular portion of the flap overlaps the underlying incision, methylene blue is used to mark this section from the point of the flap all the way to the elevated edge of the flap. This line is incised with the Bard–Parker blade and then resected with scissors, with cautery applied to the bleeding orbicularis edges.

Periosteal Fixation of the Skin–Muscle Flap

The flap is sutured to the lateral periosteum to create the desired effect of tension over the cheekbone and correct any hollowing effect in the lower lid. Multiple levels of the edge of the flap are grasped and tested for effect. Trial positioning of the flap to the lateral rim is performed until the desired tension is obtained (Fig. 8B). In many cases the lateral edges of the skin are not even in length when the desired smoothing of the malar skin is obtained. This, however, is the endpoint that must be used to fixate the flap so that the desired tension and appearance of skin over the malar bone will be present.

Once the point of purchase is determined, a 4-0 silk suture is placed through the flap. The suture is placed in the lateral periosteum at the desired position and then brought out through the skin-muscle layer of the upper incision edge (Fig. 9A). Care is taken not to place the suture too close to the canthal angle to prevent an epicanthal fold postoperatively.

Following the periosteal fixation of the skin-muscle flap, the edge of the redundant flap occurring beneath the lashes is trimmed in a piecemeal manner until the desired tension is obtained (Fig. 9B). Orbicularis fibers are then trimmed from beneath the flap in the subciliary area (Fig. 10A). These are orbicularis fibers that overlap the fibers left on the pretarsal area from the original resection. The flap is everted with cotton applicator sticks and the bipolar cautery used for hemostasis in

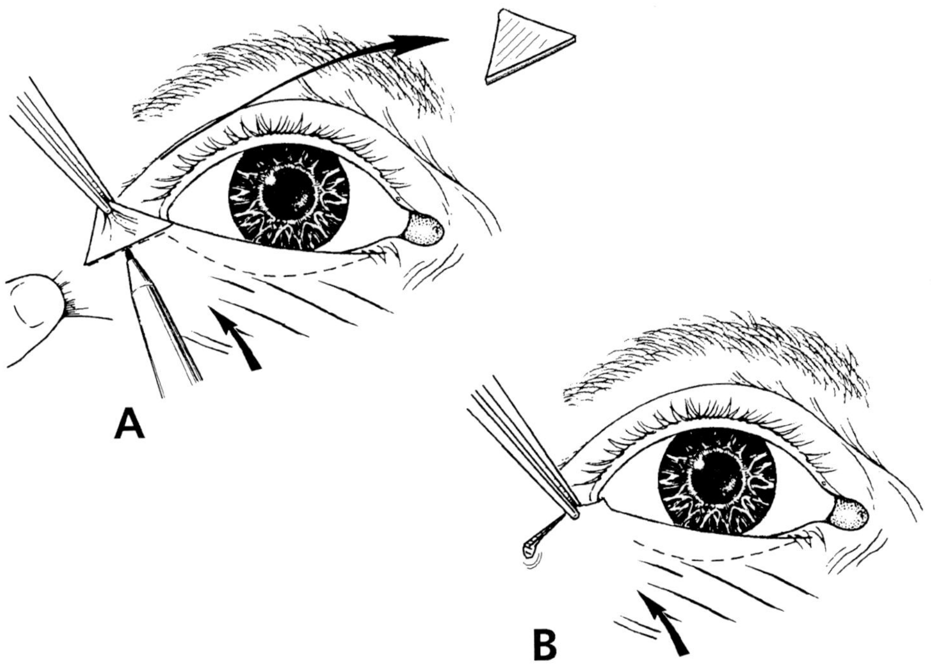

FIG. 8. A: The skin-muscle flap is rotated upward in the direction toward the upper tip of the ear. When the desired tension is obtained over the malar area, the redundant triangle overlapping the lateral wound incision is marked and excised. **B:** Forceps are used to test the desired point of purchase of the edge of the flap, which is brought to the lateral periosteum. Varying positions are tried to determine the tension over the malar area. When the desired effect is obtained, this point is used for suturing the flap to the periosteum.

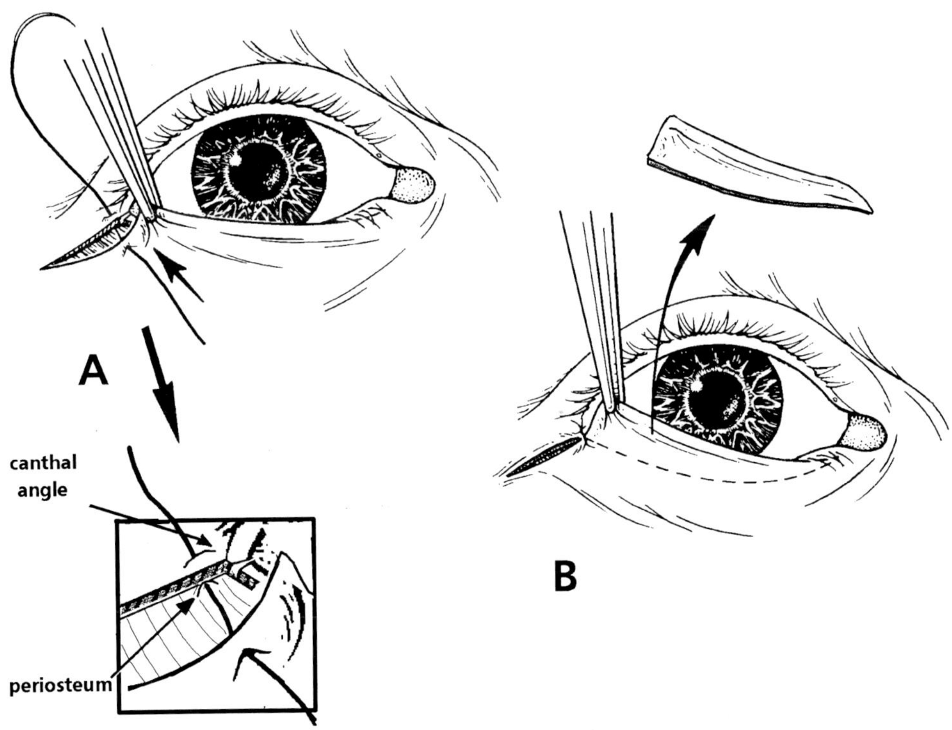

FIG. 9. A: At the desired purchase point on the flap a suture is introduced through the full-thickness skin muscle and into the periosteum at the lateral rim. The suture should not be placed too close to the canthus to prevent epicanthal fold formation. **B:** A second strip of skin and muscle is trimmed beneath the lashes. The amount needed is usually not great and can be obtained in a piecemeal manner.

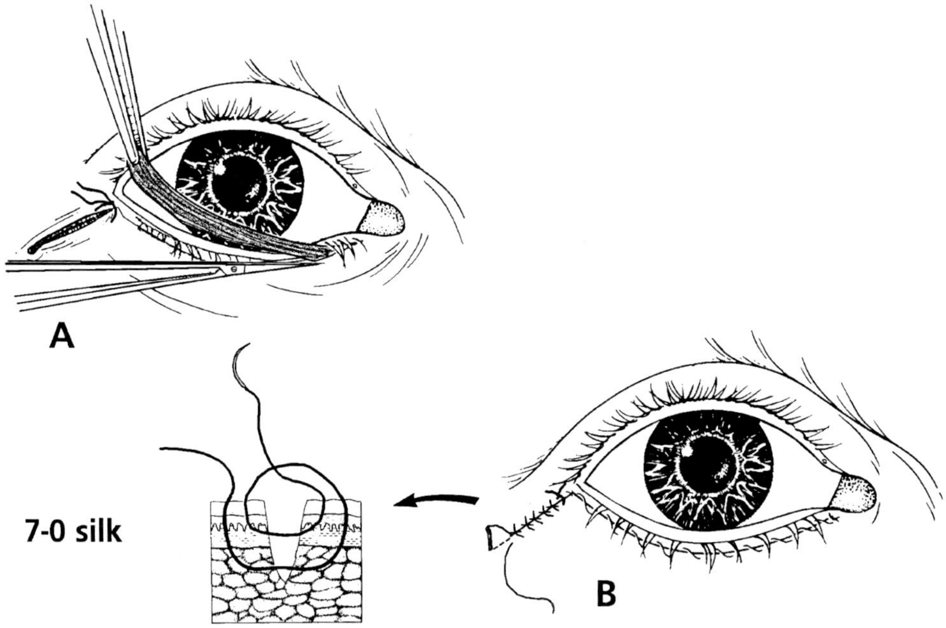

FIG. 10. A: Following removal of the skin, a strip of orbicularis is removed beneath the lash line to further thin the lid down. This seems to be an important step in women to gain a desired smoothing. It should be left in the male patient to avoid an overthinned look. **B:** The wound is closed beneath the lashes with a loose continuous suture. Laterally the closure in the visible canthal incision is highly critical. A vertical mattress 7-0 silk is used with care taken to ensure that the muscle layed is closed as well as the skin edges which are everted. There is very commonly a small dog ear formation at the end of the incision that can be excised before completing closure.

the orbicularis edges. Closure in the skin flap is then obtained with 7-0 silk sutures applied in a running manner across the lower lid. The lateral canthal angle is skipped. A vertical mattress suture is used for the lateral edge of the skin closure. Care is taken to close both the skin edge and the deep orbicularis fibers. The vertical mattress suture is placed with alternating deep bites through skin and orbicularis and shallow slanting bites through skin and subcutaneous tissue (Fig. 10B). Meticulous closure is needed in this conspicuous area to avoid scarring. There is always a small dog ear formation at the lateral edge of the incision. It is trimmed and shaved. The last loop of running suture is then placed through this and tied very loosely. A 6-0 nylon intermarginal suture is sometimes used at the lateral canthus after lateral canthoplasty to ensure alignment of the upper and lower lid edge.

CANTHOPLASTY MODIFICATION FOR PROMINENT EYE

Patients with prominent eyes, either from Graves' disease or from a familial trait, are at risk for increasing scleral show postoperatively. Cases of extreme exophthalmos are addressed by the surgical techniques described in the chapter on Graves' disease. In patients with prominent eyes, a standard lateral canthoplasty with horizontal tightening may cause a worsening of the scleral show because of a clotheslining effect. In these patients the lower lid margin can be positioned at the inferior limbus with the following modification in the lateral canthoplasty.

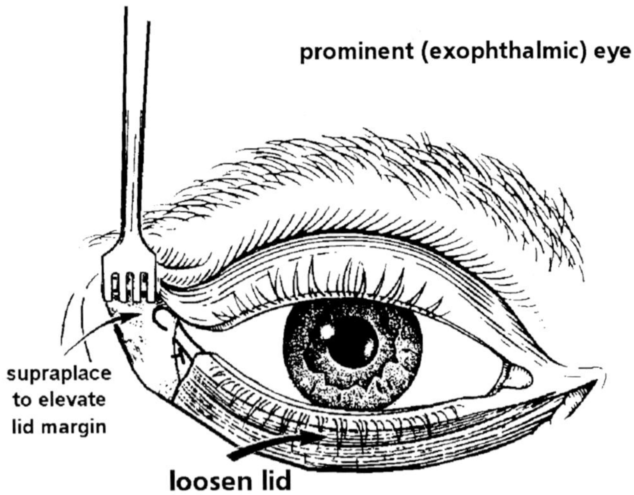

FIG. 11. Modification of the lateral canthoplasty tightening procedure in patients with a prominent eye. A clotheslining effect will occur if the lid is tightened and the lateral fixation is low in patients with prominent eyes. If this occurs, the lateral fixation sutures should be placed higher than the usual position above the pupil and then loosened to allow the lower lid to ride up so that the edge is at the inferior limbus. It is necessary to leave slack in the suture laterally.

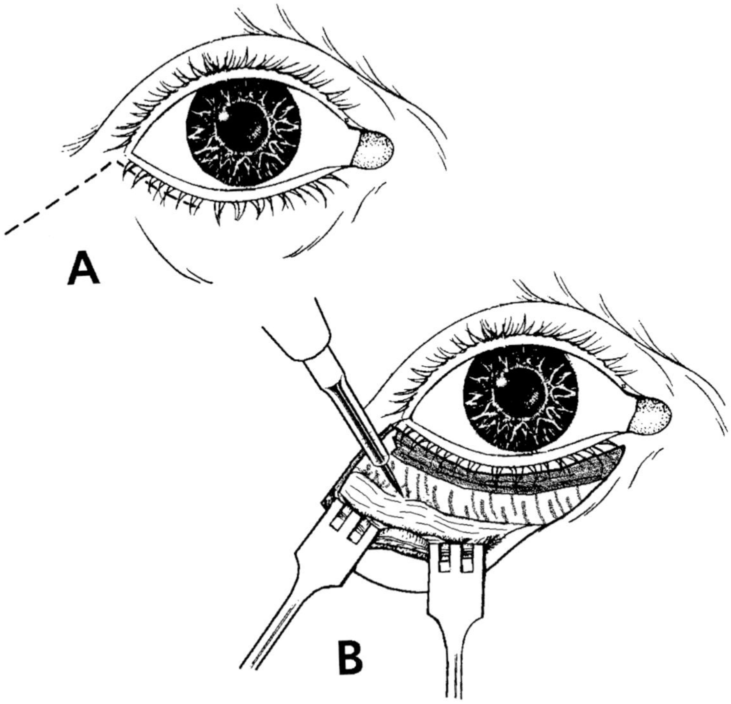

FIG. 12. Extended blepharoplasty incision for patients with malar folds. **A:** An extension of the normal lateral incision is made which can be carried slightly into the thicker skin. **B:** Following the standard blepharoplasty before the flap is rotated upward to determine redundancy, the flap is thoroughly undermined over the malar and septal areas to avoid any adherences. The undersurface of the flap in the area of malar folding can also be lightly cauterized to cause some tightening. The operation is then completed in the usual way after upward rotation of the flap.

The lateral canthotomy and cantholysis is performed. The lateral periosteum is exposed above the pupillary level by dissection. The lower limb of the canthal tendon is fixated to the periosteum at an elevated position. Slack is left in the lateral fixating suture, "loosening" the lid and allowing the lower lid to ride up to the inferior limbus, thus avoiding the clotheslining effect (Fig. 11).

EXTENDED BLEPHAROPLASTY FOR MALAR FOLDS

Folding in the malar area, usually seen in older patients, has no perfect solution. In severe cases a direct excision has been advocated but may lead to unacceptable scarring. A modification of the external blepharoplasty can improve the malar area in these patients. A longer lateral slanting incision is initially made. After elevation of the skin-muscle flap the Bovie needle is used for undermining under the malar area. With the Bovie, cautery is applied to the undersurface of the muscle, submuscular fat, and subcutaneous tissue (Fig. 12A, B). A lateral canthoplasty and periosteal fixation of the skin-muscle flap is performed. An increased dog ear is usually encountered at the inferior end of the lateral slanting incision requiring further extension of the incision. Figure 13A and B shows a patient with severe malar folds before and after and external blepharoplasty with an extended incision and undermining. Patients are told preoperatively that some dermabrasion may be necessary at a later date if the incision line is too visible. In actuality it is rarely necessary if there is good design and closure of the incision.

A 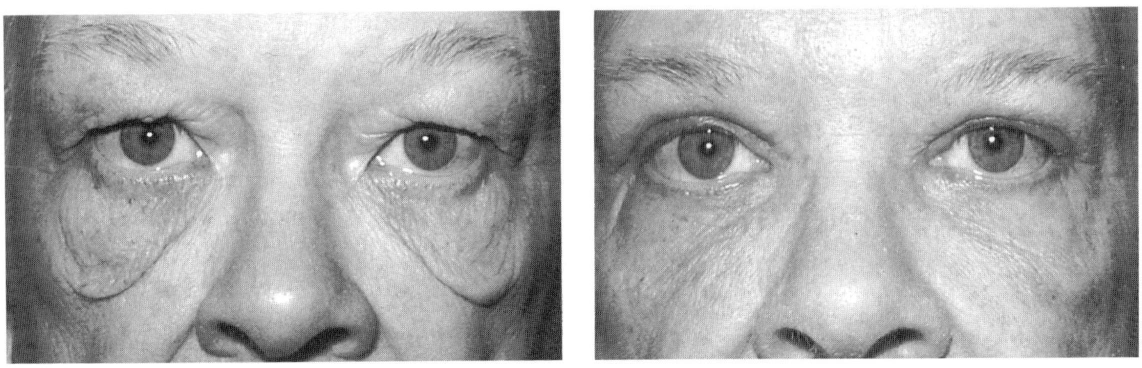 B

FIG. 13. Patient with severe malar folds. **A:** Before surgery. **B:** Six weeks following extended lower lid incision with blepharoplasty.

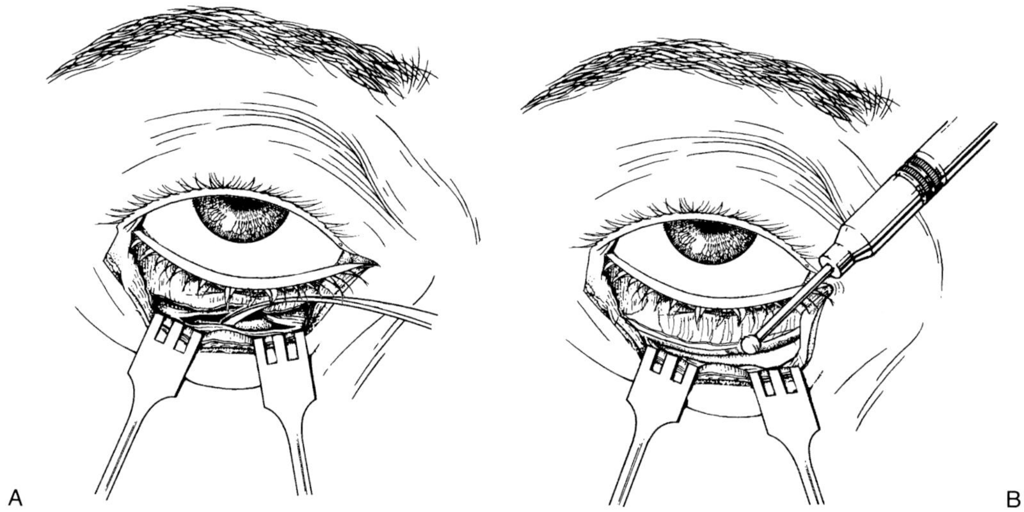

FIG. 14. Sculpting of the inferior orbital rim in patients with a protuberant and sharp inferior orbital rim. **A:** Exposure of the rim by retraction of the lower lid flap and elevation of the periosteum from the edge of the rim. **B:** Sculpting of the edge of the bone with the cutting osteotome.

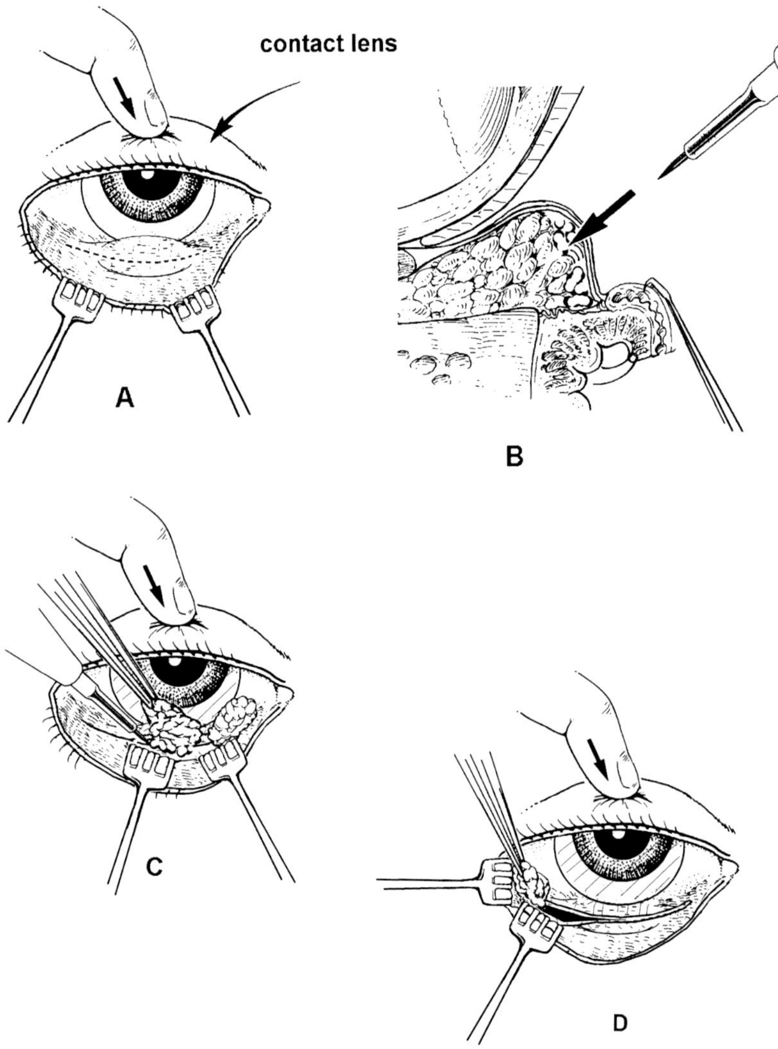

FIG. 15. Fornix fat removal. **A:** The lower lid is retracted with two Blair retractors. Pressure is used on the upper lid, transmitted to a contact lens placed over the globe. This exerts pressure in the orbital rim causing the fat pads to protrude into the inferior fornix. **B:** Cross-section showing the direction and location of the incision in the lower fornix through the lower lid retractors at the inferior edge of the tarsal plate. The incision is made with a cutting Bovie needle. **C:** Incision has been made completely through the conjunctiva and inferior retractors and the central and nasal fat pockets have been teased outward for excision. **D:** The central and nasal fat pockets have been removed and repositioning of the retractors laterally can pull the lid laterally and downward, exposing the lateral fat pocket for removal if necessary.

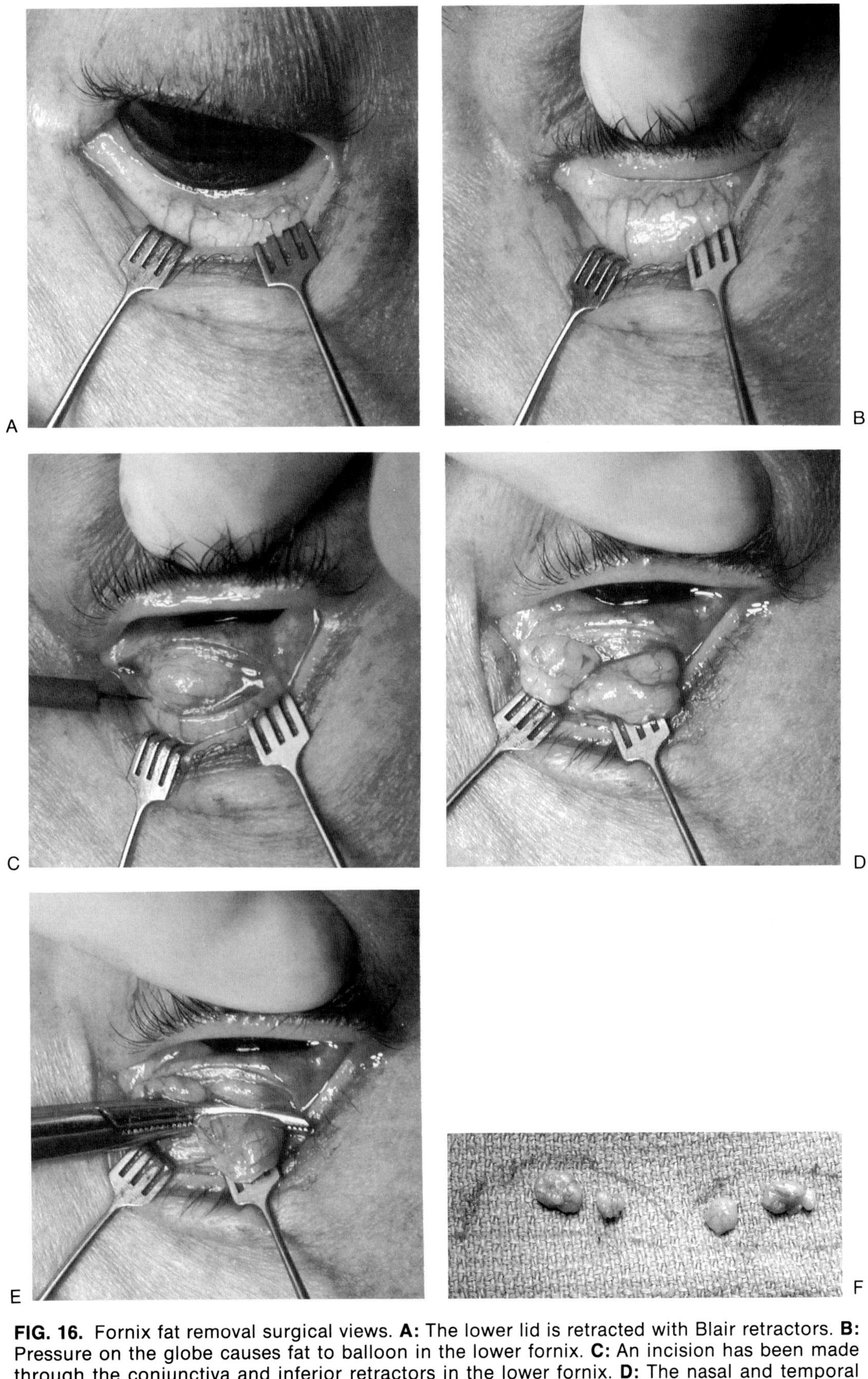

FIG. 16. Fornix fat removal surgical views. **A:** The lower lid is retracted with Blair retractors. **B:** Pressure on the globe causes fat to balloon in the lower fornix. **C:** An incision has been made through the conjunctiva and inferior retractors in the lower fornix. **D:** The nasal and temporal fat pocket have been teased outward into the wound. **E:** A central fat pocket has been clamped before excision. **F:** The nasal and central fat pockets as removed from a patient bilaterally.

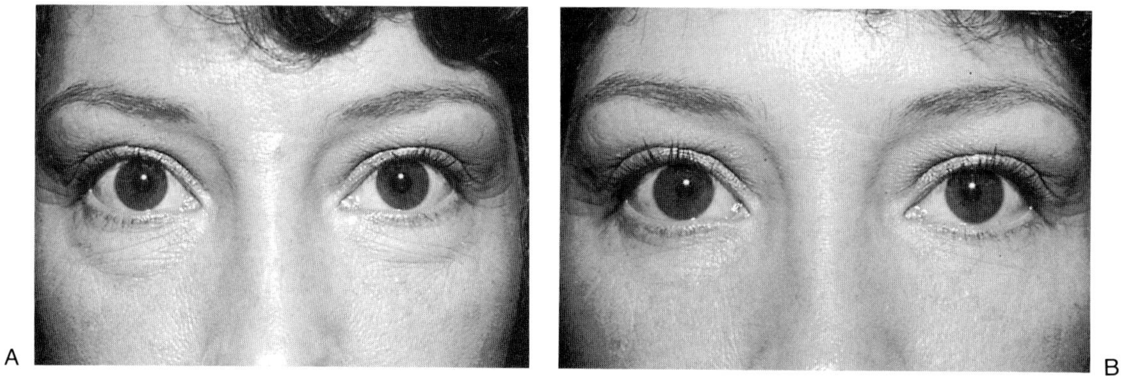

FIG. 17. Fornix fat removal. **A:** Patient preoperatively. **B:** Same patient following fornix fat removal 6 weeks postoperatively.

SCULPTING OF BONY INFERIOR ORBITAL RIM

Lateral prominence of the cheekbone is desirable but bony protrusion of the nasal inferior rim can be unattractive and simulate herniated fat. Some bony sculpting of this area can be performed if desired by the patient. The standard skin-muscle flap elevation and fat removal is performed. The flap is retracted inferiorly and dissected away from inferior orbital rim (Fig. 14A).

The periosteum is incised and elevated and the prominent bone edge sculpted with a cutting rotary osteotome (Fig. 14B). The periosteal flaps are repositioned before closure to prevent adhesions inferiorly. The blepharoplasty is completed.

SURGICAL TECHNIQUE OF FORNIX FAT REMOVAL

Anesthesia is performed with an infraorbital block, fat pad injection, and fornix injection. A protective contact lens is inserted and small rake retractors (Blair) are used to evert the lower lid. Pressure is applied to the globe through a contact lens causing the lower lid fat to balloon beneath the conjunctiva and inferior retractors in the inferior fornix (Fig. 15A). An incision is made at the apex of the bulge in conjunctiva (half the distance between tarsus and fornix) with the cutting Bovie needle through the conjunctiva and the retractor layer until the fat can be seen to protrude. Care must be taken to incise directly into the fat compartment in a perpendicular manner without veering off on a tangential plane (Fig. 15B).

The rake retractors are then repositioned to the cut edge of conjunctiva, and wider incision can be made into the retractor layer if necessary. The fat is teased out with Adson forceps and cotton swabs. The medial and nasal fat is excised with the coagulating Bovie needle (Fig. 15C). The extractors are then inserted at the lateral end of the incision and with globe pressure the lateral fat pad is excised if necessary (Fig. 15D). There is usually a need to cauterize the edge of the capsulopalpebral fascia layer for hemostasis. The conjunctiva is sutured with a 6-0 plain. Figure 16A–F shows surgical views of fornix fat removal. Figure 17A and B shows a patient before and after fornix fat removal.

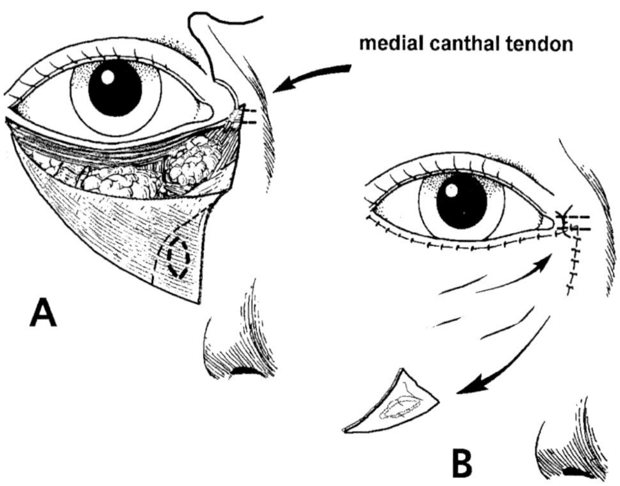

FIG. 18. A: Diagrammatic representation of a nasal-based blepharoplasty incision when performed in conjunction with excision of a lesion such as a xanthelasma. The subciliary incision has been extended to the nasocanthal area above the medial canthal tendon and then downward and reflected. The flap is everted and the lesion seen in outline. **B:** Following the standard fat removal, the flap is rotated with excision of the triangle of skin containing the lesion. The flap is fixated to the medical canthal tendon and the blepharoplasty completed.

NASAL BASED BLEPHAROPLASTY

Many patients presenting for lower lid blepharoplasty will have coincidental skin lesions in the lower lid that they wish removed while having the blepharoplasty performed. If the lesions occur in skin that is normally resected in blepharoplasty or if the lesions are very small in size, their excision with a standard external blepharoplasty presents no problem. Certain common lesions (i.e., xanthelasma) are large and occur outside of the usual resection area. For lesions that occur in the nasal skin, the skin resection of the blepharoplasty can be modified so that a triangle of skin is excised nasally instead of laterally and includes the lesion.

With this technique a subciliary incision is made to the medial canthal tendon area and then the downsloping incision is made in the nasojugal area (Fig. 18A). The skin-muscle flap is tensed as it is done laterally but in a superionasal direction creating an overlapping triangle that includes the lesion. The triangle is marked and excised with the lesion. The skin-muscle flap is anchored to the medial canthal tendon, as one would do with the flap laterally to the periosteum, fixating it with a 4-0 silk suture (Fig. 18B). The strip of skin muscle beneath the lashes is removed and the skin closed. The nasal scar is minimal if good closure is observed but in any case is less conspicuous than the original lesion.

SURGICAL TECHNIQUE FOR THE ASIAN EYELID

A specific problem that is common in the Asian lower lid is an unusual hypertrophy of orbicularis fibers, causing severe bunching when smiling, and this may be the patient's presenting complaint. This condition can be improved by an excision of the offending orbicularis fibers, more than is usual with the standard external blepharoplasty. This extra excision can take place at the end of a standard external blepharoplasty or beneath a subciliary skin incision elevated specifically for that purpose.

REFERENCES

1. Furnas DW. The orbicularis oculi muscle. *Clin Plast Surg* 1981; 8:687–751.
2. Rees TD, Tabbal N. Lower blepharoplasty. *Clin Plast Surg* 1981;8:643–662.
3. Loeb R. Necessity for partial resection of the orbicularis oculi muscle in blepharoplasties in some young patients. *Plast Reconstr Surg* 1977;60:176.
4. Rees TD, Dupuis CC. Baggy eyelids in young adults. *Plast Reconstr Surg* 1969;43:381.
5. McCord CD, Shore JW. Avoidance of complications in lower lid blepharoplasty. *Ophthalmology* 1983;90:1039.
6. Baylis HI, Sutcliff RT. Conjunctival approach in lower eyelid blepharoplasty. *Adv Ophth Plast Reconstr Surg* 1983;2:43.
7. Baylis HI, Long JA, Groth MJ. Transconjunctival lower eyelid blepharoplasty: technique and complications. *Ophthalmology* 1989;96:1027.
8. Hinderer UT. Correction of weakness of the lower eyelid and lateral canthus. *Clin Plast Surg* 1993;20:331–349.
9. Whitaker LA. Selective of the palpebral fissure form by lateral canthopexy. *Plast Reconstr Surg* 1984;74:611–619.
10. Ortiz-Monasterio F, et al. Lateral canthoplasty to change the eyelid slant. *Plast Reconstr Surg* 1985;75:1–10.
11. Carraway JH, Mellow CG. The prevention and treatment of lower lid ectropion following blepharoplasty. *Plast Reconstr Surg* 1990;85:971.
12. Custer PL, Tenzel RR. Lateral canthal sling update. *Ophth Plast Reconstr Surg* 1985;1:121.
13. McCord CD, Ellis DS. The correction of lower lid malposition following blepharoplasty. *Plast Reconstr Surg* 1993;92: 1066–1072.
14. Furnas DW. Festoons of orbicularis muscle as a cause of baggy eyelids. *Plast Reconstr Surg* 1978;61:540.
15. Small RG. Extended lower lid blepharoplasty. *Arch Ophthalmol* 1981;99:1402–1405.
16. Wilkins RB, Hunter GJ, McCord CD, Tenenbaum MT. Blepharoplasty: cosmetic and functional. *Oculoplastic surgery*. 2nd ed. New York: Raven Press; 1987:462–473.

CHAPTER 16

Subperiosteal Malar Cheek Lift with Lower Lid Blepharoplasty

In general, the process of facial aging is gradual and affects all areas of the face. However, depending on individual genetic and environmental factors, the effects of aging may become more apparent in any given facial aesthetic unit, defined as (1) upper face (brow, forehead, and upper lids), (2) orbital (upper and lower lids), (3) midface (lower lids, malar, preauricular), (4) lower face (perioral, jowl, and neck). Surgeons have traditionally considered the position of the brow when evaluating aging in the upper face and performed indicated repositioning with upper lid blepharoplasty. It is not as well appreciated but just as important to consider the position of the potentially ptotic malar soft tissue when considering lower lid blepharoplasty. The purpose of this chapter is to emphasize the relationship between the lower lid and malar soft tissues with emphasis on treatment based on accurate anatomic diagnosis of the pathology of aging as it occurs in this specific area of the face.

ANATOMY OF LOWER LID AND MALAR AGING

As aging occurs in the face, there is gradual vertical descent of the soft tissues overlying the periosteum of the malar prominence (Fig. 1). An understanding of the soft tissue topography present in the youthful vs. the aging face over the malar eminence allows the surgeon to design a more anatomically sound surgical approach for correction of soft tissue ptosis. The five distinct soft tissue layers that comprise the soft tissue component of the malar prominence are as follows:

1. Skin
2. Superficial muscular aponeurotic system (SMAS) with overlying fat: "the malar fat pad"
3. Orbicularis oculi
4. Suborbicularis oculi fat pad (SOOF)
5. Periosteum

With aging, a vertical descent of the malar soft tissue complex occurs over the fixed periosteum. The essential principle is that as descent and thinning occurs, soft tissue thickness adjacent to the inferior and lower half of the lateral orbital rim is diminished. This process gradually results in the very thin skin of the lower lid replacing thicker cheek skin over the orbital rim, loss of soft tissue prominence over the malar eminence, and deepening of the nasolabial fold. Clinically, the loss of normal soft tissue fullness over bone results in "cadaverization," the pathognomonic sign of aging in the lower orbit and malar area, which must be addressed if optimal correction is to be achieved.

CLINICAL CONSIDERATIONS AND TREATMENT PLANNING

Patients presenting for treatment of aging in the lower lid and malar area will fall into one of the following diagnostic categories.

1. Prominent postseptal fat without lower lid skin laxity or excess and without vertical descent of the malar soft tissue. These patients are usually younger and represent the only group in which conservative transconjunctival fat removal may be the only necessary treatment.
2. Laxity and/or wrinkling of lower lid skin with or without prominent postseptal fat and without vertical descent of the malar soft tissue. These patients require standard blepharoplasty and lateral canthoplasty.
3. Laxity of lower lid skin with vertical descent of the malar soft tissue with less apparent facial aging in other aesthetic units. These patients benefit from lower lid blepharoplasty and canthoplasty with superior vertical repositioning of the malar soft tissue.

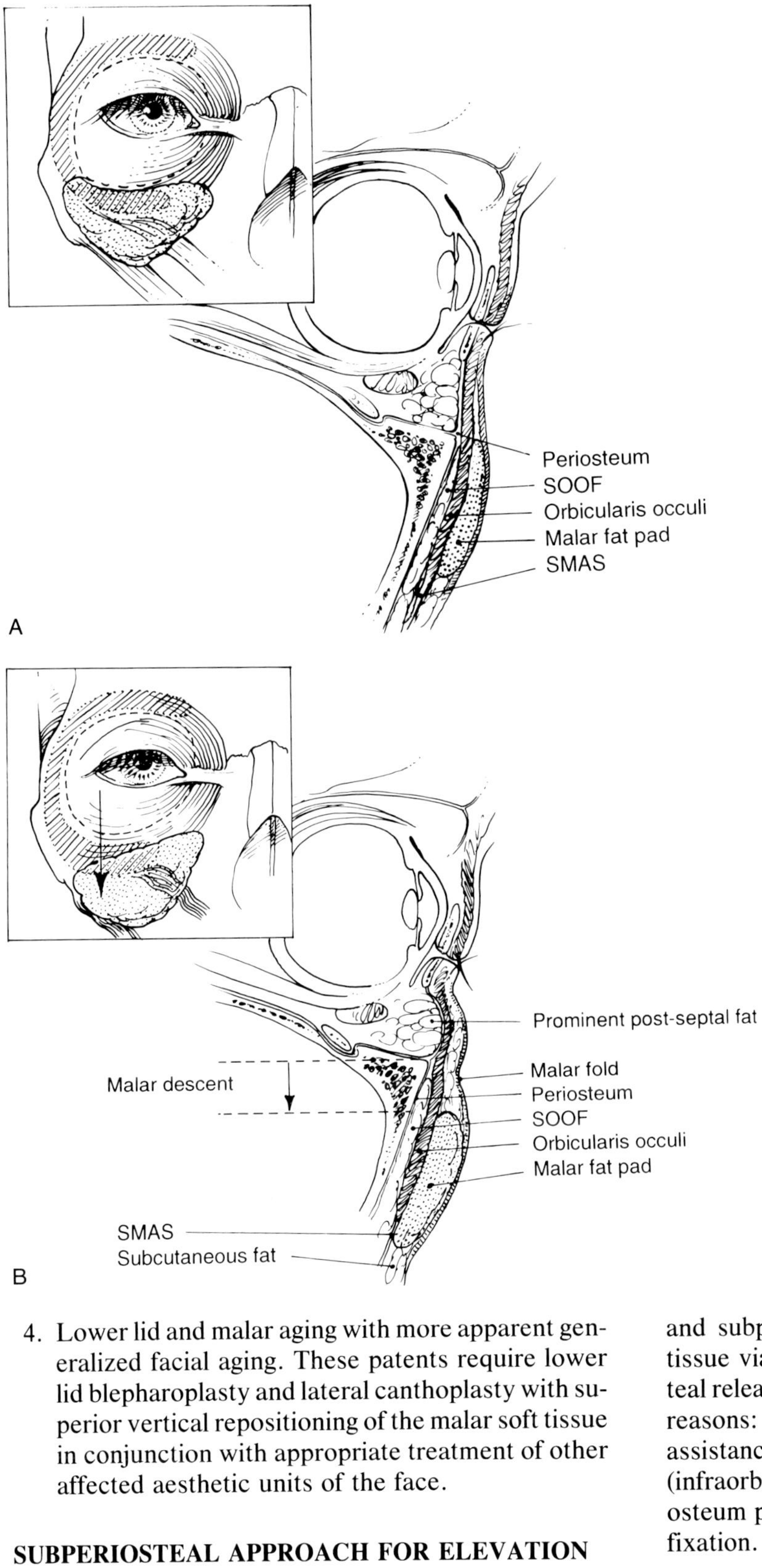

FIG. 1. (A) Cross-section and frontal view inset showing the malar soft tissue complex in the youthful face and **(B)** in the aged face with descent of the malar complex below the inferior orbital rim.

4. Lower lid and malar aging with more apparent generalized facial aging. These patents require lower lid blepharoplasty and lateral canthoplasty with superior vertical repositioning of the malar soft tissue in conjunction with appropriate treatment of other affected aesthetic units of the face.

SUBPERIOSTEAL APPROACH FOR ELEVATION OF MALAR SOFT TISSUE

Techniques suggested for rejuvenation of the aging face have proposed surgical dissection in tissue planes including subcutaneous, sub-SMAS, preperiosteal, and subperiosteal (1–9). For elevation of malar soft tissue via a lower blepharoplasty incision, subperiosteal release of malar soft tissue is used for the following reasons: (a) ease and rapidity of dissection (endoscopic assistance can be used), (b) minimal bleeding, (c) safety (infraorbital nerve easily identified), (d) elevated periosteum providing optimal strength for superior suture fixation.

TECHNIQUE

Step 1. A lower lid subciliary incision is made extending to a point just lateral to the canthus then turn-

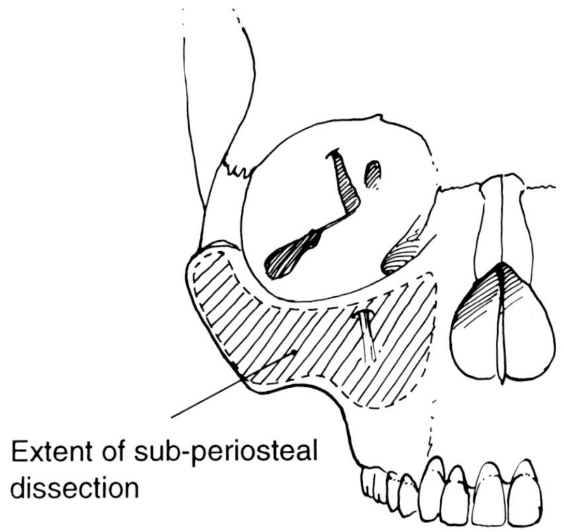

FIG. 2. Subperiosteal dissection begins 2–3 mm below the inferior orbital rim and extends medial to the inferior orbital nerve and lateral to the zygoma. Periosteal division is essential for release of the malar complex.

ing inferolateral following a natural skin crease if possible. The more inferior orientation of the lateral component of the incision, contrasted to the traditional lateral extension, allows for more effective horizontal tightening of the lower lid. Dissection is suborbicularis to the inferior and lateral orbital rims. Postseptal orbital fat reduction is conservative, based on careful preoperative evaluation.

Step 2. An incision is made along the inferior and lateral orbital rim to the level of the lateral canthus. Careful subperiosteal dissection using appropriate elevators is begun. In experienced hands, endoscopic assistance can aid in the dissection and help identify and prevent injury to the infraorbital nerve. The dissection extends in a "U"-shaped pattern across the body of the malar eminence (Fig. 2). At the extent of the dissection, the periosteum is divided using either fine-needle cautery or an appropriately designed elevator. The periosteal release has to be complete to free the soft tissue complex for elevation. During the dissection the zygomaticofacial nerve (sensory) will be encountered over the lateral dome of the malar eminence (Fig. 3). Usually the nerve is sacrificed to allow for ease and completeness of dissection. Sensory loss to the skin is minimal and temporary. The infraorbital nerve should be identified and preserved (Fig. 3).

Step 3. The malar soft tissue complex has now been freed posteriorly from its bony attachments and can be elevated. The elevation is vertical in orientation and redrapes the superior border of the malar fat pad and SOOF over the inferior and inferolateral orbital rim. In addition, ptotic cheek skin is repositioned superiorly allowing later safe removal of more skin for better correction of lower lid laxity. Elevation is maintained using a 4-0 woven nylon suture fixation placed through a composite of the periosteum, SOOF, orbicularis, and lateral aspect of the malar fat pad (Fig. 4). Superiorly, fixation is to the periosteum of the orbital rim at the level of the lateral canthus (Fig. 5). Optimal correction requires precise placement of the suture at the level of the upper border of the ptotic malar fat pad directly below the lateral canthus (Fig. 6). Experience has shown that superior traction from this point most effectively redrapes the malar soft tissues and softens the nasolabial fold. This fixation provides superior stabilization of the malar soft tissue and minimizes downward traction on the lower lid.

Step 4. Finally, control of the lower lid position is optimized utilizing a lateral canthotomy, inferior cantholysis, and canthoplasty as described in the chapter

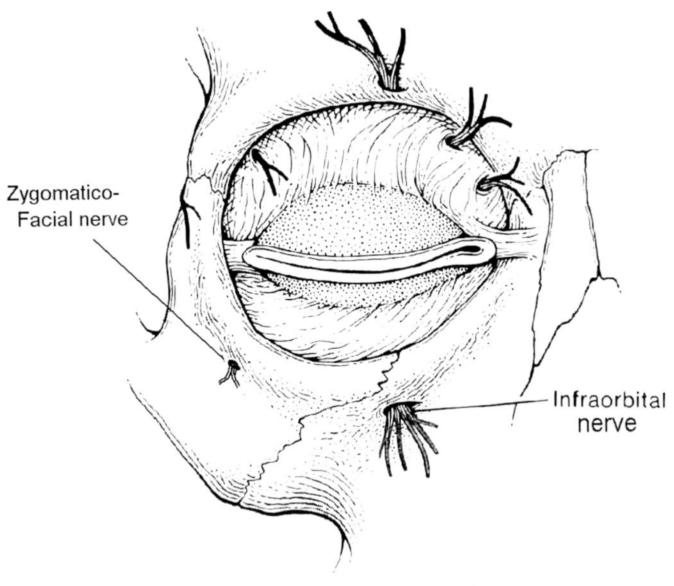

FIG. 3. Anatomic location of the inferior orbital nerve and the zygomatiofacial nerve which are encountered during subperiosteal dissection.

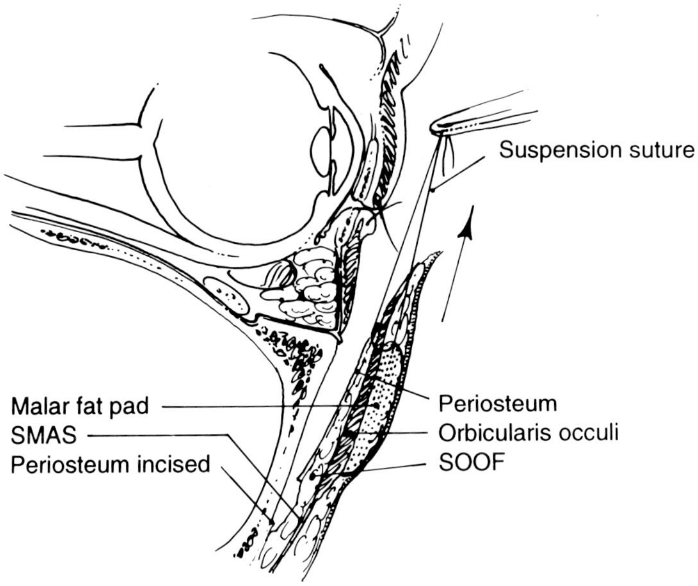

FIG. 4. Cross-section demonstrating the suspension of the malar soft tissue complex as a unit including periosteum, suborbicularis oculi fat (SOOF), orbicularis, and malar fat pad.

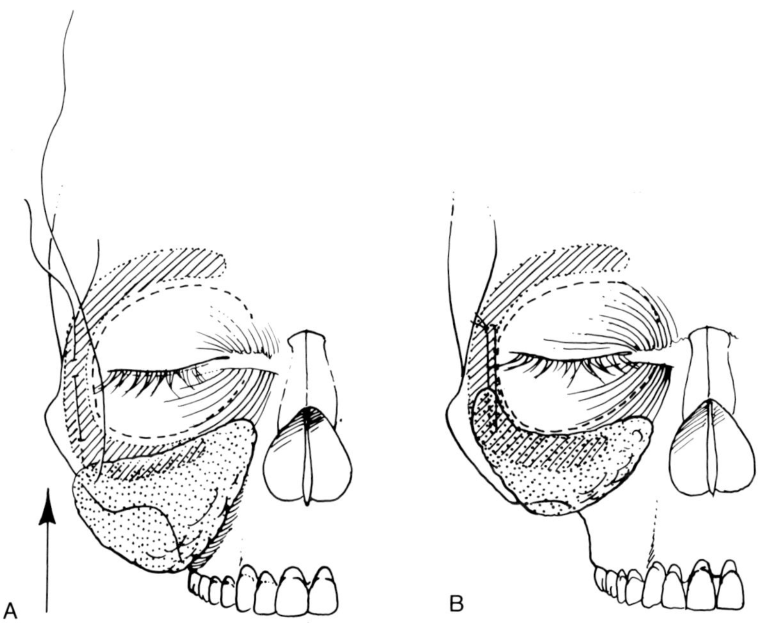

FIG. 5. A: The suspension suture is placed in the released malar complex and pulled in a vertical vector. **B:** Fixation to the periosteum just lateral to the lateral canthus maintains the elevation of the malar complex just overlying the inferior orbital rim.

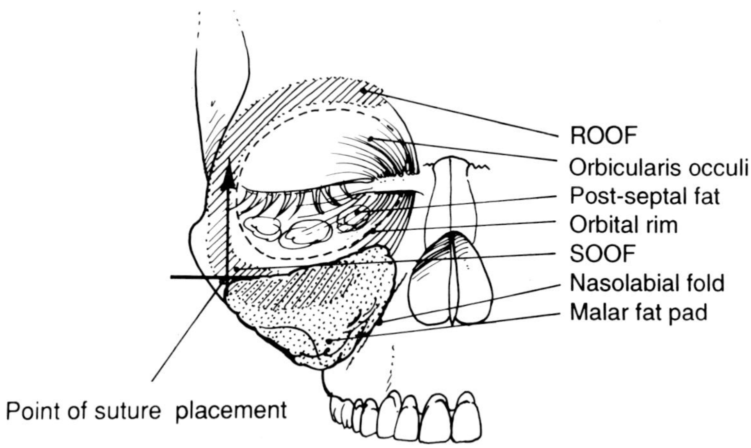

FIG. 6. Anatomy of the orbital and midfacial units include the ROOF (retroorbicularis oculi fat), the postseptal fat, and the SOOF (suborbicularis oculi fat). The location for suture placement is along the horizontal level of the descended malar fat pad and below the lateral canthus with a vertical vector of advancement.

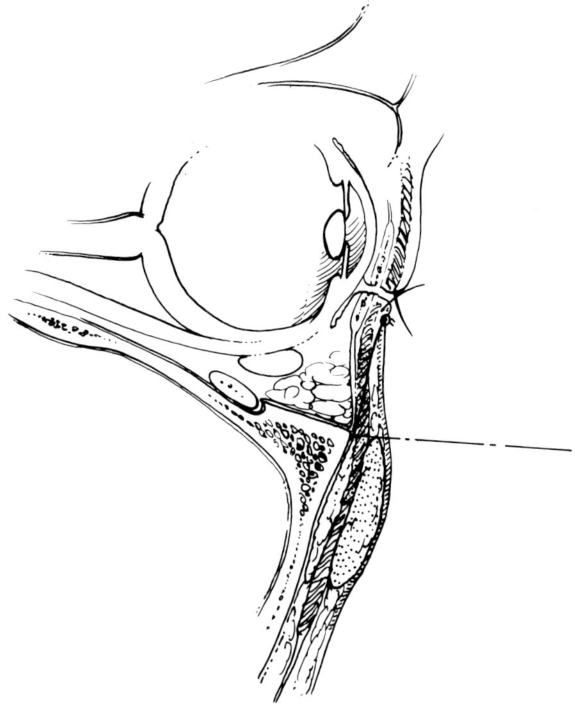

FIG. 7. Cross-section of the suspended malar soft tissue complex combined with lower blepharoplasty postseptal fat removal with resiration of a smooth transition from the orbital to the midfacial unit.

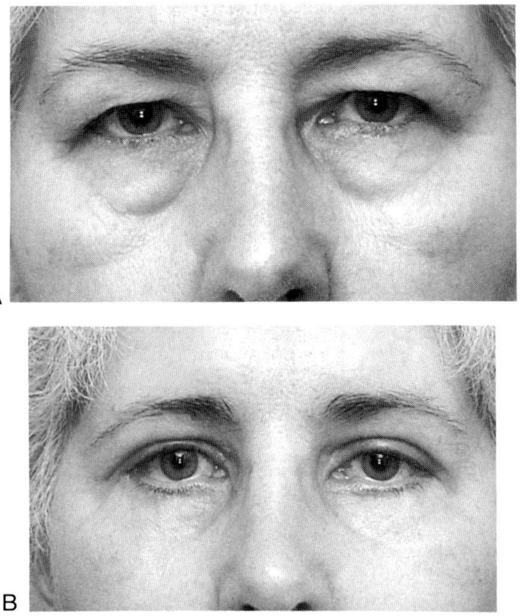

FIG. 8. Clinical examples of patients who have undergone the subperiosteal malar cheek lift with lower blepharoplasty before and after surgery.

on lower lid blepharoplasty. Excess skin and orbicularis muscle is excised and precise cutaneous closure accomplished to complete the procedure.

PREVENTING COMPLICATIONS

Complications following malar soft elevation primarily involve:

1. Soft tissue irregularities or side-to-side asymmetries that are visible or palpable along the inferior orbital rim caused by imprecise and unnecessary placement of multiple fixation sutures. Experience has shown that multiple fixation sutures along the inferior orbital rim should be avoided and that optimal symmetric superior redraping is best accomplished using single-suture fixation as described above.
2. Overresection of postseptal orbital fat. Experience has shown that overresection of prominent lower lid fat pads can result in a hollow, cadaveric appearance in any patient. It should be emphasized that in patients with malar soft tissue ptosis, thinning along the inferior orbital rim may create the illusion (rather than the actuality) of excessively prominent lower lid fat. In this setting, overresection of lower lid fat combined with the soft tissue augmentation that occurs with superior repositioning of malar soft tissue can result in the creation of an unattractive "step-off" at the infraorbital rim compared to the smooth transition between cheek and lid that occurs in the youthful face (Fig. 7).
3. There is potential for inferior displacement of the lower lid (possibly ectropion) if fixation of the elevated malar soft tissues is not secure. Stabilization of lower lid position as described in Chapter 15 on lower lid blepharoplasty is essential.

SUMMARY

When patients present with concerns regarding aging in the lower lid/malar aesthetic unit, careful evaluation of soft tissue pathology both above and *below* the inferior orbital rim is essential (Fig. 8). When significant ptosis of malar soft tissue is present, optimal correction will require superior redraping in addition to indicated treatment of the lower lid itself.

REFERENCES

1. Skoog T. *Aesthetic plastic surgery*. Philadelphia: Saunders, 1974.
2. Mitz W, Peyronie M. The superficial musculoaponeurotic system (SMAS) in the parotid and cheek area. *Plast Reconstr Surg* 1976; 58:80.
3. Owsley J. Lifting the malar fat pad for correction of prominent nasolabial folds. *Plast Reconstr Surg* 1993;91:463–476.

4. Stuzin JM, Baker TJ, Gordon HL. The extended SMAS flap in the treatment of the nasolabial fold. Presented at the annual meeting of the American Society for Aesthetic Plastic Surgery, Chicago, 1990.
5. Hamra ST. The deep plane rhytidectomy. *Plast Reconstr Surg* 1990;86:53.
6. Tessier P. Face lifting and frontal rhytidectomy. Presented at the Seventh International Congress of Plastic and Reconstructive Surgery, Rio de Janeiro, 1979.
7. Ramirez OM. The subperiosteal rhytidectomy: the third generation face-lift. *Ann Plast Surg* 1992;28:218–232.
8. Psillakis JM, Rumley TO, Camargos A. Subperiosteal approach as an improved concept for correction of the aging face. *Plast Reconstr Surg* 1988;82:383–392.
9. Vasconez LO, Grotting JC, Canasova R. The upper face in facial rejuvination: an anatomical study and a preliminary report of a new operative procedure. Presented at the American Association of Plastic Surgeons Meeting, Washington, DC, 1986.

CHAPTER 17

Postoperative Management of Complications of Cosmetic Blepharoplasty

Despite the best care of the surgeon and compliance of the patient, untoward events and complications can occur following blepharoplasty surgery. An understanding of the most common problems and a preformed plan on how to deal with them can in most cases assure a good result for the patient.

IMMEDIATE POSTOPERATIVE PROBLEMS

One of the most anxiety-producing situations that can occur in the early postoperative period is excessive bleeding. This may occur as the result of an intrinsic clotting deficiency, a drug-induced clotting deficiency, or uncontrolled high blood pressure. These tendencies can be aggravated by a vasodilating general anesthetic, such as halothane, or straining and coughing following general anesthesia. These events can result in severe swelling and hematoma formation.

Eyelid Hematoma

A hematoma confined to the eyelid itself usually is not a visual threat but may cause some secondary consequences in the surgical result. If a skin-muscle flap has been used, the blood, which acts as a foreign material, will not cause much reaction and there should occur little postoperative shrinkage as absorption takes place. If a blepharoplasty is performed under a skin flap, however, particularly in the lower lid, then the blood will act as foreign material beneath the skin and cause shrinkage and possibly an ectropion. In this situation, the hematoma should be evacuated or drained (Table 1).

Orbital Hematoma

The bleeding that produces the most anxiety in the surgeon and is the greatest threat to the patient is that occurring within the orbit with production of an orbital hematoma. Increasing pressure in the orbit can cause proptosis and possibly be a threat to vision (1,2). If the hematoma is mild, and there are no visual changes and the swelling seems to be stable, a conservative course should be followed (Table 1).

If the hematoma is severe, causing pupillary or visual changes or an extremely tense orbit, then interventional therapy must be undertaken (Table 1).

In the immediate postoperative period when the orbital hematoma is most likely to occur, it is important that the patient be observed by a trained or responsible person for a reasonable period of time. Any changes should be reported to the physician so that the patient can be examined. Severe pain following blepharoplasty is extremely unusual; if it occurs, the surgeon should think of orbital hematoma formation, corneal abrasion, or some other ocular event. It is the practice of the authors to avoid pressure bandages on the eyes and to use intermittent ice compresses. If a tight pressure bandage is applied to the eyelid and an orbital hematoma occurs, the vision will be more quickly compromised by the additional pressure. Any unusual or severe pain should be promptly evaluated.

COMPLICATIONS OF LOWER LID BLEPHAROPLASTY

A variety of untoward anatomic problems can occur in the patient's lower lids following blepharoplasty. Table 2 shows the most common problems (3–6).

TABLE 1. *Types of hematomas*

Eyelid Hematoma
Skin muscle flap—observation
Skin flap—drainage (Bard–Parker no. 11 blade or removal of stitches)
Orbital Hematoma—mild without pupillary change
Observation
Systemic steroids
Cold compresses
Orbital Hematoma—severe with pupillary and/or visual change
Remove stitches and evacuate hematoma
Large canthotomy and cantholysis
Orbital decompression if edema becomes chronic

TABLE 2. *Complications of lower lid blepharoplasty*

Lower lid retraction/ectropion
Scleral show or round eye syndrome
Phimosis or narrowing of the eyelid fissure
Residual skin folds:
Epicanthal laterally
Central
Residual fat pads (asymmetric fat removal)
Excessive fat removal—sunken appearance with prominant cheekbones
Excessive scarring (suture tracks)
Pigmentary changes—hemosiderin
Hematoma formation

These can occur because of inadequate preoperative assessment or a technical problem in surgery or judgment during the operative procedure.

Immediate Lower Lid Retraction

A downward pull of the lower lid with scleral show or eversion with ectropion can occur immediately postoperatively. This may result from the failure of the surgeon to tighten the lower lid in the presence of a lax lid or from the excessive removal of skin to override the normal lid tension.

Early Management

Immediately following surgery there may be some weighing down of the lid with retained fluid and thickening that can aggravate a lower lid malposition. Conservatism is very important in the patients who still have edema and thickening of the lower lid. Several weeks time must be given to allow the fluid to subside and the lid tissue will loosen and elevate in most cases. Upward massage is helpful. Watchful waiting and reassurance can be characterized as the approach to this problem. The patient in Fig. 1A and B shows progressive improvement 3 weeks to 2 months following surgery without surgical intervention. If little edema is present and there is tightness in the skin or subcutaneous layer, in addition to massage one can also make judicious use of injectable steroids. It is to be emphasized that steroids are to be used with caution because they can produce subcutaneous atrophy and loss of fatty tissue if overused. The patient in Fig. 2A and B shows improvement after the use of steroids and massage.

Cases of lower lid retraction or malposition that do not resolve with conservative measures will need surgical intervention for correction. The available procedures may be planned in a graded continuum depending on severity of the problem and the desire to avoid (if possible) an external skin graft in these sensitive patients.

Mild Lower Lid Retraction

Mild lower lid retraction would be used to treat mild cases of ectropion, scleral show, or round eye syndrome. If the skin deficiency is not severe and there appears to be a good bit of residual laxity of the lower lid, a tightening procedure performed at the lateral can-

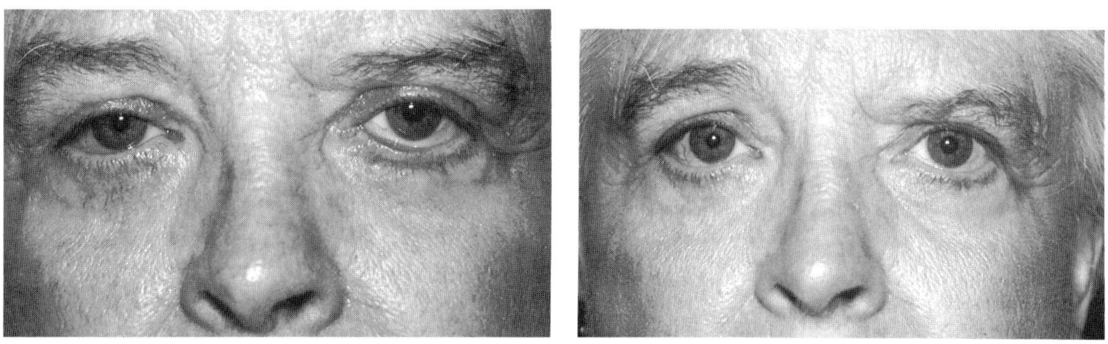

A B

FIG. 1. Early ectropion following lower lid blepharoplasty. **A:** Patient 1 month following lower lid blepharoplasty. **B:** Same patient 2 months postop following lower lid massage.

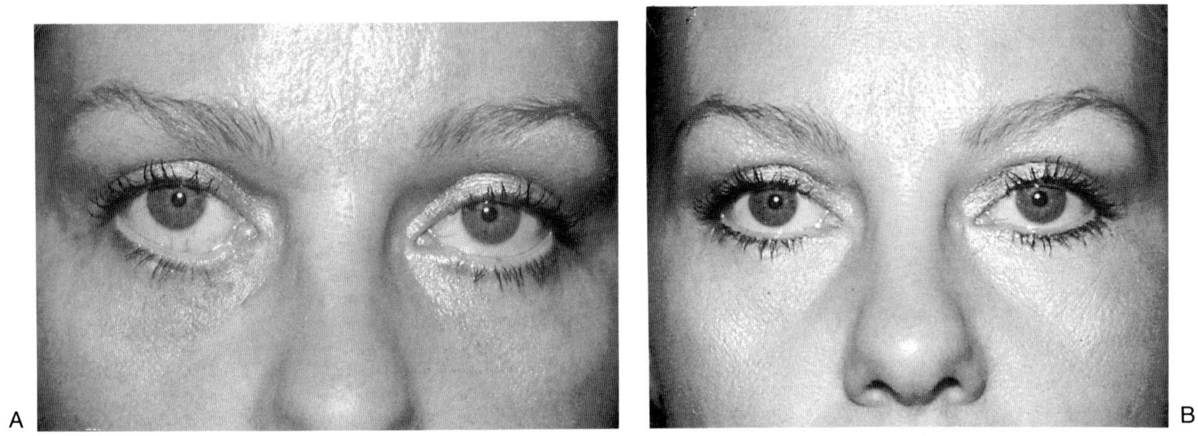

FIG. 2. Early ectropion following lower lid blepharoplasty. **A:** Five weeks following surgery with persistent lower lid retraction on the right. **B:** Same patient 6 weeks later following Kenalog injections (two) and continuing lower lid upward massage.

thus can be performed (Fig. 3A–C). The technique is described in the chapter on ectropion. Care must be taken not to overuse this procedure in cases of severe skin shortage in which little laxity is present in that it will not elevate the lid the required amount and will displace the punctum laterally. Figure 4A shows a patient referred with unresolved postblepharoplasty ectropion. Figure 4B shows the immediate result of lower lid tightening in the office.

Moderate Lower Lid Retraction and Ectropion

The preserved fascia lata sling to the lower lid has been extremely helpful in cases that require more than

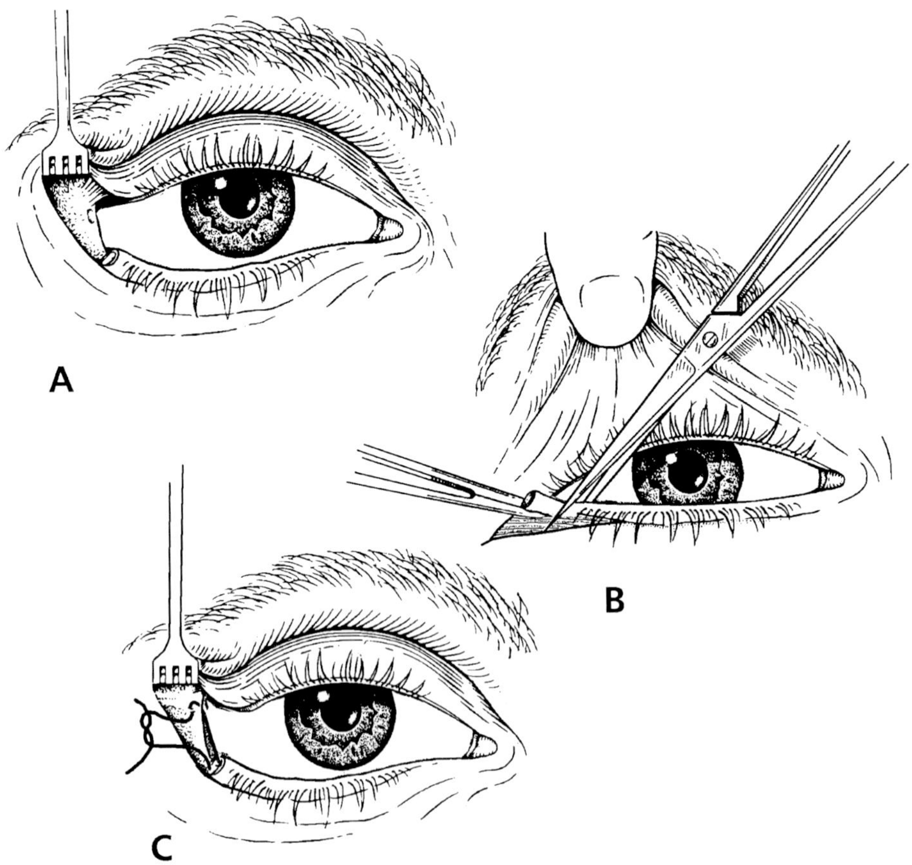

FIG. 3. Horizontal tightening with lateral canthoplasty. **A:** Canthotomy and cantholysis is performed. **B:** Trim off the edge of the tarsal plate if redundant. **C:** Plication of the lateral edge of the lid to the periosteum.

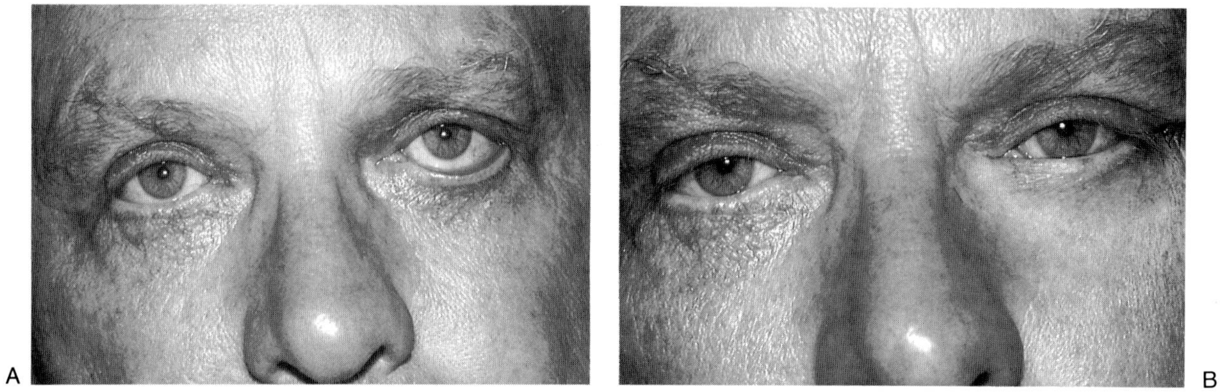

FIG. 4. Persistent ectropion following lower lid blepharoplasty. A: Patient 2 months following lower lid blepharoplasty. B: Same patient immediately following lower lid tightening at the lateral canthus as an office procedure.

a simple tightening at the lateral canthus. It has the ability to elevate the lower lid to a more normal position at the lower limbus and elevating the nasal portion of the lid (Fig. 5). The lid is not overstretched by the horizontal tightening procedure, which displaces the punctum and has a much more natural look postoperatively. This is an excellent procedure in cases of intermediate amounts of scleral show and lower lid malposition. These are cases that may ordinarily have been considered for skin grafting or posterior ear cartilage grafting. The technique is described in the chapter on ectropion. Figure 6A and B shows a patient with lower lid retraction corrected with a fascial sling.

Severe Cases of Lower Lid Malposition

Every attempt is made to correct the problem in these patients without the use of autogenous tissue grafts because of the chance of further irritating an already concerned patient. In some cases, however, the retraction cannot be remedied without the placement

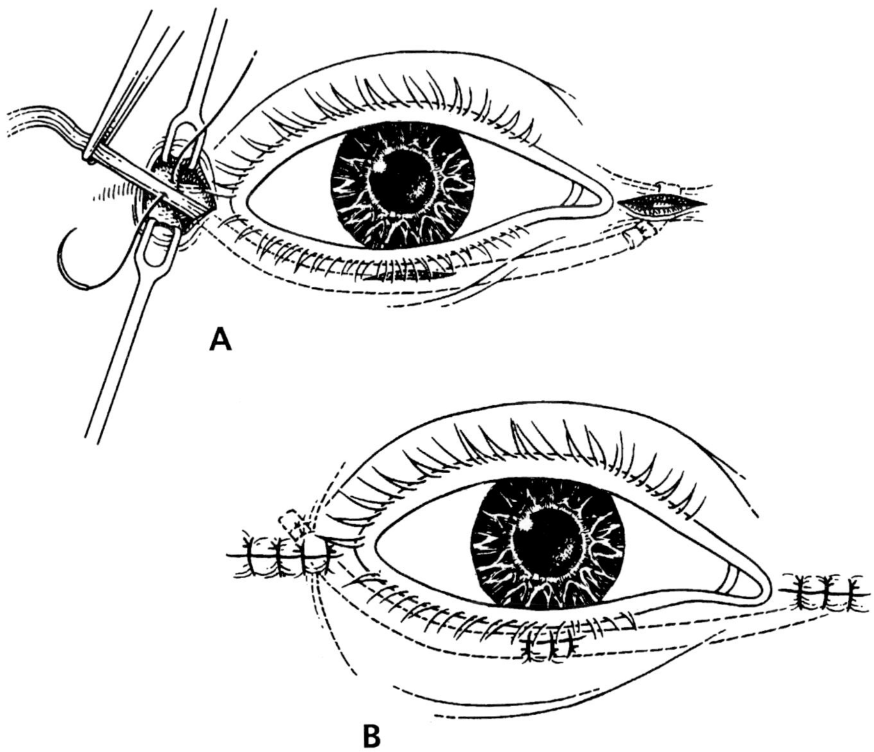

FIG. 5. Fascia lata sling to lower lid. A: Suturing of fascia sling to lateral periosteum. The fascia strip has been attached to the medial canthal tendon and threaded in the pretarsal plane. B: Final position of the sling.

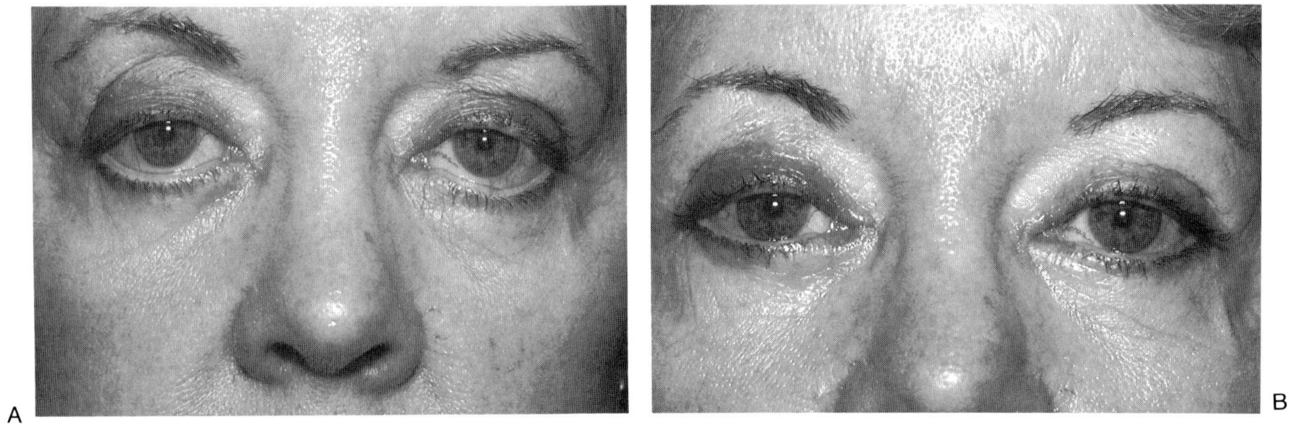

FIG. 6. Patient with lower lid retraction following blepharoplasty. **A:** Patient at 5 months following surgery. **B:** Same patient four weeks following preserved fascia sling to lower lids.

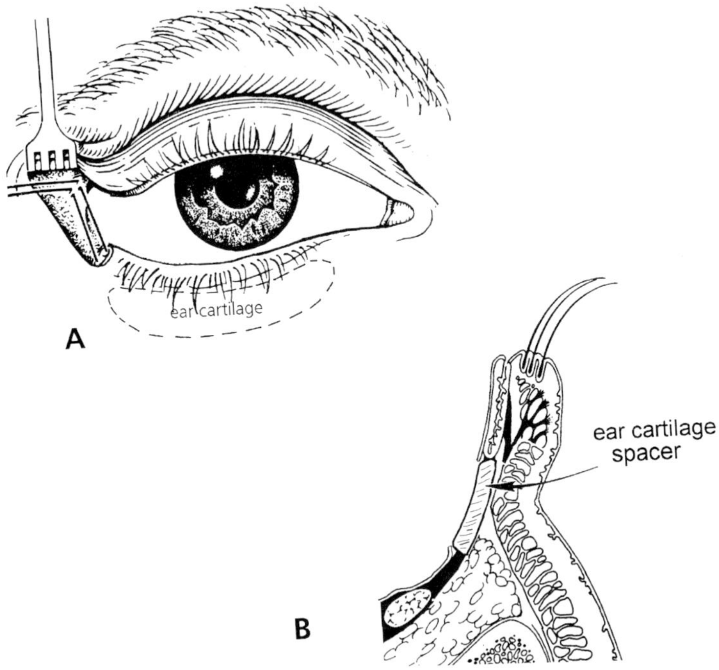

FIG. 7. Placement of spacer material (ear cartilage) in the posterior lamellar of the eyelid with horizontal tightening. **A:** Autogenous ear cartilage graft (scaphoid) placed to lengthen the internal lamella. Rigid lengthening of the posterior lamella can overcome anterior (skin) lamella shortage. A lateral canthoplasty is also needed. **B:** Cross-section view of spacer implant.

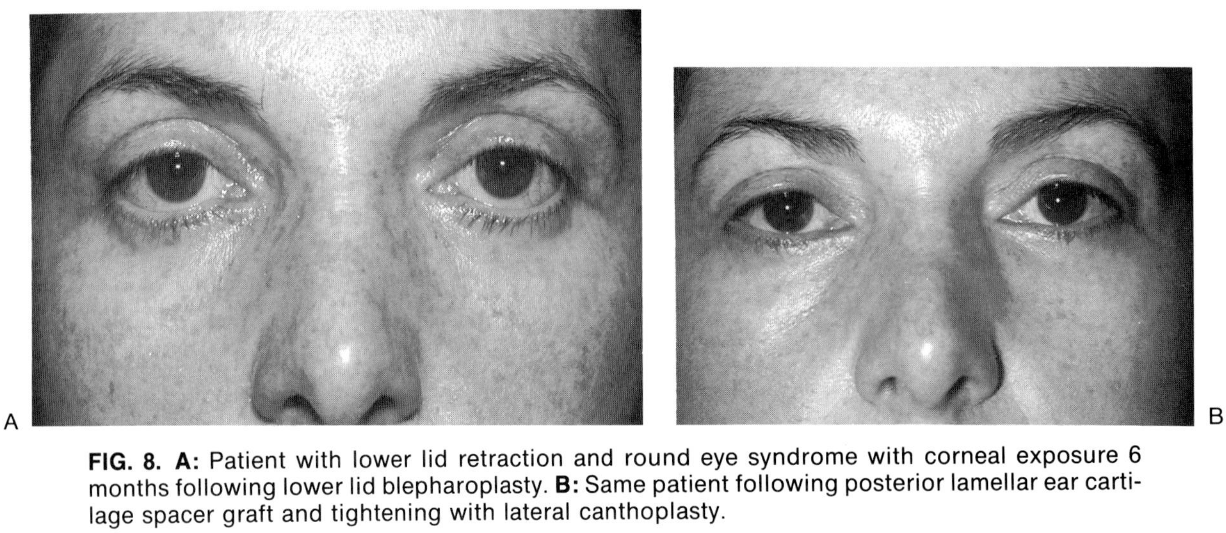

FIG. 8. **A:** Patient with lower lid retraction and round eye syndrome with corneal exposure 6 months following lower lid blepharoplasty. **B:** Same patient following posterior lamellar ear cartilage spacer graft and tightening with lateral canthoplasty.

of additional tissue in the vertically shortened lid (7). In some cases the lid margin can be elevated by insertion of rigid (usually autogenous ear cartilage) spacer material in the posterior lamella of the lid, avoiding an externally visible skin graft (Fig. 7). The placement of the ear cartilage graft is described in the chapter on Graves' disease. Figure 8A and B is an example of a patient before and after insertion of a graft.

If there is severe skin shortage, then full-thickness skin grafting must be used (Figs. 9A, B; 10A, B). The technique for placement of full-thickness skin grafts is described fully in the chapter on the correction of cicatricial ectropion. Figure 11A and B shows a patient before and after the placement of a full-thickness skin graft.

Residual Skin Folds

Residual skin folds can occur laterally in the laugh lines, which can be excised without fear of malpositioning of the lid. Additional excision of skin folds beneath the lash line should be approached with caution; many times, simple removal of the subcutaneous orbicularis will flatten the folding out.

A conservative "pinch" technique can sometimes be used to remove residual lower lid folding. Injection of the fold with local anesthetic with wydase can make the residual fold pliable and the surgeon can pinch the fold with flat forceps so that it stands up from the flattened lower lid skin. If the lower lid position is unchanged with the pinching then the fold can be trimmed with scissors. It is safer to excise folds closer to the lash line and with the patient upright.

Residual Fat Pad or Asymmetric Fat Removal

Imprecise preoperative or operative judgment of the quantity or position of the fat pads to be removed can leave displeasing asymmetries in the lower lids because of the presence of residual fat. If this is displeasing to the patient, additional fat can be removed by the fornix technique. Figure 12A and B shows a gentleman who had residual nasal fat pad that was removed from the lid during an office procedure involving a fornix incision.

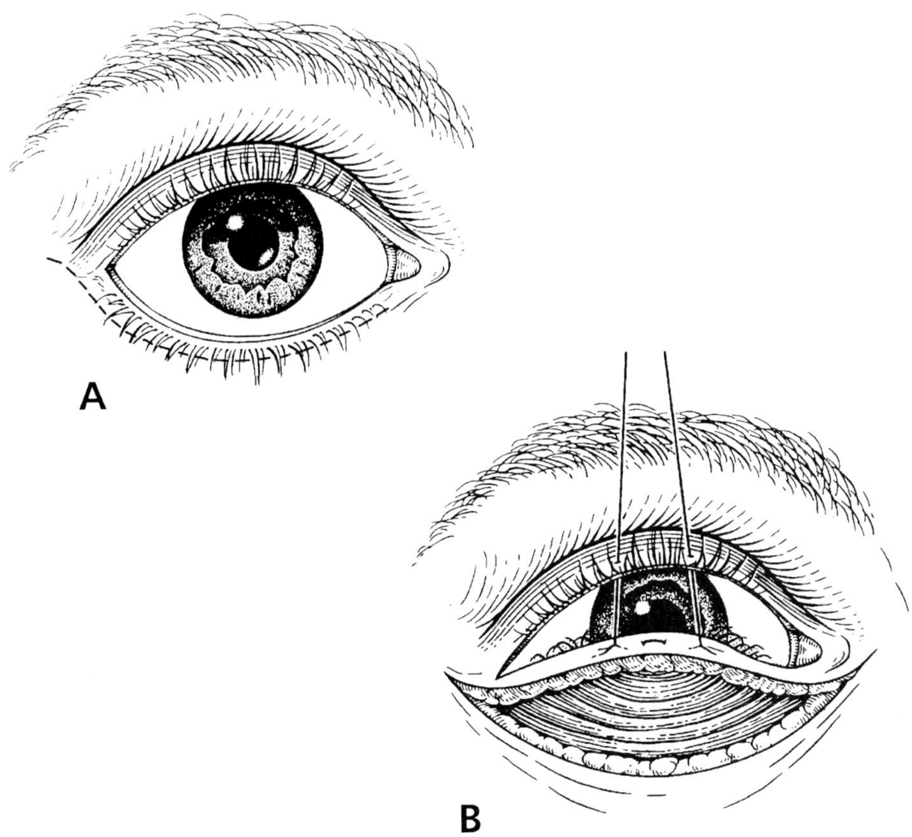

FIG. 9. Skin graft for postblepharoplasty ectropion. **A:** A subciliary incision is made in the old blepharoplasty incision line (if high enough). Should be just underneath lash line. **B:** The skin or tissue is allowed to retract to allow the lower lid to elevate.

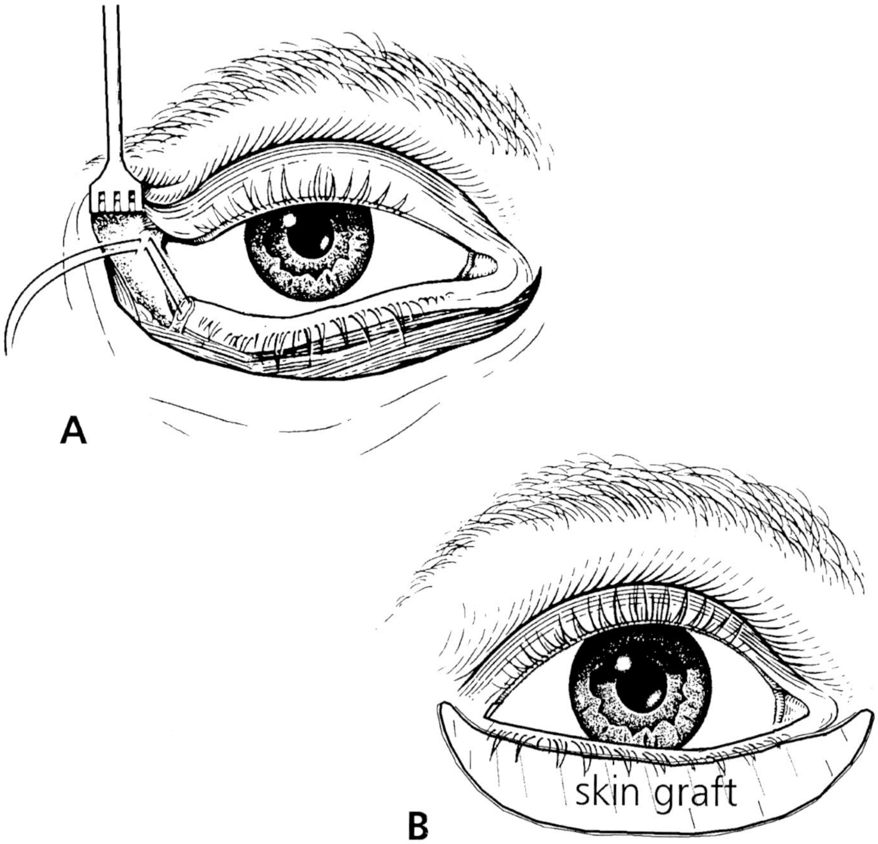

FIG. 10. Skin graft for postblepharoplasty ectropion. **A:** Lid tightening with lateral canthoplasty. **B:** Full-thickness skin graft is placed in the defect created from the incision.

Excessive Fat Removal with Sunken Eye Appearance

Overzealous removal of fat, particularly in the presence of a very prominent malar bone, can lead to a sunken appearance of the eye (Fig. 13). This unfortunate situation can only be remedied by augmentation with a dermis fat graft combined with possible sculpting of the prominent cheekbone.

Scars and Suture Tracks

Care should be taken to plan for the incision of the lower lid to be made high in the subciliary area extending to the exact canthal angle and then sloped downward laterally within a wrinkle line. Departure from these normal creases and thin skin will result in additional scarring. Improper closure with excessive ten-

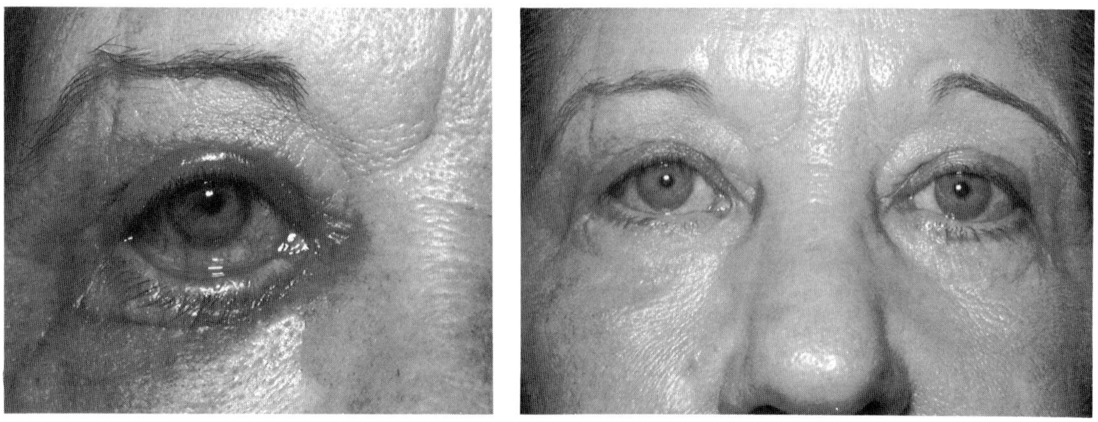

A B

FIG. 11. Severe cicatricial ectropion following lower lid blepharoplasty. **A:** Patient at 8 weeks following lower lid blepharoplasty. **B:** Same patient at 2 months following full-thickness skin graft to lower lid.

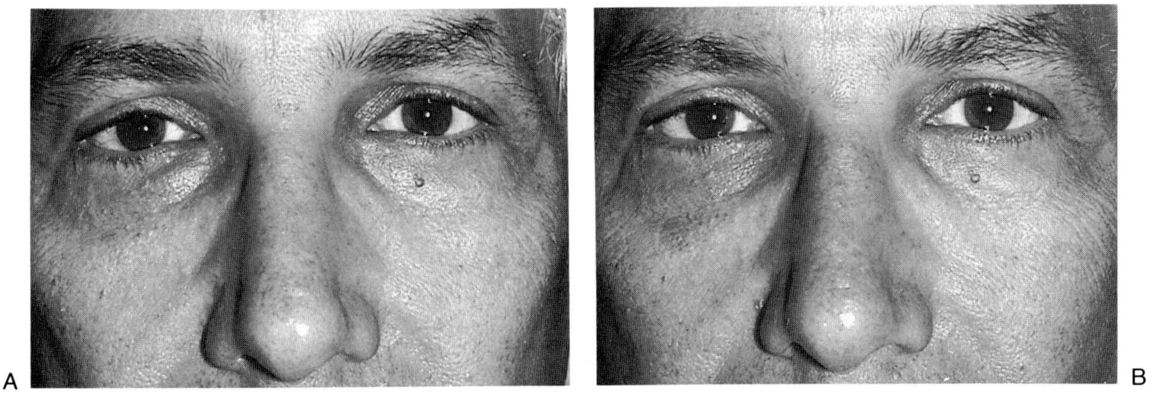

FIG. 12. Residual fat following lower lid blepharoplasty. **A:** Patient demonstrates residual fat pads nasally 4 weeks following lower lid blepharoplasty. **B:** Same patient following removal of the nasal fat pads via fornix incision.

sion and improper eversion of the skin edges will lead to excessive scarring. This is particularly true if the lateral incisions are extended ones that are carried into the thicker cheek skin (Fig. 14).

Phimosis of Eyelid Fissure

The phimosis of the eyelid fissure caused by inward pulling of the outer canthus of the lower lid seen in the round eye syndrome (Fig. 15A and B) can be corrected with the horizontal tightening procedure and reattachment of the lower lid canthal tendon to the lateral orbital rim.

Pigmentary Changes

Excessive bruising or hematoma formation following surgery will result in prolonged hemosiderin pigmentation in the tissue. Fortunately, in most cases this will wash out of the tissue with time.

Epicanthal Fold Formation

Folds may occur overlapping the lateral canthal angle if the upper lid blepharoplasty incision and the lower lid blepharoplasty incision become too close. An epicanthal fold or web usually forms at the lateral canthus. Care should be taken to keep an adequate space of skin between the lower blepharoplasty and the upper blepharoplasty excision. If folds do occur they can be corrected with a V-Y relaxation described in the chapter on lateral canthal reconstruction. Figure 16A and B shows a postblepharoplasty patient with a lateral epicanthal fold before and after correction.

Chemosis with Dellen Formation

If the conjunctiva on the surface of the eye swells, retains fluid, and becomes chemotic, a corresponding dry spot will form on the cornea next to the swelling (Fig. 17). This is much more likely in patients who have

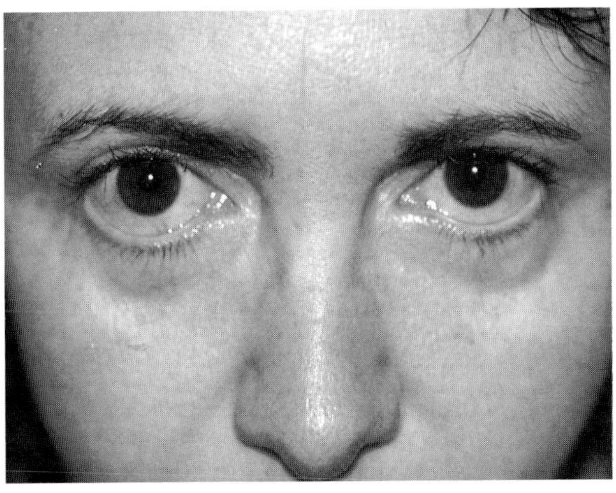

FIG. 13. Patient who has had asymmetric removal of fat from lower lids mainly in the central fat area. This is accentuated by the prominent cheekbones.

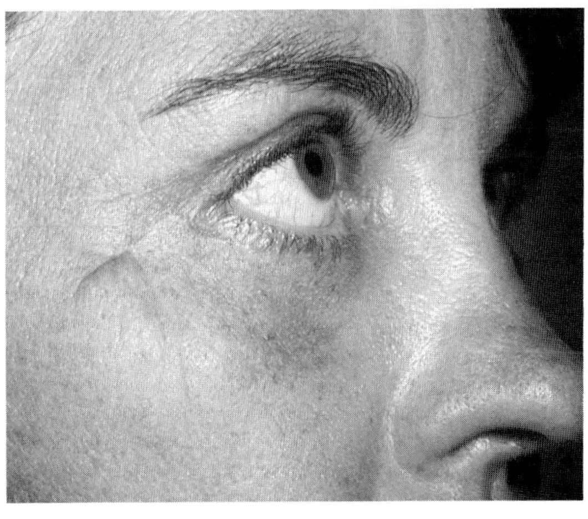

FIG. 14. Patient with excessive lateral scarring from incision carried into the thick lateral skin and failure to correct an unequal wound edge.

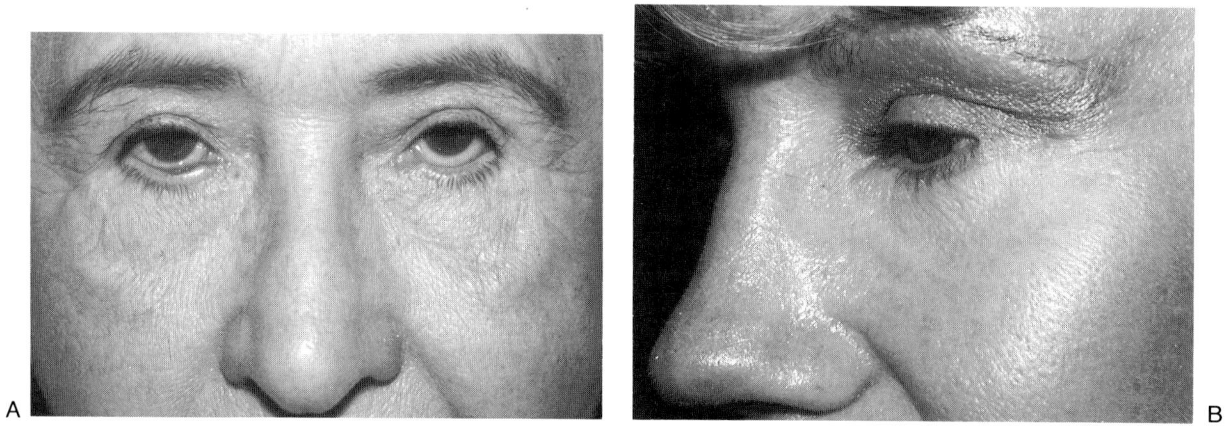

FIG. 15. A: Phimosis of the lower lid with ectropion following a lower lid blepharoplasty from failure to secure lateral canthal angle with lateral canthoplasty. **B:** Side view of a different patient with the same problem of phimosis and inward migration of the lateral canthus, which could have been prevented with lateral canthoplasty.

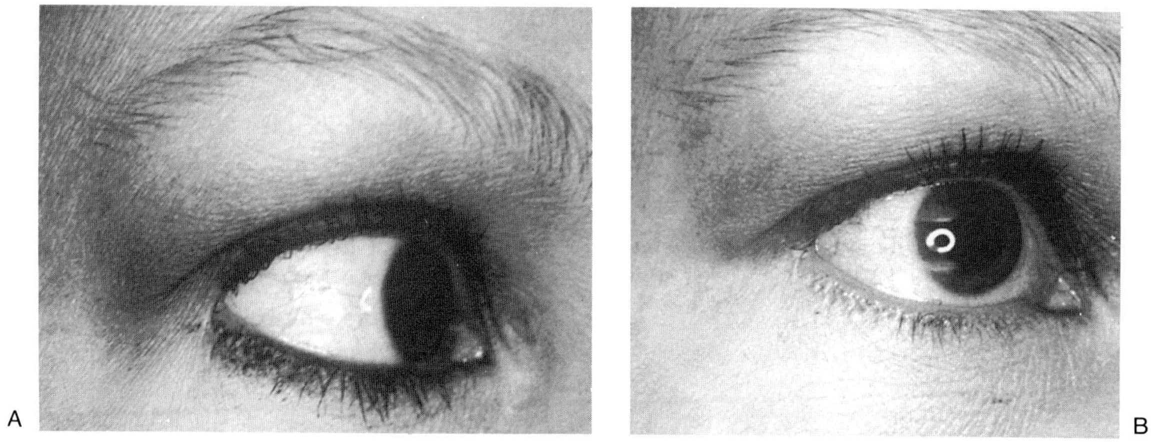

FIG. 16. Lateral epicanthal fold formation. **A:** Patient 6 months following lower lid blepharoplasty with epicanthal fold formation at the lateral canthus probably from a connection of the upper and lower blepharoplasty incisions too close to the lateral canthus. **B:** Same patient after corrective transposition flaps at the lateral canthus.

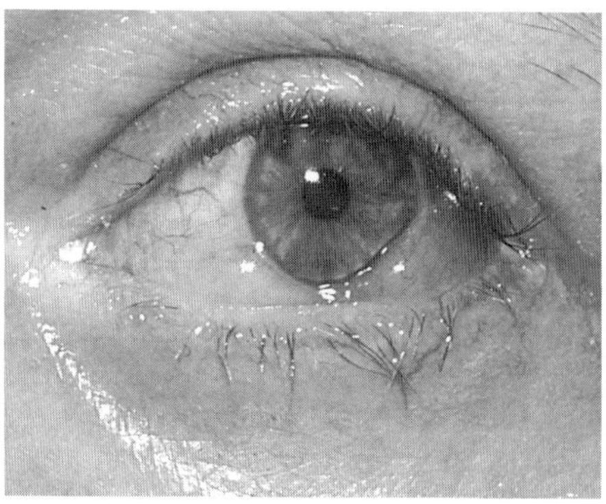

FIG. 17. Patient with chemosis of the lower lid following a lower lid blepharoplasty. A cycle of chemosis dellen (corneal dry spot) formation and increasing chemosis is set up with this situation. The cycle must be broken with lubricants, eyelid patching, or in some cases resection of the conjunctiva and patching.

preexisting conjunctivochalasis and who have a lot of reaction postoperatively or fail to use lubricants adequately postoperatively. This in most cases can be corrected with increased lubrications, patching of the eye for a period of time, and sometimes excision of the conjunctiva.

COMPLICATIONS OF UPPER LID BLEPHAROPLASTY

Complications following upper lid blepharoplasty usually are the result of failure to perform needed procedures or faulty judgment in the performance of required procedures at the time of surgery (8–10). Table 3 lists the most common complications following upper lid blepharoplasty.

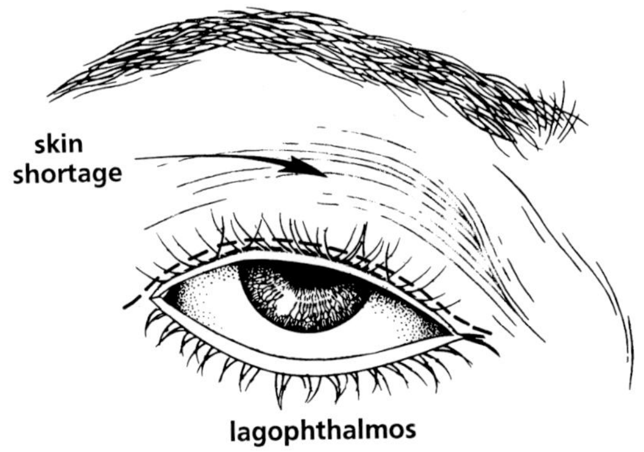

FIG. 18. Skin shortage in the upper lid following blepharoplasty causing lagophthalmos with exposure of the eye. The placement of incision in the upper lid skin for dissection for a skin graft is marked with a dotted line and is just above the lash line.

TABLE 3. *Complications of upper lid blepharoplasty*

Lagophthalmos (excessive skin removal or septal scarring)
Residual or recurrent skin folds (inadequate excision, eyebrow laxity, low lid crease)
Epicanthal folds (nasal)
Lid crease abnormalities or asymmetries
Postoperative ptosis
Asymmetric fat pad removal
Localized skin scarring or cyst
Diplopia (superior oblique paresis)
Lacrimal gland injury

Lagophthalmos

Lagophthalmos can be one of the more distressing complications of upper lid blepharoplasty, particularly if the patient has deficient eye protective mechanisms such as a dry eye or poor Bell's phenomenon. The patient in many cases will not only be prone to corneal exposure but will have discomfort to the point of incapacitation in some instances. In many cases, this is due to the overaggressive removal of skin to the point that it tethers the closure of the upper lids. Nasal skin shortage seems to produce more symptomatic lagophthalmos than temporal shortage (Fig. 18). Special care must be taken to be conservative in nasal upper lid skin removal.

Patients with good tears, good ocular motility, and good lower lid position many times can tolerate some lagophthalmos; however, a deficiency in the eye protective mechanisms can tip the scales and throw the patient into an extremely symptomatic and threatening situation. Over time, the skin may relax somewhat and with the use of lubricants and protection of the eye at night or a soft bandage contact lens the patient may improve to the point where no interventional surgery is necessary. If the patient does not improve or the lagophthalmos is more severe, then surgical intervention is necessary to protect the eye. In most cases the necessary surgery involves the replacement of skin to the upper lid to allow closure together with lysis of whatever adhesions may exist in the orbital septum. Lagophthalmos in the upper lid may occur in the presence of adequate skin for closure and exist on the basis of vertical adhesions in the orbital septal plane. Often this occurs when the surgeon attempts to close the septum following fat removal or the septum becomes foreshortened in some way. In any event, the adhesions must be lysed and adequate skin replaced if needed.

The position of skin placement is important to preserve the eyelid crease and the patient's cosmetic appearance. The upper eyelid skin is divided into two

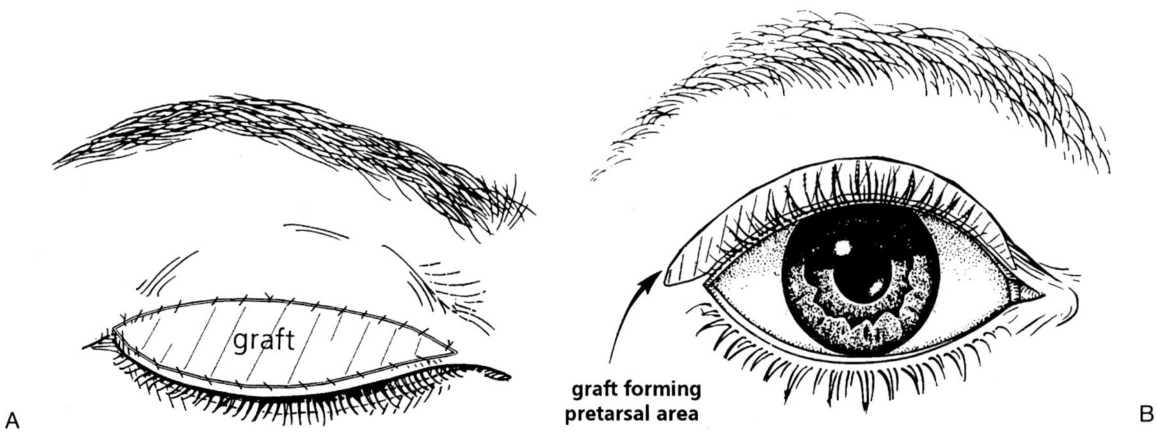

FIG. 19. Cicatricial lagophthalmos of the upper lid. **A:** After the incision is made just above the lash line, the skin is allowed to retract up to the desired lid crease. A full-thickness skin graft can then be placed between the lash line and the lid crease preserving the pretarsal unit. **B:** With this placement of skin, the lagophthalmos is improved and the position of the lid crease is maintained when the patient's eyes are open.

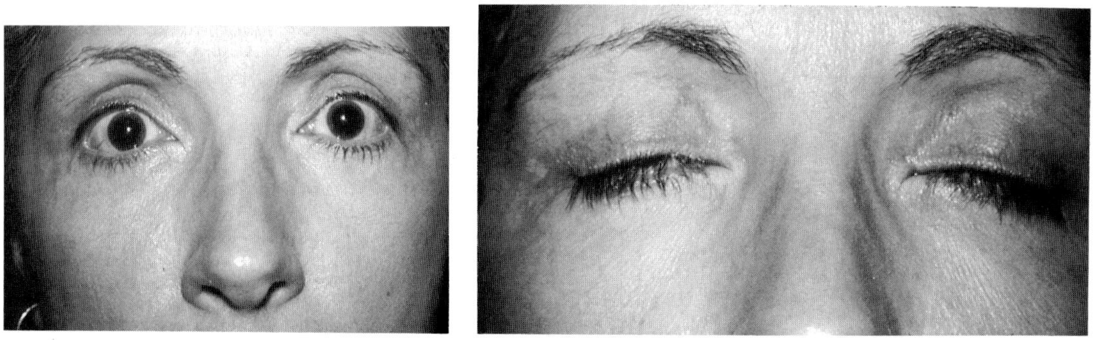

A B

FIG. 20. Skin shortage in both upper lids following upper lid blepharoplasty and coronal brow lift. **A:** Patient 2 months following surgery with corneal exposure. **B:** Same patient showing lagophthalmos of the lids and gapping of the lids with corneal exposure.

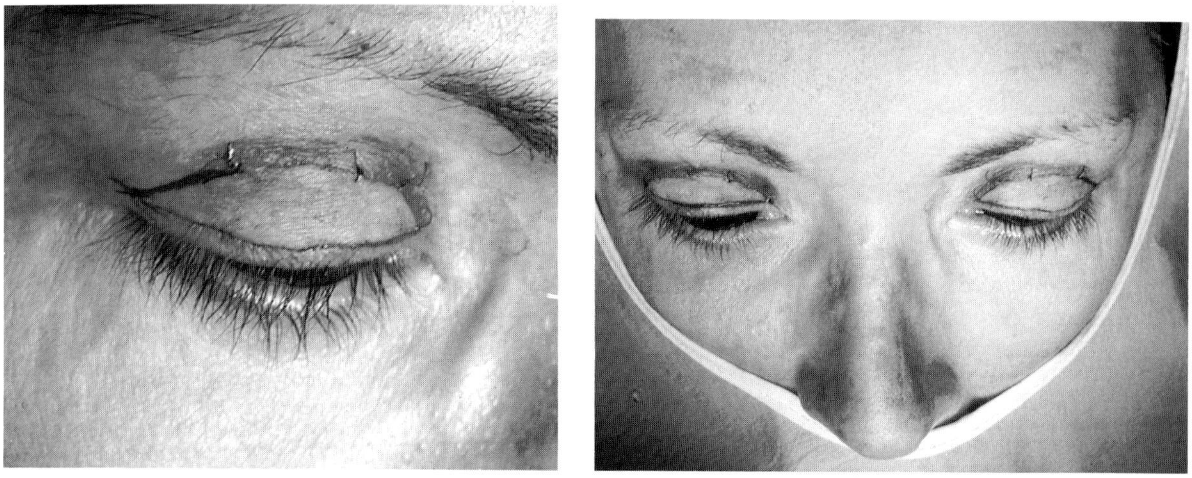

A B

FIG. 21. A: Placement of a full skin graft and pretarsal skin in the area between the lashes and the desired position of the upper lid crease. **B:** Same patient showing bilateral placement of skin grafts.

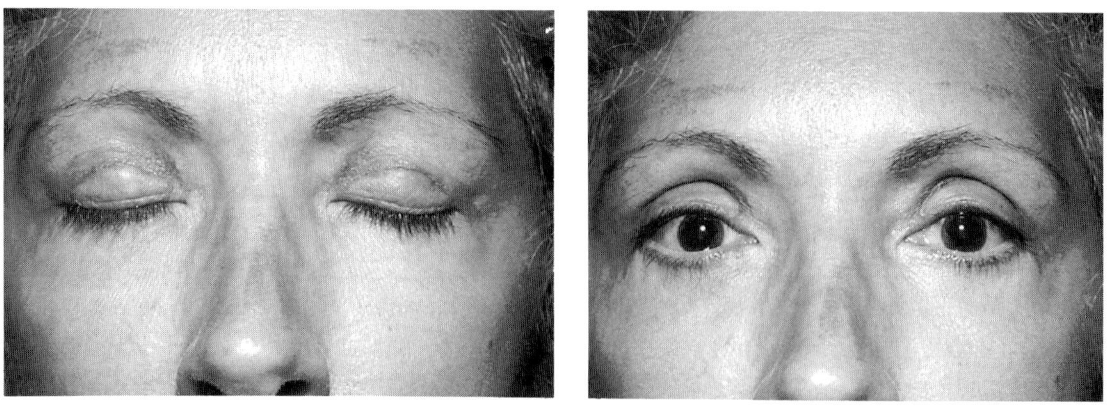

A B

FIG. 22. A: Same patient 4 weeks following bilateral skin graft with full closure of eyes. **B:** Same patient postgrafting showing retention of the lid crease in a desired position when the eyes are open.

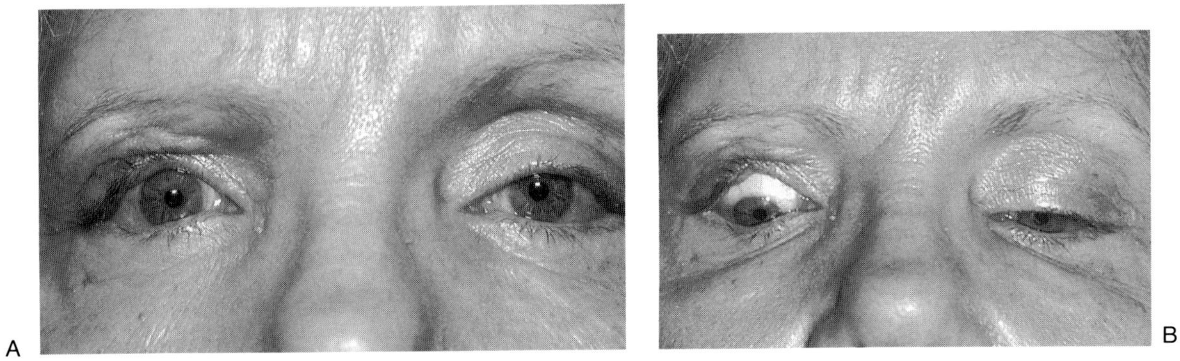

FIG. 23. Cicatricial lagophthalmos of the upper lids due to internal septal adhesions and scarring. **A:** Patient in primary field of gaze. The patient had had previous placement of the skin graft that did not improve the lagophthalmos because the skin shortage was not the main cause of lagophthalmos. **B:** Same patient in downgaze showing almost no movement of the lid downward because of internal septal adhesions. This patient required multiple surgeries of internal spacer material and skin revision to improve closure.

units: the pretarsal skin between the lash line and the crease, and the skin between the eyelid crease and the brow. No skin grafts should be placed that overlap this area. The usual placement of the skin graft is in the pretarsal area because it minimizes external visibility and allows good crease formation (Figs. 18; 19A, B). Figure 20A and B shows a patient with severe lagophthalmos and corneal damage following excessive skin removal. Figure 21A and B shows the placement of a skin graft in the pretarsal area and Fig. 22A and B the postoperative result with good closure and retention of a good upper eyelid crease formation.

Lagophthalmos of a severe type can occur postoperatively in patients with internal septal scarring who may or may not have skin shortage. Techniques that cause septal scarring are usually to blame but the postoperative lagophthalmos may be misinterpreted as skin shortage. Figure 23A and B shows a patient with internal septal scarring.

Residual Skin Folds in the Upper Lid–Brow Droppage Following Upper Lid Blepharoplasty

In most cases there is a failure to recognize preoperatively a lax eyebrow and apply an appropriate surgical treatment to either stabilize the brow or elevate it. This can result in a postoperative brow drop and a narrowed brow–lash distance. Usually when postoperative residual folds occur, the proper treatment is to perform the appropriate eyebrow procedure, either a coronal forehead lift or a direct brow pexy as a secondary procedure. Figure 24A and B shows a postblepharoplasty patient who required a coronal eyebrow lift to correct

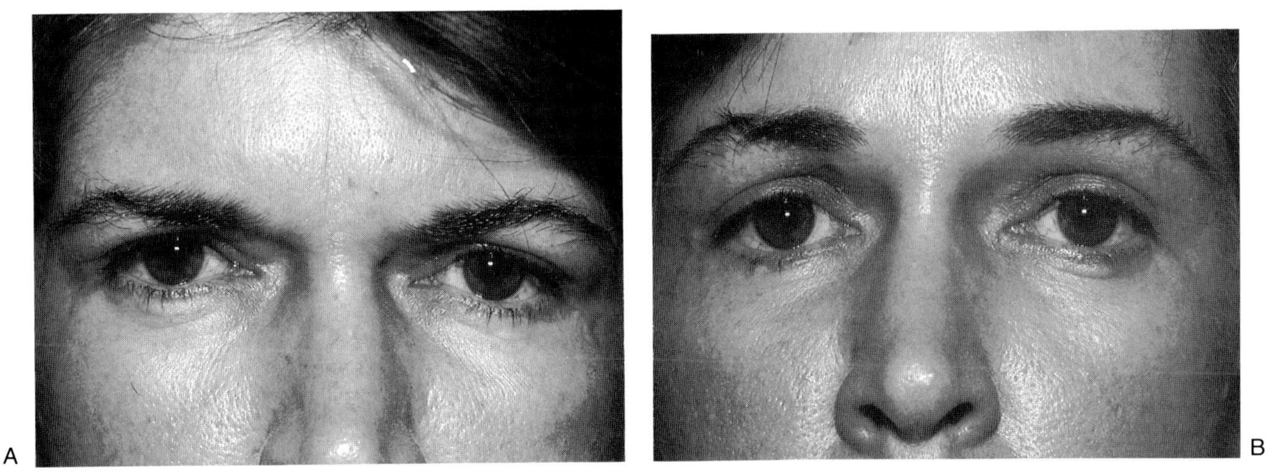

FIG. 24. Eyebrow drop following upper lid blepharoplasty. **A:** Patient following upper lid blepharoplasty at 6 months extremely displeased because of narrowing of the eyebrow distance and no visible pretarsal skin area following her surgery. **B:** Same patient following a coronal forehead lift elevating the brow and improving the brow lash distance and the visibility of the pretarsal skin.

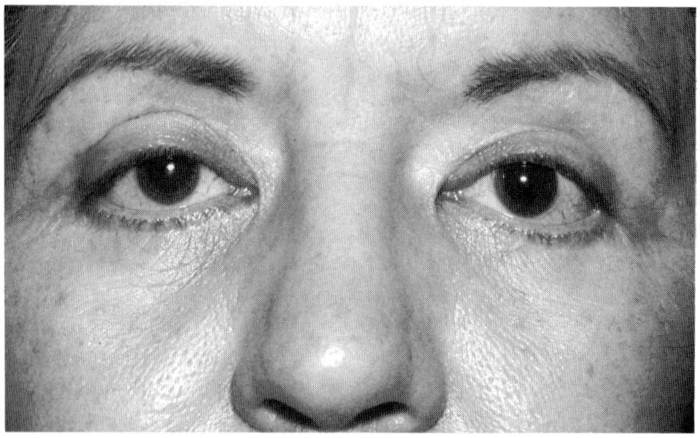

FIG. 25. Epicanthal fold formation following upper lid blepharoplasty because of extension of the nasal portion of the incision into the thick skin on the nose and over the canthal angle. This patient required correction with transposition flaps.

the brow droppage. In many of these cases, no further skin need be removed from the upper lid to reach the desired effect.

An improper position of the eyelid crease marking lower than 8 mm in females can fail to expose enough pretarsal skin and give the appearance of inadequate skin removal. In some cases, of course, the surgeon may simply have been too cautious in removing skin, particularly in the lateral area.

Epicanthal Folds

Epicanthal folds occur following upper lid blepharoplasty nasally, when the skin incision is carried too far connecting the thin skin of the eyelids to the thick skin of the nose (Fig. 25). Care should be taken to avoid connecting these two areas with the upper lid blepharoplasty incision.

Lid Crease Abnormalities

Postoperative asymmetry of the eyelid crease can be apparent if care is not taken with designing the position of the crease preoperatively and placement intraoperatively. Eyelid crease asymmetry can occur in patients with asymmetric fat removal from the upper lid (Fig. 26A). A patient who has one eye more prominent than the other (e.g., in Graves' disease) will get a higher lid crease in the more prominent eye. Asymmetric eyebrow position or eyebrow laxity can also cause crease abnormalities. Arching of the brow by the patient in an asymmetric manner can also cause this problem. Most of these conditions can be diagnosed and addressed preoperatively. Figure 26B shows an Asian patient following upper lid blepharoplasty. The patient was unhappy despite the fact that her upper lid crease positions were symmetric because they were much higher than she expected.

Postoperative Ptosis

The most preventable type of postoperative ptosis is that which exists preoperatively. It is very important to diagnose a "down" position of the upper lid margin before performing blepharoplasty because it will not be corrected by the blepharoplasty procedure alone and may even be aggravated. If this is diagnosed, then a coexisting aponeurotic repair should be performed with the blepharoplasty (Fig. 27A, B).

Asymmetry in the Fat Pads

Care must be taken to adequately plan ahead with regard to fat removal. The fat pads in the upper lid that deserve special attention are the nasal fat pad, which

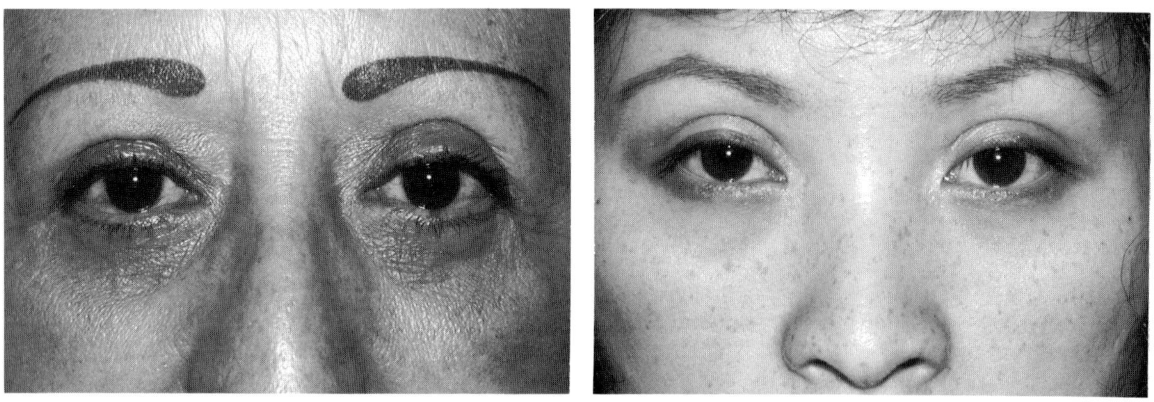

A B

FIG. 26. Eyelid crease abnormalities. **A:** Patient with asymmetric upper lid crease position. The patient felt that the left upper lid crease was excessively high. Crease position is influenced by the amount of skin removed, the amount of fat removed, and the brow laxity, which may be asymmetric. **B:** Asian patient with high occidental lid crease. This patient was quite unhappy because the height of the lid crease exceeded her expectation, which was to maintain a more ethnic Asian look.

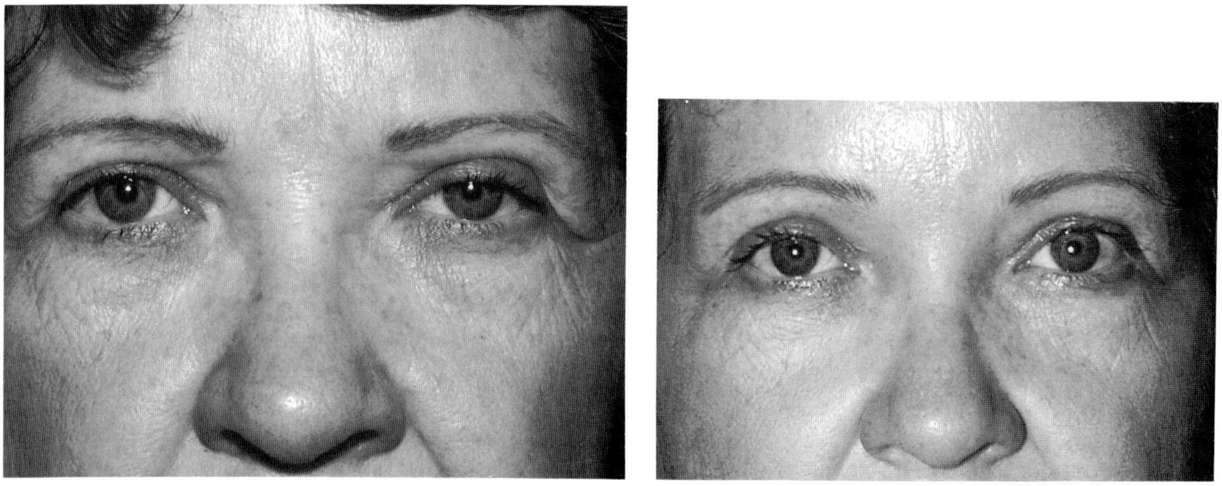

FIG. 27. Ptosis of the upper lid following upper lid blepharoplasty. **A:** A patient at 6 months following surgery with ptosis of the upper lid and some residual skin folds. **B:** Same patient following external levator repair and some additional skin excision.

produces a nasal swelling, the preaponeurotic fat pad, which become accentuated, and the subbrow fat pad, which can be seen temporally as a prominence in the lateral orbital rim.

Localized Skin Abnormalities

Interrupted silk sutures in many cases can cause suture tracks and epithelial tracks particularly in the thicker skin at the lateral portion of the upper lid and brow. A silk suture should be avoided in these areas.

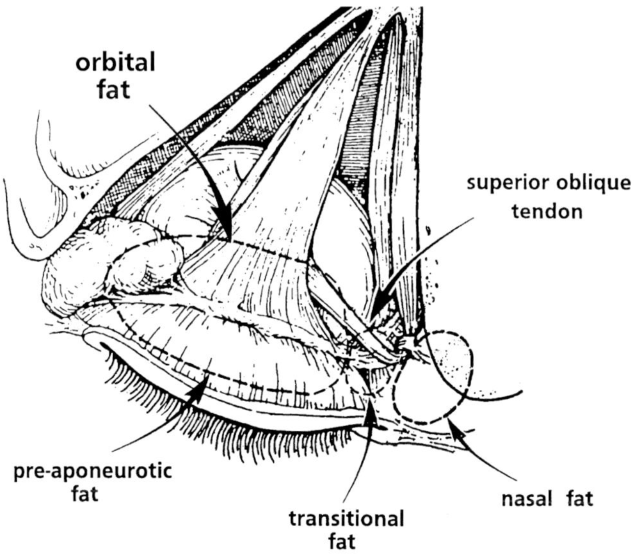

FIG. 28. Diagrammatic representation of the position of the superior oblique tendon as it traverses the lid and curves backward underneath the trochlea to become the superior oblique muscle. It is situated just behind the transitional and nasal fat pad, and blind dissection either with sharp instruments or cautery can cause damage to the tendon or its sheath.

Postoperative Diplopia

Several cases have been reported of superior oblique paresis occurring following upper lid blepharoplasty as the result of injury to the superior oblique tendon or sheath. This most commonly occurs when cautery is applied to the nasal fat pad or to control some bleeding in that area. Care must be taken when using cautery and in removing the nasal fat pad. The superior ophthalmic vein has close promixity to the transitional fat pad and the trochlea (Fig. 28). Damage to the trochlea or superior oblique tendon can cause disturbing torsional diplopia (see Fig. 29).

Lacrimal Gland Injury

The lacrimal gland may appear to protrude beneath the orbital rim laterally (11). It should not be mistaken for fat and removed. It is grayish brown in color, firmer than fat, and bleeds vigorously when cut. If it is noted to be prolapsed, it should be repositioned with a stitch underneath the rim periosteum and not excised.

PSYCHOLOGICAL MANAGEMENT OF THE PATIENT FOLLOWING BLEPHAROPLASTY SURGERY

Preoperative Counseling About Postop Course

It is important to prepare patients for their postoperative course by giving them good information before surgery on what to expect postoperatively.

It is important to mention to patients that bruising and swelling usually occur to some degree but that these will subside with time and will vary from person to person. Some people bruise more easily or more extensively than others.

It is important to mention that, for a while, vision will be blurry postoperatively because of stiffness of the eyelids, which may cause some tearing, and because of the need for ocular lubricants that are prescribed after surgery.

Patients are told that the surgical procedure itself is usually not the most annoying part of the process but that the recovery period seems to be the most frustrating. Patients must be willing to devote adequate time to using ice compresses following surgery and lubricating their eyes. They must be prepared to take some time off from activities, usually 5–7 days.

Head elevation at night and abstinence from salty foods can prevent overnight swelling.

A very important decision, as important as whether or not to have the surgery, is when to have the surgery. Patients should not schedule blepharoplasty surgery until they have a break in their activity lest they become frustrated with their inability to carry on scheduled activities.

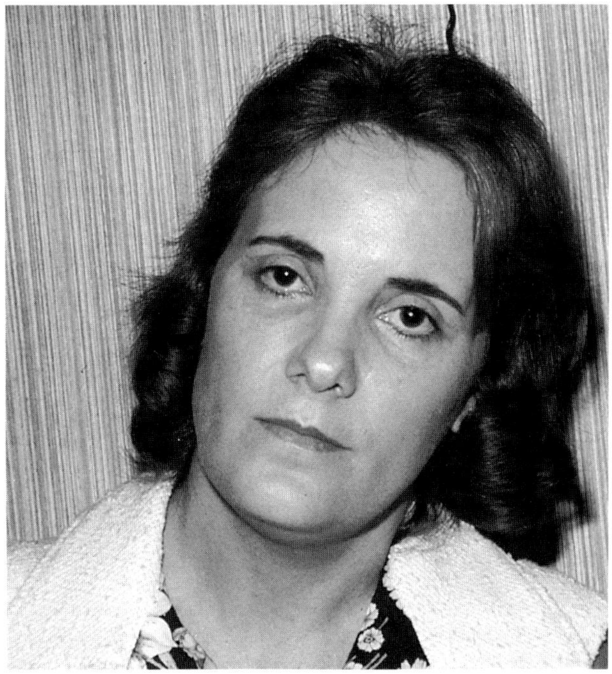

FIG. 29. A patient with an obligatory head tilt to compensate for double vision. The patient had an upper lid blepharoplasty and because of unusual bleeding underwent blind cautery with a Bovie unit in the upper nasal fat pad. The resulting damage to the tendon caused a superior oblique paralysis on the left and a compensatory head tilt to avoid constant double vision.

When Bruising and Swelling Subsides

After surgery, patients want to see what they consider to be a good result. However, they are just as interested in what you think, and most patients will ask, "How do you think I look, doctor?" The patient is obviously searching for a compliment and the surgeon must be prepared to deliver one in the appropriate way. The surgeon may be tempted to use such terms as "big improvement," "great," "beautiful," or "pretty." Many of these have been used, but certain words seem to be more effective complements postoperatively.

"Gorgeous"—This is the proper word to use with most females if done nonflippantly. It implies that the patient not only has acquired an extremely attractive appearance but now has an undefinable quality that wasn't there before. If the patient complains a bit about a residual fold or an undercorrected area, the surgeon should agree with her but say that she looks gorgeous. If the surgeon has been relating to her during the operative and postoperative period in a concerned, friendly, and positive manner, then this word will not seem inappropriate.

"Real Good"; "Great"; "Marvelous"—Many male patients will be interested in the surgeon's opinion about their appearance following surgery. The surgeon certainly doesn't want to sound effusive toward the male patients and "really good" is an expression that always seems to be effective. If there is female office staff or if the surgeon is female, the words "marvelous" and "great" tend to be well received by patients.

The Dissatisfied Patient

Most of your patients will be happy with their surgery and will say so, but you will have some complaints. This does not necessarily mean that a patient is unhappy but rather that he or she is being meticulous in the evaluation postoperatively. At this stage the before and after pictures become very important. Without question, patients forget exactly how they used to look, so it is important to show them pictures of the eyelids before surgery and the improvement in the eyelid appearance afterward. When the patient verbalizes that there has been substantial improvement, record the fact in the patient's record. In many cases it is helpful to copy the before and after pictures and give them to the patient. This can be done very easily with a photocopy machine that has enlarging capability.

Residual Folds

Probably the most common postoperative complaint refers to a residual skin fold laterally in the upper lids, which tends to occur when some brow laxity has gone untreated. It is important that the surgeon be willing to excise some of these little extra folds, or "lumps and bumps," in the office. It is important to explain to the patient that this is an aspect of the conservative safe treatment that is part of your treatment plan. It is much better to excise small amounts of skin folds in the office as a "touch-up" procedure than to remove too much skin initially. This reaffirms to the patient that you are a conscientious doctor and that you are interested in the safety of his or her eyes. Your willingness to excise extra skin folds in the office postoperatively tells the patient that you are also interested in obtaining the best possible result and that the patient is certainly getting his or her money's worth. If the surgeon does not feel that any residual skin folds need to be excised or could be excised safely, then it's important to point out to the patient that all of the skin that could be safely removed has been removed and that you would advise against any further skin removal from the standpoint of the health of the eye.

REFERENCES

1. Waller RR. Is blindness a realistic complication in blepharoplasty procedures? *Trans Am Acad Ophthalmol* 1978;85:730–735.
2. Lloyd WC, Leone CR. Transient bilateral blindness following blepharoplasty. *Ophth Plast Reconstr Surg* 1985;1:29–34.
3. McCord CD, Shore JW. Avoidance of complications in lower lid blepharoplasty. *Ophthalmology* 1983;90:1039.
4. Hamako C, Baylis HL. Lower eyelid retraction after blepharoplasty. *Am J Ophthalmol* 1985;89:517.
5. Carraway JH, Mellow CG. The prevention and treatment of lower lid ectropion following blepharoplasty. *Plast Reconstr Surg* 1990;85:971.
6. Neuhaus RW, Baylis HL. Complications of lower eyelid blepharoplasty. In: Putterman A, ed. *Cosmetic oculoplastic surgery*. New York: Grune and Stratton; 1982:276–306.
7. Lisman RD, Hyde K, Smith B. Complications of blepharoplasty. *Clin Plast Surg* 1988;15:309.
8. Tenzel RP. Surgical treatment of complications of cosmetic blepharoplasty. *Clin Plast Surg* 1978;5:517–523.
9. Rafaty FM. Complications of cosmetic blepharoplasty. *Cosmet Surg* 1983;2:17–29.
10. Levine M, Boyton J, Tenzel RR, Miller GR. Complications of blepharoplasty. *Ophth Surg* 1975;6:53–57.
11. Smith B, Petrelli R. Surgical repair of prolapsed lacrimal glands. *Arch Ophthalmol* 1978;96:113–114.

CHAPTER 18

Concepts of Impaired Vision from Upper Lid Malposition

When evaluating patients with upper lid malposition it is important to recognize the effect that upper lid position and function may have on visual activity. As a corollary, it is also important to recognize that patients who have visual symptomatology (asthenopia, difficulty reading, limited range of vision) may have unrecognized upper lid malposition or heaviness of the upper lids causing fatigue.

Ptosis, or abnormal weighting down of the upper lid from redundant lid tissue, may be masked in patients by chronic arching of the brow. Patients, compensating for upper lid ptosis or dermatochalasis with involuntary brow arching, can tolerate the effort in the early hours of the day, but as the day does on they become fatigued. By the end of the day patients will not usually tolerate the need to sustain their "brow-lifting" effort and will relax the brows resulting in blockage of vision. It is very important to recognize the possibility of upper lid relaxation, malposition, or heaviness in patients with visual fatigue symptoms.

It is also important to define this situation to permit certification of patients for provider coverage of their corrective upper lid surgery. In today's climate the surgeon must document the impaired visual function by plotting the amount of actual blocked vision on a visual field or produce graphic evidence of the deformity with photographs.

VISUAL FIELD BLOCKAGE

Documentation of upper visual field blockage with visual fields (devices vary from tangent screen to automated perimeter) in the lid-relaxed and lid-raised position is most commonly used to demonstrate actual occlusion of vision and arrive at the amount of blockage deemed to be significant. The amount of blockage determined to be "visually impairing" is arbitrary, but current criteria usually require that nearly 30% of the upper field of vision be blocked for certification. The exact methods for testing visual field blockage, whether tangent screen or perimeter, have not yet been defined by the agencies involved. It is important when testing by whatever method to get true representation of the blockage and to this end all brow arching should be avoided, if possible.

WEIGHTING-DOWN EFFECT

There is excellent evidence that there is usually more impairment in visual function than is reflected in the upper field blockage method as described above. The actual field blockage may not give a complete picture of visual impairment in that it does not measure the amount of compensatory effort required for visual function in each patient. The weighting-down effect may be much more severe in one patient than another who has the same visual field blockage.

IMPAIRMENT OF DOWNGAZE VISION

It has been shown that upper lid laxity can cause a disproportionate blockage in downgaze vision and in the reading area (1–3). In many cases of involutional ptosis, the ptosis is greater in downgaze. In some patients (in the early stages of ptosis) the increased lowering of the lid is only present in downgaze and may not yet be visible in the primary position. This type of impairment has been corrected by aponeurotic surgery in the upper lid (1). It is felt that the earliest sign of loss of aponeurotic integrity occurs in downgaze because the patient loses the ability to exert compensatory mechanisms that are present in the straight-ahead position of gaze. This form of visual impairment obviously is not detected in upper visual field measurements.

MARGIN–REFLEX DISTANCE

Visual field measurement can be imprecise and very subjective, particularly in inattentive elderly patients or in the very young. There is a very precise correlation between the distance of the upper lid margin from the light reflex seen in the pupil (margin–reflex distance, or MRD; see Fig. 1) and the amount of blockage of the upper field of vision (4–6).

This correlation has been documented by studies that occlude the pupil with a series of partially opaque contact lenses simulating a lowered lid margin (4) or actually lowering the upper lid margin by degrees with a gold weight (6). The amount of visual field defect is correlated with the narrowing of the margin reflex distance. The pupil reflex can be produced with a penlight or photographic flash. The MRD measurement can be taken directly from the patient or, with a reduced scale, from photographs. Figure 2 shows the plotted correlation of superior field blockage and the MRD. A more graphic portrayal of the findings in the studies are shown in Figs. 3–6. The value of this measure can be seen clinically in the patient in Fig. 7A and B.

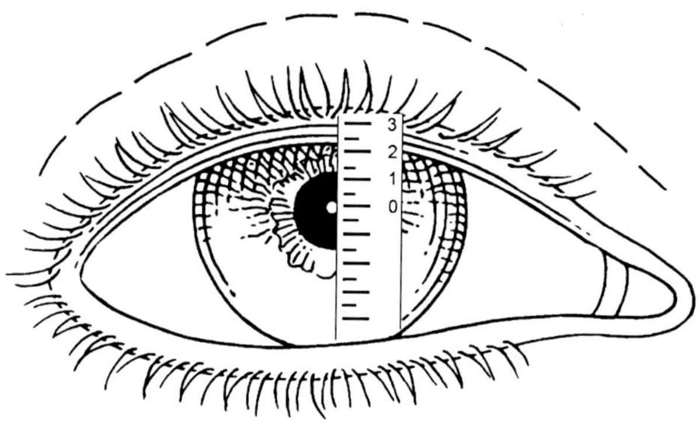

FIG. 1. Measurement of the margin–reflex distance (MRD). This shows the light reflex centered in the visual axis. The light reflex can come from either a photographic flash or a flashlight. A millimeter scale is centered and zeroed in on the light reflex and the distance from the margin is measured in millimeters. A reduced scale is used when measuring the MRD in photographs.

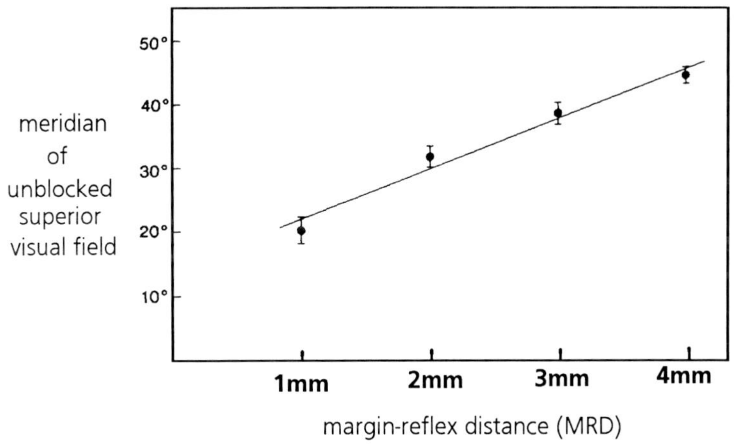

FIG. 2. Correlation between blockage in the visual field and a narrowing margin–reflex distance (MRD). The study was performed measuring visual fields in a series of patients with partially opaque contact lenses that simulated different MRDs. From Meyer et al. (4).

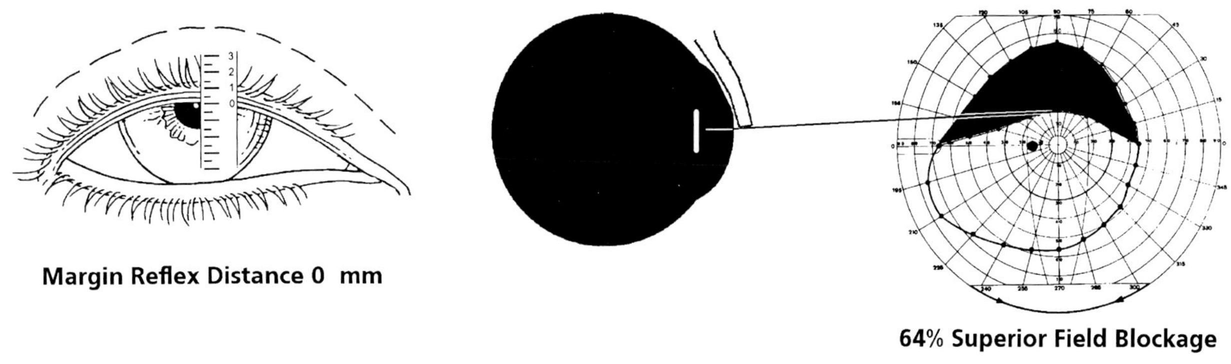

FIG. 3. Margin–reflex distance (MRD) correlated with the amount of visual field blockage. MRD = 0 mm, correlating with 62% upper field blockage. From Meyer et al. (4).

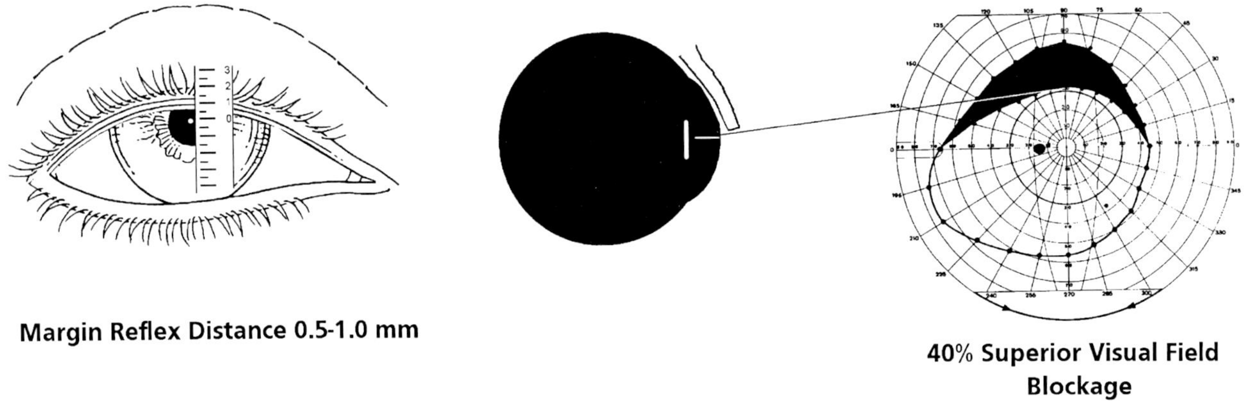

FIG. 4. Correlation of upper visual field defect with margin–reflex distance (MRD) showing the MRD of 0.5–1.0 mm produces 40% superior visual field blockage. From Meyer et al. (4).

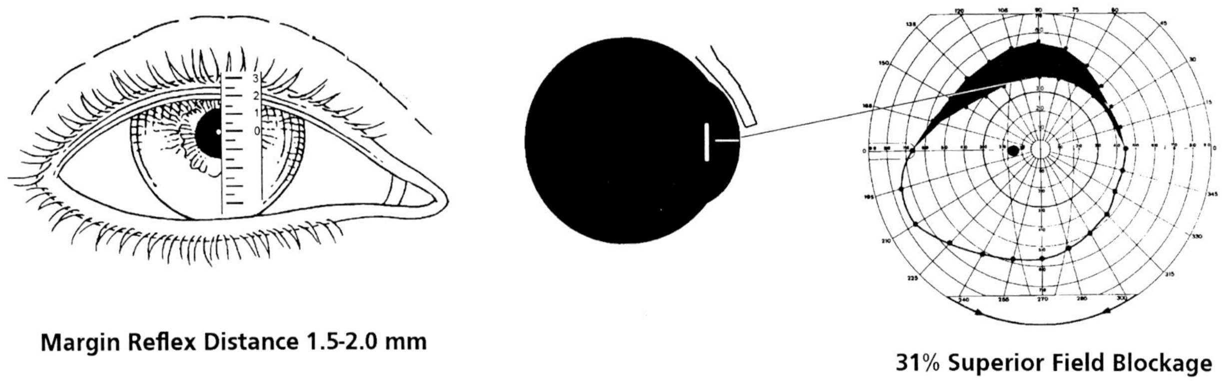

FIG. 5. Correlation of upper visual field defect with a margin–reflex distance of 1.5–2.0 mm producing 31% of superior visual field blockage. From Meyer et al. (4).

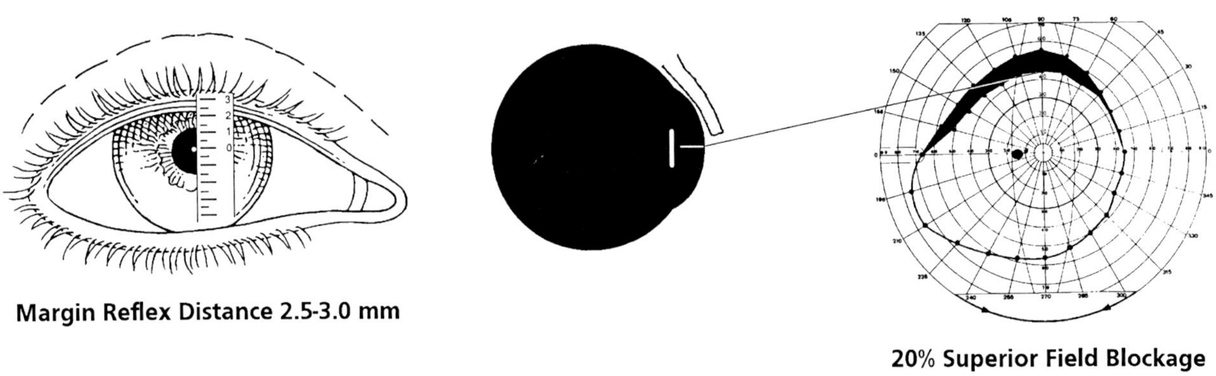

FIG. 6. Correlation of upper visual field defect with a margin–reflex distance of 2.5–3.0 mm producing 20% of superior visual field blockage. From Meyer et al. (4).

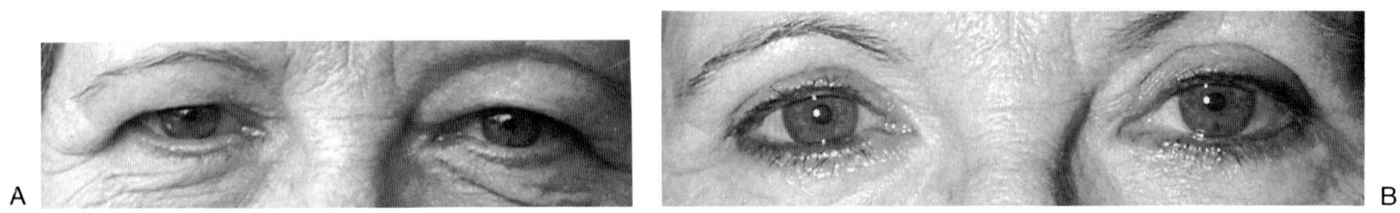

FIG. 7. A: Patient with severe dermatochalasis of the upper lids showing an extremely narrow (0–0.5) margin–reflex distance (MRD) on the right and a 0.5–1 MRD on the left. **B:** Same patient following upper lid blepharoplasty showing an increase in the margin–reflex distance with a corresponding improvement in the superior visual field.

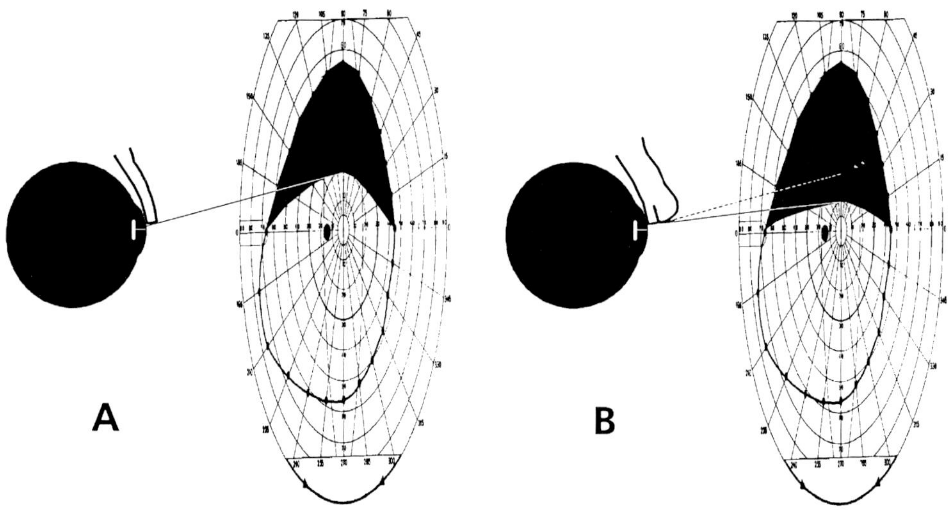

FIG. 8. Visual field blockage in addition to that caused by narrowing of the margin reflex, caused by protrusion of skin—the "shelf effect." **A:** Visual field blockage from the margin of the eyelid alone (narrow MRD). **B:** Margin position (MRD) the same as in Fig. A except the protruding shelf has further increased the visual field blockage.

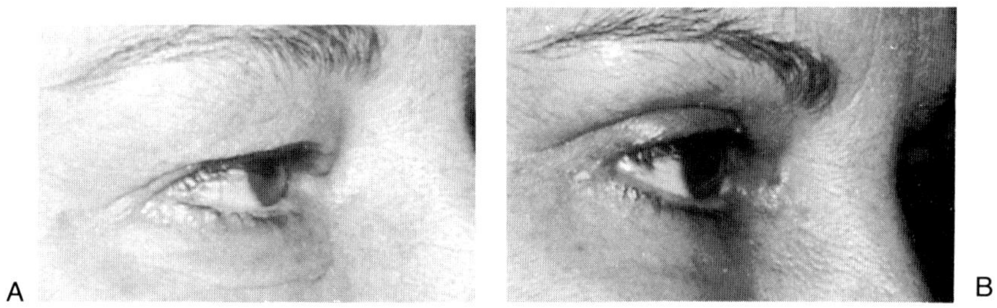

FIG. 9. **A:** Patient with dermatochalasis with protruding skin over the lashes demonstrating a shelf effect. **B:** Same patient. Postoperative upper lid blepharoplasty with removal of the shelf with corresponding increase in the superior visual field area.

SHELF EFFECT

The measurement of the MRD may actually underestimate visual impairment in some patients because this measurement does not take into consideration the "shelf effect" of protrusion of a skin fold from the upper lid, which may block the upper field vision. The actual blockage is more than that produced by a decreased MRD because the MRD measurement only takes into account blockage by the upper lid edge. The MRD does not take into consideration field blockage from forward protrusion of skin, which is commonly seen in patients with dermatochalasis (Fig. 8) (7). Patients with a shelf deformity can have a significant improvement from surgery as shown in Fig. 9.

It is clear that the position and integrity of the upper lid tissue must be evaluated in patients with impaired visual function. Quantitation of the amount of visual impairment from upper lid abnormalities is important for documentation, both to evaluate the effectiveness of treatment and to certify the patient for insurance coverage. Present methods of evaluation routinely used are somewhat rudimentary and may not truly reflect the amount of impairment that upper lid abnormalities may be producing.

More sophisticated testing will probably evolve in the future. It is felt that the photographic evidence (frontal view, side view) more reliably quantitates the impairment effect in the upper lid because it is less subjective, consistently reproducible, and graphic. Because of this it is hoped that agencies will be trained to use this method for quantitation.

REFERENCES

1. Wojno T. Downgaze ptosis. *Ophth Plast Reconstr Surg* 1993;9:83–89.
2. Patipa M. Visual field loss in primary gaze and reading gaze due to acquired blepharoptosis and visual field improvement following ptosis surgery. *Arch Ophthalmol* 1992;110:63–67.
3. Dryden RM, Kahanic DA. Worsening of ptosis in downgaze. *Ophth Plast Reconstr Surg* 1992;8:126–129.

4. Meyer DR et al. Quanting the superior visual field loss associated with ptosis. *Arch Ophthalmol* 1987;107:840–843.
5. Cahill KV, Burne JA, Weber PA. The effect of blepharoptosis on the field of vision. *Ophth Plast Reconstr Surg* 1987;3:121–125.
6. Meyer DR et al. Evaluation of the visual fields effects of blepharoptosis using automated static perimetry. *Ophthalmology* 1993;100:651–659.
7. Hachler HD, Hollsten DA. Investigation of automated perimetry in the evaluation of patients for upper lid blepharoplasty. *Ophth Plast Reconstr Surg* 1992;8:250–255.

CHAPTER 19

Thyroid Eyelid Disease: Correction of Upper and Lower Lid Retraction

(Graves' Disease)

Graves' disease is an inflammatory process of orbital tissue. It is associated with a thyroid disorder and primarily affects extraocular and eyelid muscles, lacrimal gland, and perhaps orbital fat. This process causes stiffness and contracture of the eyelids, causing them to be retracted from the globe and resulting in corneal exposure. Surgical correction of this problem often is necessary for adequate protection of the cornea and preservation of sight but can also have the side effect of restoring to the patient a more standard appearance.

Several considerations must be given before undertaking eyelid surgery on an elective basis. Graves' disease has an active, inflammatory, "hot" phase, in which the tissue is not stable and surgery undertaken during this time is difficult. Frequently, further changes in the tissue will take place that may negate the effect of the surgery. It is best to wait until the process of active inflammation has subsided and the patient has reached the "cold," inactive phase before subjecting him or her to surgery. Tissue changes in this condition are not caused by the thyroid hormone and progressive changes can take place in patients who are hyperthyroid, euthyroid, or hypothyroid. There is no test currently available to measure the causative substance, so there can be no specific way to guarantee that the patient will not have further changes. In general terms, active inflammatory changes can take place from 6 months to a year so a stable period of several months must be reached to lessen the chance of further changes taking place. If there are threatened visual changes or if the patient is experiencing discomfort, some surgery can be undertaken; however, the patient must be advised that further changes may still take place. Patients with Graves' disease who have been treated for hyperthyroidism, have been placed on replacement thyroid medication, and have had no eyelid changes for 6 months usually have no further changes.

Another consideration is the timing of eyelid surgery in terms of other types of rehabilitative surgery. In patients with extreme exophthalmos, orbital decompression may be considered; in patients who have severe restrictive myopathy with double vision, extraocular muscle surgery may also be considered. The sequence of these procedures is based on the fact that one procedure can affect the results of other procedures. Specifically, orbital decompression can affect both extraocular muscle positioning and eyelid positioning. Extraocular muscle surgery can affect eyelid position. Eyelid surgery seems to affect neither of the above, so in view of this situation, it is generally recommended that eyelid surgery be considered the last in the line of rehabilitative procedures (Table 1) (1).

EVALUATION OF UPPER LID RETRACTION

Graves' disease is the most common cause of true retraction of the upper lid. Other causes of true upper lid retraction are not as common and are listed in Table 2. Figure 1A–C shows unusual examples of causes of upper lid retraction.

In patients who have unilateral upper lid retraction, unconscious compensatory efforts to lower the retracted lid because of Herring's law of equal innervation to the eyelids cause a pseudoptosis in the normal side. True retraction from Graves' disease will cause

TABLE 1. *Proper sequence of rehabilitative procedures in patients with Graves' disease*

1. Orbital decompression
2. Upper lid surgery
3. Extraocular muscle surgery
4. Lower lid surgery (combined upper and lower lid surgery)

TABLE 2. *Causes of upper eyelid retraction*

Graves' disease
Posttraumatic or postinflammatory eyelid scarring
Hydrocephalus (Collier's sign)
Liver disease
Sympathetic irritation
Synkinetic upper lid movement
Innervation abnormalities: jaw winking syndrome, aberrant third nerve regeneration

lagophthalmos in the higher lid, confirming the fact that Graves' disease is present and a thyroid workup is necessary. Figure 2A and B shows a patient with retraction with pseudoptosis in the contralateral upper lid. Conversely, some patients with unilateral ptosis, because of an effort to elevate the ptotic lid, may cause retraction in the normal side. Lagophthalmos will not be present in the normal, higher lid.

The anatomic or physiologic reasons for upper lid retraction in Graves' disease are listed in Table 3. Figure 3 shows focal areas of adhesions and fibrosis that are commonly seen in the upper lid in Graves' patients. The sympathetic stimulation elevating the upper lid is seen only in patients who are hyperthyroid and elevation on this basis will subside when the hyperthyroidism is under control or can be treated with sympatholytic eyedrops (2,3). The mechanical changes listed form in the active inflammatory phase of the disease but persist even when the patient reaches the cold phase and are the problems that are addressed by rehabilitative surgery.

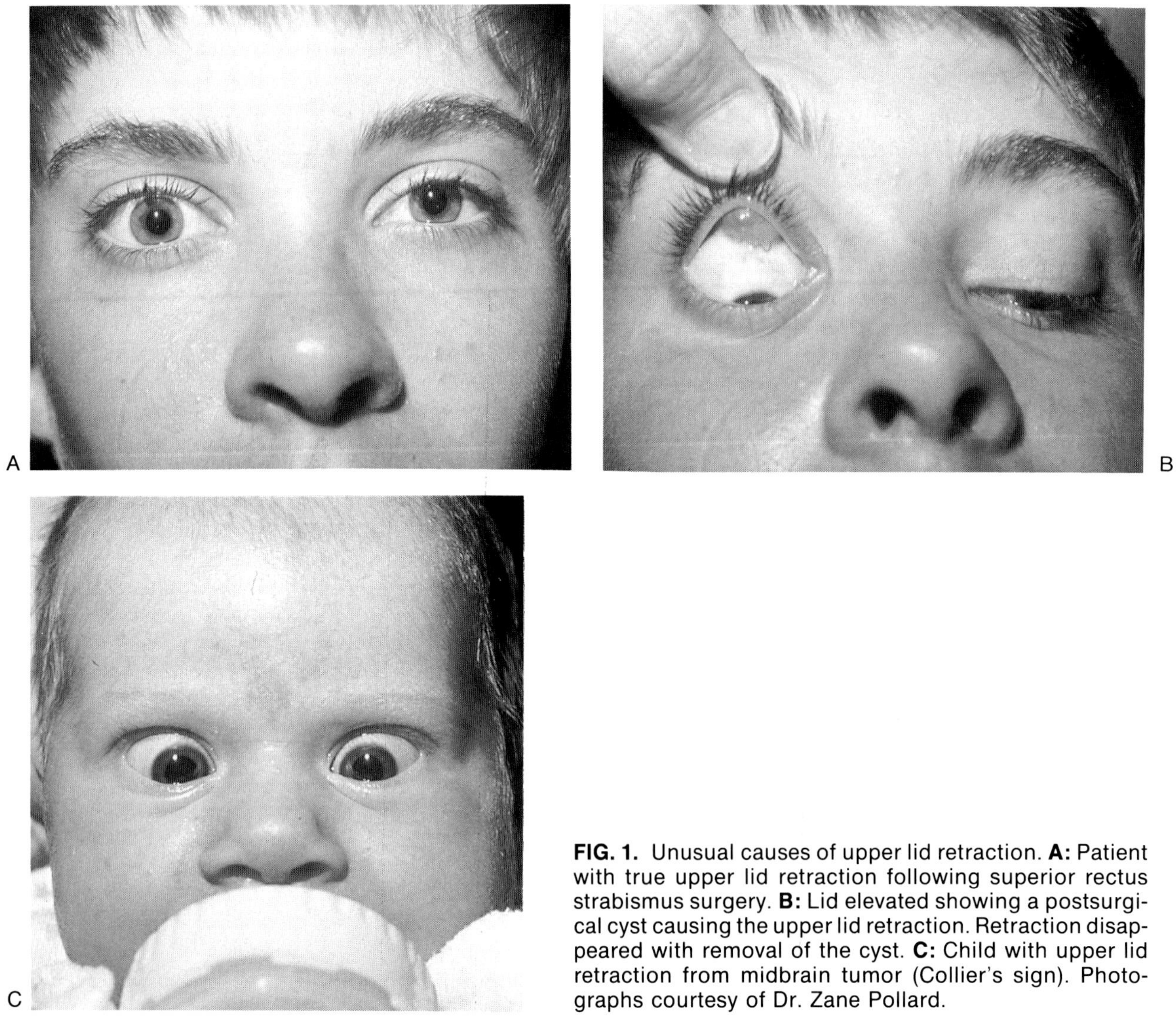

FIG. 1. Unusual causes of upper lid retraction. **A:** Patient with true upper lid retraction following superior rectus strabismus surgery. **B:** Lid elevated showing a postsurgical cyst causing the upper lid retraction. Retraction disappeared with removal of the cyst. **C:** Child with upper lid retraction from midbrain tumor (Collier's sign). Photographs courtesy of Dr. Zane Pollard.

TABLE 3. *Anatomic causes of upper eyelid retraction in Graves' disease*

Sympathetic stimulation of Müller's muscle
Infiltrative myopathy of the levator muscle with contracture
Adhesions of the levator muscle-to-fat septum
Overaction of the levator muscle (restrictive myopathy of the inferior rectus)

When evaluating the patient for upper lid surgery, the surgeon must be aware of compensatory squeezing or frowning commonly seen in these patients as a way of lessening their exposure and discomfort. This may cause the surgeon to underestimate the true amount of retraction in the upper lids or miss milder retraction of the "normal"-appearing contralateral side. Giving topical anesthetic drops and encouraging the patient to relax the eyes will unmask this situation in most cases. Patients who have asymmetric globe position, if receiving symmetric upper lid surgery, will get a higher lid crease on the side of the more prominent eye because of indentation of the globe on the eyelid. This must be recognized preoperatively and compensated for during surgery (Table 4).

TABLE 4. *Problems in evaluating and management of upper lid retraction in Graves' patients*

Eyelid "squeezing" (masks retraction)
Asymmetric retraction (may mask bilateral retraction)
Asymmetric globe position (asymmetric exophthalmos lid crease)
Active, inflamed, or "hot" phase (or hyperthyroid)

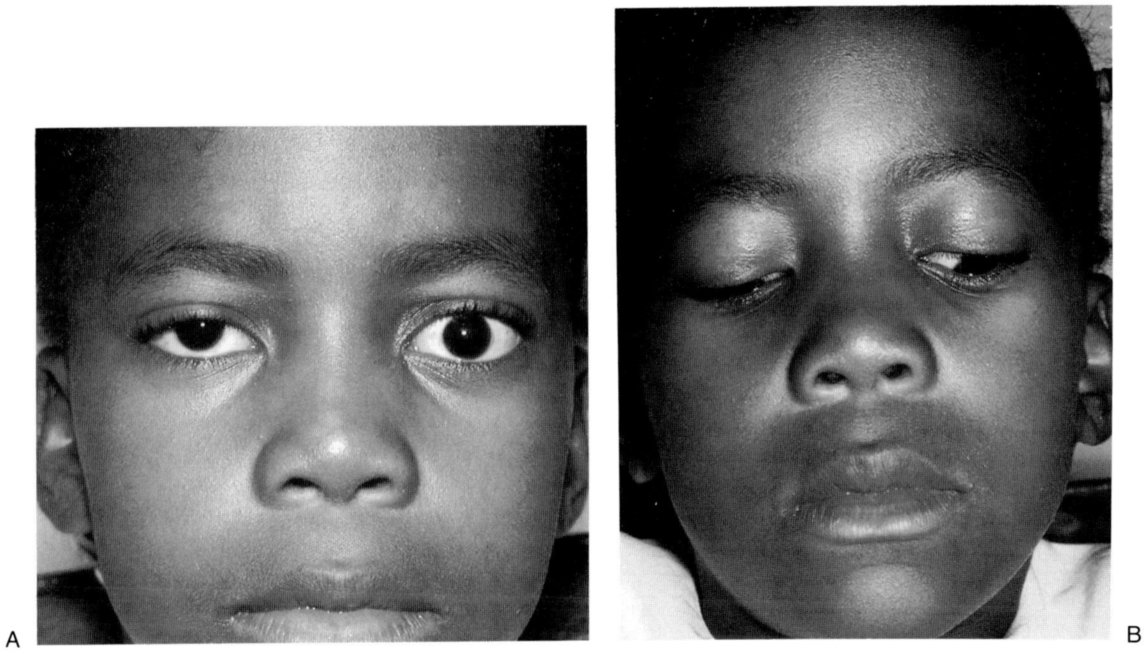

FIG. 2. Graves' disease presenting as pseudoptosis. **A:** Child with known hyperthyroidism and eye changes due to "squeezing" to protect the retracted eye has lowered the retracted upper lid to a normal level and caused a pseudoptosis in the contralateral side. **B:** Lagophthalmos of the "normal" upper lid in downgaze confirming retraction and Graves' disease.

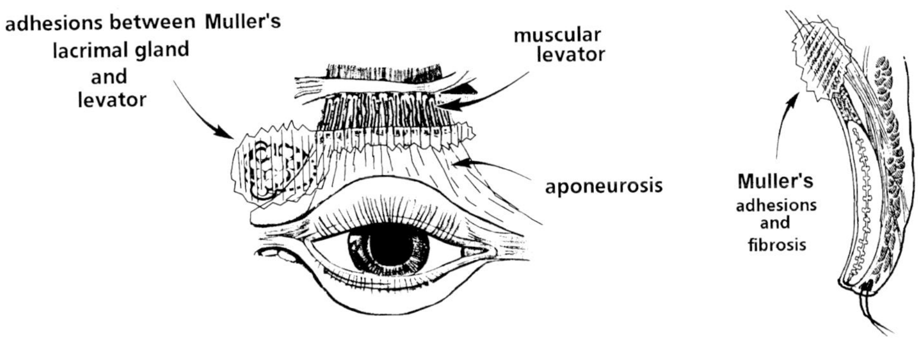

FIG. 3. Diagrammatic representation of eyelid anatomy showing areas of adhesions and fibrosis in Müller's muscle and lacrimal gland area in patients with Grave's disease. Frontal view and cross-section.

The inflammatory stage of Graves' disease must be planned for in order to avoid surgery during that phase, except in acute situations.

TECHNIQUES OF UPPER LID RECESSION

In the past a wide variety of surgical techniques for recession of the upper lid in thyroid retraction were proposed (4–8). Over the years, most differences in opinion have revolved around whether or not to use "spacer" material in the upper lids. In the past, spacer material of varying types was used: donor eye bank sclera, fascia lata, temporalis fascia, or ear cartilage. Harvey and Anderson (9) proposed a technique of recession of the upper lid with dissection and the use of no spacer material. This technique has been modified and used over the years, and it is felt to be superior to the use of spacer material (10,11).

The basis of the technique is a complete detachment of Müller's muscle from the levator's aponeurosis and muscular portion. Lysis of the lateral horn of Müller's muscle and the levator aponeurosis. No spacer material is used but a central suspender suture stabilizes the upper lid level and eyelid crease fixation adjusts the crease level.

SURGICAL TECHNIQUE

The upper lid is infiltrated with a frontal block with care taken to locally infiltrate the area of the lacrimal gland and Müller's muscle. A protective contact lens is inserted.

A lid crease incision is marked as in a blepharoplasty (Fig. 4A, B). If there is significant exophthalmos, the lid crease incision should be marked lower 7–8 mm because there will be a tendency for the lid crease to migrate higher postoperatively. If asymmetry of globe position is present, the crease should be marked lower on the side of the more prominent eye for compensation. Less fat should be removed on that side as well to compensate for the tendency of a higher crease on that side if more fat is removed. A modified blepharoplasty can be performed with excision of skin. Preaponeurotic and nasal fat can be removed, but in the presence of significant exophthalmos conservatism must be used in removal of skin and fat because it will exaggerate the prominence of the eye postoperatively.

Methylene blue is used to mark a line at the superior tarsal edge where the levator aponeurosis is to be incised. The aponeurosis and tissue is grasped with the forceps and the incision is made through the aponeurosis, just within the superior edge of the tarsal border (Fig. 5). Downward traction on the lid with a retractor allows tensing of the tarso–Müller's complex so that the levator aponeurosis can be dissected free from the underlying Müller's muscle. At the juncture of Müller's muscle and the undersurface of the levator, dense fibrous adhesions will be found and it is felt that this is the primary nidus of inflammation in the levator Müller's complex.

With traction on the levator aponeurosis and downward retraction of the tarsolevator Müller's layer, an incision is made under the undersurface of the levator completely severing Müller's muscle from the undersurface of the levator muscle and aponeurosis, until the lid can be fully retracted (Fig. 6A, B). Thin adventitial strands of tissue just above Müller's muscle on the conjunctival surface should also be severed to allow complete relaxation, but avoidance of buttonholes in the conjunctiva is observed.

Lateral dissection of the Müller's muscle, horn, and levator aponeurotic horn around the palpebral lobe of the lacrimal gland is very important (Figs. 7A–C; 8). In the past, poor dissection in this area caused the most common deficiency in upper lid levator recession, i.e., undercorrection of the temporal portion of the lid. In the past when spacer material was used, one noted that

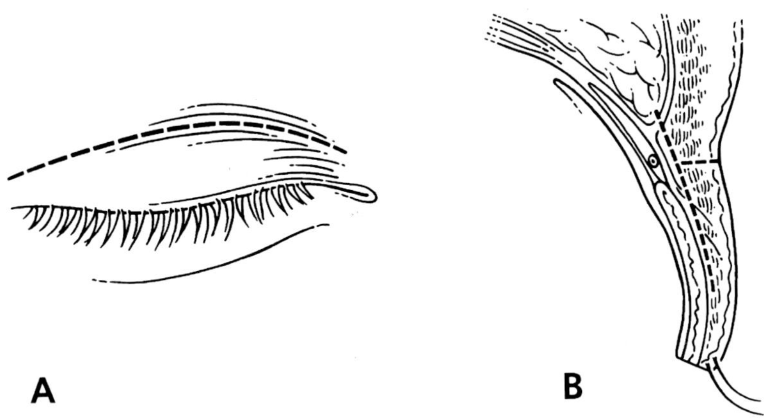

FIG. 4. Levator recession of upper lid. **A:** Eyelid crease incision. **B:** Eyelid crease incision and dissection plane.

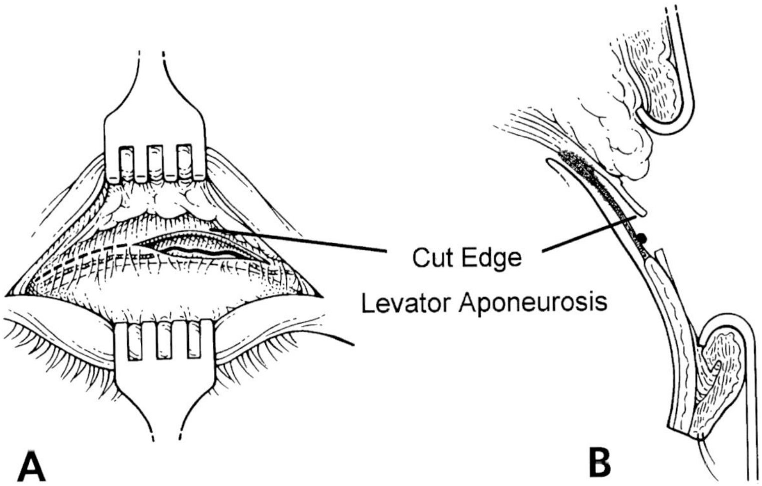

FIG. 5. Levator recession of upper lid. **A:** Incision through levator aponeurosis. **B:** Plane of dissection under levator to adhesions of Müller's muscle.

twice as much spacer material was used temporally as centrally to fully correct the lid. This is an obvious attempt to compensate for failure to dissect the adhesions and horns in the lateral portion of the lid. Many adhesions are found in this area, which also points out the lacrimal gland area as a nidus of the inflammatory reaction of Graves' disease. The lateral horn of the levator can be easily cut; however, it is a vascular area and care must be taken in a dissection of the lateral horn of Müller's muscle from around the nasal portion of the palpebral lacrimal gland. This can, however, be done satisfactorily with the cutting Bovie needle, and the lid can then be fully retracted downward laterally. When this dissection is finished, the protective contact lens is removed to allow the surgeon to view the position of the pupil.

A single, central "suspender" suture is then placed inside the superior edge of the tarsal border in line with the pupil (Figs. 9; 10A, B). A double-lock stitch is used to secure the suture to the tarsal substance and the suture should not be full-thickness tarsus. A double-arm 6-0 silk is used and the two arms are then brought up into the recessed edge of the levator aponeurosis enough to ensure that no cheese wiring or pulling loose takes place postoperatively. The suture is then tied temporarily and the amount of recession desired is estimated by measurement of the distance of the superior edge of the tarsus to the cut edge of the levator. In most cases the exact amount of desired recession is measured between the cut edge of the levator and the superior tarsal edge with calipers. The patient can be aroused and asked to focus on a cotton applicator stick

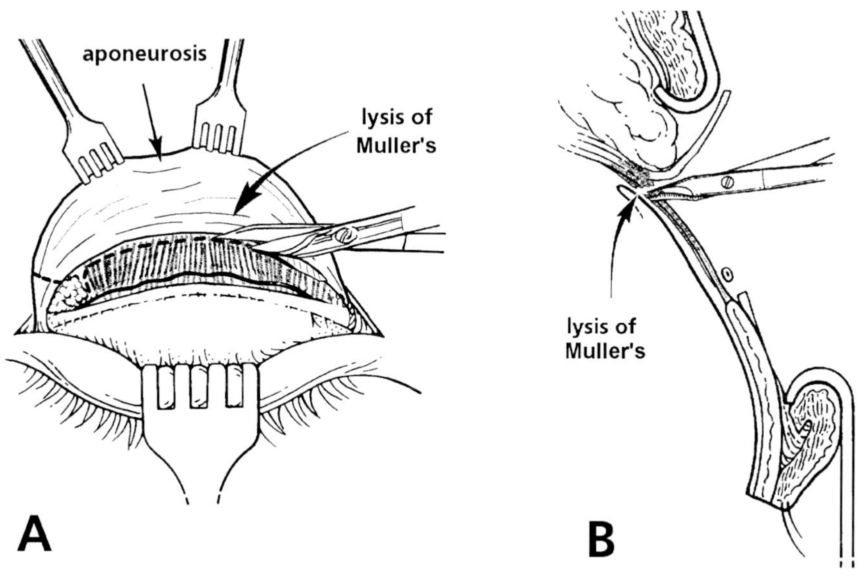

FIG. 6. Levator recession. **A:** Levator aponeurosis has been retracted showing attachment of Müller's muscle to undersurface in area of fibrosis. Müller's muscle is being dissected from the undersurface of levator. **B:** Cross-section showing plane of dissection, lysing Müller's muscle from the undersurface of the levator.

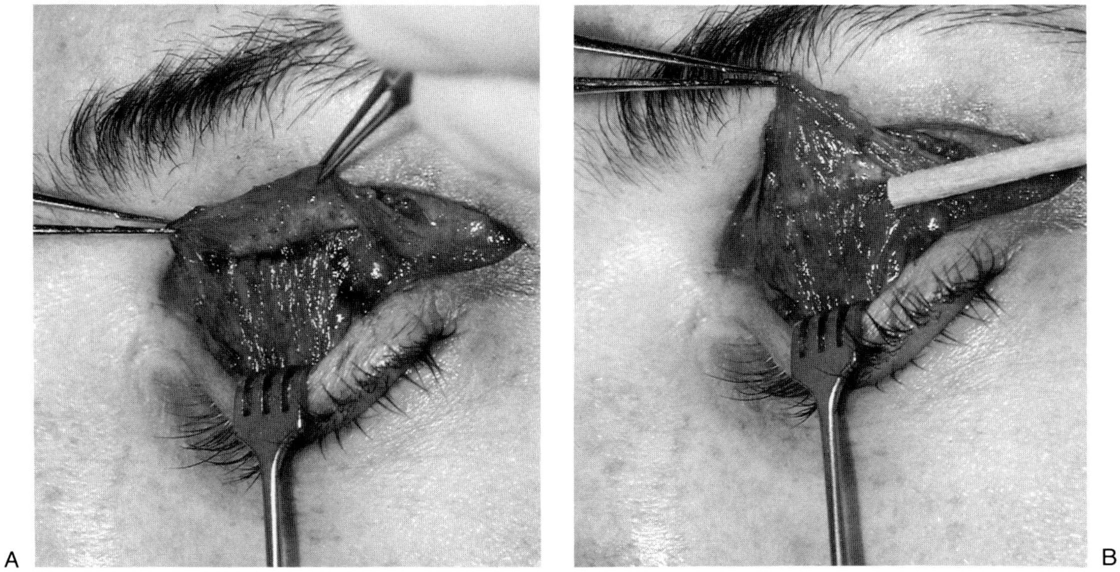

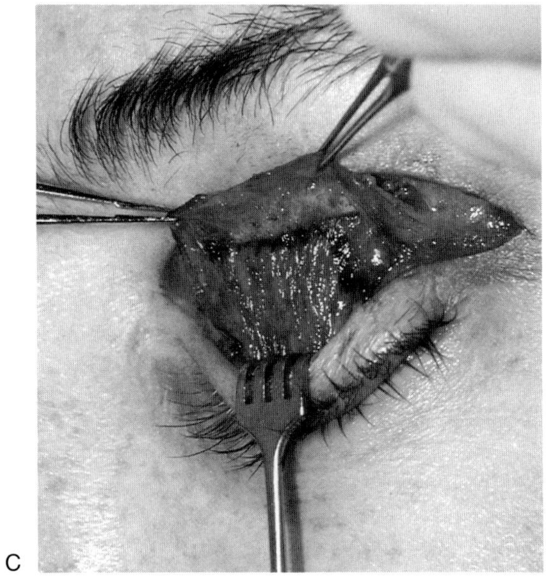

FIG. 7. Levator recession. **A:** Surgical view showing levator aponeurosis retracted and exposing Müller's muscle and adhesions. **B:** Cotton applicator stick pointing to area of thickening fibrosis and adhesions of Müller's muscle at its attachment on the undersurface of the levator. **C:** Area of lysis of Müller's muscle from the undersurface of levator and lysis of the lateral horn of Müller's muscle around the palpebral lobe of the lacrimal gland.

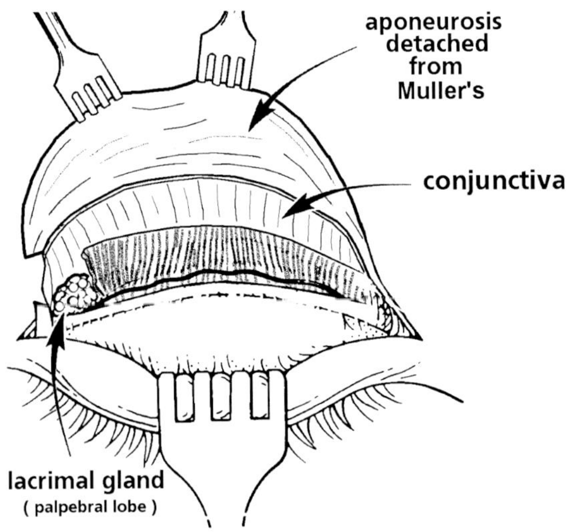

FIG. 8. Levator recession. Müller's muscle has been detached from the undersurface of the levator muscle and the lateral horn of the levator aponeurosis has been incised as has the lateral horn of Müller's muscle in the area of the palpebral lobe of the lacrimal gland.

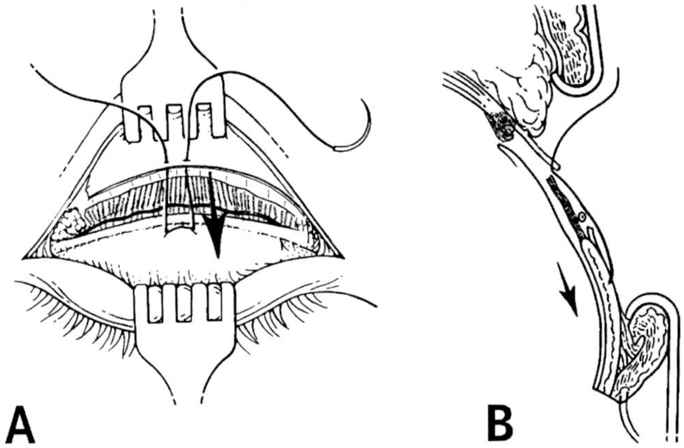

FIG. 9. A: Levator recession. A 6-0 silk suture has been placed at pupillary level in the superior edge of the tarsal plate and through the cut edge of the levator aponeurosis, allowing a downward movement of the lid and recession of the levator. **B:** Cross-sectional view of above.

and the lids can be adjusted accordingly. If the anesthesia and block has affected lid position too much, then the lid is adjusted by the gapping method to reduce the gap by the desired amount over what was noted after the local anesthesia had taken effect before the operation began. When the desired level of the upper lid is reached, the sutures are tied permanently (Figs. 11 and 12).

If the patient has exophthalmos or if the surgeon is worried about upward migration of the crease, no eyelid crease sutures are used at this point. If the patient has no exophthalmos and a crease at a desired position is needed, the transcutaneous sutures are used to fixate the pretarsal skin to the superior edge of the tarsus to ensure that the crease forms at that position. Before closure, the tissue is flushed with Kenalog solution. In the judging upper lid position, it is better to undercorrect the lid (have the lid slightly too high postopera-

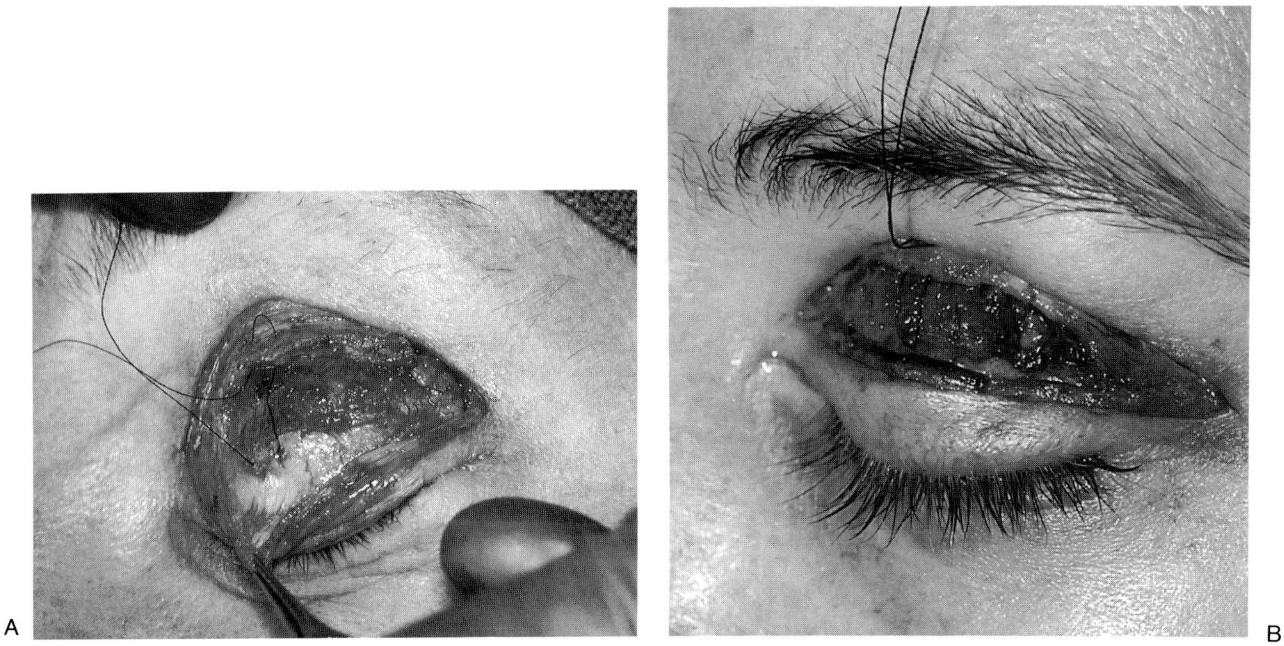

FIG. 10. Levator recession. **A:** The levator aponeurosis has been detached from underlying Müller's muscle and the suture spans from the superior edge of the tarsal plate to the cut edge of the levator. **B:** The upper lid has been recessed to the desired amount with a 1-mm for 1-mm correction for recession of the upper lid.

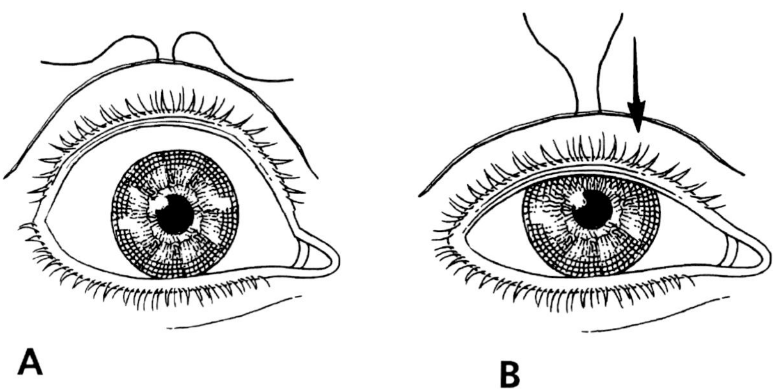

FIG. 11. Levator recession. **A:** Lid retraction before the suture is relaxed to allow recession of the upper lid. **B:** After adjustment and loosening of the sutures so that the upper lid level reaches the normal position halfway between the top of the pupil and the limbus. If anesthesia can be obtained without akinesia, this can be done with voluntary opening during surgery.

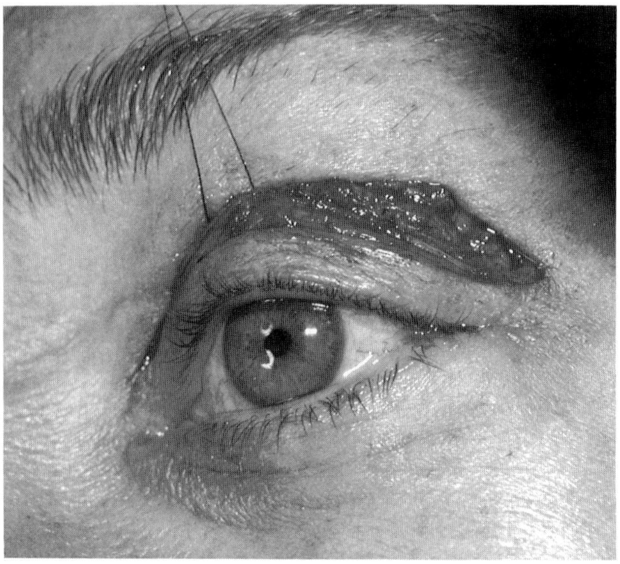

FIG. 12. Patient during surgery showing proper adjustment of the upper lid level with levator recession.

tively) than to overcorrect the lid (have the lid too low postoperatively). The slightly undercorrected lid can be very easily massaged downward for a full correction. Since there is only a central suspender suture, the rest of the tissue is held in place at 1 week only by "tissue glue," which is quite malleable and sensitive to massage.

Figure 13A and B shows a patient seen preoperatively and 1 week postoperatively at the time of suture removal with undercorrection of the temporal portion of the lid on the left. With massage over the next 2 weeks the lid was brought down to the desired position (Fig. 14A and B).

COMPLICATIONS OF LEVATOR RECESSION

Undercorrection

If recognized early, postoperative undercorrection of the temporal portion of the lid or the entire lid can

A 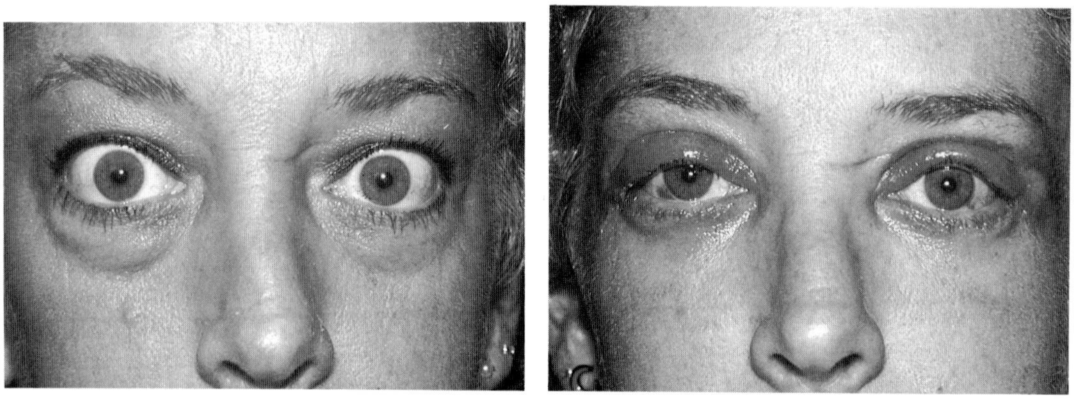 B

FIG. 13. Levator recession. **A:** Patient preoperatively with upper lid retraction, with herniated fat in the lower lids. **B:** Same patient following recession of the levator in the upper lids and lower lid blepharoplasty with tightening and supraplacement of the lateral canthal tendon. The left upper lid is too high and undercorrected.

A 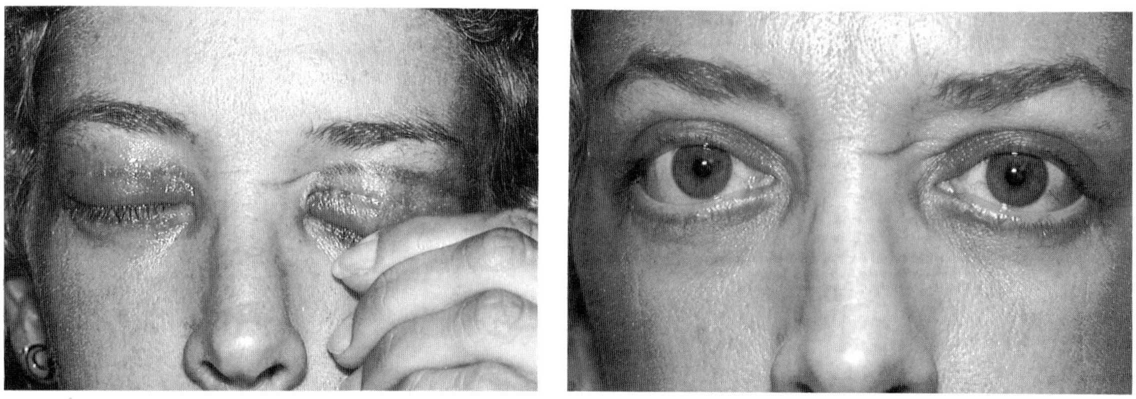 B

FIG. 14. Levator recession. Same patient as in Fig. 13 at 1 week postop stretching the lid with downward traction for early correction of undercorrection. **A:** The patient grasps the lashes with downward traction and looks toward the ceiling several times. **B:** Same patient 2 weeks later with good lowering of the left upper lid to the desired position following postoperative stretching.

be corrected by a downward stretching, as seen in Figs. 13 and 14. If over a period of several months the lid continues to be undercorrected or if a previously adequately positioned lid retracts, it will most likely retract in the temporal portion, and additional revisional surgery can be done. Further recession of the levator can be performed but it has been common experience that simple additional lysis of tissue with a suspender suture is not enough. The tissue will tend to retract and elevate again with healing and it is in this situation that spacer material such as ear cartilage should be inserted to prevent the re-retraction of the lid.

Overcorrection

Overcorrection or a downward pull at the position of the lid can occur from faulty intraoperative judgment or severe postoperative swelling, which can stretch the levator–tarsal complex and cause overcorrection. Sometimes late overcorrections occur that may be related to the natural course of the underlying Graves' in which levator myopathy can occur. The levator initially can be quite fibrous and retractive but can undergo a further fatty degeneration and loosening with time.

Management of the overcorrected lid can be more of a problem because the levator behaves very commonly as a patient with severe congenital ptosis with poor levator function. If the surgeon feels that adequate levator function is present, he or she can attempt to reattach the tarsal plate to the levator complex to elevate the lid. In some cases of severe overcorrection that do not respond to levator advancement, a frontalis suspension procedure may be needed.

GRAVES' DISEASE: CORRECTION OF LOWER LID RETRACTION

Some of the principles of corrective lower lid surgery are the same as those of the upper lid in that the patient should have obtained the noninflamed or cold phase of Graves' disease before undertaking lower lid surgery if possible. In addition, the corrective lower lid surgery should be placed in the context of other rehabilitative surgical procedures for Graves' disease as previously

TABLE 5. *Causes of lower lid retraction in the Graves' patient*

Contracture of the inferior retractors (capsulopalpebral fascia)
Adhesions in the fat–orbital septum
Exophthalmos with forward protrusion of the globe
Re-retraction following eye muscle surgery (recession of inferior rectus with retraction of capsulopalpebral fascia)

TABLE 6. *Classification of Graves' patients with lower lid changes (with recommended procedure)*

Puffy lids, little or no retraction (standard blepharoplasty with lateral canthoplasty)
Retraction—mild to moderate proptosis (recession of retractor muscles; supraplacement of lateral canthal tendon; insertion of spacer material–ear cartilage)
Retraction—severe proptosis (loosening of lower lid, transverse blepharotomy; intermarginal adhesion to upper lid; spacer material insertion; supraplaced periosteal fixation of skin muscle flap)

described. It is common that orbital decompression may improve lower lid retraction because of settling of the globe (hypoophthalmos) following decompression with relative elevation of the lower lid margin.

The causes of the lower lid retraction in Graves' disease are shown in Table 5 and there may be a combination of causes in each patient. The patients can be placed in three groups with regards to the application of surgical procedures: those with little or no lid retraction, those with moderate retraction and proptosis, and those who have retraction and significant proptosis (Table 6).

The underlying principle between the two last groups is that in the usual patient without severe exophthalmos the lower lid can be elevated by tightening the lid with some supraplacement of the lateral tendon with spacer material nasally (Fig. 15). If, however, the patient does have a significant amount of exophthalmos, this tightening and supraplacement will not work and a clotheslining effect will occur. As one attempts to tighten and supraplace the lateral edge of the lid toward the orbital rim, which has been recessed in relationship to the front surface of the eye, the lid margin will clothesline and slide underneath the globe and an ad-

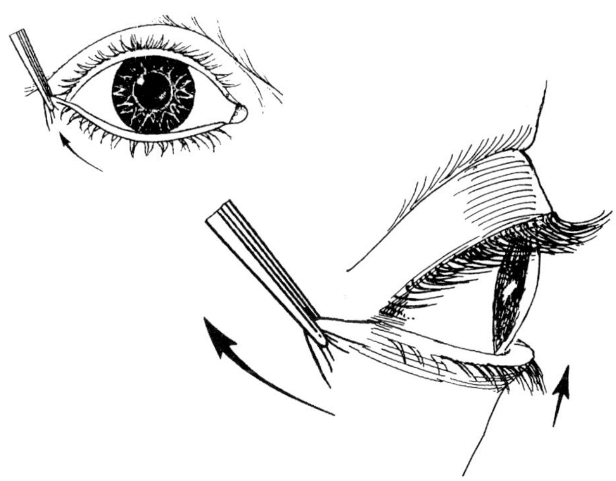

FIG. 15. Patient with Graves' disease with mild exophthalmos showing the ability to elevate the lid with general upward traction. Patients in this category can be helped with a standard blepharoplasty and supraplacement of the lateral canthal tendon.

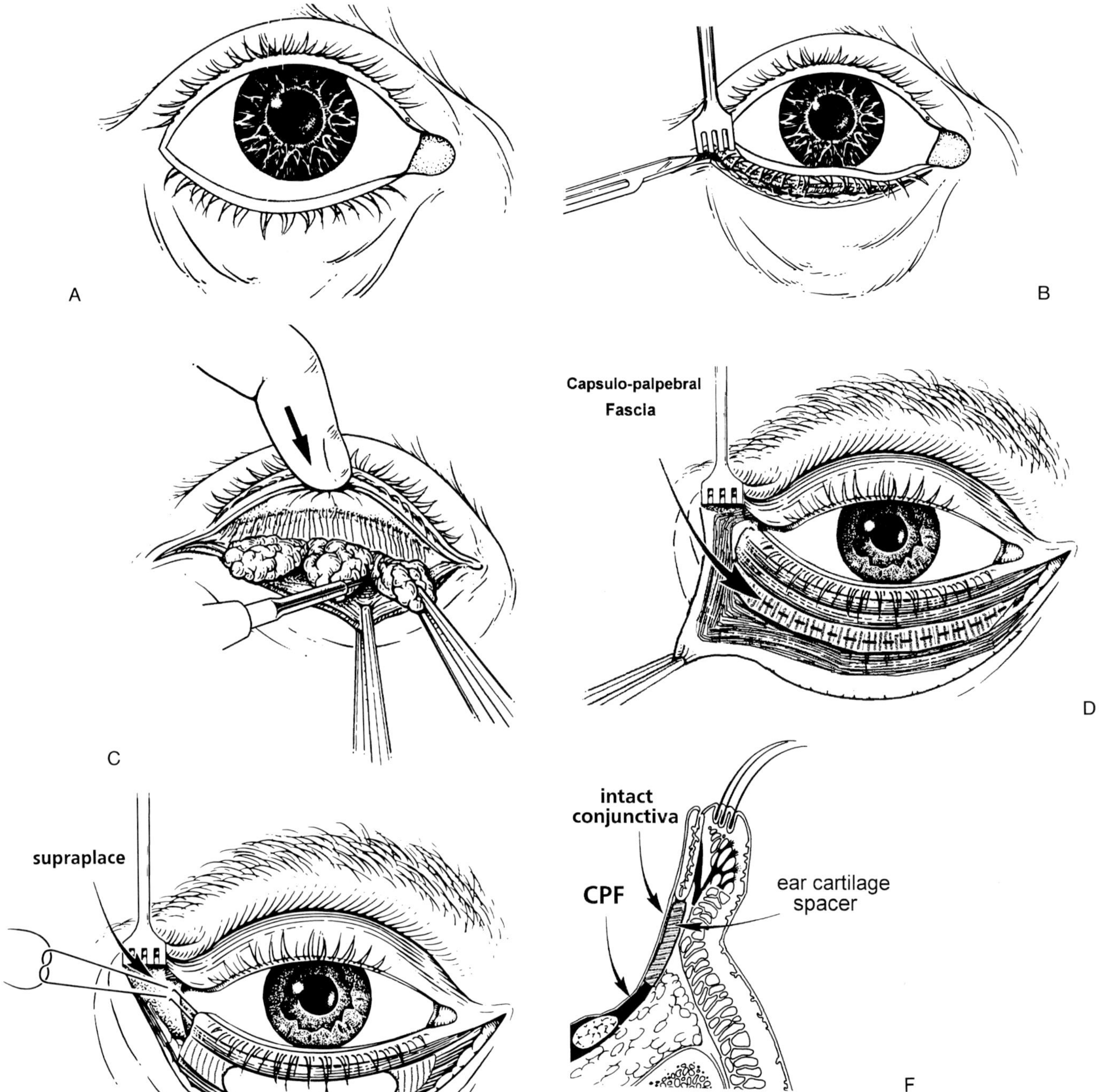

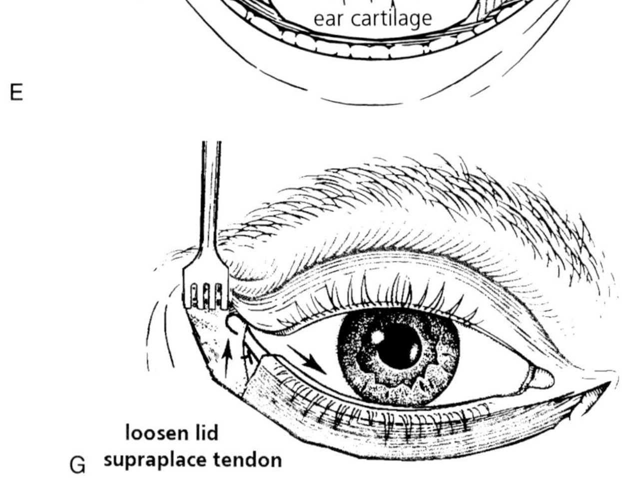

FIG. 16. Correction of lower lid retraction with supraplacement of lateral canthal tendon and spacer implant. **A:** Patient with lower lid retraction and mild proptosis. **B:** Subciliary skin muscle incision and elevation of flap. **C:** Removal of fatty pads. **D:** Incision of the capsulopalpebral fascia of the lower lid to allow spacer implant. Ear cartilage spacer material is placed in the area dissected in the capsulopalpebral fascia. **E:** A canthotomy and cantholysis with horizontal tightening has been performed with suture placed to supraplace the lateral lid. **F:** Cross-section showing position of the spacer implant in the lower lid. **G:** The lateral suture, which has been supraplaced to elevate the lid, may need loosening to allow the lid edge to elevate in patients with more exophthalmos. In general terms, increasing exophthalmos requires a loosening of the lower lid to allow it to elevate and to avoid clotheslining of the lid underneath the globe.

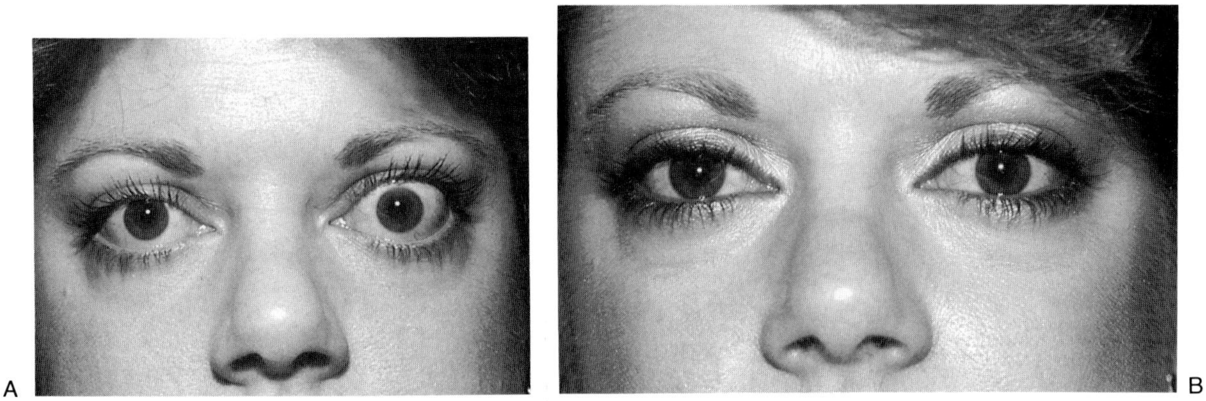

FIG. 17. A: Patient with lower lid retraction before recession of the upper lid and lower lid lateral canthal tendon supraplacement with spacer implant. **B:** Same patient postoperatively. The patient has had supraplacement of the lateral canthal tendon and an ear cartilage spacer implant. The patient has also had recession of the levator in the left upper lid.

verse effect will be obtained (Fig. 18). This clotheslining effect can be lessened with lateral orbital bony wall advancement because the point of purchase of the canthus becomes more anterior. In some patients, however, eyelid surgery may be the only chosen course, or some patients may have significant residual exophthalmos despite reconstructive efforts. This can be compensated for by loosening the eyelid instead of tightening the eyelid and allowing the lower lid margin to ride up to the inferior corneal limbus. This new position of the eyelid can be sustained with spacer material together with reformation of the canthus, plus supraplacement of a skin-muscle flap for an added elevating effect.

Patients with Minimal or No Retraction

Standard blepharoplasty technique is used as described in the chapter on lower lid blepharoplasty. A supraplacement and loosening of the lateral canthal tendon may be needed.

Surgical Technique for Correction of Lower Lid Retraction in Patients with Mild to Moderate Proptosis

In these patients, a standard external blepharoplasty approach is used with excision of appropriate fat pads (Fig. 16A–C). More extensive removal of fat has been described (12,13). The capsulopalpebral fascia is then dissected from the inferior tarsus and freed up from the underlying conjunctiva and its attachments until the lid can be easily passively elevated upward (Fig. 16D). Spacer material, usually ear cartilage from the scaphoid area, is inserted and sutured to the inferior edge of the tarsal plate (Fig. 16E, F). Other material has been used as spacer (14–17). Spacer is more commonly needed in the nasal portion of the lid and may be sutured to the conjunctiva for fixation when the desired elevation and contour is obtained. The lateral canthotomy, cantholysis, and supraplacement of the lateral edge of the lid is performed. If enough proptosis is present that the beginning of a clotheslining effect is noted, then it is appropriate to loosen the lateral suture fixation to allow the lid to ride upward (Fig. 16G). The operation is completed with fixation of the skin-muscle flap and closure. Figure 17A and B shows a patient with little exophthalmos before and after surgery with the described technique.

Surgical Technique for Correction of Lower Lid Retraction in Patients with Significant Proptosis

A different technique must be used in patients with increasing exophthalmos because of the clotheslining effect as shown in Fig. 18.

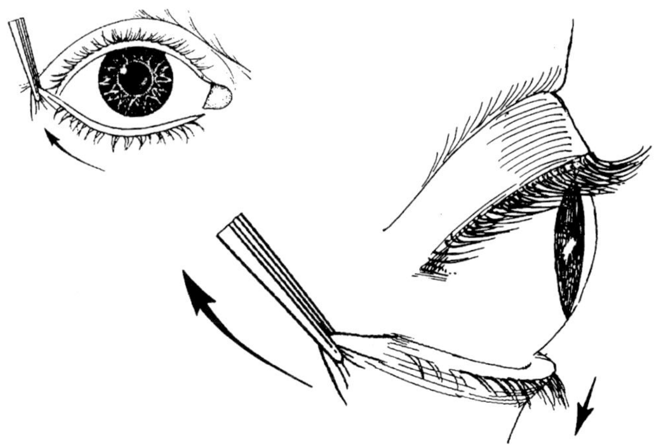

FIG. 18. Patient with moderate to severe proptosis. A tightening of the lid despite supraplacement will cause a clotheslining of the lid under the globe increasing the scleral show. In these patients with lower lid retraction and severe exophthalmos, an additional modification in surgical technique is needed to elevate the lid.

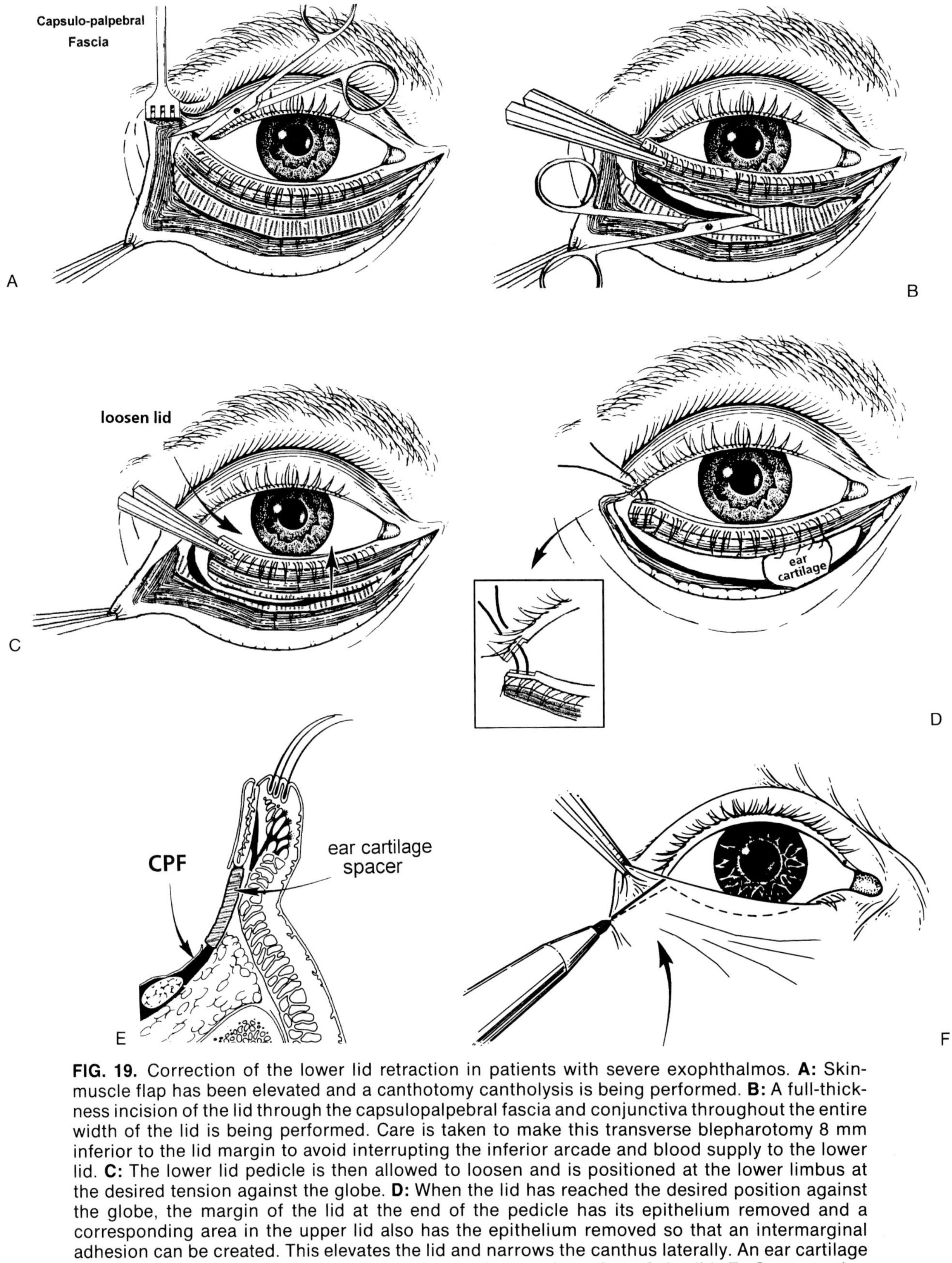

FIG. 19. Correction of the lower lid retraction in patients with severe exophthalmos. **A:** Skin-muscle flap has been elevated and a canthotomy cantholysis is being performed. **B:** A full-thickness incision of the lid through the capsulopalpebral fascia and conjunctiva throughout the entire width of the lid is being performed. Care is taken to make this transverse blepharotomy 8 mm inferior to the lid margin to avoid interrupting the inferior arcade and blood supply to the lower lid. **C:** The lower lid pedicle is then allowed to loosen and is positioned at the lower limbus at the desired tension against the globe. **D:** When the lid has reached the desired position against the globe, the margin of the lid at the end of the pedicle has its epithelium removed and a corresponding area in the upper lid also has the epithelium removed so that an intermarginal adhesion can be created. This elevates the lid and narrows the canthus laterally. An ear cartilage spacer graft must be placed nasally to elevate the nasal portion of the lid. **E:** Cross-section showing the positioning of the nasal ear cartilage spacer. **F:** The skin-muscle flap is rotated outward and tensed to determine redundancy in the lateral portion of the flap and a triangular excision is performed. *(Figure continues.)*

An external blepharoplasty-type incision is made in the subciliary and lateral canthal area. The skin-muscle flap is elevated and appropriate amounts of tissue from the fatty packets are removed if needed. A complete canthotomy and cantholysis is performed (Fig. 19A). With the edge of the lid grasped at the lateral end and the skin-muscle flap retracted, a complete and full-thickness incision is made through the lid (capsulopalpebral fascia and conjunctiva) beneath the inferior arcade with sharp scissors. Care is taken to ensure that the incision is well beneath the blood supply to the lid margin. The vertical height of the tarsus is approximately 4 mm and the arcade is just below that, so that 5–6 mm should be used for the blepharotomy site (Fig. 19B). The protective contact lens is removed so that the surgeon can see the cornea and inferior limbus. The lower lid pedicle flap is then brought up and allowed to ride up on the surface of the globe until the inferior margin is at the lower limbal position (Fig. 19C). It is then tensed enough to have it conform to the globe without altering vertical position, and the position where the cut edge of the lower lid margin touches the upper lid is noted. At this point, the posterior surface of the upper lid margin is removed with sharp scissors as well as the corresponding position on the lower lid margin, on its posterior edge with care taken to preserve the lashes. The lower lid pedicle is then attached to the upper lid edge with translid 6-0 vicryl suture,

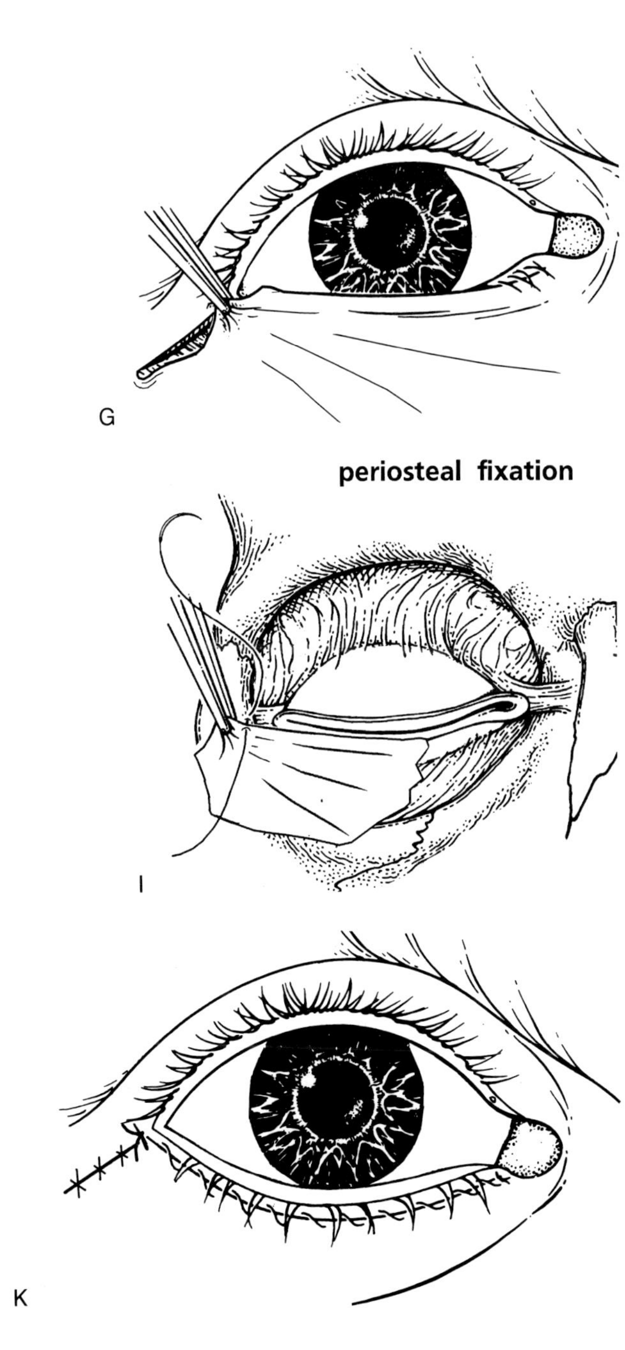

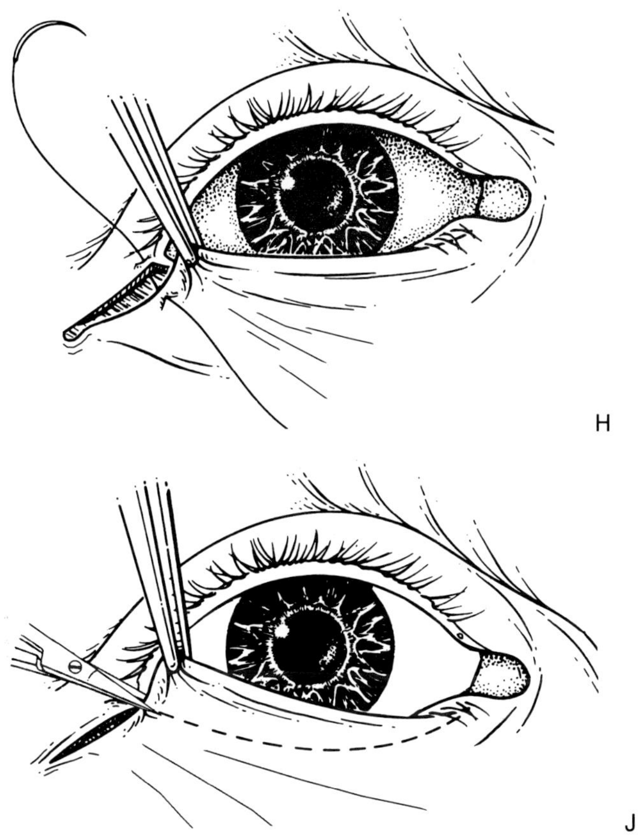

FIG. 19. *Continued.* **G:** The edge of the skin-muscle flap is tensed toward the lateral periosteum in such a way as to act as a supporting element for the lower lid. The lower lid margin is observed and the proper grasping and tensing of the flap can further elevate the lower lid margin. Care must be taken to provide the right tension in that too much tension can cause an outward buckling of the lower lid margin. **H:** Once the desired location of fixation with proper tension is obtained, the flap is sutured to the lateral periosteum with a 4-0 silk suture. **I:** A cutaway diagram showing the position of the flap sutured to the lateral rim so as to create tension across the lid edge to further approximate the lid margin against the globe. **J:** Redundant tissue beneath the lash line margin is trimmed. **K:** Final closure is then accomplished with sutures positioning the lower lid margin at the inferior limbus.

with the knot tied on the anterior surface of the upper lid skin. This will noticeably move the lateral canthal formation in closer to the lateral limbus. The position change should not be so extreme as to cause a phimotic appearance (Fig. 19D). The margin pedicle should not be overly loose.

After suturing of the pedicle, the lower lid position is again noted. If the nasal portion of the lower lid still is not as high as desired with scleral show present, a portion of ear cartilage is sutured to the inferior edge of the tarsal plate and then the retractors as an ear cartilage strut to elevate the nasal portion of the lid (Fig. 19D, E). The amount of cartilage needed is not great and can generally be obtained by bisecting the ellipse of ear cartilage as taken from one ear in the scaphoid fossa area and turned vertically.

Following the positioning of the lower lid margin, the skin-muscle flap is stretched toward the lateral orbital rim. With the stretching, it should be brought across the lower lid pedicle so that the position of the lower lid margin can be noted while the flap is being stretched. There is always redundant skin laterally and a triangular portion of skin should be excised as it overlaps the lateral skin incision as in the blepharoplasty procedure (Fig. 19F). The lateral edge of the skin-muscle flap is then attached to the periosteum of the lateral orbital rim with the desired amount of tension. With proper tension the tightening and elevation of the skin-muscle flap will also have an added effect of elevating the lower lid margin (Fig. 19G–I). Care must be taken not to have too much tension on the skin-muscle flap with its attachment to the periosteum as it can also have a clotheslining or margin everting effect. Once the surgeon is satisfied that the skin-muscle flap is on the desired tension it is sutured with 4-0 silk to the lateral rim periosteum. Closure is then accomplished in the standard blepharoplasty manner. The wound is irrigated with a dilute Kenalog solution (Fig. 19J, K). Figure 20 A–C shows a patient after orbital decompression with recurrent lower lid retraction and exophthalmos following inferior rectus recession. Correction of lower lid retraction was obtained with the blepharotomy technique described.

POSTOPERATIVE CARE

Ice compresses are used continuously for 2 days following eyelid surgery in Graves' disease. There is much more of a swelling tendency in Graves' patients than in routine blepharoplasty patients, and they are told so preoperatively. The use of local steroid solutions have replaced systemic steroids in most cases to control some of the swelling tendency. It is common

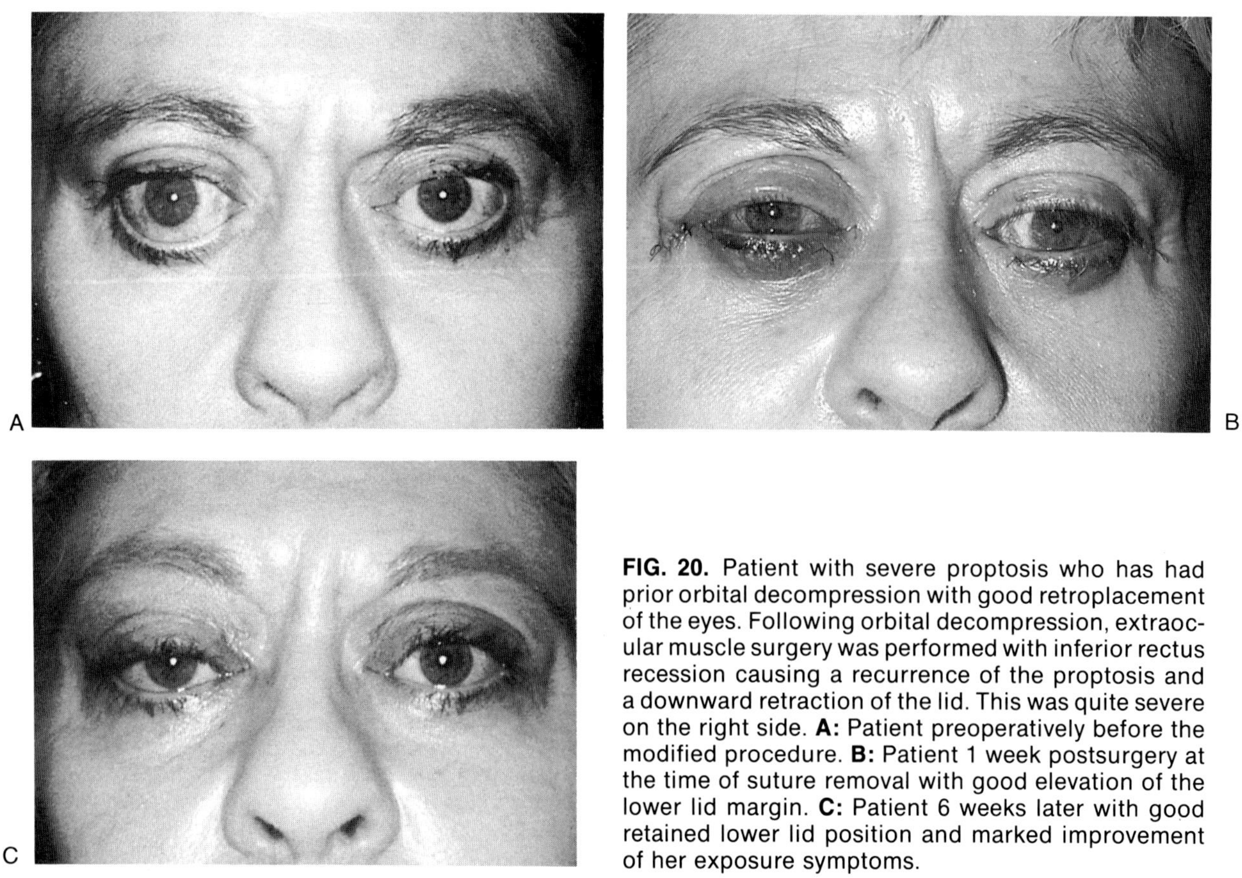

FIG. 20. Patient with severe proptosis who has had prior orbital decompression with good retroplacement of the eyes. Following orbital decompression, extraocular muscle surgery was performed with inferior rectus recession causing a recurrence of the proptosis and a downward retraction of the lid. This was quite severe on the right side. **A:** Patient preoperatively before the modified procedure. **B:** Patient 1 week postsurgery at the time of suture removal with good elevation of the lower lid margin. **C:** Patient 6 weeks later with good retained lower lid position and marked improvement of her exposure symptoms.

to need "touch-up" adjustments in the upper lid position but lower lid revisions are usually not necessary.

REFERENCES

1. McCord CD Jr. Current trends in orbital decompression. *Ophthalmology* 1985;92:21–33.
2. Walstein SS, West GH Jr, Lee WY, et al. Guanethidine in hyperthyroidism. *JAMA* 1964;189:609–612.
3. Dixon RS, Anderson RL, Hatt MU. The use of thymoxamine in eyelid retraction. *Arch Ophthalmol* 1979;97:2147–2150.
4. Henderson JW. Relief of eyelid retraction: a surgical procedure. *Arch Ophthalmol* 1965;74:205–216.
5. Chalfin J, Putterman AM. Müller's muscle excision and levator recession in retracted upper lid. *Arch Ophthalmol* 1979;97: 487–491.
6. Putterman AM. Surgical treatment of thyroid-related upper eyelid retraction. *Ophthalmology* 1981;88:507–510.
7. Doxanas MT, Dryden RM. The use of sclera in the treatment of dysthyroid eyelid retraction. *Ophthalmology* 1981;88:887–894.
8. Putterman AM, Fett DR. Müller's muscle in the treatment of upper eyelid retraction: a 12-year study. *Ophth Surg* 1986;17: 361–367.
9. Harvey JT, Anderson RA. The aponeurotic approach to eyelid retraction. *Ophthalmology* 1981;88:513–524.
10. McCord CD Jr. Surgery of the eyelids. In: Duane TD, ed. *Clinical ophthalmology*. vol 5. New York: Harper and Row; 1986: 28–29.
11. Tanenbaum M, McCord CD Jr. Graves' ophthalmopathy. In: McCord CD Jr, ed. *Oculoplastic surgery*. New York: Raven Press; 1981:169–196.
12. Trokel S, Kazin M, Moore S. Orbital fat removal. *Ophthalmology* 1993;100:674–682.
13. Olivari N. Transpalpebral decompression of endocrine ophthalmopathy (Graves' disease) by removal of intraorbital fat: experience with 147 operations over 5 years. *Plast Reconstr Surg* 1991; 87:627–643.
14. Waller RR. Lower eyelid retraction: management. *Ophth Surg* 1978;9:41–47.
15. Baylis HL, Perman RL, Fett DF, Sutcliffe RT. Autogenous auricular cartilage grafting for lower eyelid retraction. *Ophth Plast Reconstr Surg* 1985;1:23–27.
16. Karesh JW, Fabrega MA, Rodrigues MM, Glaros DS. Polytetrafluoroethylene as an interpositional graft material for the correction of lower eyelid retraction. *Ophthalmology* 1989;96:419–423.
17. Crawford JS, Easterbrook M The use of a blank sclera to correct lid retraction. *Can J Ophthalmol* 1976;11:304–309.

CHAPTER 20

Upper Eyelid Reconstruction

Full-thickness upper eyelid defects are most often those caused traumatically or created by the removal of eyelid tumors. Less commonly encountered defects are caused by loss of tissue from irradiation, burns, or inflammatory conditions such as herpes zoster or congenital colobomas. In most cases, upper eyelid defects should be reconstructed immediately, although patients who exhibit an adequate Bell's phenomenon and tear film may tolerate an upper eyelid defect temporarily.

A number of procedures are available for upper lid reconstruction and are usually chosen on the basis of the ease or convenience to the patient combined with the desire to give the patient the best-looking final result. In some cases, convenience will take priority over final cosmetic appearance, and age of the patient influences the choice of procedure. In general terms, the procedure that produces a functional improvement and gives the best-looking result that is the easiest for the patient to go through is the proper one. In certain older patients or in some patients with severe or traumatic defects, a less cosmetic procedure is necessary to produce a functional result acceptable to the patient. The surgeon should prioritize the choice of procedure on the basis of these factors and the patient's expectations (see chapter on decision making in eyelid reconstruction).

DIRECT CLOSURE

Upper eyelid defects resulting from tumor, trauma, or congenital defects, that are as large as one third of the lid can be closed directly in younger patients. The increased laxity of tissues in older persons may allow direct closure of defects of up to 40% of the upper lid or more with the use of lateral cantholysis to allow relaxation of tissue for approximation of the lid margin. Postoperatively these lids may appear tight and ptotic, but over several weeks the lid will undergo relaxation and possible intussusceptive growth to provide a normal appearance and opening of the upper lid. Direct closure minimizes discontinuity of the lashes and avoids multiple-stage procedures. The most important part of direct closure is reapproximation of the tarsal plate, in which the residual edges of the tarsus or "skeleton" of the upper eyelid are sutured together in as exact an approximation as possible. Use of magnification facilitates this closure. In traumatic cases an irregular or traumatized tarsus should be trimmed perpendicularly for the full vertical height of the tarsus to help this reapproximation. With tumor removal these vertical incisions can be made electively. Hesitation on the part of many surgeons to perform a full vertical excision of a tarsal segment extending to the superior tarsal border before closure results in notching or buckling of the upper lid with an abnormal lid contour. The margin does not close evenly if a superior bridge of tarsus is left (1) (Fig. 1).

Technique

The wound edges are made perpendicular to the lid margin. Before closure of the tarsal plate proper, an initial lid margin suture of 7-0 silk is passed through the gray line (mucocutaneous junction) and pulled, temporarily, to determine if the margin can be brought together directly with a moderate amount of tension on the eyelid. This suture must pass exactly through the gray lines of each wound edge with bites equidistant from the wound on each side of the defect (Fig. 2A).

If the eyelid tension is excessive with the trial suture, lateral cantholysis must be performed. A blade is used to make an incision horizontally at the lateral canthus through the skin down to the orbital rim. Sharp scissors are used to detach the upper limb of the lateral canthal tendon from the bony orbital rim in a nibbling manner to obtain the desired laxity. With larger defects the

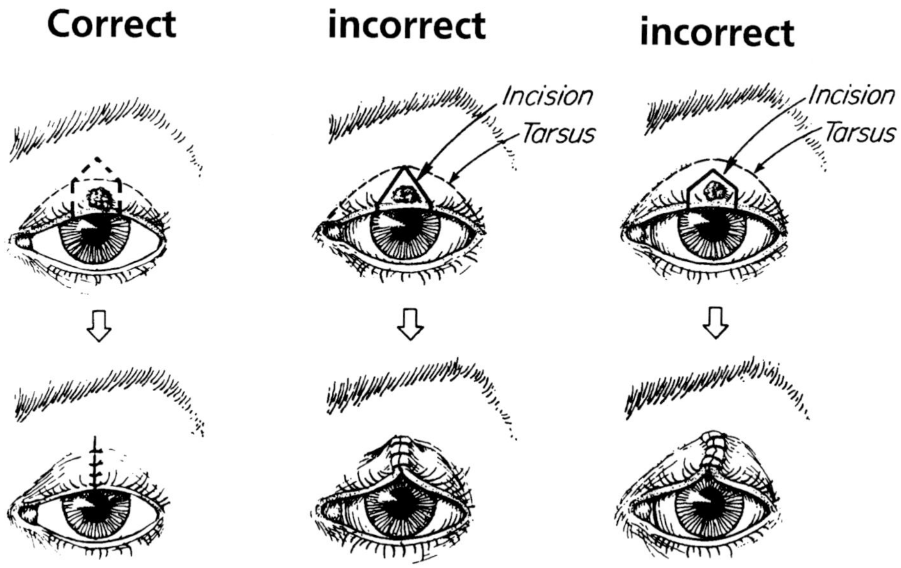

FIG. 1. Diagram showing proper design of incision for full-thickness resection of the lid and margin as well as also incisions and configurations that can cause postoperative notching and irregular contour. The full-thickness defects in the upper lid must have parallel edge-to-edge closure of tarsus that extends to the full vertical width of the tarsal plate.

entire upper lateral canthal tendon and septal strands must be severed to allow the edges of the upper lid defect to close without undue tension.

The vertical cut edges of the tarsal plate are now closed using three 7-0 silk sutures on a small needle placed half-thickness through the tarsus so that the knots are buried on the anterior surface of the tarsus (Fig. 2B). The separation of the orbicularis muscle from the tarsal plate, before the sutures are passed, ensures that only the tarsus is included in this initial part of the layered closure. Absorbable sutures such as vicryl and Dexon can be used, but the ease of tying

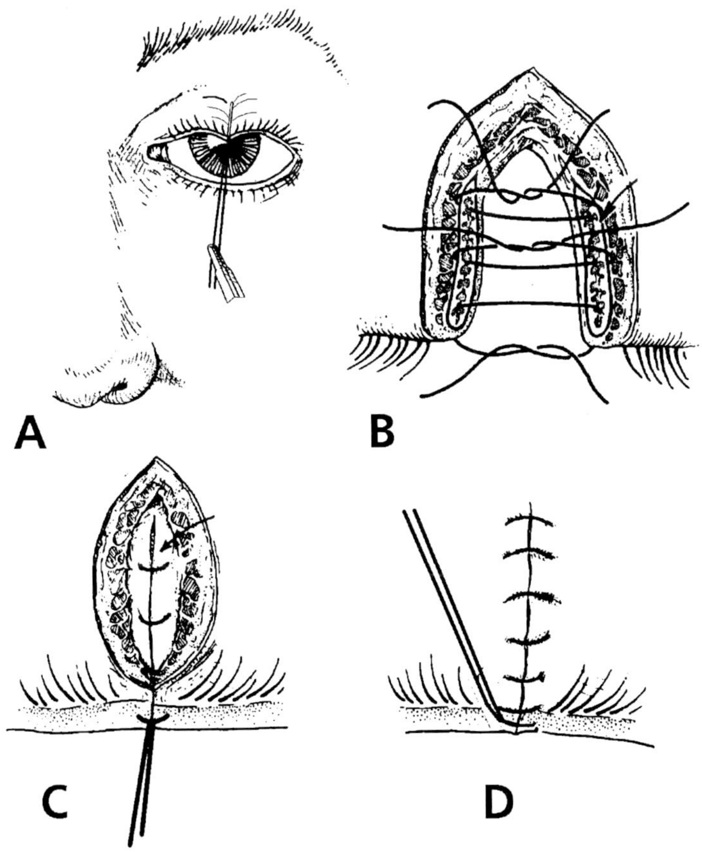

FIG. 2. Technique of direct closure of full-thickness defect of the upper lid. **A:** An initial suture is placed through the gray line of the lid for traction to align the two sides of the tarsal defect. **B:** Intratarsal sutures are placed to create stability of the posterior lamella of the lid and contour. **C:** The intratarsal sutures have been tied. **D:** A skin-muscle layer is then closed. Commonly only one suture is used in the margin of the eyelid. The ends are left long so as not to invert and abrade the cornea.

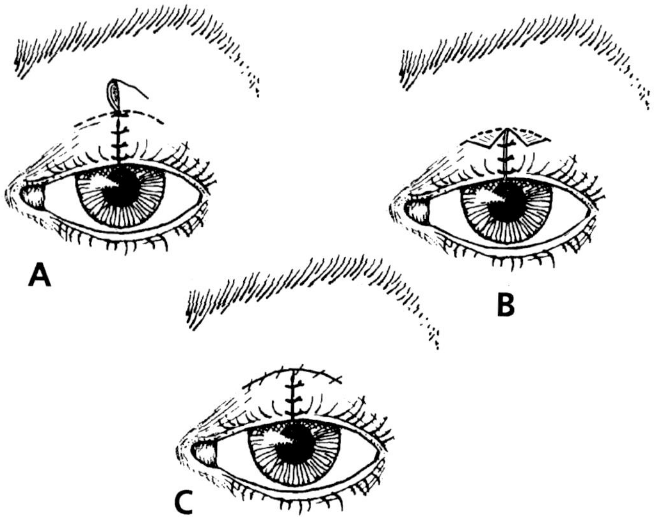

FIG. 3. Management of redundant skin above the eyelid resection. In many cases full-thickness resection and closure of the lid will cause a redundant dog ear formation above the crease. **A:** Relaxing incisions are made nasally and temporally in the dog ear in the crease line. **B:** The skin-muscle is undermined creating an overlap of Burow triangles. **C:** The triangles are excised and the crease closed.

7-0 silk is unequaled. The small silk sutures have caused no tissue reaction when left permanently and maintain approximation of the lid margin. One sutures of 7-0 silk is then placed in the eyelid margin itself approximating the lash line and the posterior edge of the eyelid. These are tied separately and left long so that they can be draped anteriorly over the lid surface (Fig. 2C, D).

A dog ear formation frequently occurs above the upper lid crease. This is best smoothed with two horizontal incisions in the fold in the line of the crease. This will produce two Burow triangles that are trimmed and the upper lid crease is closed horizontally. The resulting contour is quite cosmetically acceptable (Fig. 3A–C). The skin is then closed using interrupted or running 7-0 silk sutures. Ointment is placed on the skin edges daily. Sutures can be removed 7 days later under normal healing conditions.

The tight postoperative appearance after direct closure of larger defects will resolve in subsequent weeks and with relaxation of the tissues the lid will develop good mobility and cosmetic appearance. The necessity of sharp, vertical margins in the surgically created defects and the careful approximation of the tarsal plate so that an even upper lid contour will be produced is to be emphasized.

In problem cases, with tissue deficiency or a tendency to retraction, an additional step may be used at the time of closure to prevent notching. A reversed Frost suture may be placed at the suture line, creating downward traction on the upper lid in this area for 1 week to provide additional downward traction along the suture line.

ROTATIONAL FLAP FOR UPPER LID (TENZEL) RECONSTRUCTION

Central upper lid defects of up to 40–60% of the original lid margin can be closed in the upper lid by a semicircular skin-muscle flap rotated into the lid defect area as described by Tenzel (2) for upper and lower lid defects of a similar type.

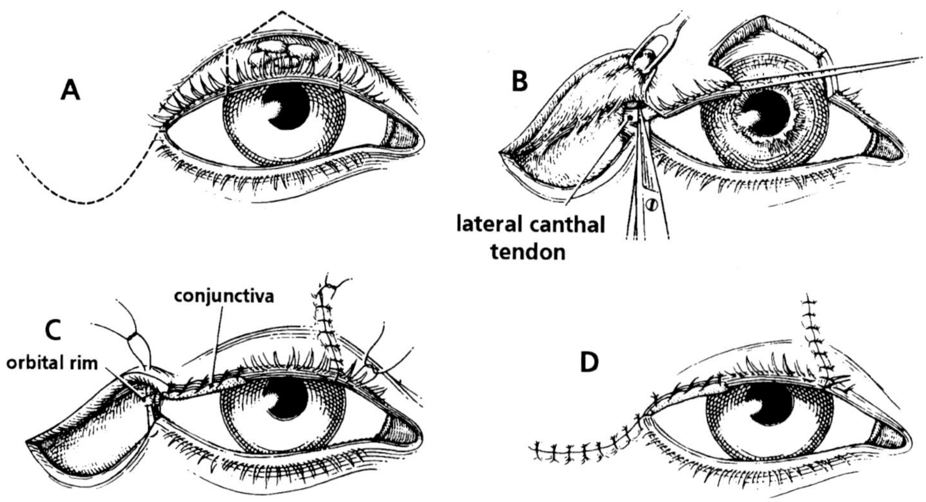

FIG. 4. Reconstruction of upper lid defect with rotational myocutaneous flap (Tenzel). **A:** Area of defect to be created in outline of semicircular flap. **B:** Development of skin-muscle flap laterally and lysis of the lateral canthal tendon and septum. **C:** The flap has been advanced with direct closure of the upper lid defect. The advanced flap has been fixated at the appropriate position to the lateral orbital rim. The margin of the advanced flap is lined with advanced conjunctiva. **D:** Position of final sutures.

Technique

The upper lid defect should be fashioned so that the tarsal edges are perfectly perpendicular to the lid margin as described under the section on direct closure. An inferior arching semicircular line is drawn with methylene blue at the lateral canthus (Fig. 4A). The diameter of the flap can be from 2 to 6 cm in diameter, extending inferiorly and temporally to the lateral extension of the hairline. The musculocutaneous flap incision is made with a blade and the needle cutting Bovie is used to cut through the muscle fibers for hemostasis. A lateral canthotomy incision is made beneath the semicircular skin incision and dissection is carried out to the lateral orbital rim. The superior ramus of the lateral canthal tendon is cut and the upper lid mobilized completely at the lateral aspect, detaching it from the lateral orbital rim (Fig. 4B). Care should be taken to preserve the inferior ramus of the lateral canthal tendon. The flap is then undermined and rotated inward. The edge of the flap is advanced to the medial edge of the defect and repaired with layered closure as described in the direct closure section (Fig. 4C). Lateral lid support is obtained and canthal formation is accomplished by suturing the edge of the flap to the inner periosteum of the lateral orbital rim with fixation to the inferior ramus. This step of lateral canthal fixation is necessary to allow the new upper lid to curve inward and follow the contour of the globe. Conjunctiva can be undermined and advanced to the edge of the flap margin and sutured with a 7-0 silk running suture (Fig. 4D). The lateral incision is closed directly with mattress sutures and standard skin closure. If a dog ear is encountered because of unequal edges, a small triangle may have to be excised temporally.

SLIDING TARSAL (TARSOCONJUNCTIVAL) FLAP

Isolated medial or lateral defects of the upper lid too large to close with direct closure or those occurring in children susceptible to amblyopia can be reconstructed without the bridge flap technique, which involves eyelid closure and lid sharing. This is accomplished by horizontally sliding a section of tarsus from the remaining lid segment into the defect and covering the external surface with a skin graft (1).

Technique

To reconstruct the defect shown in Fig. 5A, the lid remnant is everted over a Desmarres retractor. A horizontal incision is made in the tarsal plate with a blade

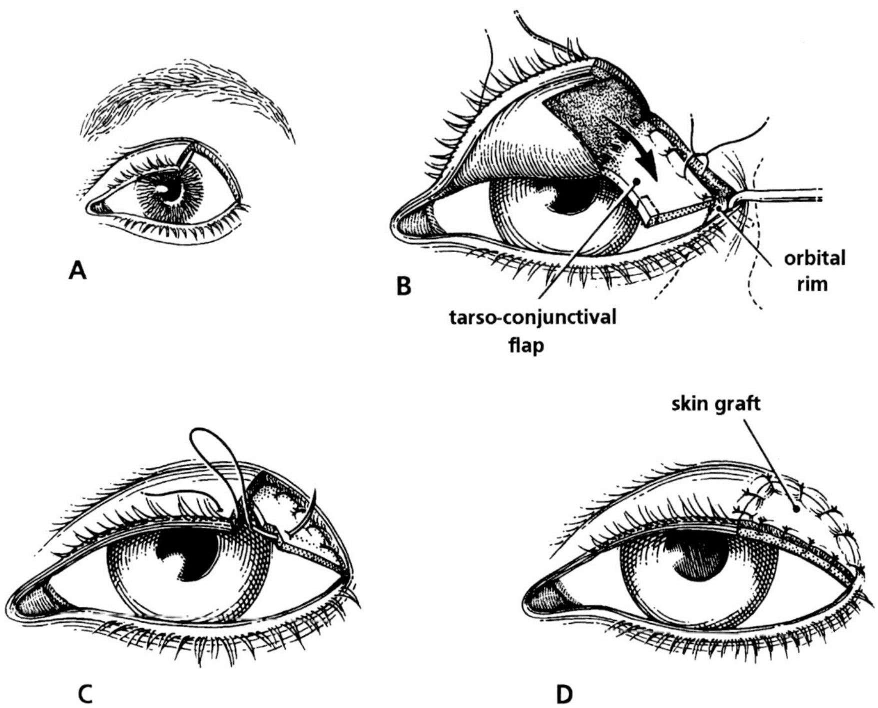

FIG. 5. Reconstruction of a temporal upper lid defect with sliding tarsoconjunctival flap. **A:** Area of temporal upper lid defect. **B:** Development of tarsoconjunctival flap from under surface of the upper lid advancing laterally and suturing the periosteum for lateral fixation inside the orbital rim. The flap is developed 4 mm above the margin to avoid margin deformity. **C:** Attachment of the edge of the flap to the residual lid edge for alignment. **D:** Covering of the defect with a skin graft. An advancement skin-muscle flap can also be used.

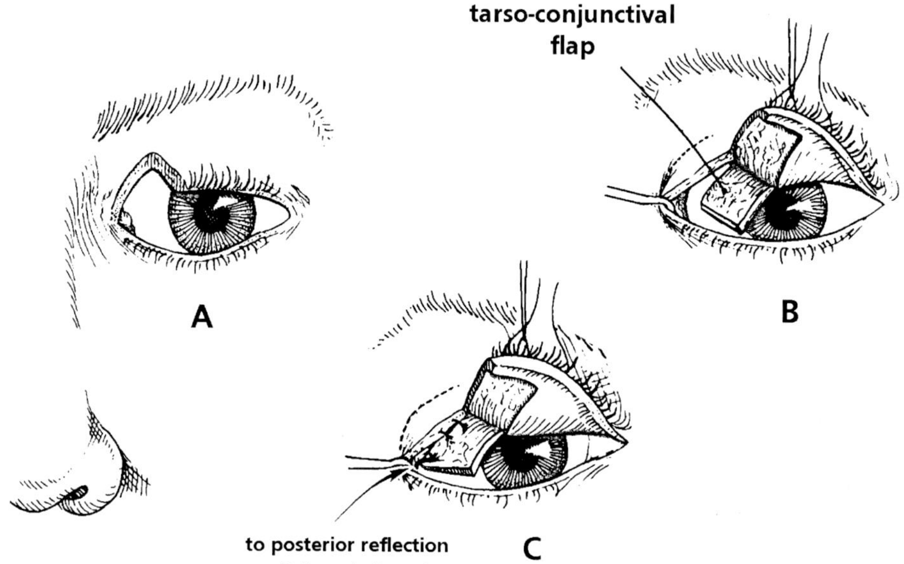

FIG. 6. Reconstruction of nasal upper lid full-thickness defect with sliding tarsoconjunctival flap. **A:** A nasal upper lid defect. **B:** The lid has been everted in the flap developed from the undersurface of the lid as into the lateral technique. **C:** The flap is fixated medially with proper medial fixation to the posterior reflection of the medial canthal tendon. The temporal edge of the flap is attached to the residual lid edge. The skin defect can be covered with a skin graft, an advancement flap, or a glabellar flap.

4 mm above the lid margin and approximately the width of the defect. An additional relaxing incision is then made vertically in the tarsus with a blade to the superior border of the tarsus and into the upper fornix (Fig. 5B).

This tarsal-conjunctival flap is horizontally moved into the defect. One edge is attached to the periosteum or remnants of the lateral canthal tendon inside the orbital rim with a permanent suture such as 4-0 prolene. A half-circle P–2 needle makes this placement easier. The superior border of the tarsal flap is sutured to the cut edges of the levator aponeurosis. The edge of the tarsal flap next to the remaining upper lid margin is anchored to the margin with a 6-0 silk suture. The suture is placed at half-tarsal thickness so as not to be exposed on the undersurface of the lid, to prevent corneal irritation (Fig. 5C). A full-thickness graft from the retroauricular area is placed over this tarsoconjunctival flap and sutured into place with interrupted 7-0 silk (Fig. 5D). The eyelids are closed with mattress sutures that are left in place for 1 week before removal. Dressing of the graft is important. Telfa is placed directly over the graft, then moist cotton applied over the Telfa. Finally, a moderate pressure dressing of eyepads is placed over the wound. The eyelid closure sutures immobilize the lid and prevent shrinkage; the dressing keeps gentle pressure to ensure better grafting results from the full-thickness graft.

Defects in the upper lid occurring at the inner canthus are repaired similarly, sliding a tarsoconjunctival flap into the defect in a horizontal manner and covering the surface with a full-thickness skin graft. It is important that fixation of the sliding flap at the inner canthus be made to the posterior reflection of the canthal tendon (Fig. 6A–C). If the flap is fixed too anteriorly, the resultant lid will not follow the contour of the globe and separation of the lid from the globe will occur.

Loss of upper lid lashes is more conspicuous nasally than temporally and conversion of a nasal defect to a lateral defect can overcome this problem. In appropriate cases with nasal defects, a vertical incision is made at the lateral canthus and the lid segment containing lashes is moved close to the nasal defect. The resulting temporal defect is then reconstructed as previously described.

The full-thickness skin graft over the fixated tarsal flap should be sutured carefully to the newly created lid margin or tarsus and conjunctiva, but should not be rotated underneath the margin, which would result in irritation of the cornea by the keratinized epithelium. Failure to use an intermarginal traction suture or a reverse Frost suture at the junction of the flap and eyelid margin can result in shrinkage of the graft and notching of that area of the upper eyelid.

LOCAL MYOCUTANEOUS FLAPS WITH POSTERIOR LAMELLAR GRAFT

In patients who have laxity or redundancy of skin in the upper lid and periorbital area, skin-muscle flaps

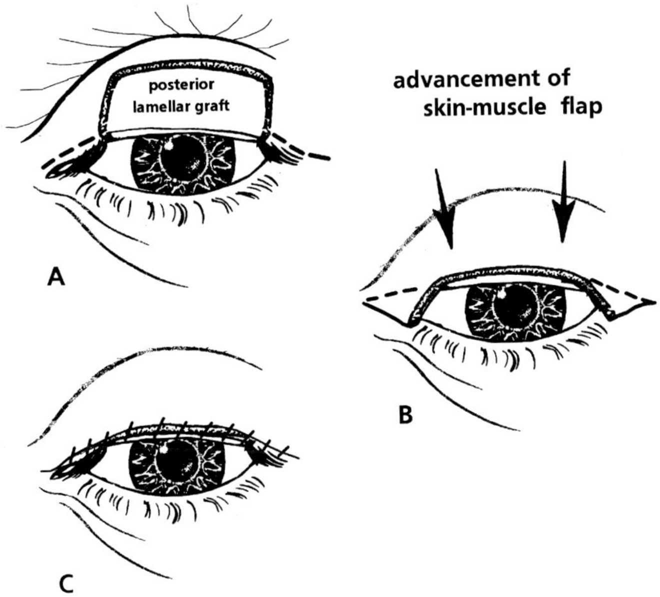

FIG. 7. Reconstruction of upper lid defect in patients who have skin muscle laxity with an advancement myocutaneous flap and a posterior lamellar graft. **A:** A central upper lid defect showing placement of a posterior lamellar graft. The graft must have a mucous membrane line surface or, if not, placed on top of an advanced conjunctival flap. **B:** Following placement of the graft the skin is undermined and advanced vertically to the lid edge and the redundant skin removed. **C:** Final closure.

can be brought in to cover the external lamellar defect (3). This technique, if it can be performed, has the advantage of being a one-stage procedure and avoids an intermediate stage of eyelid closure. The flaps can either be advancement or rotational. These must be

TABLE 1. *Grafts and flaps for construction of posterior lamella of upper lid*

Free tarsoconjunctival graft
Palatal mucoperiosteal graft
Buccal mucous membrane graft
Conjunctival advancement from upper fornix
Conjunctival advancement flap from lower lid
Composite eyelid graft (including margin and lashes)
Nasal mucoperichondrial graft

backed with a posterior lamellar lining or graft to create a posterior lamella for the upper lid. In many cases conjunctiva from the upper lid fornix or an advancement flap of conjunctiva from the lower lid can be used to supplement the posterior lamellar lining. Fornix conjunctival advancement can be combined with an ear cartilage graft. Free grafts of rigid mucous membrane–lined tissue such as tarsoconjunctiva or palatal mucoperiosteum are ideal for this purpose (Table 1).

In lax-skinned older patients with centrally placed upper lid full-thickness defects, a posterior lamellar graft can be placed in the defect and covered with the redundant skin and muscle that is present in the upper lid. This is particularly convenient with residual tarsus remaining nasally and temporally, or if there is a remaining bridge of tarsus remaining superiorly.

If adequate upper lid and brow skin laxity is present, a posterior lamellar graft can be placed in the defect and a skin-muscle flap dissected in a superior direction. The flap can then be brought inferiorly to cover the lid surface. There will usually be an uneven edge to the flap and revisions of the edge with trimming is needed for smooth contour (Fig. 7A–C).

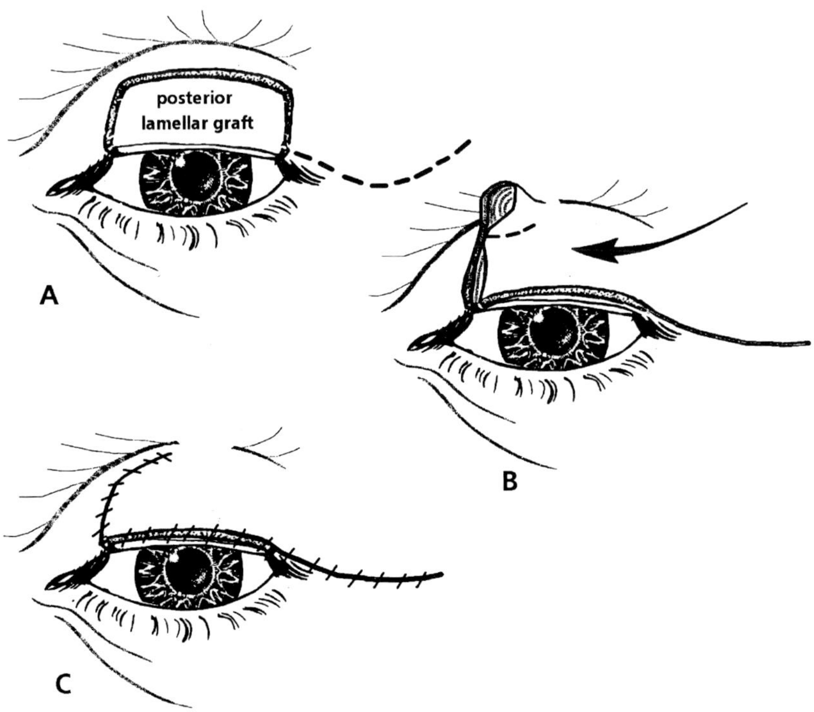

FIG. 8. Reconstruction of full-thickness upper lid defect in patients with laxity of the skin-muscle layer. **A:** Shows defect with outline and placement of a rotational myocutaneous advancement flap. **B:** The myocutaneous flap has been advanced laterally and sutured. There is always a redundant dog ear formation, which is corrected with Burow triangle formation and excision. **C:** Final suturing of the flap into position.

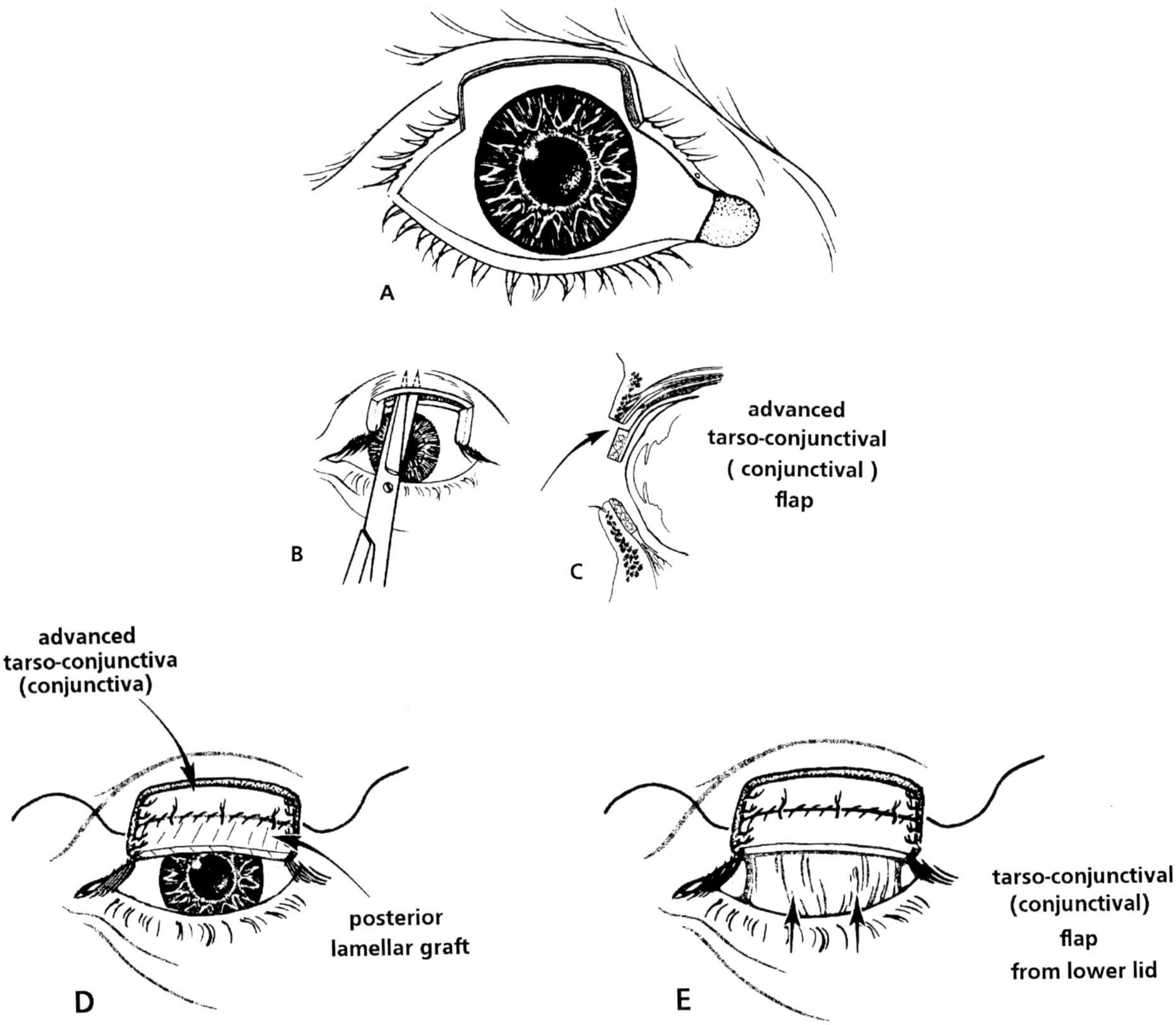

FIG. 9. Reconstruction of central upper lid defect with residual tarsus by advancement of tarsus or tarsoconjunctiva to create posterior lamella. **A:** Upper lid defect. **B:** Residual tarsus and/or conjunctiva is undermined vertically and advanced downward. **C:** Sagittal view showing downward advancement of tarsoconjunctiva. **D:** Advanced tarsoconjunctiva is sutured to the new eyelid margin edge. It must be completely dissected free from the retractors of the upper lid. If there is not enough tarsoconjunctiva in the upper lid to advance, it can be supplemented with a posterior lamella graft. **E:** With deficient tarsoconjunctiva in the upper lid, supplementation of the mucous membrane of the posterior lamella can be accomplished with an advancement tarsoconjunctival flap from the lower lid in lieu of a mucous membrane–lined free graft. The resulting skin-muscle defect is then closed with one of the advancement flap techniques.

In some cases it may be more convenient to cover the posterior lamellar graft with a rotational skin-muscle flap. A semicircular incision is made in the skin-muscle layer laterally and a flap developed and brought across the defect (Fig. 8A). After horizontal closure of the inferior portion there will usually be a redundant dog ear formation above the crease (Fig. 8B). A relaxing incision and excision of a Burow triangle will equalize the edges for smooth closure (Fig. 8C).

In some cases the size of the posterior lamellar defect can be lessened by advancing tarsoconjunctiva from above if there is residual tissue present (Fig. 9A–C). An additional source of lining for the posterior lamella of the upper lid is conjunctiva (tarsoconjunctiva) from the lower lid. This source of mucous membrane can be used to supplement any of the other methods of posterior lamellar replacement (Fig. 9D, E).

LOWER (OPPOSING) EYELID FLAPS

The technique of sharing a lid flap from the lower lid provides a good functional result in patients with large defects who do not have enough skin laxity for local closure. These flaps have the disadvantage of requiring two stages and an intermediate stage of eyelid fusion, but they must be used in patients who do not have a lot of laxity or in patients with laxity but very large defects.

BRIDGE (CUTLER–BEARD) FLAP

The Cutler–Beard (4) or bridge flap (5) technique is used to reconstruct larger full-thickness eyelid defects, including total loss of the upper lid. The technique consists of advancing a full-thickness flap from the opposing normal lower lid. A full-thickness flap of skin, muscle, and conjunctiva is developed beneath the intact lower lid margin and advanced into the defect. The incision to create the flap is made 4–5 mm below the lower lid margin to reserve the vascular supply and prevent devitalization of the remaining bridge of the lower lid margin (Fig. 10A). Because this flap contains little or no tarsus (6), we have modified the original Cutler–Beard procedure (7) by inserting ear cartilage between the skin, muscle, and conjunctiva, to be used as a tarsal replacement in reconstructing a more stable upper lid.

Technique

The upper lid defect is created in a rectangular fashion, with adequate excision of the tumor mass or, in traumatic and congenital defects, by "freshening" of the epithelialized border (Fig. 10A). If the defect includes the entire upper lid, the lateral borders will contain no tarsal plates but rather the medial or lateral canthal tendons. The flap of tissue to be used from the lower lid should be approximately the same width as the upper lid defect. In very lax upper lids the flap of tissue from the lower lid may be narrower because the upper lid edges may stretch to reduce the size of the defect.

A horizontal full-thickness incision is made in the lower lid 5 mm below the margin (just below the base of the tarsus and the marginal artery) (6) using a blade, with a corneal protector or lid plate between the lower lid and globe for protection. At the end of the horizontal incision, full-thickness incisions with a blade are carried vertically downward to the lowest aspect of the inferior fornix on the conjunctival side of the flap. The skin is undermined over the malar eminence. Once the

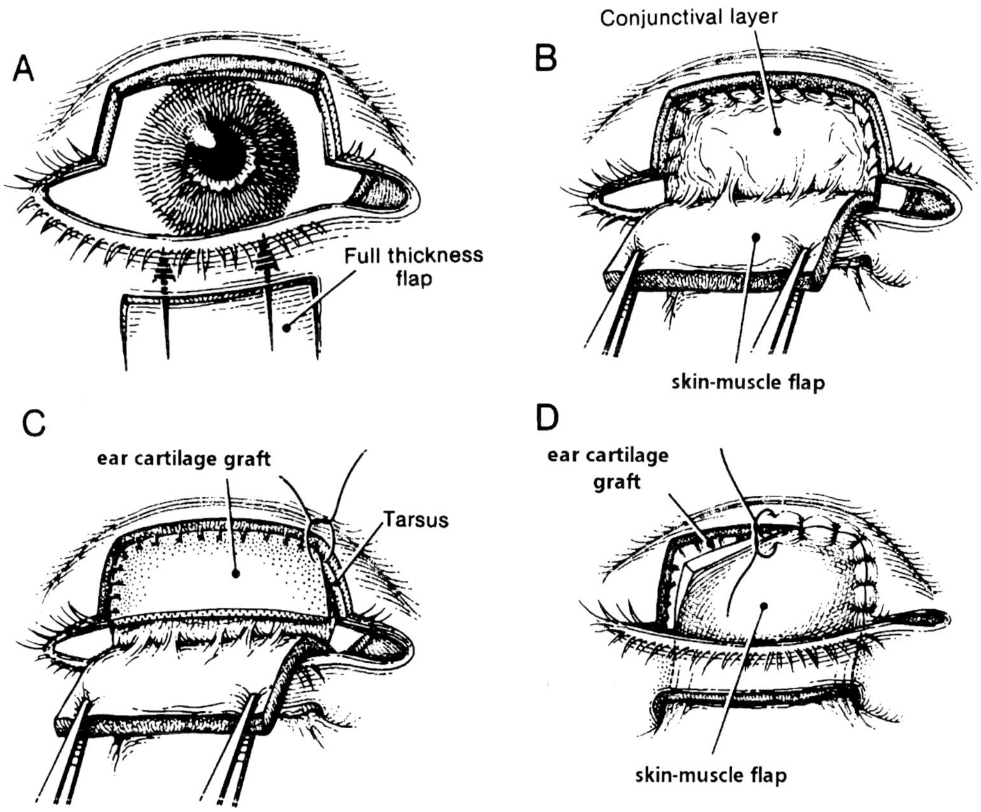

FIG. 10. A lid-sharing bridge flap technique for reconstruction of larger upper lid defects (Cutler–Beard). **A:** Upper lid defect and outline of skin-muscle flap to be advanced beneath the eyelid margin into the upper lid. **B:** The posterior lamella of the advancement flap has been sutured to the posterior lamella of the upper lid. **C:** An autogenous ear cartilage graft has been inserted in front of the advanced posterior lamella and will be covered by the anterior lamella (skin-muscle) in a sandwich manner. **D:** The anterior lamella (skin-muscle) has been sutured over the graft.

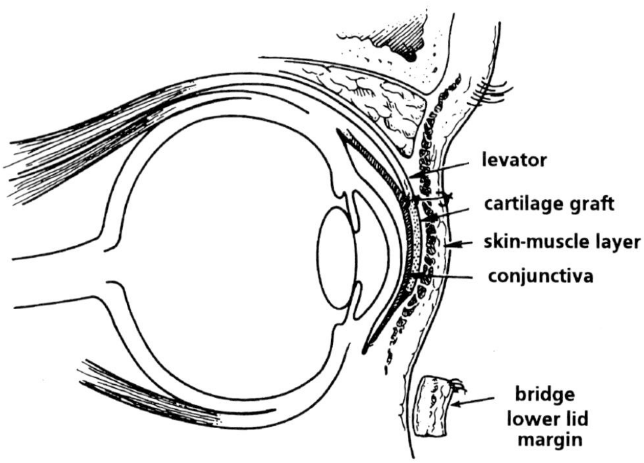

FIG. 11. Sagittal view of the interim stage of the bridge flap technique showing the flap in position containing the ear cartilage graft. The tissue is left in this position for approximately 6–8 weeks.

flap is incised, contraction of the orbicularis muscle and elastic tissue gives the appearance that inadequate horizontal dimension has been prepared; however, this will stretch to fit the defect in the closure to be described.

The flap is then put on a stretch with skin hooks, and sharp Westcott scissors are used to dissect the conjunctival layer of the flap from the musculocutaneous layer. Some relaxing incisions in the capsulopalpebral fascia may be needed. This flap of conjunctiva is pulled up under the bridge of the lower lid margin. The conjunctival layer of the flap is sutured to the conjuctiva of the upper lid defect with a running 6-0 plain gut suture (Fig. 10B).

An autogenous ear cartilage graft is harvested as described in the chapter on grafts. It is fashioned to fit the upper lid defect. Ear cartilage is then sutured with interrupted 7-0 silk medially and laterally to the tarsal remnants (medial or lateral canthal tendons if all the tarsus has been excised) and superiorly to the cut edge of the levator aponeurosis. If this has been excised the cartilage should be attached to the levator muscle itself (Fig. 10C).

Finally, the musculocutaneous flap from the lower lid is advanced under the bridge of the lid margin and sutured into the skin edges of the upper lid defect with interrupted 7-0 silk (Fig. 10D). Additional undermining of the skin flap may be necessary to allow it to advance into place. The orbicularis muscle in this flap of tissue will fit the shape of the defect without undue tension as the skin is closed. The cartilage graft has now been interposed in a sandwich manner between the flap of conjunctiva and the musculocutaneous layer from the lower lid (Fig. 11).

Separation of the flap is carefully carried out 8 weeks later. Premature separation may result in shrinkage. The flap should be left longer in cases of irradiated tissue or alkaline burns. Methylene blue is used to mark the incision to separate the flap approximately 2 mm below the desired position of the new upper lid margin. The assistant provides downward retraction on the bridge and a grooved director is placed under the flap so that a blade can be used to make an incision through the skin (Fig. 12A). Scissors are used to make the incision full thickness. One to two millimeters of keratinized skin and muscle is trimmed, leaving 2 mm of extra conjunctiva to rotate anteriorly over the lid margin, so that the lid margin will be composed of mucous membrane rather than keratinized epithelium (Fig. 12B). Failure to "overcorrect" the amount of mucous membrane on the lid margin can result in corneal erosion from keratinized (skin) epithelium or trichiasis of hairs of the skin.

Attention is then directed to the lower lid, where the inferior aspect of the lower lid margin bridge is deepithelialized. The lower lid conjunctiva can be left

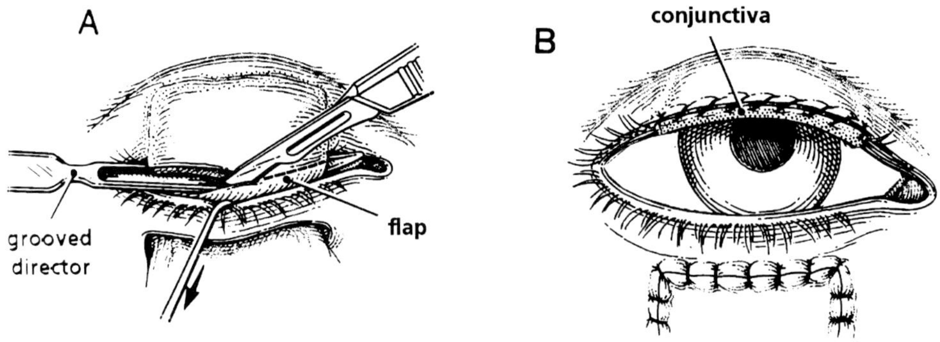

FIG. 12. Bridge flap technique with second-stage opening of the flap. **A:** A groove director is inserted beneath the flap to protect the eye and the flap is completely incised. Care is taken to incise the flap far down enough to allow for adequate tissue for the new upper lid. **B:** The upper lid margin has been reformed. Some subconjunctival tissue is usually trimmed to allow the conjunctiva to rotate outward to form a new lid margin. The skin should not be on the edge of the lid in order to avoid trichiasis. The lower lid flap has been repositioned after revision of edges and sutured in position.

open. The lower lid skin edges are closed with running 7-0 silk. The lower aspects of the cheek incision may need to be undermined and redundancies excised to promote smooth closure and prevent lower lid malposition. Full-thickness mattress sutures of 4-0 silk can be used to form a lid fold at the time the bridge flap is separated. All sutures are removed 1 week after separation of the flap. Edema is usually present in the upper lid for 4–5 weeks and then the reconstructed eyelid resumes a more normal appearance, with a stable lid margin and good vertical mobility.

If cartilage or eyebank sclera is not available for a tarsal replacement, the flap from the lower lid is sutured into the defect in two interrupted layers as originally described by Cutler and Beard in the manner described, omitting the placement of eye bank sclera or cartilage. Other materials, such as Gore-tex, have been used instead of autogeneous material (8).

Shortcomings of Bridge Flap

The absence of lashes from the reconstructed segment may be treated with artificial lashes or lash grafts. Although hair-bearing grafts can be placed, they generally do not have a normal appearance.

Should a notch develop where the reconstructed segment meets the lid margin, revision can be accomplished by excising the notch, followed by direct closure. Corneal irritation from trichiasis of skin hairs can be eliminated with application of lid cryotherapy or excision.

A shortened upper lid with resultant lagophthalmos can be prevented by suturing upper lid remnants as far down on the advanced flap as possible to include the greatest amount of musculocutaneous flap in the reconstructed defect. Consequently, when the flap is finally separated, the upper lid will have a greater vertical dimension.

PEDICLE FLAP FROM LOWER LID MARGIN

The technique of rotating a pedicle flap from the lower lid margin to the upper lid is a modification of Mustarde's technique for total upper lid reconstruction (9). This modification is thought to be useful in cases with broad shallow defects. It is also useful in cases in which an abnormal eyelid margin is encountered that resists reconstruction by conventional methods or if the patient simply wishes to have intact lashes restored to the upper lid. In this technique, the margin of the lower lid is transferred to the upper lid in a two-staged procedure with placement of the pedicle into the upper lid during the first stage and separation of the pedicle and revision of the lower lid during the second stage.

Technique

A full-thickness pedicle taken from the central portion of the lower lid margin is developed as shown in Fig. 13A. It is important to outline the pedicle in the central portion of the lower lid because it makes subse-

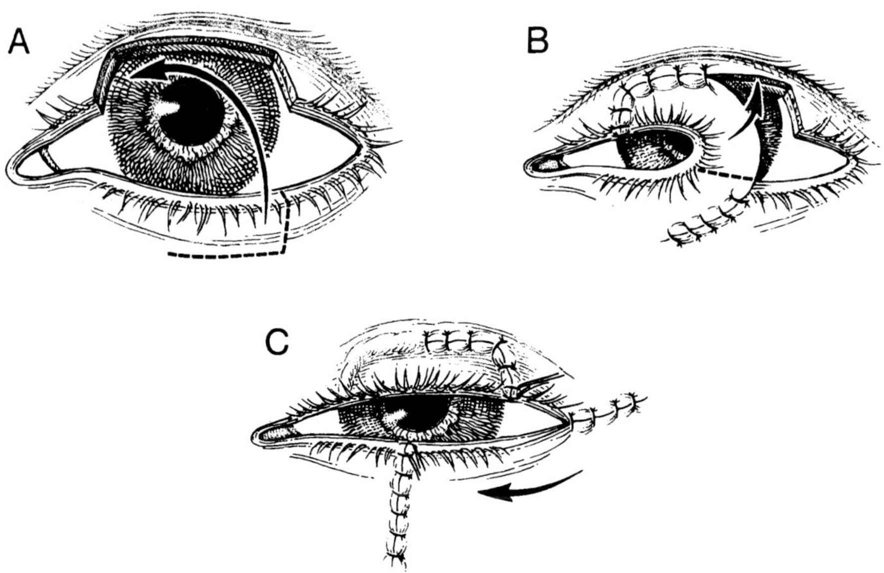

FIG. 13. Reconstruction of a shallow margin upper lid defect with eyelash-bearing pedicle from lower lid. **A:** Upper lid defect showing rotation of a pedicle flap including eyelid margin to the upper lid. The flap is usually based in the central portion of the lid so that closure can be facilitated by the stretchability of the canthal tendons. **B:** Flap being rotated into position and sutured for the intermediate stage. **C:** Final position after flap has been severed from the lower lid and revision of the lower lid if needed. A 6-week interval is required before separation.

quent closure of the lower lid defect easier in the second stage. It is possible to outline the pedicle closer to the canthal angles if the upper lid defect is off midline; however, it should be emphasized that closure of the lower lid defect is much easier if the pedicle is rotated from the central portion of the lower lid. Care is taken after developing the pedicle to ensure that the marginal artery is included, and this means including the entire tarsus of the lower lid in the pedicle flap. The vertical width of the tarsal plate in the lower lid averages 3.8 mm in most people (6), and the peripheral arcade is approximately at the base of the tarsus, so that a flap at least 5 mm in height should be designed. It should be rectangular and not elliptical as in Mustarde's original technique. The end of the flap is then rotated and margin-to-margin attachment made from the flap and lower lid margin to the upper lid (Fig. 13B). Some kinking may be encountered, but if the peripheral arcade from the lower lid is intact, good blood supply will ensue. It is impossible to suture the flap entirely in position in the upper lid, but the end of the flap and the edge must be approximated to establish blood supply in the upper lid. This is done with multiple sutures of 7-0 silk. Care is taken not to cauterize vessels near the base because this may compromise the flap. A pressure bandage is not applied but rather a shield, so as to avoid any compression so the flap retains its blood supply. The flap will stay pink. In about 4–6 weeks it should gain a blood supply from the upper lid so that it can be severed from the lower lid.

The second stage of the pedicle flap is the separation of the base of the flap from the lower lid, its rotation to the upper lid defect, and closure of the lower lid. A slanting wedge is designed that encompasses the base of the flap in the lower lid. This is excised full thickness and the lower lid is then closed in a manner described in the chapter on closure of full-thickness lower lid defects (Fig. 7C). A slanting musculocutaneous wedge precludes in most cases the need for much dog ear correction in the lower lid closure (see chapter on lower lid reconstruction). If marked tension is encountered, a cantholysis should be performed to close the lower lid. In most cases the resulting lower lid shows a reduction in the number of lashes, but if closure is accomplished in a precise manner the resulting contour is excellent. The defect in the upper lid commonly has to be modified to accept the full flap. Some additional tarsus may be trimmed from the upper lid so that the flap can be incorporated in an even manner.

When the flap is rotated in position, initially and over the next few weeks it may seem that too much tissue is present. As weeks go by, however, there will be a tendency for some shrinkage, and although revisional excision may be necessary it should be delayed as long as possible to allow this shrinkage to take place. In most cases the result is excellent as far as restoring

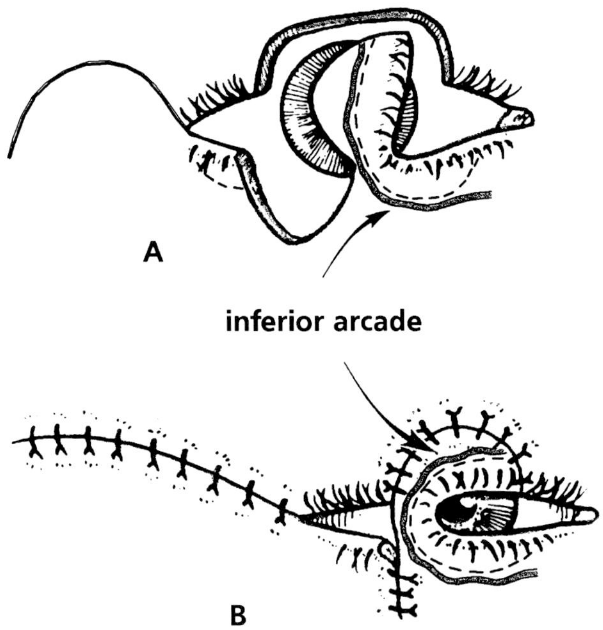

FIG. 14. Reconstruction of a large upper lid defect with a pedicle from lower lid (Mustarde). **A:** A large pedicle segment of lower lid is rotated into upper lid defect following canthotomy, cantholysis, and advancement of the lower lid. **B:** Closure of lower lid defect with advancement myocutaneous flap. The pedicle segment is sutured into the upper lid defect. A 6- to 8-week interval is required before separation.

the contour of the lid. The lashes, although somewhat shorter than normal upper lid lashes, appear to be adequate from a cosmetic standpoint. This procedure is the best corrective procedure for margin defects including lashes but does require some skill on the part of the surgeon and patience on the part of the patient.

Larger margin deficiencies in the upper lid may require larger and wider flaps from the lower lid. The original method described by Mustarde in which a large segment pedicle flap to the upper lid is combined with a lower lid lateral rotational myocutaneous flap may be used (9). This technique is easier if the pedicle flap is based nasally (Fig. 14A). The same important principle of sparing the inferior vascular arcade in the base of the lower lid pedicle applies with this technique. The lower lid defect is much larger and a more formal lower lid reconstructive procedure is needed after the flap is rotated. The lateral rotation flap is described in the chapter on lower lid reconstruction (Fig. 14B).

FREE GRAFTS: SPLIT LEVEL EYELID GRAFTS (FOR VERTICAL FULL-THICKNESS DEFECTS SPARING MARGIN)

A defect of full-thickness vertical shortening of the upper eyelid with an intact lid margin is usually caused by cicatricial changes following burns, trauma, irradia-

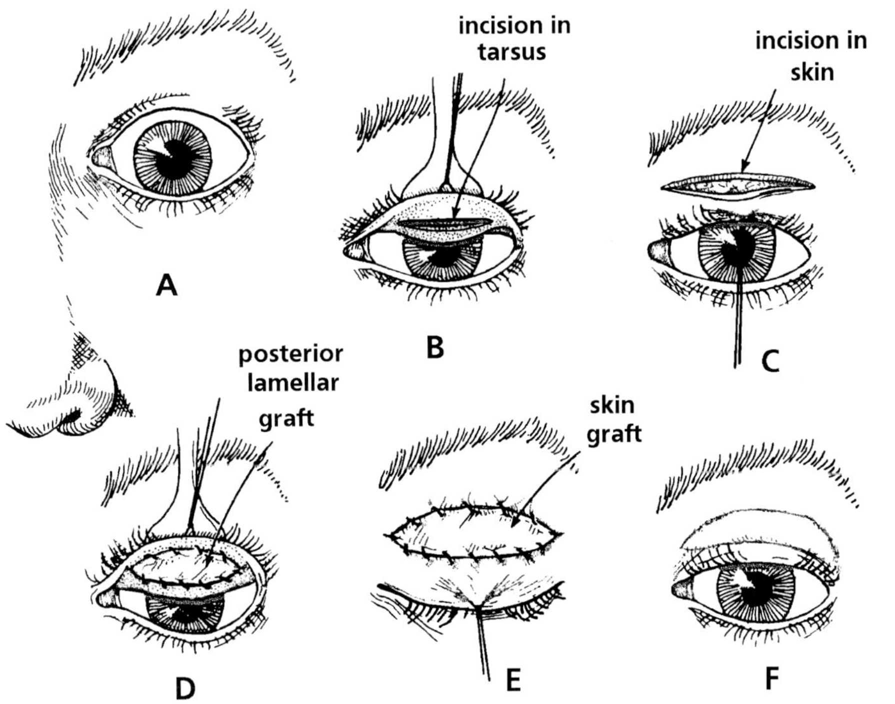

FIG. 15. Repair of full-thickness upper lid shortening (defect) sparing eyelid margin with split level grafting technique (Brown–Beard). **A:** Vertically retracted upper lid from shortage of anterior and posterior lamella with intact margin. **B:** The upper lid inverted with a relaxing incision in the posterior lamellar and retractor layers. **C:** Incision in the anterior lamella (skin-muscle of the upper lid) offset from the lower incision. **D:** Eversion of the lower lid showing placement of a mucous membrane graft to the posterior lamella lengthening the posterior lamella. **E:** Anterior view of skin graft to the anterior lamella lengthening the anterior lamella. **F:** Final lowered position of the upper lid margin following the split level grafting.

tion, or severe inflammation, such as herpes zoster. Brown and Beard (10) developed a method to correct full-thickness defects of this type in the upper lid using split level full-thickness eyelid grafts of skin and mucous membrane. Each graft is furnished a vascularized bed. In this method postauricular skin is used for the anterior lamella; buccal mucous membrane (or nasal chondromucosa) is used for the posterior lamella. The upper lid is split and separated so that the two grafts are laced at different levels in the eyelid, with each graft resting on its own vascular bed to ensure survival. Because this technique is usually employed with severely cicatrized upper lids, the grafts may undergo some shrinkage. The addition of a few millimeters of vertical lengthening of the upper lid with this procedure, however, may add an adequate margin of corneal protection to eliminate exposure in cases of diseased corneas.

Technique

The vertically shortened upper lid (Fig. 15A) is everted, if possible, over a Desmarres retractor and a horizontal incision made through the tarsal surface approximately 5 mm above the eyelid margin (Fig. 15B). The retractor is removed, the lid pulled downward with mattress suture through the margin, and a horizontal skin incision made across the upper lid above the superior edge of the tarsal border (Fig. 15C) with a blade. If eversion of the upper lid is not possible because of ridigity, the external skin incision is made first; after retraction of the skin edge, eversion is easier and the tarsal incision is made. Sharp scissors are used to undermine the skin superiorly and inferiorly, releasing any traction bands holding the eyelid in the retracted position.

The lower edge of the skin incision is then joined with the upper edge of the tarsal incision (see Figs. 16A–C). With the upper lid everted over a Desmarres retractor a full-thickness buccal mucous membrane or chondromucosal graft is sutured into the posterior incisions between the cut edges of the tarsal conjunctiva with a continuous G-O plain gut suture (Fig. 15D). With the lid retracted downward, a retroauricular full-thickness skin graft is placed into the anterior incision with either interrupted or running 7-0 silk sutures (Fig. 15E). The pattern of graft placement may be revised if new mucous membrane is needed on the lid margin. Margin sutures of 7-0 silk are used to perform a temporary

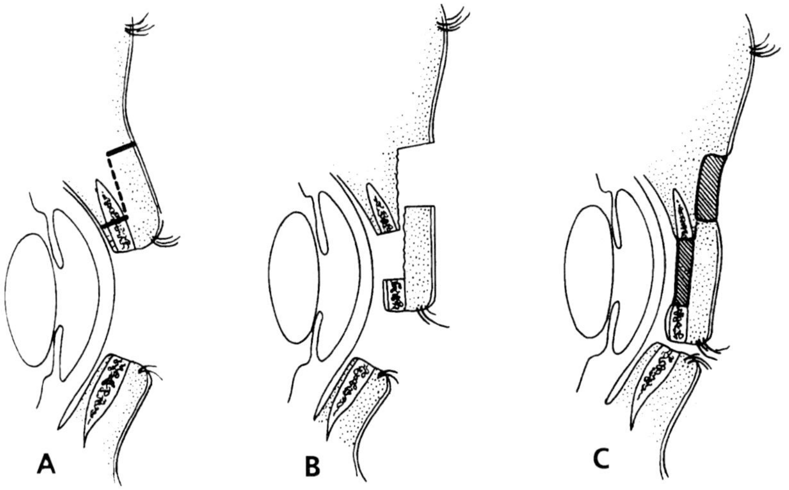

FIG. 16. Sagittal view of split level grafting. **A:** Incisions made in the anterior and posterior lamella. **B:** Dissection has been made through the full-thickness lid allowing lowering of the lid margin but creating defects in the anterior and posterior lamella. **C:** Position of the anterior and posterior lamellar grafts.

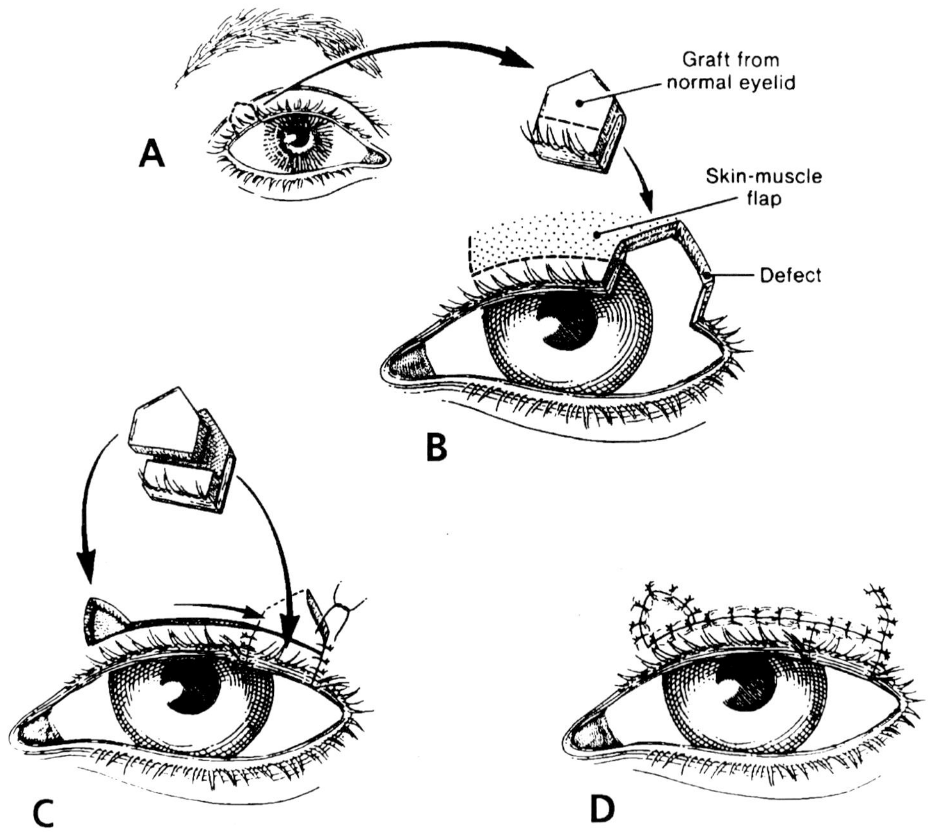

FIG. 17. Repair of upper lid defect with composite eyelid graft (Putterman). **A:** A full-thickness resection of the donor (contralateral) eyelid including the margin with closure is performed. **B:** The graft from the donor eyelid is placed in the defect in the recipient eyelid and a skin-muscle flap is developed. **C:** The skin-muscle tissue from the donor composite graft is excised leaving only a small strip of the lashes and the graft is placed in the defect. The skin-muscle flap is then advanced horizontally to cover the exposed tarsus of the graft. If needed, the skin excised from the graft can be placed nasally. **D:** Final position of the composite graft skin-muscle flap and skin graft if needed.

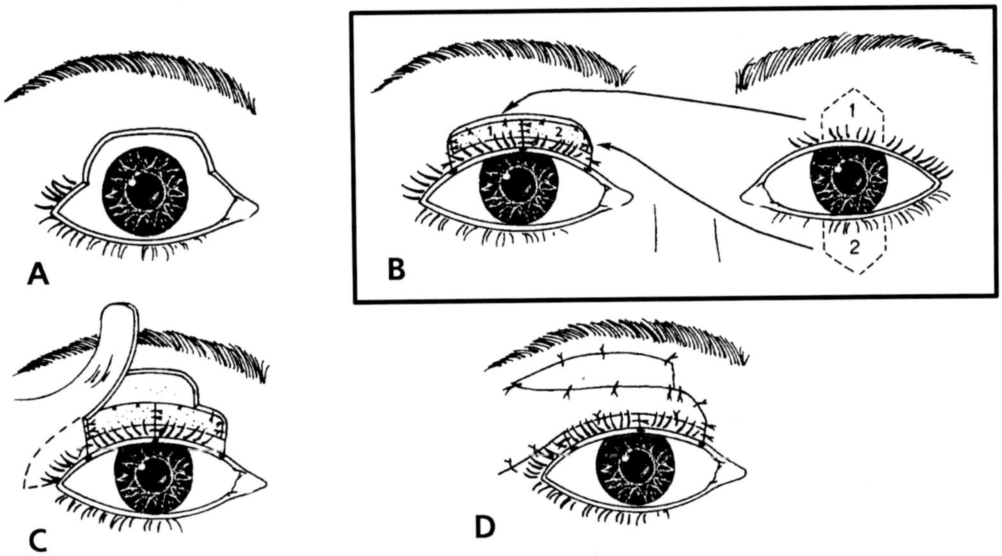

FIG. 18. Repair of upper lid defect with tandem composite grafts to upper lid (Beyer–Machule). **A:** Full-thickness upper lid defect. **B:** Composite grafts from the upper and lower lids of the donor eyelids have been placed in a tandem manner in the upper lid defect to create the posterior lamella. **C:** A skin-muscle flap has been developed to cover the composite grafts. **D:** If there is skin shortage, a skin graft can be taken to place above the defect created with the advanced skin-muscle flap. Patients with redundant upper lid skin may not require grafting.

tarsorrhaphy for 1 week to keep the lid stretched and prevent retraction. The skin graft is stented with Telfa, dental wax, and eyepads as mentioned in the section on sliding tarsal grafts. The graft is immobilized until all sutures are removed 1 week postoperatively (Fig. 15F).

An alternative method of suturing the mucous membrane graft in place on the undersurface of the lid is to utilize through-and-through mattress sutures of 6-0 silk, which are brought through the lid and tied externally.

COMPOSITE GRAFT

An alternative technique of upper lid reconstruction that may be used when precise margin reconstruction is necessary or when other methods cannot be used is the full-thickness composite graft from the opposite eyelid.

Technique

Full-thickness sections of the upper and sometimes lower eyelid are harvested from the contralateral eyelid. Closure of the donor area is performed as previously described. The musculocutaneous layer is removed from the graft down to a level just above the lashes. The donor graft may then be covered with a skin-muscle flap in the recipient area for maximum vascularization (Fig. 17A–C). Minimal cautery must be used and meticulous suturing of the graft under minimum tension is necessary for a good take. Even though the soft tissue take is excellent with good margin restoration, in many cases (approximately 50%) the lashes will not be retained. Although in most cases it is not necessary, the skin excised from the donor graft may be used to supplement the recipient upper lid skin (Fig. 17D). Putterman (11) described this technique well, and Beyer–Machule et al. (12) described the use of two composite grafts in tandem (Fig. 18A–D).

PERIORBITAL FLAPS

Periorbital flaps, which are derived from tissue above the eyebrow area, must usually be lined with a suitable posterior lamellar graft.

MEDIAN FOREHEAD FLAP

The median forehead flap, although rarely used, is needed with massive tissue loss of the upper eyelid when tissue cannot be borrowed from the lower lid or adjacent areas to reconstruct the defect (13). This technique is used to reconstruct an upper eyelid when no other technique is available.

Technique

A flap of vertically oriented skin is outlined with methylene blue (Fig. 19A), ideally to a length not exceeding four times the width. The flap is incised and elevated. The surrounding tissue is extensively undermined in the forehead area to allow the flap to rotate into the defect (Fig. 19B) and to allow direct closure of the donor site. The vertical donor site incision is closed with subcutaneous 6-0 plain gut sutures or spanning 6-0 silk mattress sutures in interrupted fashion; 6-0 nylon sutures are used for skin closure. The undersurface of this flap, which opposes the globe, must be lined with a posterior lamellar graft or remnants of the conjunctiva from the lower fornices, which can be advanced upward. The free grafts in most cases will "take" on a well-vascularized flap. If the situation is not urgent, a free graft of mucous membrane may be placed in the forehead area in an additional stage and allowed to take prior to transposition of the flap (14). The ideal lining of the flap is conjunctiva from the lower lid or fornix, if available.

The forehead flap is attached to the levator aponeurosis or remnants of the levator muscle with 6-0 silk mattress sutures through the flap to give the appropriate vertical mobility to the upper lid. Laterally the tip of the flap is attached with 4-0 sutures to the remnants of the lateral canthal tendon. The graft of mucous membrane is carefully rotated around the lid margin and sutured in place with running 7-0 silk to ensure that mucous membrane rather than keratinized epithelium will be in contact with the cornea (Fig. 19B). If the undersurface of the forehead flap has been lined with conjunctiva from the lower lid, it can be separated in 2 weeks, leaving enough conjunctiva to cover the lower margin of the forehead flap, which becomes the new upper eyelid margin.

Eight weeks later the base of the flap is separated and the base of the pedicle replaced into the donor (glabellar) area to prevent a narrowing of the eyebrows. The remaining donor incisions are closed with interrupted 6-0 nylon sutures (Fig. 19C).

A flap of sufficient width should be prepared to provide adequate vertical width of the resulting upper lid. With some contraction occurring during the postoperative period, vertical shortening is generally more of a problem than excessive length of the upper lid. Excess bulk tissue can be trimmed later if necessary. The lid will appear tight for many weeks before the levator muscle begins to provide vertical mobility. The resultant eyelid skin is thicker than normal and may be "thinned" with caution at a later date.

TEMPORAL FOREHEAD (FRICKE) FLAP

An additional technique used to supply tissue for very large upper lid (and sometimes lower lid) defects when no adjacent tissue or tissue from the opposing eyelid is available is the transposition of a temporally based flap from the suprabrow area (15). Frequently this flap can be a true axial one in that the superficial branch of the temporal artery can be included within the flap.

The temporal forehead flap provides tissue for the upper lid and lateral canthal area and is suited for large

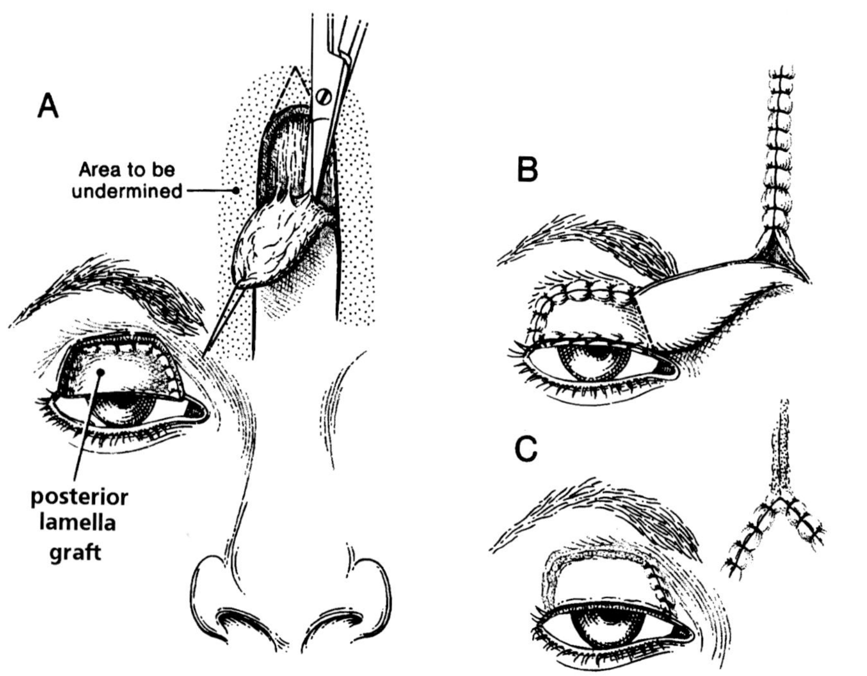

FIG. 19. Repair of full-thickness upper lid defect with a median forehead flap and posterior lamellar graft. **A:** The upper lid defect has been partially reconstructed with a mucous membrane–lined graft to the posterior lamella. A conjunctival flap from the lower lid can also be used. The median forehead flap is being developed. **B:** The median forehead flap has been transposed to cover the defect in the upper lid. The donor site is closed and the interim stage with the connected flap in position is approximately 6–8 weeks. **C:** The median forehead flap has been severed and the base reposited to the glabellar area with closure.

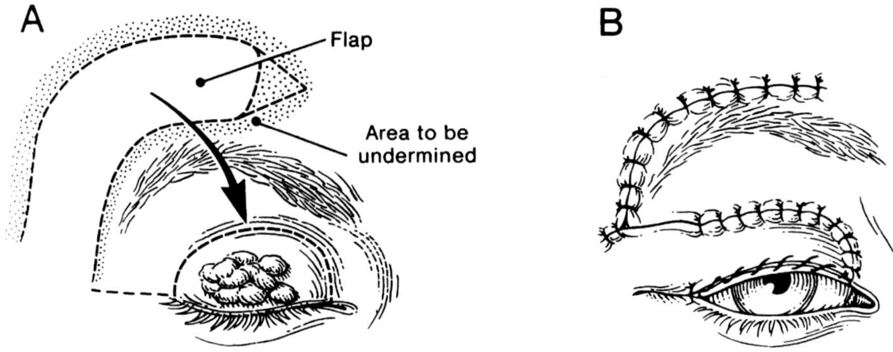

FIG. 20. Repair of upper lid defect with transpositional forehead flap to upper lid (Fricke). **A:** Outline of defect to be created in upper lid and outline of flap to be developed and transposed to defect. **B:** The forehead flap has been transposed to the eyelid defect. Before positioning the flap, the posterior lamella of the upper lid defect has been recreated with advanced conjunctiva, a mucous membrane–lined free graft, or a conjunctival flap from the lower lid.

defects in that area; however, it does introduce skin of a much greater thickness than is normally found in the upper lid area and should be reserved as a last-resort procedure. In many cases the flap is a bridge of tissue that spans normal skin and requires a second revisional procedure.

Technique

Methylene blue is used to outline the design of the flap above the brow as seen in Fig. 20A. The flap is designed to be based temporally and the base of the flap to angle as close as possible to the lateral canthus for good transposition. Incisions are then made through the skin down to the subbrow fatty pad. Very little muscle is included in this flap, so it is mainly a cutaneous flap. Undermining should be carried out temporally; however, one must remember that the superficial branch of the temporal nerve supplying the brow is in this area and only subcutaneous undermining should be carried out. The flap is then transposed into the upper lid or canthal defect, with closure of the original site of the flap performed with deep and cutaneous sutures. The flap is anchored into position in the recipient skin (Fig. 20B). If there is a full-thickness defect present the flap must have a mucous membrane lining, which can be derived either by bringing down existing mucous membrane in the upper fornix and suturing it to the undersurface of the flap, or by using a buccal mucous membrane graft to line the portion of the flap that will oppose the cornea. Care must be taken to attach the upper lid retractors to the flap to establish movement.

In 6–8 weeks the flap can be trimmed at its temporal aspect if there is a pedicle present. If the defect extended in such a way that a complete transposition was possible, no revision is needed. The thicker skin in many cases provides adequate movement but produces a tethering effect on the lid. It can be thinned down and crease formation obtained. The resulting lid is functional but far from normal.

TOTAL EYELID DEFECTS

Certain cases of "total" eyelid loss can occur following severe trauma, Moh's microscopic control excision of tumors, or severe burns. In the more severe cases, there may be loss of the upper and lower lid anterior and posterior lamella. In many burn cases there may be sparing of parts of the tarsoconjunctiva. The priority in these cases is protection of the cornea from exposure and possible corneal ulceration. The conventional procedures previously described may not be useful in many cases because of unavailability of tissue from the local or remote areas. In burn cases there may be elements of the posterior lamella (tarsoconjunctiva) that are intact.

A reparative technique to provide corneal protection and furnish the basis for further eyelid reconstruction consists of advancing residual conjunctiva or tarsoconjunctiva from the upper and lower fornix over the cornea reforming a conjunctival sac preserving the moisture and protection of the cornea (Fig. 21A–D). In more severe cases inversion of residual conjunctiva may be all that can be accomplished. After providing the cornea with a conjunctival mucous membrane lined flap, if there is skin (skin-muscle) available to form a flap from the facial area, a flap can be brought into position. In many cases, particularly burns, the local flap tissue is not available. In some cases in severe systemic burns only split skin can be found, but it can be used to cover this area.

If a flap can be used, then an ear cartilage graft can be interposed between the flap and the inverted conjunctiva to form the basis of eyelid structure for later procedures (Fig. 21E). If this is not the case, then after the initial take of the skin graft, cartilage can be inserted in a plane beneath the grafted skin and the conjunctiva at a later date to form a basis for lid structure and stability. With cases of severe trauma, particularly burns, there may be greater contracting forces and the lids should remained fused longer, 2–3 months if possible, to compensate for this problem. The fused lids can be separated at that time to allow vision (Fig. 21F); however, in many cases revisional procedures are necessary for optimum results.

BROW

The tissue around the eyebrow is mobile and can be arranged with a variety of flaps either advancement or transpositional. The problem with reconstruction of the brow area is maintaining the proper position and alignment of the brow hairs with proper contour to give a pleasing result. With resections of lesions in the brow a technique recommended by Carraway seems to provide the easiest way to resect brow hairs, repair the surrounding tissue, and maintain brow hair alignment (16). Figure 22A–C shows the technique of rectangular

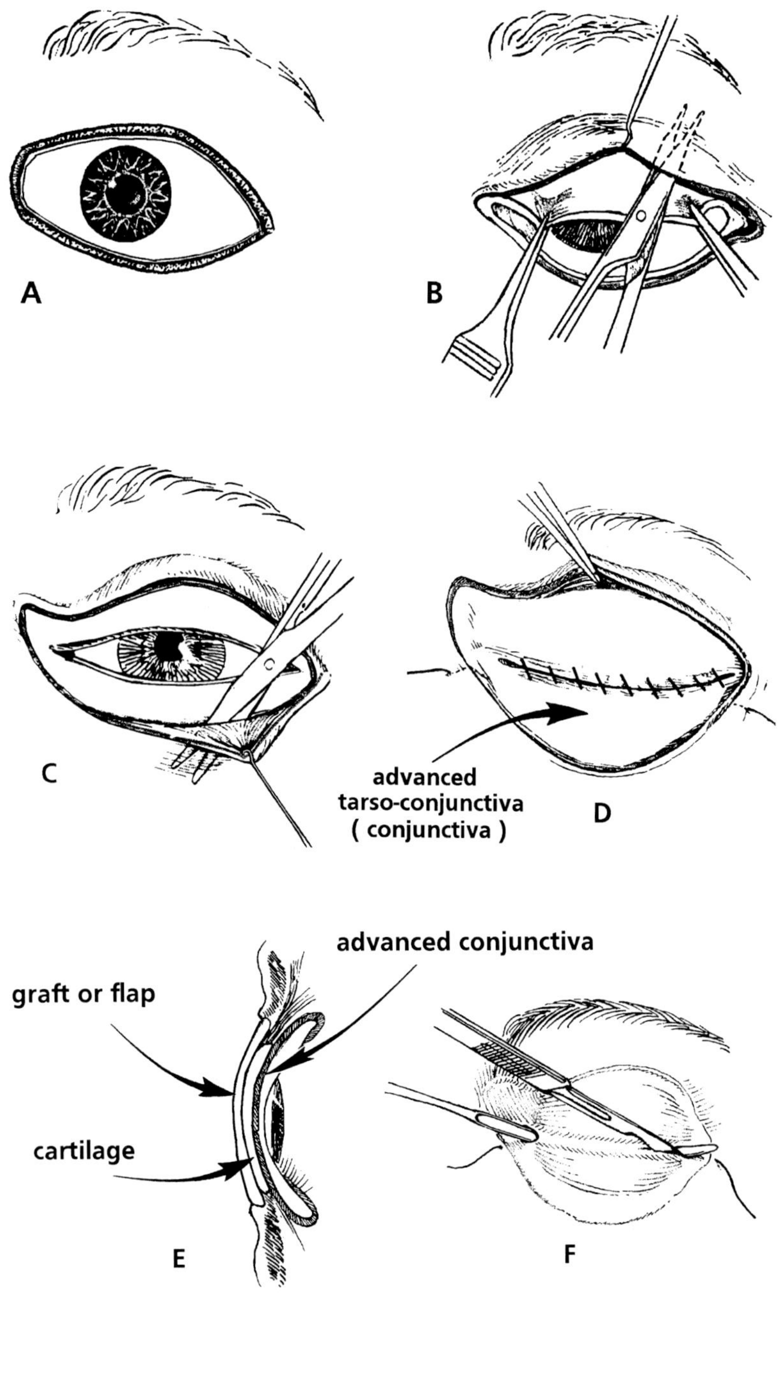

FIG. 21. Reconstruction of total upper lid and lower lid defect. This deformity is commonly seen in severe burn patients. **A:** Defect of upper lid, lower lid, and partial inner and outer canthus. **B:** The posterior lamella of the upper lid is being dissected free. Relaxing incisions in the retractor muscles are needed in many cases. **C:** The posterior lamella of the lower lid is being dissected and incision of the retractors of the lower lid are also needed for advancement of the posterior lamella. **D:** The two posterior lamella flaps have been advanced and sutured together to cover the cornea. **E:** On the anterior surface of the advanced conjunctiva, if there is no residual tarsal plate present, a free autogenous cartilage graft can be placed to create stability in the flap. If a free graft is used, then the anterior lamella must be covered with a flap to provide blood supply. If a cartilage graft is not needed, a skin graft can be placed for the external layer. **F:** After 6–8 weeks a separation of the anterior and posterior lamella can be performed at the desired position of the fissure. A longer period of closure must be observed if there are unusual contracting forces that may be present postoperatively.

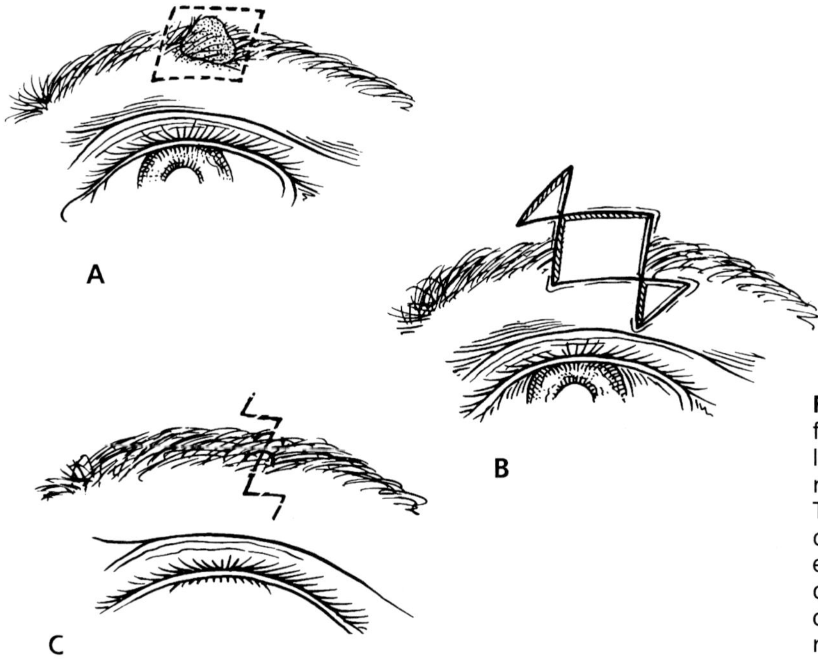

FIG. 22. Repair of full-thickness eyebrow defects (Carraway). **A:** Full-thickness rectangular resection of the eyebrows. **B:** A double-rhomboidal advancement flap is designed. **C:** The advancement flaps have been shifted to close the defect and provide continuity to the eyebrow hairs. In many cases additional vertical resection are needed because of resulting dog ear formation above and below the closed rhomboids.

resection with triangular extension for resection of redundancies created by closure of the rectangle. Not uncommonly, further redundancies beyond the original triangles will occur vertically but can be easily trimmed.

REFERENCES

1. McCord CD, Wesley R. Reconstruction of upper eyelid and medial canthus. *Oculoplastic surgery*. New York: Raven Press; 73–91.
2. Tenzel RR. Reconstruction of the central one half of an eyelid. *Arch Ophthalmol* 1975;93:125–126.
3. Anderson RL, Edwards JJ. Reconstruction by myocutaneous eyelid flaps. *Arch Ophthalmol* 1979;97:2358–2362.
4. Cutler N, Beard C. A method for partial and total upperlid reconstruction. *Am J Ophthalmol* 1955;39:1–7.
5. Smith B, Obear MF. Bridge flap technique for reconstruction of large upper lid defects. *Plast Reconstr Surg* 1966;38:45–48.
6. Wesley RE, McCord CD Jr. Height of the lower tarsus of the lower eyelid. *Am J Ophthalmol* 1980;90:102–105.
7. Wesley RE, McCord CD Jr. Transplantation of eyebank sclera in the Cutler–Beard method of upper eyelid reconstruction. *Ophthalmology* 1980;87:1022–1028.
8. Steinkogler FJ. A sandwich technique for reconstruction of the lower lid. *Orbit* 1989;8:37–43.
9. Mustarde JC. Eyelid reconstruction. *Orbit* 1982;1:33–43.
10. Brown BZ, Beard C. Split level full thickness eyelid graft. *Am J Ophthalmol* 1979;87:388–392.
11. Putterman AM. Viable composite grafting in eyelid reconstruction. *Am J Ophthalmol* 1978;85:237–241.
12. Beyer-Machule CK, Shapiro A, Smith B. Double composite lid reconstruction: a new method of upper and lower lid reconstruction. *Ophth Plast Reconstr Surg* 1985;1:97–102.
13. Kazanjian VH, Roopenian A. Median forehead flaps in the repair of defects of the nose and surrounding areas. *Trans Am Acad Ophthalmol Otolaryngol* 1956;60:557–566.
14. Smith BC, Nesi FA. Upper lid reconstruction: a new technique for the use of mucous membrane lined pedicle flaps. *Ophth Surg* 1979;10:17–19.
15. Fricke JCG. Die Bildung neuer Augenlider (Blepharoplastik) nach Zerstorungen und dadurch hervorgebrachten auswartswendungen derselben. Hamburg: Perthes and Bessler; 1829.
16. Carraway J, Dean JA. The brow slide: a technique for the aesthetic treatment of eyebrow tumors. *Plast Reconstr Surg* 1992; 89:554–557.

CHAPTER 21

Lower Eyelid Reconstruction

This chapter deals with full-thickness tissue loss of the lower eyelid. As in the upper lid, the large majority of defects in the lower lid result from skin cancer removal, trauma, surgery, or congenital deformities. Before one decides on a specific reconstruction procedure, the patient's age and elasticity of tissue must be taken into account. The elderly patient's tissue has increased laxity, allowing the lid substance to stretch and reducing the size of any defect. The young person's skin because of its elasticity is less able to stretch to reduce the size of defects (see chapter on decision making in eyelid reconstruction). When considering specific reconstructive procedures, it should be remembered that for proper function the lower lid should contain a mucous membrane–lined eyelid margin, a rigid support supplied anatomically by the tarsal plate, skin covering, and mucosal backing. Adequate reconstruction must deal with all of these components to achieve an acceptable functional and cosmetic result. Although the literature is replete with alternative procedures that have value in some situations, the procedures described are standard and, either singly or in combination with other procedures described, can be counted on for repair of a wide variety of lower lid defects (1).

DIRECT CLOSURE

As in the upper lid, the most commonly used of all reconstructive procedures in the lower lid is direct, end-to-end closure of the lid margin. This surgical technique should be considered initially for repair of central eyelid defects affecting less than 40% of the original lid margin in older individuals. In younger patients with greater tissue elasticity, it may be practical to close only a wound of 30% or less of the lid margin with simple direct closure. In borderline cases, the added relaxation of a lateral cantholysis may provide sufficient relaxation to allow closure. A pair of skin hooks or fine-toothed forceps should be used to grasp and reapproximate the margins of the defect. This will provide a good estimate of the adequacy of direct closure.

When creating a defect, a slanting of the external musculocutaneous layer excision can be performed in the lower lid to reduce inferior redundancy and dog ear formation, which is common with lower lid closure. By slanting the incision temporally, the tension and length of the upper and lower edges remain more comparable, thereby lessening redundancy. The borders of the tarsus should be squared to create perpendicular defect edges, from the lid margin to a level below the tarsus (Fig. 1A).

A single 6-0 silk traction suture is placed through the gray line (mucocutaneous junction) (Fig. 1B) of the margin on either side of the defect to draw the wound together and provide sufficient retraction to allow approximation of the edges. Two- or three interrupted 7-0 silk sutures are placed intratarsally, or in the inferior retractor, in a vertical line for closure. Conjunctiva should not be included in these sutures. Closure of the tarsus is the most important aspect of direct closure, and great care should be taken to reapproximate the perpendicular edges precisely. 7-0 silk can be left permanently with no ill effects to the tissue.

The original aligning suture is tied and a second margin suture may be needed for better alignment. The ends of these sutures are left long and draped externally over the skin to avoid corneal irritation (Fig. 1C). If a lateral cantholysis is needed to reduce tension on the wound edges, this is done by making a horizontal incision at the lateral canthal angle and extending approximately 5 mm on the skin surface. Sharp dissection is carried down to the periosteum of the lateral orbital rim, and the lower arm of the lateral canthal tendon is severed from the rim (Fig. 2). Increased laxity will immediately be noted in the lower lid. Lateral orbital septum fibers are also lysed to further loosen the lid. The lateral margin of the wound can then be mobilized nasally to close the lid margin defect.

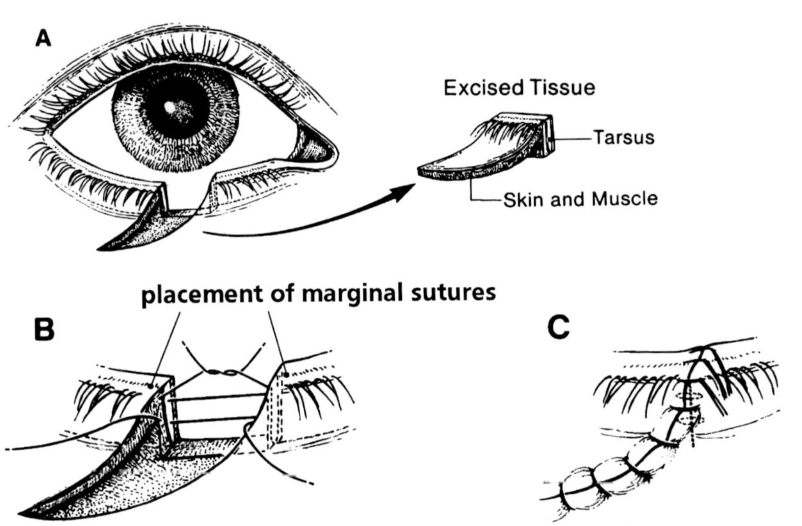

FIG. 1. Direct closure of lower lid full-thickness defect. **A:** Full-thickness defect with vertical tarsal resection but slanting skin-muscle resection. **B:** Closure of the tarsal plate with intratarsal sutures. **C:** Closure of the skin-muscle layer.

Redundant skin, which commonly occurs at the inferior limits of the skin defect, is excised next. This is best accomplished by making a full-thickness oblique skin cut with straight scissors, in a line parallel to the skin lines of the cheek (see Fig. 3). Skin medial to this incision is draped in an overlapping manner, marked with methylene blue, and excised. The skin-muscle layer is then closed with vertical mattress sutures. Vertical mattress sutures provide for maximal wound edge eversion and alignment of the epithelium. The conjunctiva surface will have been well approximated and need not be sutured.

Because the main support to the eyelid repair consists of the nonabsorbable silk intratarsal sutures, all external sutures, including margin sutures, may be removed in 5–7 days.

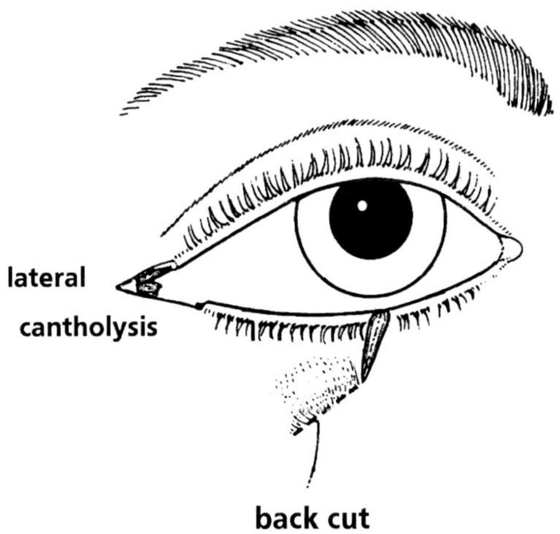

FIG. 2. Direct closure of the lower lid following canthotomy and canthal lysis laterally. When the lower lid is advanced, despite slanting of the incision some redundancy of tissue and dog ear formation is encountered requiring revision.

ROTATIONAL FLAP (TENZEL)

Lower lid defects of 40–60% of the original lid margin can be closed by a lateral, semicircular myocutaneous flap rotated into the lid defect (2). The lower lid defect must first be fashioned so that the tarsal edges are perfectly perpendicular to the lid margin and the tissue beneath the tarsal defect is excised in a slanting triangular manner as described in the section on direct closure. A superior arching line is drawn with methylene blue, beginning at the lateral canthus (Fig. 4). The diameter of the flap can be from 2 to 5 cm and it extends superiorly and temporally to the lateral extension of the brow line.

The cutaneous incision is made with a blade and the muscle layer incision is made with the cutting Bovie needle. A lateral canthotomy incision is made beneath the semicircular skin incision. Dissection is carried down to the lateral orbital rim. The inferior ramus of the lateral canthal tendon is cut to mobilize completely the lateral aspect of the lid. Septal fibers must also be severed to allow freedom of advancement. Care should

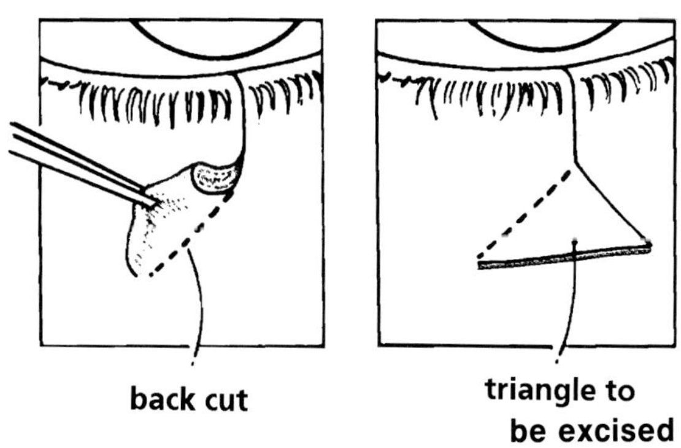

FIG. 3. A–D: Revision of dog ear following advancement of lower lid with direct closure.

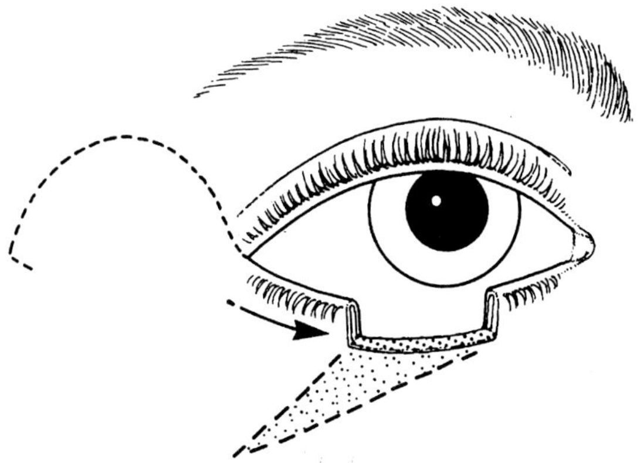

FIG. 4. Repair of lower lid defect with myocutaneous semicircular flap. Outline shows the area of skin-muscle tissue that is usually needed to be resected to approximate lid edges after the flap has been rotated.

be taken to preserve the superior ramus of the lateral canthal tendon. The semicircular flap is thoroughly dissected in the submuscular plane and rotated inwardly (see composite of steps in Fig. 5).

The lateral lid defect edge is advanced to the medial edge of the defect and joined in the manner described under direct closure. The lateral lid support must be recovered by suturing the muscular plane of flap tissue to the periosteum of the inner aspect of the lateral orbital rim (Fig. 6). This step of lateral canthal fixation is necessary for support of the lid to conform to the curvature of the globe.

Additional fixation of the flap to the periosteum outside the rim higher than the canthal angle is also needed to prevent lateral sagging of the lid. The fornix conjunctiva is then undermined, advanced to the skin edge of the lid margin, and sutured with 7-0 silk running marginal sutures. The lateral incision is closed directly with mattress sutures, i.e., standard skin closure. If the sides of the lateral incision are not equal, a small dog ear may be excised at the temporal portion of the wound edge (Fig. 7).

The rotational flap is excellent by itself for moderate-sized full-thickness lower lid defects. As the defects enlarge, there is a tendency for deficiency in the temporal portion of the lower lid because there is no "sup-

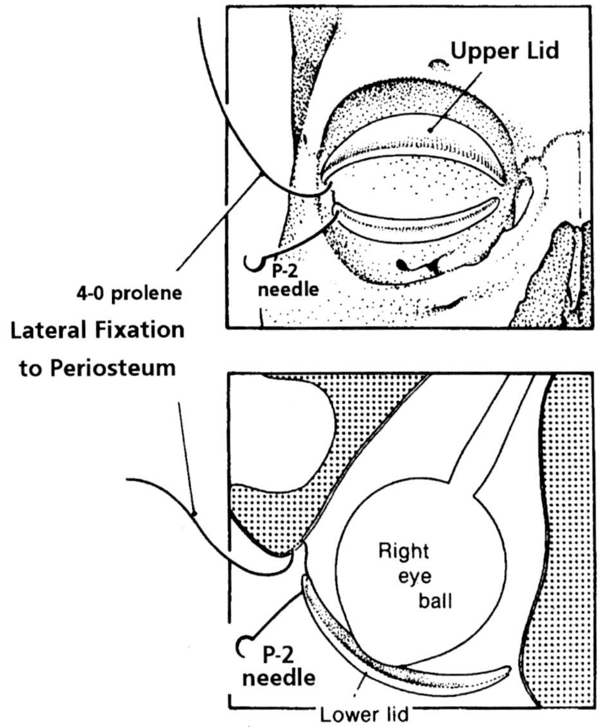

FIG. 6. Diagrammatic representation of lateral canthal fixation. It is emphasized that the attachment of the lower eyelid is made inside the orbital rim to the periosteum at the lateral tubercle to create the normal curvature of the globe. This fixation is best accomplished if a sturdy half-circle needle is used.

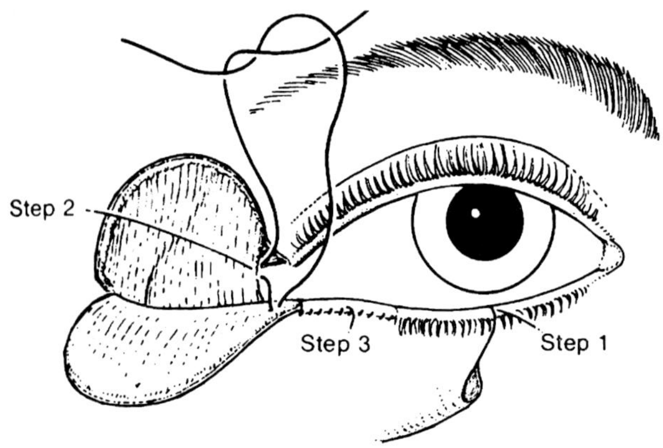

FIG. 5. Direct closure of lower lid defect with rotational myocutaneous flap. The sequence of steps are shown after the flap has been developed and the lid advanced. Step 1: Direct closure of the lid margin. Step 2: Fixation of the flap to the lateral canthus inside the rim with the proper tension. Step 3: Eversion of the conjunctiva to recreate margin.

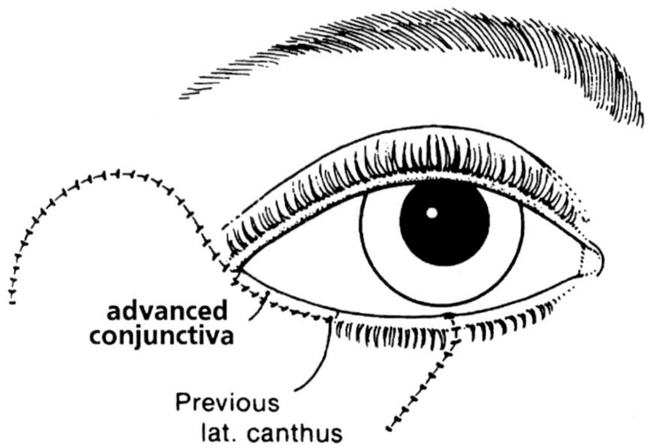

FIG. 7. Reconstruction of the lower lid with myocutaneous semicircular flap. The flap has been sutured into position showing the final fixating sutures.

port structure" for the flap. An attempt to push the flap too far will lead to inevitable complications such as lower lid retraction and lateral sagging of the lid with irritation of the eye. As the size of the defect one wishes to repair increases, additional techniques can be used to enhance and extend the rotational flap to prevent these problems and allow the closure of the larger defects in the lower lid.

ROTATIONAL FLAP WITH PERIOSTEAL FLAP

The first supplemental procedure that can be performed on larger defects is the periosteal strip from the lateral orbital rim that is hinged at the orbital rim (1,3). The rotational flap is first developed in the usual manner. Then, before closure, methylene blue is used to outline the periosteal flap, based or hinged at the edge of the rim, at the lateral canthal. This rectangular strip of periosteum is elevated from the rim as shown in Fig. 8A. Care must be taken to base the flap high enough on the orbital rim to ensure upward pull of the lid. The flap should be placed at least at the midpupillary level. The flap should be slanted with its base upward, so that it will pull the lid upward postoperatively. As the periosteal flap is elevated it is stretched across and anchored as far as possible inside the advanced myocutaneous flap (Fig. 8B). In smaller defects the periosteal flap can be sutured to the edge of the tarsus; however, in some larger defects it is simply tacked to the inner surface of the advanced musculocutaneous flap. Following the periosteal flap addition the Tenzel flap is closed in the usual manner.

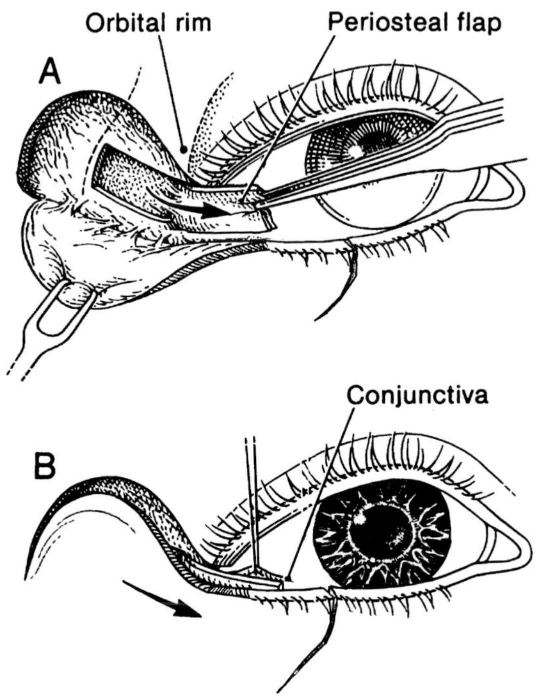

FIG. 8. Repair of lower lid defect with rotational myocutaneous flap augmented with a periosteal flap. **A:** The myocutaneous flap has been advanced to provide further support at the canthus. A periosteal flap, hinged on the rim, is rotated inward to line the inner surface of the flap. **B:** The flap is then sutured and the periosteum incorporated.

ROTATIONAL FLAP WITH SUPPLEMENTAL EAR CARTILAGE

With larger lower lid defects, in which the lateral edge of the tarsus is pulled further away from the lateral orbital rim as the Tenzel flap is advanced, supplemental procedures of a larger magnitude must be performed to ensure the stability of this lateral portion of the lower lid (1). In these larger defects even the addition of a periosteal flap may not furnish enough support and a supplemental ear cartilage graft must be used to "back" the advanced Tenzel flap. The ear cartilage graft is taken (as described in the chapter on free grafts) and the graft is squared off so that it can be approximated to the edge of the residual tarsal plate in the eyelid. The cartilage should be secured to the edge of the tarsal remnant with two or three 6-0 vicryl sutures (Fig. 9). The lateral canthal fixation of the cartilage to the periosteum can be trying because a needle can be successfully passed through the cartilage only one or two times before the cartilage tends to fragment. Wider initial bites must be taken in the cartilage to avoid multiple punctures of the cartilage with the needle. After placement of the cartilage and tensing at the lateral canthal area so that the lower lid has reached the desired position, tension, and contour, the Tenzel flap procedure is completed in the usual manner. The ear cartilage does not have to be covered with conjunctiva and, indeed, in many cases this is impossible because of the amount of resection. In over 3–4 weeks the cartilage will reepithelialize, but it can produce some temporary follicular conjunctivitis, which can be con-

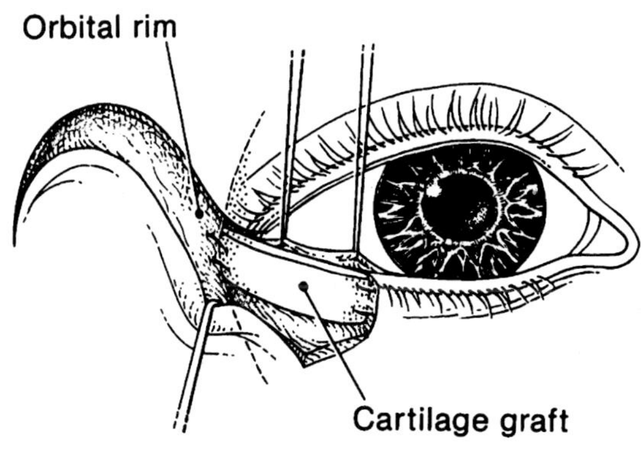

FIG. 9. Reconstruction of lower lid defect with myocutaneous flap augmented with an ear cartilage graft. This shows the graft sutured in position to the lateral rim before fixation of the myocutaneous flap over the graft.

trolled with steroid-antibiotic ointment in the ensuing weeks.

ROTATIONAL FLAP WITH PERIOSTEAL FLAP AND "EXTENDER" GRAFT

Even more extensive defects of the lower lid, particularly if they are "shallow," can be corrected with the rotational flap, a periosteal extension flap, and an additional graft applied to the end of the periosteal flap (Fig. 10A, B). This serves as a reconstructive procedure for the posterior lamella. Either autogenous ear cartilage or a "free" tarsal conjunctival graft from either of the upper lids can be attached to the end of the periosteal flap as an extender. This technique does presume that there is enough local skin-muscle tissue in the lower lid and cheek area to be rotated across the lid to cover the extended periosteal flap and graft.

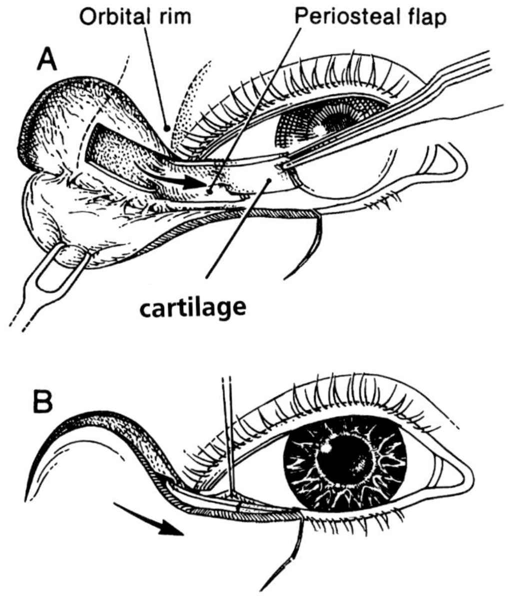

FIG. 10. Reconstruction of lower lid defect with rotational myocutaneous flap augmented with a tandem periosteal flap and ear cartilage graft. This amount of support is needed in patients who have more extensive defects and greater need of lateral support of the rotated flap. **A:** The periosteal flap has been rotated inward with the ear cartilage graft attached to the end of the flap. The cartilage is brought to the cut edge of the residual lid. **B:** The myocutaneous flap is closed over the periosteum and cartilage.

LOCAL MYOCUTANEOUS FLAP WITH FREE TARSOCONJUNCTIVAL GRAFT

Broad-shallow defects can be corrected without lid sharing techniques if there is an adequate skin-muscle layer present in the lid and cheek area. This technique is particularly useful in older patients who have redundancy in the skin-muscle layer (4,5).

With temporally located defects, the skin-muscle flap is elevated in the manner of an extended blepharoplasty with extensive undermining. An incision is made in the residual subciliary area with the incisions placed in the skin-muscle flap so that it can be rotated outward when developed. Dissection of the flap exposes the inferior orbital rim and the extent of the posterior lamella defect. The temporal posterior lamella defect can then be repaired with the use of a free tarsoconjunctival graft from the upper lid, taken from either the ipsilateral or the contralateral eye (Fig. 11A, B) (6,7). In

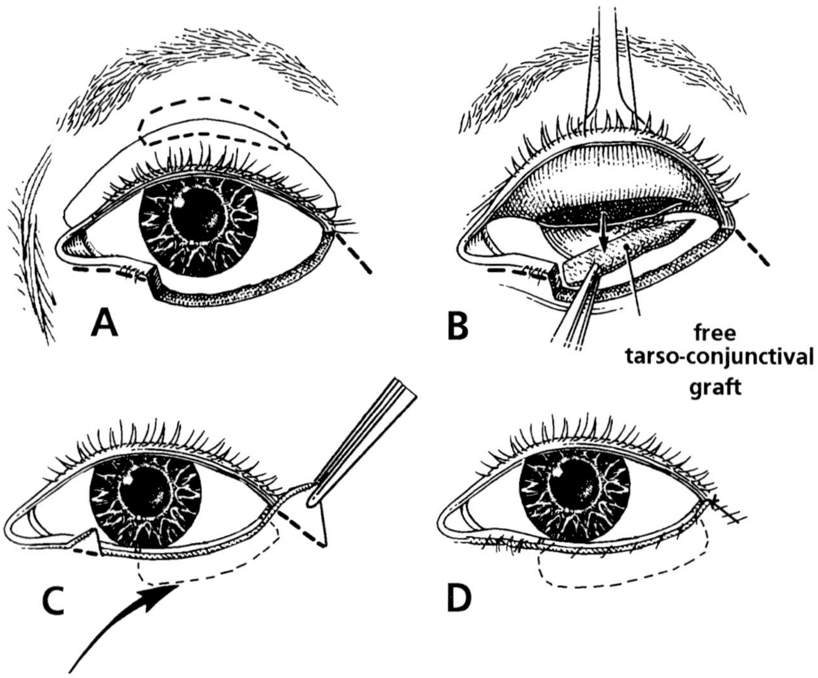

FIG. 11. Reconstruction of broad-shallow defect in the lateral portion of the lower lid with free tarsoconjunctival graft from the upper lid and outwardly rotated myocutaneous flap. **A:** Outline of defect and incision lines to develop the skin-muscle flap in the lower lid, outline of tarsoconjunctival graft from upper lid. **B:** The upper lid is everted with excision of the free tarsoconjunctival graft that straddles the upper edge of the tarsus. The tarsoconjunctival graft is placed so that the cuff of conjunctiva can be used to rotate over the lid margin. **C:** The tarsoconjunctival graft has been sutured to the posterior lamella with the proper tension and the myocutaneous flap rotated outward as in a blepharoplasty procedure. Redundant edges are resected. **D:** The myocutaneous flap has been anchored to the periosteum at the lateral orbital rim with enough tension to support the lid.

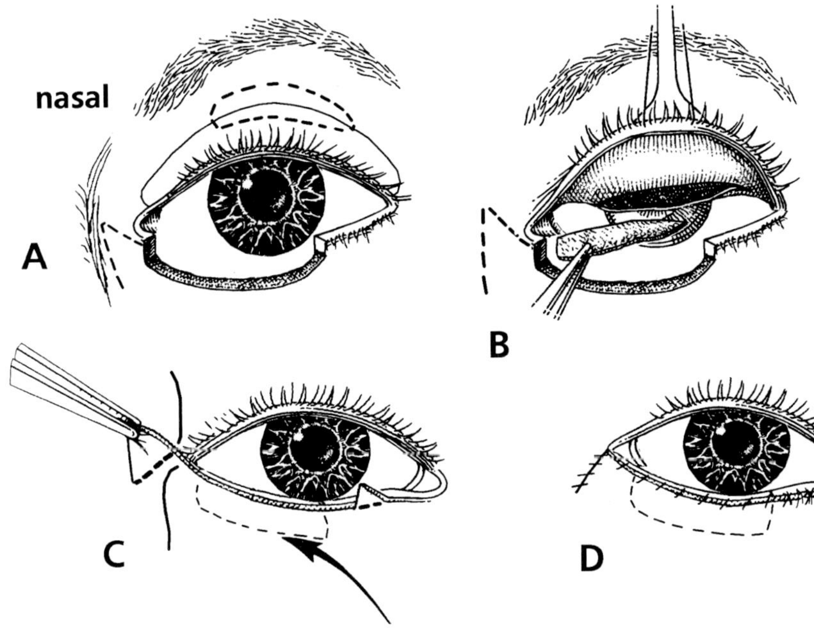

FIG. 12. Repair of shallow, nasally positioned defect in lower lid with rotational myocutaneous flap and free tarsoconjunctival graft. **A:** Position of the defect and the incisions needed to elevate the myocutaneous flap in the lower lid. **B:** The free tarsoconjunctival graft has been excised from the superior edge of the tarsal plate and positioned so that the cuff of conjunctiva can be brought up over the edge of the new lid. **C:** The free tarsoconjunctival graft has been sutured to the posterior lamella with desired tension. The lower lid myocutaneous flap has been rotated up and inward, and a fixation suture is taken through the anterior reflection of the medial canthal tendon. Edges of redundant skin are excised. **D:** Final position of the lid.

patients with adequate fornix conjunctiva and skin-muscle layer, Gore-tex implants have been used as a tarsal substitute in a sandwich manner for reconstruction of this type of defect (8). Once the posterior lamella has been reformed, the flap is rotated upward and attached to the periosteum laterally so as to act as fixation and support for the lower lid. Proper fixation of the skin-muscle flap in this area is needed so that the lower lid position will be stable and the margin placed at the inferior limbus. In many cases, removal of fatty pads in the inferior orbital rim area is needed to provide slack to allow the flap to be rotated up adequately. Triangles of skin are resected in the areas that overlap the lower lid margin. An overlapping redundant triangle occurs laterally when the flap is tightened to position the lid margin and is resected (Fig. 11C, D). In many cases the final result causes a smoothing effect to the lower lid more than to the contralateral side and should be mentioned to the patient preoperatively.

If the defect is nasally located, then the myocutaneous flap will require rotation in a nasal direction. The subciliary incision is made in the residual lid but the vertical incision should be made in the nasolabial fold as in the case of a nasally based blepharoplasty incision (Fig. 12A, B). The steps are the same as with the lateral defect; however, when the flap is rotated inward, it should be fixated to the anterior reflection of the medial canthal tendon to stabilize the lid (Fig. 12C, D).

With the local myocutaneous flap the tension of the lid margin is determined by the tensing of the flap. It is important when the flap is laterally rotated that the skin-muscle flap be attached with proper tension to the lateral periosteum. If the flap is inwardly rotated, it is important that the flap be attached to the medial canthal tendon with adequate tension (Fig. 13).

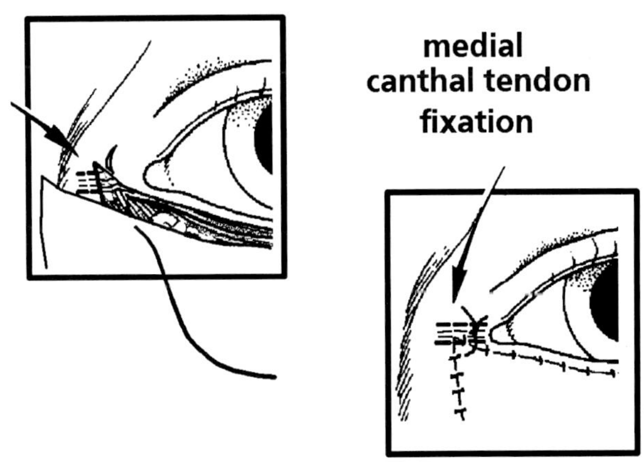

FIG. 13. A more detailed view showing the fixation of the nasal myocutaneous flap to the anterior reflection of the medial canthal tendon.

ROTATIONAL CHEEK FLAP (MUSTARDE)

The Mustarde flap is a large rotational skin-muscle cheek flap that can, if necessary, be relied on to cover virtually any lower lid defect (9). It may be considered a progression in size from the smaller Tenzel-type rotational flaps. It has the advantage of allowing a complete lower lid reconstruction in one operative procedure. The Mustarde flap is most useful for vertically deep defects, especially those in which the vertical dimension is greater than the horizontal dimension. Nasal defects are better suited to the rotational flaps. Objections to this procedure are the excessively long scar line on the face and the adynamic nature of the reconstructed lower lid. There is the necessity of excising a triangle of normal tissue underneath a lesion for rotation and closure of the flap.

Because of these inadequacies, the very large rotational cheek flaps are reserved for specific situations: a large, vertically deep nasal defect that may extend to include most of the lower lid, the undesirability of keeping the eye closed for a prolonged period (because of ocular disease such as glaucoma, active corneal disease, or risk of amblyopia in a child), and patients who are unable to tolerate staged surgical procedures (poor surgical risk).

Technique

The rotational cheek flap is begun by infiltrating the cheek and lid area with local anesthetic and 1:100,000 epinephrine. If a lesion is to be excised, a large superiorly based triangle with the medial edge in the nasolabial fold is outlined (Fig. 14A). A semicircular flap beginning at the lateral canthus and extending to the area immediately adjacent to the auricular tragus is then outlined. The most important requirement of this outlined flap is that the superior limit extend at least to the level of the brow or above. Obtaining sufficient height of the flap will help to counteract the inevitable sagging of the lateral lid margin. The medial triangle is excised. The vertical length of the medial triangle may vary with the amount of tissue that needs to be rotated to cover the lid defect. The semicircular flap is then developed in the submuscular plane. With the dissection it is important to obtain hemostasis and to avoid branches of the facial nerve.

Prior to rotation of the undermined tissue, a graft must be obtained to reconstruct the posterior lamella. This will provide the internal support and mucous membrane components of the reconstructed lower lid. The nasal septum contains cartilage with its own mucosal backing and historically has been the site for donor material. Autogenous ear cartilage can be used because it will epithelialize over a 6-week period. Ocular irritation will be present during this epithelialization period and can be controlled with ointment. Palatal mucoperichondrium is also a good alternative. Alternatives to posterior lamella replacement are listed in Table 1.

The graft is then placed with the mucosa inward facing the inferior cornea. The inferior margin of the mu-

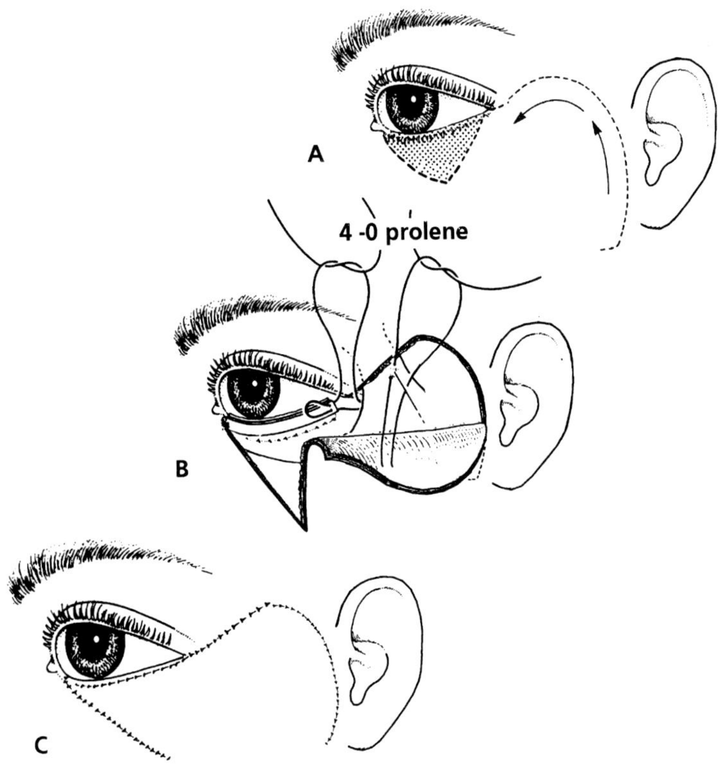

FIG. 14. Repair of full-thickness lower lid defect with large (Mustarde) myocutaneous flap rotation and posterior lamella reconstruction. **A:** Outline of defect and incisions for development of the flap. **B:** The posterior lamella of the eyelid has been reconstructed with a free mucous membrane–lined graft. The flap will be rotated and the temporal portion of the flap fixated to the periosteum laterally for support. **C:** The flap has been rotated and fixated into position. Lateral support of the canthus is critical and deep fixating sutures to the lateral periosteum are needed.

TABLE 1. *Posterior lamella lining for lower lid reconstruction*

Ear cartilage graft
Free tarsoconjunctival graft
Palatal mucoperiosteum
Nasal mucoperichondrium
Buccal mucous membrane
Conjunctival advancement from fornix
Composite eyelid graft including margin (includes lashes)

cosa is sutured to the cuff of conjunctiva in the inferior fornix if present (Fig. 14B). The graft is left temporally free at its lateral and medial margins. The rotational cheek flap is then mobilized nasally to fill the nasal triangular defect. Medial canthal fixation is accomplished by placing a 4-0 prolene suture through the cheek flap and anchoring it to the posterior ramus of the medial canthal tendon or to the periosteum of the medial orbital rim as described in the chapter on medial canthal reconstruction. If indicated, the lacrimal drainage system should also be addressed.

After fixating the flap in the medial canthus, the posterior lamellar graft is sutured to the posterior margin of the flap at the new lid margin. Running 6-0 plain gut suture is placed at the mucosal–epithelial border and tied externally to avoid corneal irritation. The lateral canthus is reformed with lateral canthal fixation of the flap to the inner aspect of the lateral orbital rim. Additional deep 4-0 nonabsorbable sutures should be used to attach the flap to the rim periosteum laterally and apply upward traction at the apex of the flap. The skin is then closed (Fig. 14C). The lateral edge of the flap may need a triangular excision of redundant skin for even closure. Finally, the eyelids are sutured together with a tarsorrhaphy stitch to provide additional upward tension on the flap and to evert the mucosa–skin interface during the initial healing period. The tarsorrhaphy and skin sutures may be removed in 5 days.

OPPOSING EYELID FLAPS

Advancement Tarsoconjunctival Flap (Hughes Procedure)

Large defects affecting more than 50% (depending on lid laxity) of the lower lid margin can be reconstructed with a tarsoconjunctival flap from the upper eyelid. This technique was originally described by Hughes but has since been modified (10,11). This lid-sharing technique is superior for both cosmesis and lid function, produces a dynamic, movable lower lid. The disadvantage of the lid sharing procedure is that it is a two-stage procedure, the first stage requiring that the eye be kept closed for several weeks. After that time, a second procedure is needed to open the lid margins.

The margins of the defect are made perpendicular from the lid margin to below the tarsus (Fig. 15A). The lower extent of the wound is cut in a rectangular shape. The margins of the defect are gently pulled toward the center until the desired tightness against the globe is achieved. Calipers are then used to measure the horizontal length of the defect in order to determine the correct width of tarsal flap to take from the upper lid. If the lower lid is loose or inelastic, a narrower flap may be used.

The upper eyelid is everted over a Desmarres retractor and methylene blue is used to mark a superiorly based, three-sided advancement flap on the tarsal conjunctiva (Fig. 15B). The horizontal margin of the flap must be at least 4 mm away from the lid margin. If less than 4 mm of intact upper lid marginal tarsus remains after the procedure, upper lid deformities such as entropion, ectropion, and trichiasis can result. The outlined flap is incised through conjunctiva and tarsus to a plane between tarsus and orbicularis muscle.

Dissection is continued superiorly between Müller's muscle and levator aponeurosis. Conjunctiva and Müller's muscle can be left attached to the tarsal segment in cases when a superior blood supply is needed

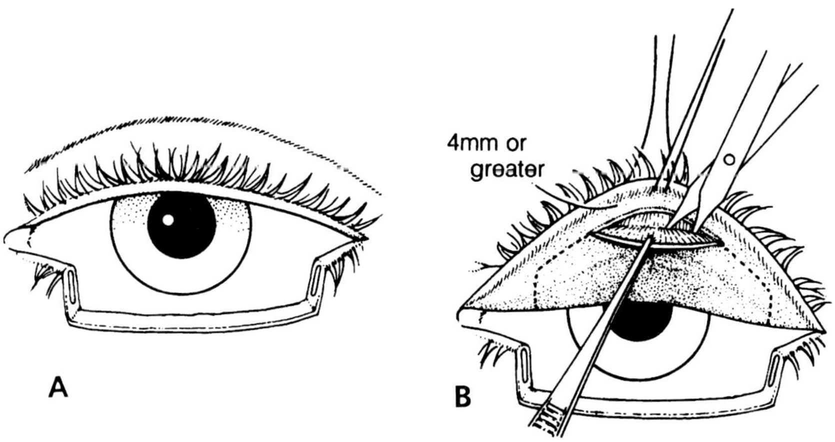

FIG. 15. Repair of lower lid defect with eyelid sharing tarsoconjunctival flap from the upper lid (modified Hughes). **A:** Defect in lower lid encompassing almost full width of lid. **B:** The upper lid is everted and a tarsoconjunctival flap is developed from the undersurface of the lid sparing the margin by 4 mm.

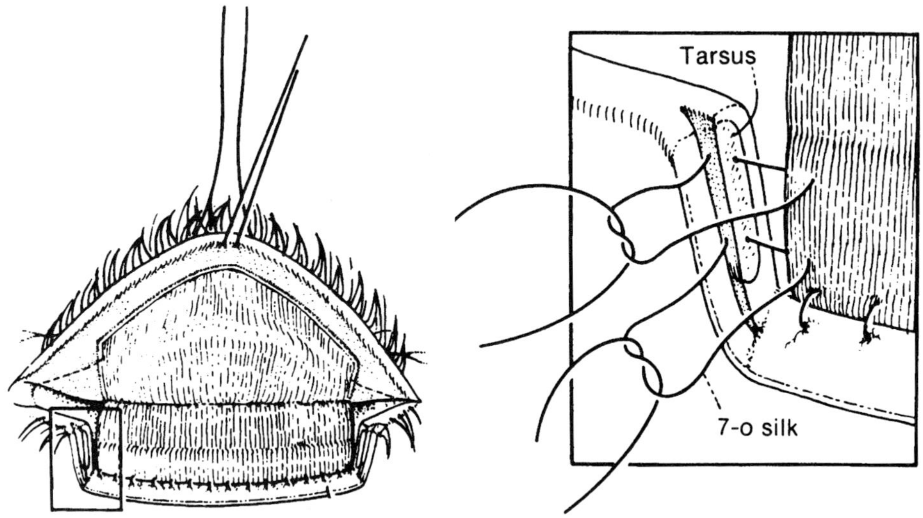

FIG. 16. The flap has been dissected from the upper lid. In most cases Müller's muscle is dissected free leaving only conjunctiva attached. The flap is attached to the retractor layer inferiorly, nasally, and temporally, to the edges of the tarsus, with intratarsal sutures.

(e.g., irradiated cases). Blunt dissection with a wet cotton–tipped applicator may facilitate dissection between Müller's muscle and levator aponeurosis. If Müller's muscle is used in the flap, care must be taken when separating the flap at the second stage to dissect it fully free to avoid upper lid retraction.

Most surgeons prefer to exclude Müller's muscle from the flap. Although this allows greater ease in separating the lid later, it may compromise the graft vascularity in marginal cases. When the flap is sufficiently mobilized from the upper lid it is advanced into the lower lid defect and the lateral and medial margins of the tarsal flap are sutured to the cut edges of residual lower lid tarsus with direct intratarsal suturing (Fig. 16). The previous upper lid superior tarsal border becomes the lower lid tarsal margin. If no residual lower lid tarsus at the lateral margin of the defect is available, the tarsal flap from the upper lid can be anchored to the periosteum using lateral canthal fixation. If there is an absence of residual lower lid tarsus nasally, the flap must be fixed to the posterior reflection of the medial canthal tendon with medial canthal fixation (see Chapter 22 on reconstruction of medial canthal defects). The inferior margin of the flap is sutured to the remaining conjunctiva below with a running 5-0 plain suture. By advancing the upper lid tarsus and conjunctiva on a pedicle flap, the lower lid defect will have been restored with two of its necessary ingredients. The third ingredient is supplied by a full-thickness skin graft over the composite pedicle flap (Fig. 17A). Donor skin may be obtained, in order of preference, from either upper eyelid if sufficient redundancy exists, postauricular skin, or supraclavicular skin.

A skin graft is taken as described in the chapter on free grafts and the dermal surface thinned with sharp scissors. The skin graft is sutured over the flap with

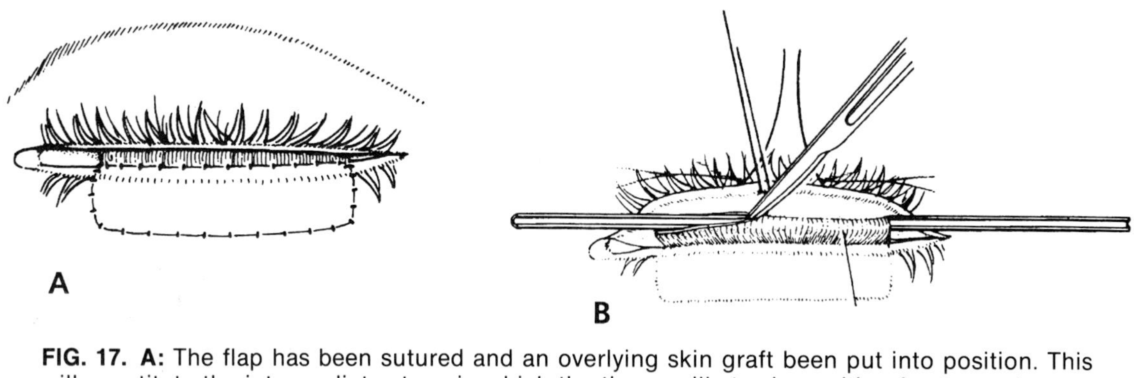

FIG. 17. A: The flap has been sutured and an overlying skin graft been put into position. This will constitute the intermediate stage in which the tissue will stay in position for approximately 4–6 weeks. **B:** The flap is separated protecting the eye with a grooved director. A redundant cuff of mucous membrane is needed to overlap the lower lid margin and adequate release of the superior retractors is needed to prevent upper lid retraction.

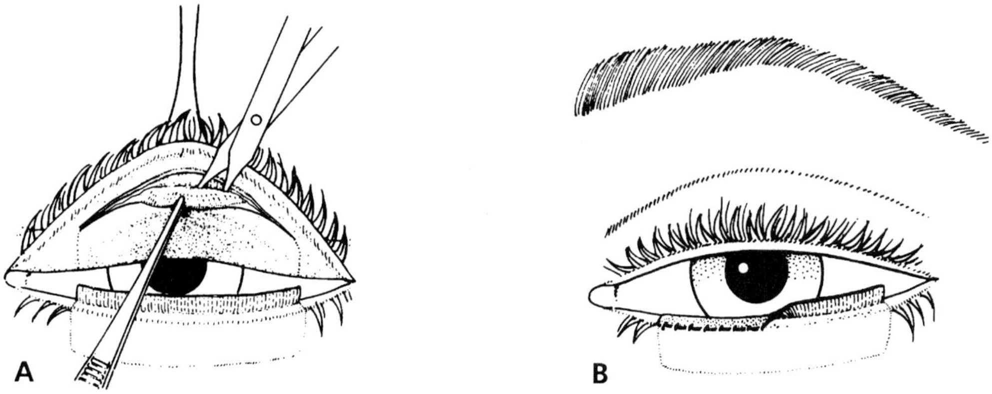

FIG. 18. A: Dissection of advanced tissue releasing the superior retractors with separation of the flap. A cuff of conjunctiva is present in the lower lid. **B:** Final lower lid position suturing the cuff recreating the lower lid margin.

7-0 silk. The superior edge of skin is sutured to the conjunctival flap 1–2 mm higher than the future lower lid margin. The grafted area is covered with Telfa. This, in turn, is covered by a light pressure dressing that will prevent tenting of the wound edges, which may cause later prominence of the tissue interface. The dressing should be left undisturbed for 7 days until the time of suture removal.

The flap and skin graft are left undisturbed, with the lids fused, for a period of 6–8 weeks and then can be separated (Fig. 17A).

Separation of the Hughes Flap

The flap is infiltrated with a local anesthetic containing epinephrine. A grooved director is inserted beneath the flap to protect the cornea, and the flap is severed flush or as close as possible to its origin under the upper lid (Fig. 17B).

If Müller's muscle was included and advanced in the flap, the released upper lid is everted over a Desmarres retractor. The bed of the flap is undermined into the superior fornix. The dissection is carried out in a plane between Müller's muscle fibers and the levator aponeurosis. Müller's muscle and the levator should be allowed to retract to their original level and prevent lid retraction secondary to Müller's muscle advancement (Fig. 18A). Less dissection is necessary if Müller's was not included in the flap.

After release of the upper lid, a skin incision is made along the desired position of the new lower lid margin. Excess grafted skin is trimmed, but care is taken not to excise the excess conjunctiva from the released flap. The conjunctiva is then everted over the new lid margin and sutured to the anterior cutaneous edge with a running 6-0 plain suture. The conjunctiva must completely cover the margin of the new lower lid or entropion and corneal irritation may occur. The excess conjunctiva on the lid margin will keratinize with time, or it can be cauterized at a later date to give a more normal appearance.

Transposition Tarsoconjunctival Flap (Hewes' Procedure)

A valuable procedure for repair of shallow lower lid defects in the temporal half of the lower lid is a transposition flap of tarsoconjunctiva from the superior edge of upper lid tarsus brought into the lower lid defect and covered with either a full-thickness skin graft or a flap (12). The procedure is somewhat limited in application but is quite excellent for defects not including the entire length of the lower lid margin at the lateral canthal area.

The steps of the procedure are shown in Fig. 19A–D. The upper lid is everted and methylene blue is used to outline a flap encompassing tarsoconjunctiva at the superior tarsal border and the conjunctiva above the superior tarsal border, and is based at the lateral canthal angle. The flap, designed in this manner, is a true axial flap because the peripheral vascular arcade at the superior tarsal edge is included and gives an intact blood supply to the flap. The flap is then dissected into the canthal angle until it moves freely; however, care is taken to spare the arcade as it enters the base of the flap. Stretching of the lower lid to reduce the size of the defect is performed to estimate the true length of flap that is needed to produce the proper tension in the lower lid. The flap is brought down and is sutured to the tarsus and conjunctiva in the lower lid with the tarsal edge in the downmost position, using absorbable sutures. Care must be taken so that too long a flap is not brought down, which may cause laxity in the lower lid postoperatively and a possible ectropion. The transposed tarsoconjunctival flap is then covered with a full-thickness skin graft from a suitable donor site. It is also

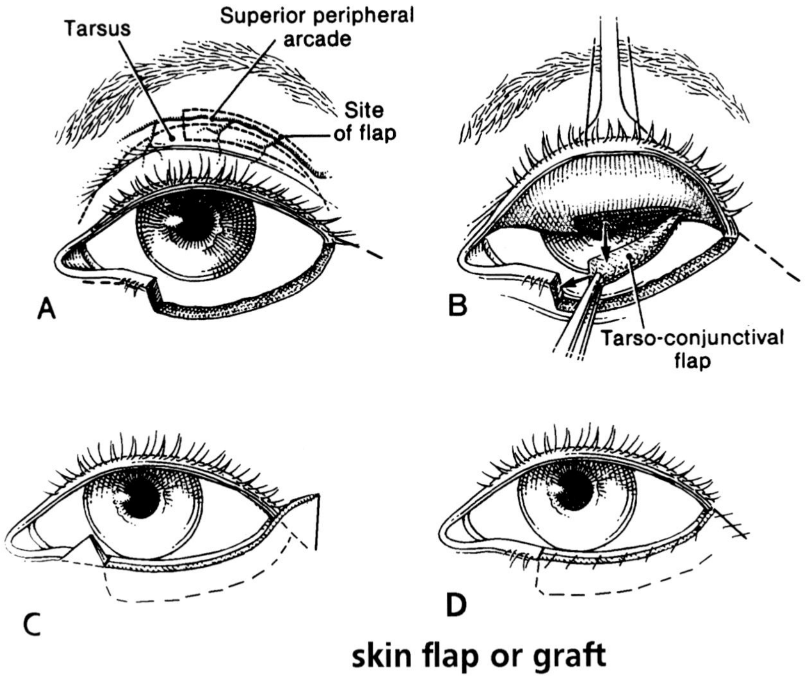

FIG. 19. Reconstruction of broad-shallow defect in the lateral portion of the lower lid with a transpositional tarsoconjunctival flap (Hewes). **A:** The position of the lower lid defect is seen and the outline of the flap from the undersurface of the lid based on the superior arcade is seen. **B:** The flap is transposed into the lower lid with the conjunctival surface inward and sutured. **C:** The myocutaneous flap is rotated up and outward with resection of redundancy and lateral periosteal fixation. **D:** Final position of the reconstructed lid. A skin graft can be used in patients instead of a flap if desired since blood supply is present in the pedicle flap.

possible to cover the transposition flap with a musculocutaneous transposition flap from the same upper lid based at the lateral canthal angle. This works particularly well in older individuals with much laxity of the musculocutaneous layer. This has the advantage of a one-stage procedure and furnishes adequate support and tension to the lower lid at the lateral canthal angle. The procedure has a cosmetically satisfactory effect, particularly in older individuals.

PERIORBITAL FLAPS

In many cases of eyelid reconstruction the surgeon is faced with situations in which local tissue adjacent to the eyelid or in the opposing upper lid is not available. This may be in patients who have had repeated surgery, or patients who have undergone extensive resection producing unusually large defects such as the patients who have had Mohs' histologic controlled excision of tumors. The stiffer skin in the forehead/lower cheek area flaps can be used for replacement, but they are best used in older people who have looser and redundant skin that is less elastic and contractile. In any of the flaps that are described subsequently, it is important that the flap be done with medial canthal fixation and lateral canthal fixation, if needed, to avoid postoperative sagging of the lower lid. The flap itself generally is skin or skin-muscle and has no mucous membrane lining. In most cases the flap should be lined with mucous membrane obtained from the inferior fornix (if available), a free tarsal conjunctival graft from an upper lid, a mucoperichondrium from the hard palate, or buccal mucous membrane from the lip or cheek.

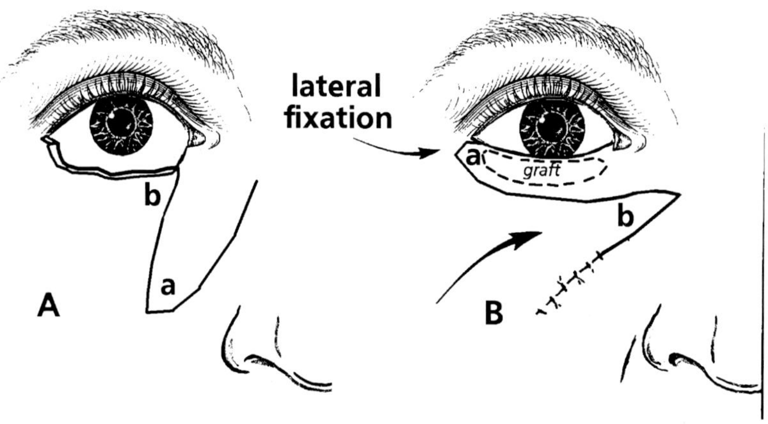

FIG. 20. Reconstruction of full-thickness lower lid defect with transpositional nasolabial flap. **A:** Lower lid defect and outline of transpositional flap from the nasolabial area. **B:** The nasolabial flap has been transposed to form the outer surface of the lower lid. The flap is lined with a free mucous membrane–lined graft.

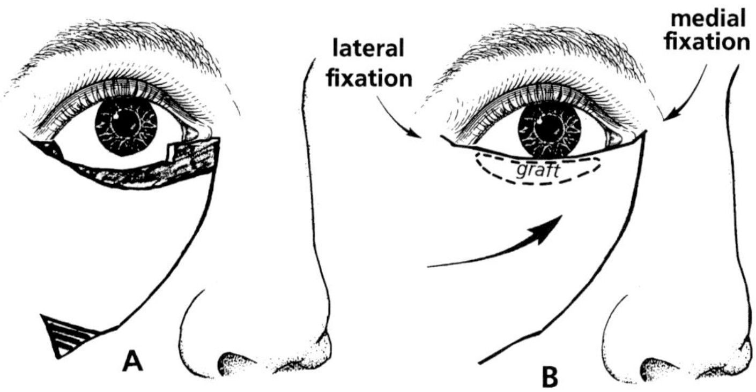

FIG. 21. Reconstruction of lower lid with advancement cheek flap. **A:** Defect in lower lid and outline of cheek flap to be rotated upward. **B:** Cheek flap has been rotated upward and fixated to the anterior reflection of the medial canthal tendon. The posterior surface of the flap has been lined with a mucous membrane–bearing free graft.

Transposition Cheek Flap

A transposition flap can be hinged at either the medial or the lateral canthus but is more commonly hinged medially (Fig. 20A, B). The thicker tissue is rotated upward to form the outward support of the lid and is fixated in the medial and lateral canthus with a fixation procedure and lined with a posterior lamella graft or conjunctival advancement (13).

Rotational Cheek Flap

The rotational cheek flap is an upward-rotated cheek flap facilitated by inferior incisions above the mouth and cheek area with undermining and upward advancement. It must also be fixated medially and laterally as previously described and provided with posterior lamella mucous membrane (Fig. 21A, B).

Temporal Forehead Transposition (Fricke) Flap

The Fricke is a transposition flap that has been used in the upper lid but also can be transposed further down to a lower lid defect to form the basis for support in the lower lid (14). The principles of canthal fixation and lining also apply to this flap (Fig. 22A, B).

Composite Grafts

It is not as common to use full-thickness eyelid composite grafts in the lower lid as it is in the upper lid because the need for lashes and a perfectly formed margin is not as great. A single composite graft taken from the contralateral lower lid (or upper lid) can be used, or two can be used in tandem and covered with a local myocutaneous flap as previously described in the chapter on upper lid reconstruction. In patients who demand the chance to have eyelashes, this is the best way to attempt that. Composite grafts will lose eyelashes in 40–50% of the cases despite good take of the soft tissue.

Staged Grafting

In extreme cases of total eyelid loss resulting from trauma, severe burns, or Mohs' excision of tumors, the primary goal is protection of the cornea and therefore the inverting conjunctival procedure with on-laid flaps of grafts can be performed. Many times the initial flap or graft can only be a skin and conjunctiva and a secondary ear cartilage graft must be inserted once the flap or graft has taken. This technique is described in the chapter on upper lid reconstruction.

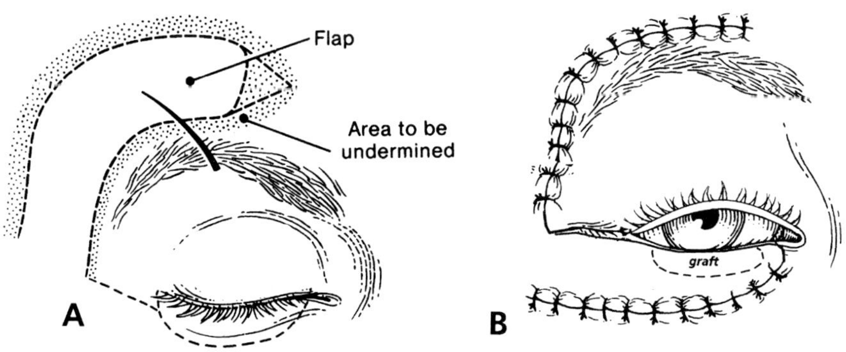

FIG. 22. Reconstruction of lower lid defect with transpositional temporal forehead flap (Fricke). **A:** Outline of defect in lower lid and outline of temporal forehead flap to be transposed. **B:** The temporal forehead flap has been transposed to the lower lid and sutured. The posterior surface of the flap is lined with a free mucous membrane–surfaced graft or advanced conjunctival.

COMPLICATIONS OF LOWER LID RECONSTRUCTION

Eyelid margin positional abnormalities are usually not a serious complication, but they can be annoying to both the patient and the surgeon. They may also require further surgery for correction. The most common complication of lower eyelid reconstruction is lower lid sagging or ectropion.

Lower Lid Ectropion

The most common reasons for postoperative ectropion are a vertical shortage of eyelid skin, residual lower lid laxity because of excessive horizontal length, and inadequate canthal fixation.

Vertical shortage of lower lid skin is accentuated by the natural downward pull of gravity and altered lid mobility. The surgeon should not hesitate to use full-thickness skin grafting to the lower lid at the original reconstruction to ensure vertical lower lid skin adequacy. After most lower lid reconstructions, a tarsorrhaphy suture left in place for a week helps to counteract the natural tendency for graft shrinkage. Other authors have performed reconstructive techniques using vertical advancement flaps of cheek skin to the lower eyelid defect. Descriptions of these procedures have been omitted deliberately in this chapter because only rarely can an upward advancement be employed successfully without resulting in contracture and lower lid ectropion.

Ectropion caused by laxity of the lower lid margin may result from the use of tarsoconjunctival flaps that are too wide. Measuring the correct length of horizontal tissue needed to fill a defect should be done with calipers and with the lower lid stretched to approximate the desired tension on the lower lid margin. The ability of the lower lid to stretch and cover defects, particularly in the older patient, must not be underestimated.

Proper lateral canthal and medial canthal fixation is an important part of any reconstruction involving the lower lid. Nonabsorbable sutures should be used. If the suture does not actually engage the periosteum laterally or a reflection of the canthal tendon medially, incompetence will result in lid laxity.

Lateral Lid Sag

Sagging of the lateral lower lid in the late postoperative course occurs for many of the same reasons as ectropion. If a rotational flap technique such as the Mustarde or Tenzel flap is used, the apex of the semicircle must be sufficiently high to exert an exaggerated upward pull on the lateral lower lid. Nonabsorbable sutures from the repositioned flap to the temporalis fascia can augment this effect. The use of the supplemental periosteal flap and autogenous ear cartilage will augment this support.

Upper Eyelid Abnormalities

Upper eyelid abnormalities are related to the use of the upper lid sharing with the Hughes procedure. Some degree of upper eyelid retraction can occur with the modified Hughes procedure after separation of the flap in the second stage. This can be minimized by careful dissection between Müller's muscle and the levator aponeurosis. At the time of separation of the flap, any advanced Müller's muscle or advanced levator must be tenotomized. If significant retraction persists, it can be corrected with a levator recession and a spacer material implant from an external approach. Tenting of the margin or entropion and trichiasis can occur if the tarsoconjunctival flap is developed too close to the upper lid margin (as in the originally described procedure). A minimum of 4 mm of intact tarsus along the margin of the upper lid is essential for upper lid stability.

REFERENCES

1. McCord CD, Nunery WR. Reconstruction of the lower llid and outer canthus. *Oculoplastic Surgery*. 2nd ed. New York: Raven Press; 1987:93–115.
2. Tenzel RR, Stewart WB. Eyelid reconstruction by semi-circular flap technique. *Trans Am Soc Ophthalmol Otolarygol* 1978;85: 1164–1169.
3. Weinstein GS, Anderson RL, et al. The use of the periosteal strip for eyelid reconstruction. *Arch Ophthalmol* 1985;103:357–359.
4. Anderson RL, Edwards JJ. Reconstruction by myocutaneous eyelid flaps. *Arch Ophthalmol* 1979;97:2358–2362.
5. Beyer CK, Bathrick ME. One stage lower lid reconstruction. *Ophth Surg* 1982;13:551–554.
6. Stephenson CM, Brown BZ. The use of tarsus as a free autogenous graft in eyelid surgery. *Ophth Plast Reconstr Surg* 1985; 1:43–50.
7. Leone CR Jr, Hand SL Jr. Reconstruction of the medial eyelid. *Am J Ophthalmol* 1979;87:797–801.
8. Steinkogler FJ. A sandwich technique for reconstruction of the lower lid. *Orbit* 1989;8:37–43.
9. Mustarde LC. *Repair and reconstruction in the orbital region*. Edinburgh: Churchill–Livingstone; 1971: Chaps. 7 and 8.
10. Hughes WH. Reconstruction of the lids. *Am J Ophthalmol* 1945; 28:1203–1211.
11. Hughes WH. Total lower lid reconstruction: technical details. *Trans Am Ophthalmol Soc* 1976;74:321–329.
12. Hewes EH, Sullivan JH, Beard C. Lower eyelid reconstruction by tarsal transposition. *Am J Ophthalmol* 1976;81:512–514.
13. Blasius E. *Beitrage zur praktischen Chirurgie*. Berlin: A Forstner; 1848.
14. Fricke JCG. *Die Bildung neuer Augenlider (Blepharoplastik) nach Zerstorungen und dadurch hervorgebrachten auswartswendungen derselben*. Hamburg: Perthes and Bessler; 1829.

CHAPTER 22

Medial Canthal Reconstruction

Defects of the medial canthal region occur most commonly following excision of skin tumors or trauma. If the defect in the canthus detaches the tarsoligamentous sling from the nasal wall, the repair procedure must include a refixation of the tarsoligamentous sling to the posterior reflection of the medial canthal tendon (as previously described in the chapter on lower lid reconstruction). Techniques for repair of the anterior lamella such as natural granulation, full-thickness skin graft, and glabellar flap must include this repair to restore the direction of the normal canthal angle. A permanent suture such as 4-0 prolene is used to obtain the desired posteriorly directed pull to the medial canthal angle. Braided nylon sutures have been used in the past but have produced granuloma formation in a high percentage of patients. Attachment to the posterior reflection of the medial canthal tendon is necessary not only to create a normal appearance but to facilitate the later placement of a Jones tube, which requires a normal medial canthal angle to function properly.

Defects in the medial canthal area that are diamond-shaped, as shown in Fig. 1, are most easily closed, and surgically created defects should be fashioned in this manner if possible. A strong permanent suture such as 4-0 prolene is placed through the tarsal remnants of each upper and lower lid and then attached to the posterior reflection of the medial canthal tendon. The half-circle P2 needle facilitates the placement of this suture (1).

With a defect such as that shown in Fig. 1, the lid defect remnants are first pulled over and attached with a permanent suture to the tarsal plate and to the posterior section of the medial canthal tendon. The remaining skin (anterior lamella) defect can be closed by any of three methods.

GRANULATION

The defect can be allowed to granulate spontaneously over several weeks with daily dressing changes. Some contraction will take place and in larger defects may displace the lid and canthus requiring secondary surgical revision. Cleansing with peroxide and lubrication with ointment will promote smooth closure.

FULL SKIN GRAFT

A full-thickness skin graft can be sutured in place with interrupted 7-0 silk as shown in Fig. 1, with a dressing of Telfa, molded dental wax, and cotton pads placed over this to stent the graft. Sutures are removed 1 week postoperatively.

GLABELLAR FLAP

A transpositional glabellar forehead flap can be used for immediate reconstruction. The flap is drawn with methylene blue (Fig. 2A) and incised. The flap and skin around the area are extensively undermined to allow the flap to rotate into the defect as well as to permit closure of the donor site (Fig. 2B). A small triangle may need to be excised for the flap to fit the defect. This technique may cause some postoperative narrowing of distance between the eyebrows requiring plucking. The redundant triangular tip can be used for filling in of defects not covered with the flap. A quilting suture passed through the flap externally, plicating the flap to the medial canthal tendon, will shape the flap for a more normal canthal contour.

The use of direct closure, full-thickness skin graft or closure by granulation in the medial canthal defects tends to leave a normal concavity and contour to the medial canthal area. The glabellar flap tends to fill this area, giving less concavity, and may require additional debulking.

Unless clear margins are obtained with frozen sections in the removal of skin malignancies, defects in the medial canthal region should be allowed to granulate rather than receive full-thickness grafts or flaps in

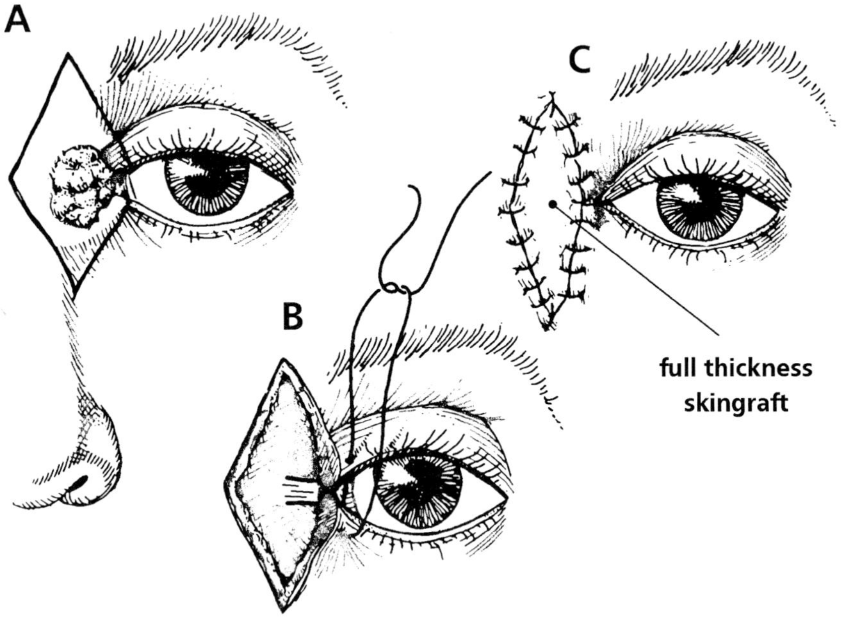

FIG. 1. Reconstruction of medial canthus with full-thickness skin graft. A: Outline of proposed defect triangulated for better closure. B: Attachment of lid edges to residual anterior reflection of medial canthal tendon (if present). C: Full-thickness skin graft in place.

order to allow inspection and rebiopsy for tumor recurrence. Only after clear edges and deep margins are obtained should a medial canthal defect be covered with a flap or full-thickness graft. Covering unsuspected residual tumor with a flap or graft can allow the tumor to extend insidiously into the orbit.

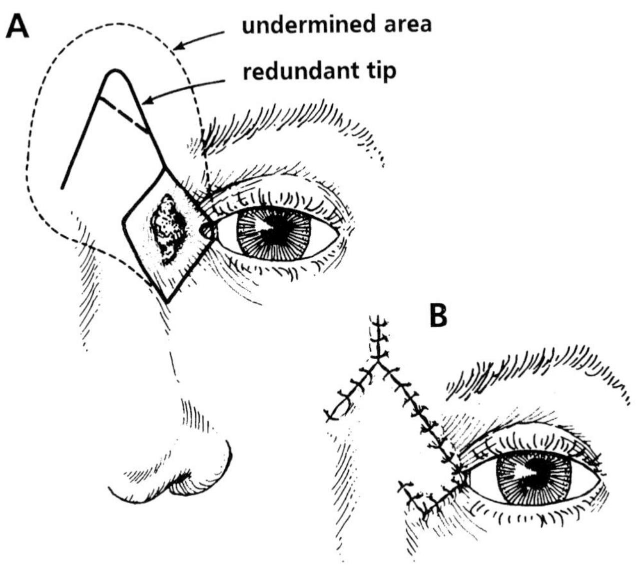

FIG. 2. Reconstruction of medial canthus with glabellar rotational flap. A: Outline of flap in midforehead area. B: Transposition of flap into inner canthus. The flap is usually fixated to the anterior reflection of the medial canthal tendon with a 4-0 prolene quilting suture. Redundant tip can be used as graft if needed.

TARSAL (TARSOCONJUNCTIVAL) FLAP (WITH SKIN GRAFT OR FLAP)

When the posterior lamella of the lid is missing from the canthal area, one cannot simply repair the anterior lamella with a skin graft or flap and have adequate canthal reformation; the posterior lamella must be repaired as well. This can be accomplished with a horizontally sliding section of tarsus or sliding tarsal conjunctival flap (as described in the chapter on upper lid reconstruction) (Fig. 3A–C). In cases in which the defect in the canthus encompasses a section of upper and lower lid, the sliding tarsal flap must be positioned and be shared between the upper and lower lids when fixated to the canthus. The tarsal conjunctival flap can then be covered with either a full-thickness skin graft, a local skin-muscle flap, or a glabellar flap (Fig. 3D–F).

INNER CANTHAL FIXATION

Deep Periosteal Suture

In patients with a medial canthal defect, which in most cases includes a section of the upper and lower lids, the proper reattachment of the tarsoligamentous sling should be made to the posterior reflection of the medical canthal tendon positioned behind the lacrimal sac (Fig. 4). If there is residual tissue in this posterior sac area, either periosteum or residual reflected tendon, direct fixation of the edge of the upper and lower lid to this posterior reflection can be performed with a 4-0 prolene suture. The suture must have a very small but sturdy half-circle needle in order to take the poste-

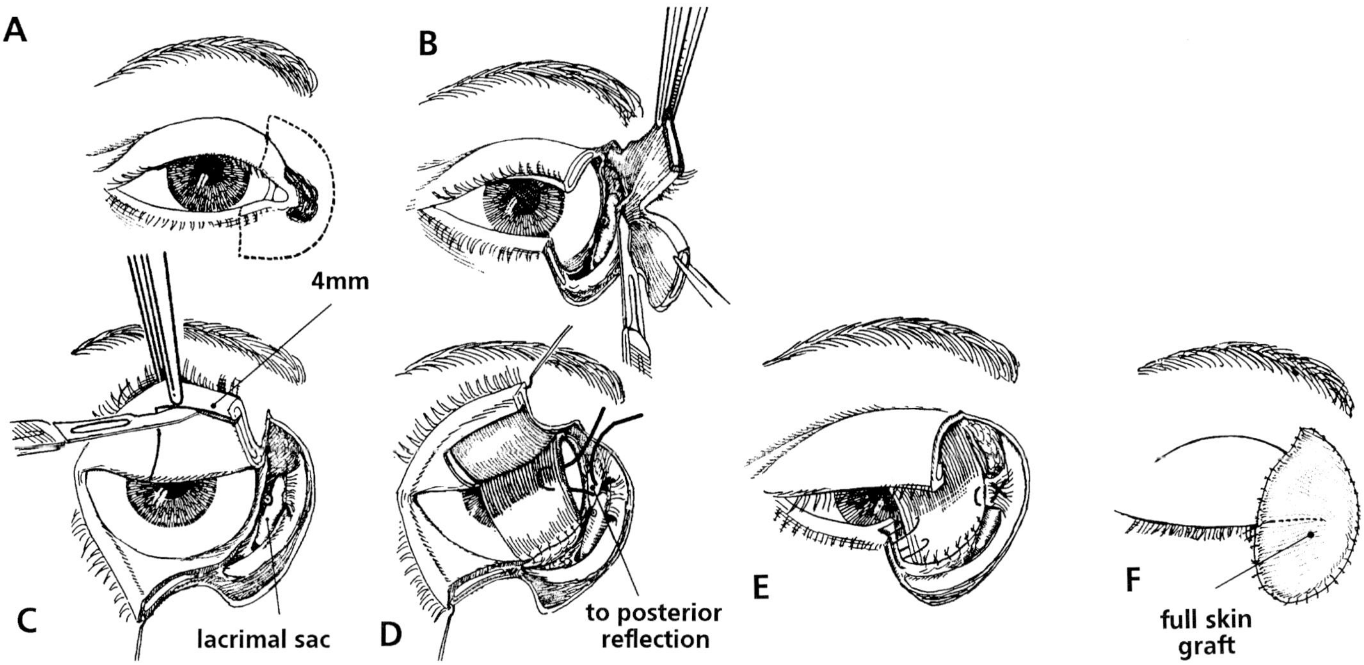

FIG. 3. Reconstruction of medial canthus with sliding tarsoconjunctival flap. **A:** Lesion in medial canthus for excision is outlined showing size of defect. **B:** Tissue is removed including the portion of the anterior reflection of the medial canthal tendon and canalicular system. **C:** Upper lid everted showing development of a tarsoconjunctival flap from the undersurface of the upper lid. **D:** Tarsoconjunctival flap has been advanced medially and inferiorly and fixated to the posterior reflection of the medial canthal tendon posterior to the lacrimal sac. **E:** The flap is then fixated to the temporal edge of the lower lid defect for alignment of the posterior lamella structures. **F:** Defect is covered with a full skin graft. Advancement flaps from the eyelid or rotational flaps from the glabellar area can also be used.

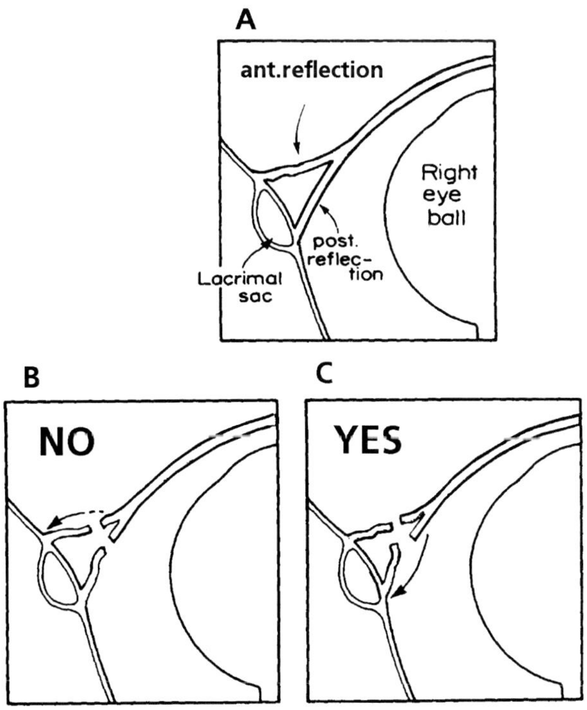

FIG. 4. Diagrammatic representation of the medial attachment of the eyelids with the anterior and posterior reflection of the medial canthal tendon. **A:** The posterior reflection of the medial canthal tendon follows the insertion of the tarsoligamental sling (posterior lamella). The anterior reflection of the medial canthal tendon is the point of insertion of the myocutaneous (anterior lamella). **B:** If there is interruption of the tarsoligamental sling, the edge of the lid should not be attached to the anterior reflection alone. **C:** The proper attachment of the tarsoligamental sling is made to the posterior reflection behind the lacrimal sac in order that the lower lid curvature follow the curve of the globe and to prevent space forming between the lid and the globe.

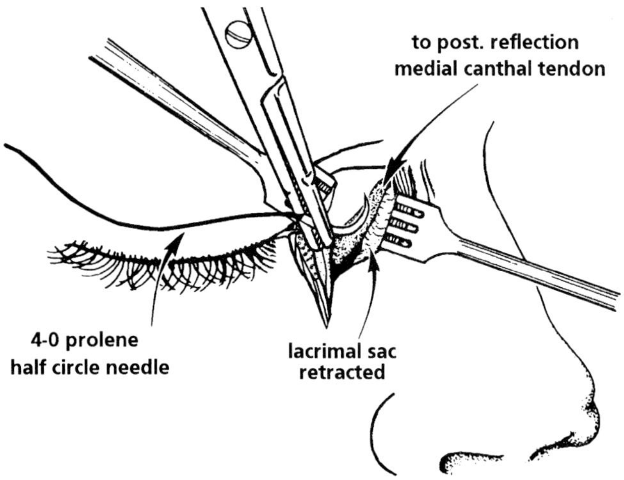

FIG. 5. Placement of the fixating suture to the posterior reflection of the medial canthal tendon. This requires adequate exposure with retraction of the lids laterally and the lacrimal sac anteriorly. A malleable retractor can be used. In order to be able to take a "bite" in the posterior reflection, a sturdy half-circle needle should be used.

rior bite. The posterior area is exposed with a malleable retractor reflecting the lacrimal sac forward and another retractor protecting the globe. The suture can then be taken in this posterior tissue (Fig. 5). The attachment of the suture should be in firm, preferably periosteal tissue. A test of its adequacy can be done by tugging on the suture once it is inserted and feeling its rigidity or observing a slight movement of the head when it is gently pulled. It is important to place the suture on a level with a pupillary plane so that when the upper and lower lids are attached through the resected edges of the tarsal plates the canthal angle will be reformed in its desired location. The suture of choice is a 4-0 prolene on a P2 needle. The ME-2 needle on braided nylon is another half-circle needle that can be used for this purpose. However, the braided nylon has been shown to form granulomas in a large percentage of cases when buried in this area.

Nasal Periosteal Flap

If lost from trauma or tumor resection, the anterior reflection of the tendonous lid attachment can be recreated with a periosteal flap (2). An incision is made through the skin in an arcuate manner, medial to the remaining medial canthal tendon or area where it existed previously. The length of the incision will vary depending on the size or periosteal rotation flap needed for reconstruction. The dissection is carried through subcutaneous and muscular tissue down to periosteum. Some overlying muscular tissue may be left attached to periosteum to add bulk to the rotation flap. A rectangular flap is fashioned that is hinged laterally at the remaining stump of medial canthal tendon or, if all of the tendon has been removed, as close to the area as possible (Fig. 6A). The width of the flap should be 6–10 mm if possible. A sharp periosteal elevator is used to elevate the flap with care taken not to weaken the nasal attachment. Once elevated and rotated laterally, the flap is sutured to the remaining portions of lateral upper and/or lower eyelid with permanent 4-0 suture (Fig. 6B, C). The periosteal rotation flap forms the foundation for a new medial canthal tendon. Conjunctival mobilization may be necessary to form a new canthal angle. Unfortunately, the direction of pull is more anterior than desired for the tarsoligamentous sling but furnishes a good attachment for the anterior lamella of the lid. In some cases anterior attachment is better than no attachment.

Ipsilateral Nasal Drill Holes

Nasal and nasolacrimal bony irregularities anterior to the anterior lacrimal crests, if present, are smoothed with a high-speed dental burr. Two perforations sepa-

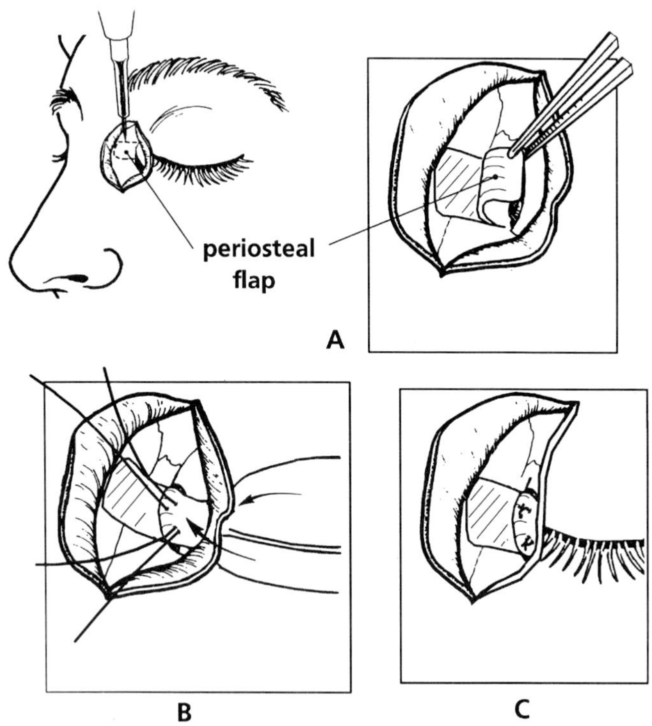

FIG. 6. Reconstruction of the medial canthal tendon (anterior reflection) with periosteal flap. In cases in which bone and posterior reflection are absent, lid fixation, although not ideal, can be accomplished with a posteriorly rotated periosteal flap. **A:** Shows outline and development of the periosteal flap. **B:** The edge of the upper and lower lid have been attached with sutures to the posterior surface of the flap. **C:** The suture is tightened with reformation of the canthus before closure of the skin.

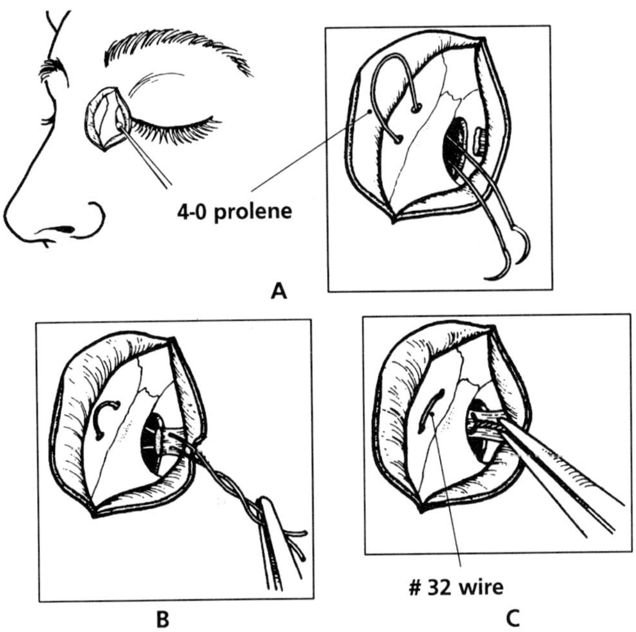

FIG. 7. Reconstruction of the medial canthus with direct fixation to bone. In cases in which there is absence of the posterior reflection of the tendon or bone and the anterior periosteum is not available for a periosteal flap, direct fixation of the medial corner of the upper and lower lid can be accomplished with drill holes and direct attachment. **A:** Drill holes have been created in the remaining bone anterior to the lacrimal sac fossa and sutures passed in a posterior direction. The fixation can be done with wire or with 4-0 prolene suture. **B:** The wire or sutures have been passed through the edge of the tarsal plate in the upper and lower lid or remnant of the anterior medial canthal tendon. **C:** The wire is tightened or the sutures snugged into the nasal corner of the orbit. Care is taken to create the attachment as posteriorly as possible.

rated by a minimum of 1 cm are made through the unaffected nasal bone 3–4 mm anterior to the anterior lacrimal crest. A single 30-gage stainless steel wire (or 4-0 prolene suture) is then placed from through the bony perforations and brought out behind the anterior lacrimal crest (Fig. 7A). This wire is then sutured to the edge of the eyelids with a curved needle and tightened in order to bring about the appropriate medial placement of the eyelids (Fig. 7B, C). It is difficult to position the wire posteriorly enough (particularly if there is a deficiency of bone) and the exact posterior fixation needed may not be obtained. However, this is a useful technique in some cases when the other techniques cannot be used.

Miniplate

The miniplate technique allows more posterior fixation but presumes the presence of enough anterior bone to affix the miniplate (3).

The nose should be packed with vasoconstrictors. In the exposed area the periosteum is first reflected anteriorly toward the dorsum of the nose, to expose the thicker nasal bone, which will provide the anterior fixation site of the miniplate. Periosteum is then reflected posteriorly toward the lacrimal sac fossa. Care must be taken to avoid damaging the canaliculi and lacrimal sac. It is essential to dissect all soft tissue from bone before proceeding.

Bony irregularities can be sculpted with the high-speed dental drill. Care must be taken not to avulse bony fragments out of the area with a rongeur because this may damage either the anterior ethmoidal artery or the cribriform plate, with resultant hemorrhage or cerebrospinal fluid leak. Rather, the comminuted fragments are excised sharply.

Once exposure of the lacrimal crest and sac fossa is achieved, a five-holed, Y-shaped miniplate is placed against the lateral aspect of the nose with forceps and bent with pliers to closely mirror the normal bony contour. Contouring of the miniplate is necessary to adjust its final position because the plate will conform to the bone once the screws are tightened. The long arm of the Y also must be bent to the correct position to allow for the proper posteriorly directed cantilever effect. The posterior arm should rest in the plane of the lamina papyracea just inferior to the frontoethmoidal suture and should extend toward the apex of the orbit to the position of the anterior ethmoidal artery. Pilot holes are then drilled into bone through the holes in the short arms of the plate while the globe is protected with a malleable retractor. Removal of the nasal packing sponges before drilling the holes prevents them from becoming engaged by the drill or the screws.

The inferior hole of the short arm of the Y or the apex of the short arm is initially drilled. Usually a 6-mm screw is placed and not fully tightened to provide a more stable fixation while the remaining two holes are drilled. When the superior hole of the short arm of the Y plate is being drilled, care should be taken to direct the drill in a slightly inferior direction, away from the cribriform plate. As an additional precaution, only a 4-mm screw is placed through this most superior hole (Fig. 8A).

A 4-0 prolene suture is passed through the edge of the eyelids or the residual medial canthal tendon. Both ends of the suture are then passed through the appropriate hole of the long arm of the miniplate (Fig. 8B). Usually one of the two most posteriorly positioned holes provides the appropriate site for the posterior fixation of the medial canthal tendon, corresponding to the level of the posterior lacrimal crest. One screw that has not been previously tightened serves as an anterior fixation site for the suture. The sutures are passed around this screw and tied. The assistant provides firm medial and posterior pressure to the medial

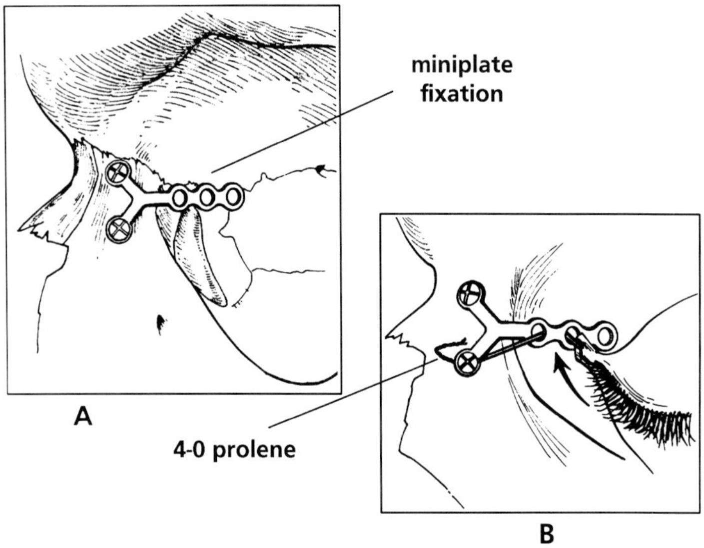

FIG. 8. Reconstruction of the medial canthus with the use of miniplate [after Shore et al. (3)]. **A:** Miniplate has been fixated to the anterior lacrimal crest and the straight portion curved posteriorly. **B:** The edge of the upper and lower lid, or residual distal remnant of the medial canthal tendon, has been directed posteriorly to a middle or posteriorly placed hole. The suture is then brought anteriorly for fixation producing a cantilevered effect directing the lid edge posteriorly and recreating its curvature against the globe.

canthal tendon as the sutures are tightened and tied. The medial canthal tendon will move into correct position. A lateral canthotomy and cantholysis may be performed if tension on the lids is too great. Nose pads may be incorporated at this point with a 4-0 double-armed prolene suture passed around a hole in the miniplate with the ends extending through the skin incision. Once skin is closed around the prolene suture, one silicone pad is threaded over each suture and the suture is then tied over a dental roll to compress skin in this area, flattening out any epicanthal folds. The nose pads and external prolene suture are removed 7–10 days later.

Transnasal Wires

The passage of a fixating wire from the contralateral canthus is the most effective way to fixate the eyelids to a canthus, particularly in patients with deficient bone. Repositioning of the medial canthal angles with transnasal wires also corrects the deformity of posttraumatic telecanthus. In posttraumatic cases anterior tomography of the orbital bones and medial aspects of both orbits may be needed in problem cases to identify the extent of underlying bony abnormalities. This information is necessary to determine if enough bone is present to support the posterior placement of the transnasal wires, although in some cases the intranasal septum can play a role in furnishing a posterior edge to hold the wires back. The possible complication of herniation of central nervous system tissue via the area of bony defect should be ruled out utilizing anterior tomography.

Unilateral Transnasal Wiring

In medial canthal defects, for fixation of the lid edges to the area behind the lacrimal sac fossa, a stainless steel wire must be passed from the opposite side (Fig. 9A, B) (4,5). The superior aspect of each nasal cavity is packed with cottonoid sponges moistened with a mixture of oxymetazoline hydrochloride (Afrin) 0.05% and phenylephrine hydrochloride (NeoSynephrine) 0.25%. The medial canthal angle is infiltrated with lidocaine 2% with epinephrine 1:100,000 and hyaluronidase (Wydase). The local anesthetic mixture is injected into the ethmoid air cells by passing the needle through the medial orbital wall. This in conjunction with the nasal packing will greatly aid hemostasis during surgery. The skin and subcutaneous tissue just anterior to the medial canthus on the unaffected or normal side is likewise injected.

In cases in which a defect is not already present and a secondary reconstruction is being done, a crescent-shaped skin incision is made 2 mm anterior to the canthal angle on the affected side. The incision is carried down to include the periosteum. Any abnormal subcutaneous tissue is excised before reflecting the periosteum temporally. Hypertrophic scar tissue is usually found following trauma to this area and must be trimmed to get a good result. Damage to the lacrimal canaliculi and sac must be avoided during the dissection, which is continued until the anterior and posterior lacrimal crests and the superior portion of the lacrimal sac fossa are exposed. The periosteum may be quite adherent to bone in this area following nasoorbital fractures, making the dissection difficult; however, the periosteum and adherent scar tissue must be dissected off the bone before proceeding.

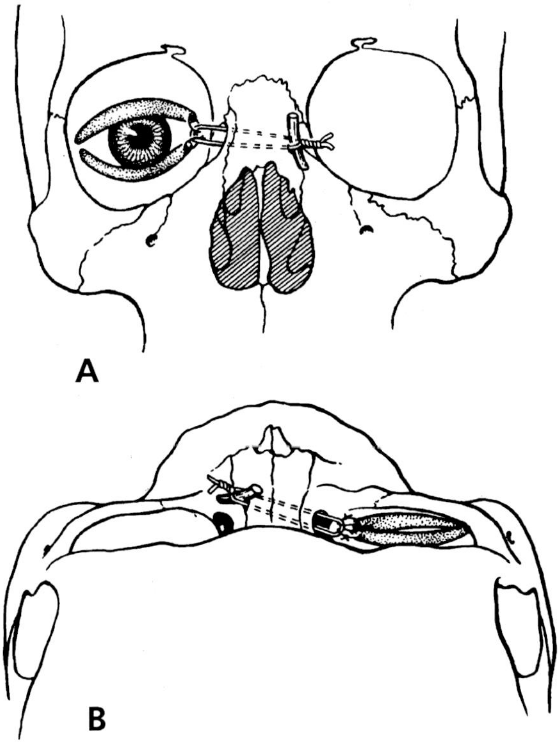

FIG. 9. Medial canthal reconstruction with fixation with transnasal wiring. This is the most precise method for canthal fixation but is more technically involved. **A:** Frontal view showing wires that have been passed through drill holes using a trocar from the contralateral side in a posterior direction for fixation. The wires have been fixated on the contralateral side with a bolster that is usually formed from a segment of the stylet of an 18-gage spinal needle. A 32-gage wire is used. **B:** Axial view showing the proper direction for passage of the wires to create a posterior fixation for canthal reconstruction. This technique is effective for use in patients in whom bone and tissue is not available for direct posterior fixation. It also is the only method of fixation in extreme cases in which supporting structures are not available for fixation on the side of the canthal deformity.

In posttraumatic cases hyperostotic bone is formed during the healing of nasoethmoidal fractures and may extend inferiorly into the lacrimal sac fossa and nasolacrimal canal. A medium-sized dental burr on a rotary osteotome is introduced into the area and the splayed-out bone in the region of the posterior lacrimal crest is thinned down completely to the level of the ethmoidal air cells. Adequate bone removal must be accomplished by thinning to restore the bony canthal configuration prior to transnasal wiring. In order to reform the canthal angle properly, the direction of pull on the eyelids must be toward the posterior lacrimal crest, and that must be the level of passage of the transnasal wires. There must be intact bone present anterior to this level to prevent the wires from migrating to a more forward position. The bone anterior to the posterior lacrimal crest can be thinned a great deal to restore contour; however, it must not be completely removed as that might allow forward migration of the wires, although occasionally an intact nasal septum will stabilize the wires posteriorly. Anterior migration can result in poor eyelid apposition to the globe postoperatively.

Before passage of the wire the nasal packing is removed. A small hole is drilled in each lateral nasal wall where the wires will subsequently be passed. A 14-gage trochar is passed transnasally from the normal to the abnormal side through the holes previously created in the side of the nose.

In most cases the trochar must be tapped through the septum with the help of a small mallet. It is important to protect the globes during the passage of the trochar, and an assistant must watch for the appearance of the tip of the trochar. The trochar should be aimed as well as possible to appear at the desired position of posterior fixation. Protective scleral contact lenses should be placed on the globe and a malleable retractor positioned to prevent possible penetration of the globe by the point of the trochar. When the trochar has been passed, the stylet is removed; a 32-gage stainless steel wire is then bent on itself and the loop of the wire passed through the lumen of the trochar transnasally so that the loop of the wire is present on the abnormal side. The trochar is then removed leaving the loop of wire in place. The wire has usually been pinched at the apex of the loop during passage through the trochar creating a weak spot in the wire. The ends of the wire should be adjusted to bring this kink back through the nose to the normal side where it is cut off leaving a smooth loop of wire for suture fixation to the eyelids.

The tissue in the area of the medial canthal tendon is sutured to the wire on the looped side with 4-0 nonabsorbable suture, e.g., prolene. The wire is now ready for tightening. To fixate the wire, a metal bolster pin is fashioned by cutting of an 8-mm length from the central portion of the stylet of a 19-gage angiocath. The pin is bent slightly in the middle and held against the lateral nasal bone with a vertical orientation resting between the ends of the wire, which are now twisted over the pin, anchoring the pin against the bone and giving excellent purchase for further tightening to the wire. Simultaneously pulling on the ends of the wires and twisting them over the pin until the telecanthus is slightly overcorrected tightens the wire loop. The twisted wire is cut and bent into the hole in the lateral nasal bone. The skin is closed with 6-0 nylon sutures.

Nose pads are usually not required in unilateral cases; however, if necessary they can be applied. A transcutaneous 4-0 prolene suture can be looped under the wire loop and used to anchor a tie-over cotton bolster for compression postoperatively. After the wiring tightening has been completed, the skin sutures are left in place for 7–10 days. The deep, looped transnasal wire remains in place permanently.

Epicanthal Folds

Epicanthal folds in the medial canthal area occur most commonly as a congenital deformity or may occur with trauma to soft tissue in the canthal area. The congenital epicanthal folds have been classified in the past by Johnson as epicanthus supratarsalus, epicanthus supraciliaries, epicanthus palpebralis, and epicanthus inversus depending on the position of the fold around the inner canthal angle (6). Regardless of its position, the correction consists of removal of subcutaneous tissue and rearrangement of the skin in the canthal angle so that the fold is flattened. This can be accomplished with excision of subcutaneous tissue and rearrangement of the skin with transposition flaps and external compression or quilting sutures. The design of successful flaps for correction of lateral canthal displacement requires that there be traction in one set of flaps pulling the inner canthus toward the nose. The flaps can be single or double transposition. In cases that are combined with a severe telecanthus deformity, transnasal wiring with external compression with nose pads is necessary.

In general, the important steps in the correction of epicanthal folds, regardless of what kind of skin flap is used, are the adequate removal of abnormal subcutaneous tissue and external compression of the skin postoperatively.

TRANSPOSITION FLAPS

Single Transposition

A Z-plasty transposition can be useful in folds that are less severe and span the vertical or higher part of the eyelid. One arm of the Z is inside the fold and one is outside (Fig. 10A–D) (7).

Double Transposition

In more severe cases, particularly in those folds that extend to the lower lid, the double Z configuration is more effective. Plication of the tendon with nasal traction improves lateral canthal displacement in cases without bony deformity (Fig. 11A–D) (6).

Neither flap type produces a good result unless there is debulking of subcutaneous tissue in the canthal area anterior to the anterior reflection of the medial canthal tendon. After closure of the flaps, a 4-0 prolene suture may be passed through the skin, under the anterior reflection of the medial canthal tendon, to serve as fixation for an external nose pad. External compression of the canthal flaps can be accomplished postoperatively with quilting fixation sutures to get adequate flattening and smoothing of the area.

Bilateral Transnasal Wires with Nose Pads

This technique is used specifically if there is a severe bilateral deformity, particularly if there is a bony ab-

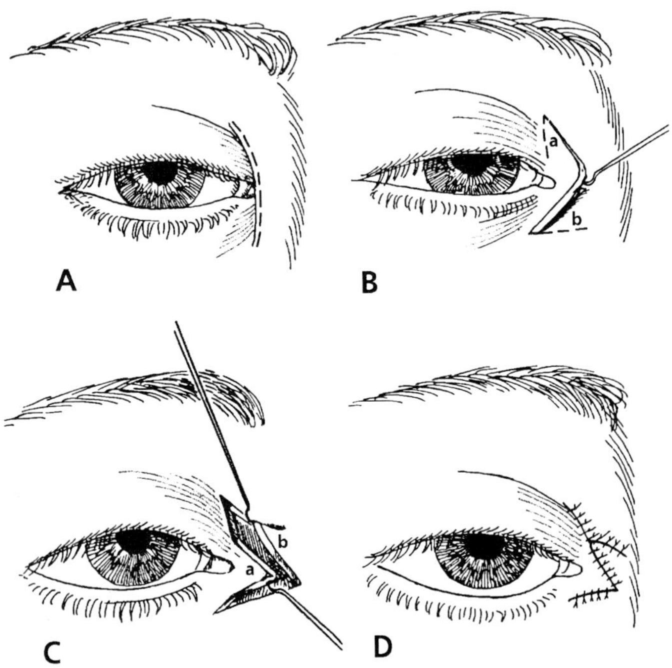

FIG. 10. Epicanthal fold repair. Transposition flaps with the technique of Blair, Brown, and Hamm (7). **A:** Epicanthus palpebralis with outline of incision on the edge of the fold. **B:** The fold has been retracted showing additional incisions for development of transposition flaps. **C:** The flaps have been undermined, subcutaneous tissue or scar tissue removed, and the flaps transposed. **D:** Final position of the transposed flaps.

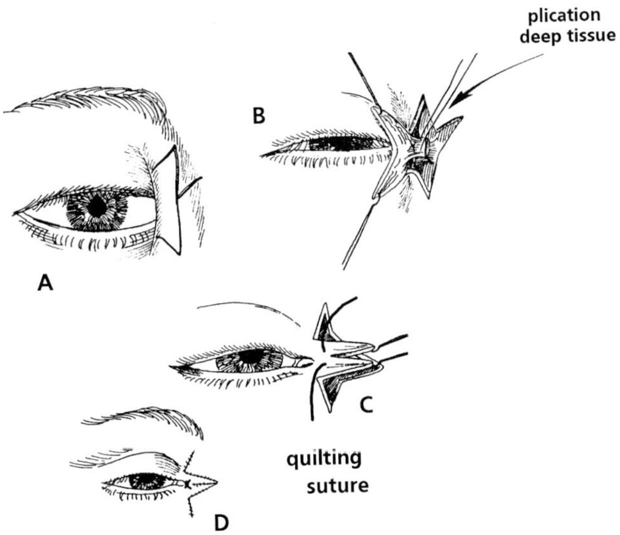

FIG. 11. Medial canthoplasty for repair of epicanthal fold and mild telecanthus [modified from the method of Carl Cordes Johnson (6)]. **A:** Epicanthal palpebrallis showing marking of skin incisions for remedy of flap and to improve telecanthus. **B:** The flaps have been incised and elevated and the medial canthus plicated with direct suturing. **C:** The flaps have been brought forward with traction to further improve the canthal position. A quilting suture can be used to suture through the flap to the anterior reflection of the medial canthal tendon. Some redundancy of the flaps may be excised. **D:** Final suture line following transposition of flaps, fixation, and closure. A tie-over bolster is sometimes used for compression.

normality. Very firm nasal pad compression is required postoperatively (4,5).

The surgical technique for bilateral transnasal wiring differs from that described for unilateral cases. The crescent-shaped skin incision is made bilaterally just

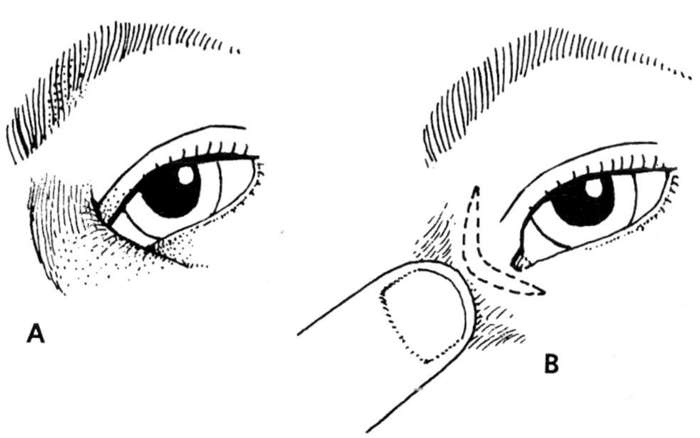

FIG. 12. Medial canthoplasty for epicanthal fold and telecanthus as a preliminary for an external compression procedure, usually transnasal wiring. **A:** Diagrammatic representation of epicanthus palpebralis or inversus and telecanthus. **B:** Area of excision of tissue. Subcutaneous tissue including fibrous tissue, fatty tissue, and other anomalous tissue in the anterior lacrimal crest area is excised.

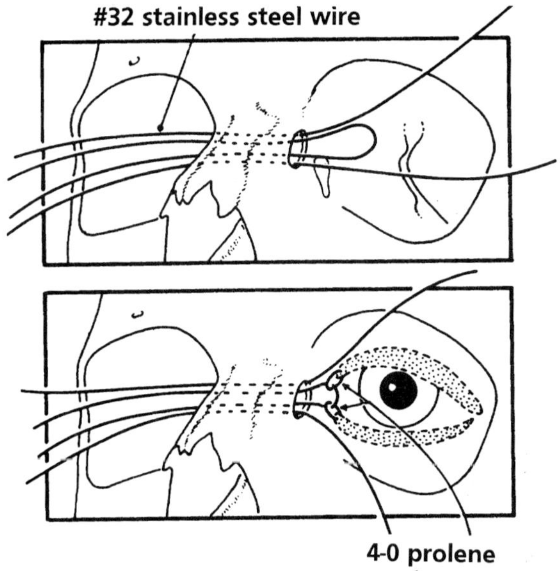

FIG. 13. Diagrammatic representation of placement of transnasal wires used for fixating the eyelids to the medial canthus and for external compression of the canthal area. The wires can be passed from one side to the other with the use of a 16-gage trocar through a single hole. For canthal fixation the edge of the lids are attached to the loop of wire or looped wire with 4-0 prolene sutures.

anterior to the canthal angles (Fig. 12A, B). If an epicanthal fold exists, a small amount of skin may be excised; the subsequent dissection and removal of excess subcutaneous tissue and the thinning of hyperostotic bone is completed bilaterally just as described for unilateral cases.

Penetration of the bone must be near the level of the posterior lacrimal crest bilaterally, and intact bone should be left anterior to that position if possible to avoid forward migration of the wires postoperatively.

Once the trochar has been passed and the stylet removed, one looped and two straight 32-gage stainless steel wires are threaded through the trochar, which is then removed, leaving the wires in place (Fig. 13). The two straight wire ends on opposite sides are tagged with hemostats and become the external fixation wires. The loop and its ends fix the canthal tendons bilaterally. The tissue in the medial canthal area is now sutured to the wire on the looped side with a 4-0 nonabsorbable suture such as prolene. The two ends of the wire opposite the loop are twisted on themselves forming a second loop that is sutured to the medial canthal tendon on that side with 4-0 nonabsorbable suture. By tightening the looped wire each canthal angle will be pulled toward the base of the nose reforming the canthal angles bilaterally. The external wires will protrude through the skin and be tied over nose pads to restore concavity to the soft tissues in the canthal angles. The tightening of the looped wire, which repositions the

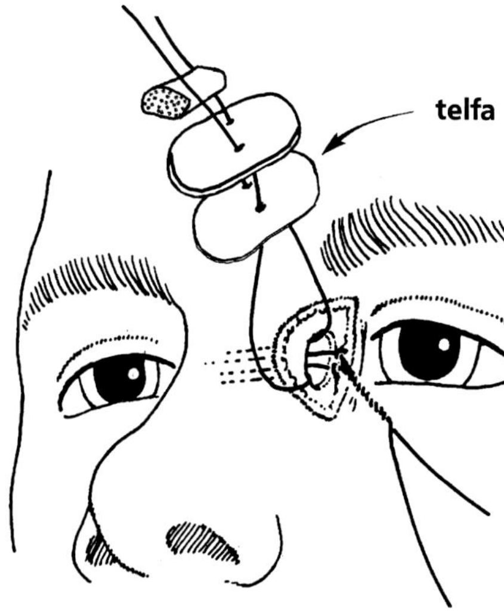

FIG. 14. Canthal fixation has been obtained of the edge of the lid to the medial orbit to the loop of wire, which will remain internal. The external wires are then threaded through nose pads for external compression to the soft tissue and skin to compress the epicanthal fold. The nose pad is composed of a layer of Telfa, silicone pad (soft conformer), and a cotton bolster.

tendons in the canthal angles of the base of the nose, is performed by three manipulations taking place simultaneously. As the twisted wires are tightened, countertraction pulls the loop on the opposite side tight; at the same time, the nonabsorbable sutures on the twisted side are pushed inward toward the base of the nose with forceps sliding the attached lids down the wire. The sutures will slide very easily down the wire toward the base of the nose as the twisting takes place. After proper tightening of the canthal tendons corrects the telecanthus, the twisted wire is cut short and the ends are inverted in the deep tissue. The skin is closed with 6-0 nylon. The two free wires are used to fixate the silicone nose pads (Fig. 14). The external wires and nose pads are removed in 7–10 days. The deep transnasal wire is left in place permanently. Skin sutures are removed 7 days following removal of the nose pads. A modification of the procedure omitting the deep looped wire can be used when there is primarily soft tissue deformity without telecanthus. Only the skin wires are passed to use with external nose pads for very firm compression in more severe cases.

LACRIMAL

Canalicular Reconstruction and Canaliculostomy

The punctum and a portion of the inferior canaliculus are often a part of the full-thickness defects of the lower lid and inner canthus. Reconstruction of the lower canaliculus in combination with eyelid reconstruction can sometimes preclude postoperative epiphora and the later need for secondary Jones tube placement (8).

Reforming lower lacrimal drainage apparatus is possible when as little as one fourth of the original canaliculus is present. The distal end of the severed canaliculus is identified. The tissue surrounding the canaliculus is undermined with sharp scissors to allow stretching of the canaliculus and intubation of both canaliculi is then carried out. The Crawford tubes are preferred (Fig. 15).

The medial eyelid margin can now be positioned. If a sliding or rotational lower eyelid flap is employed, the cut edge of the remaining tarsal plate is sutured to the posterior reflection of the medial canthal tendon. The direction of the lid margin must be toward the posterior lacrimal sac crest, behind the lacrimal sac. A suture in the area of the anterior reflection of the medial canthal tendon will cause medial separation of the lid from the globe.

The medial canthal fixation is best carried out with a 4-0 prolene suture on a half-circle needle (P2). The caruncle is first excised to allow greater accuracy in the placement of the medial canthal suture. The lacrimal sac must be retracted anteriorly and the suture placed in the firm tissue posterior to the sac. It is a difficult placement. Some extra dissection must expose the posterior tendon and a small half-circle needle must be used.

Following the reattachment of the medial canthal tendon, a notch on the posterior tarsal plate must be

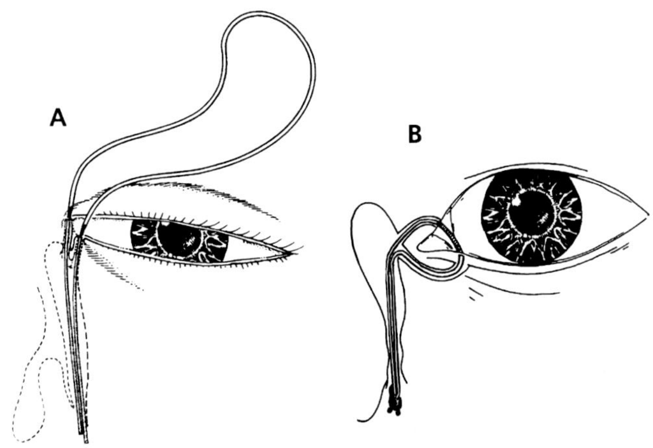

FIG. 15. Intubation of lacrimal drainage apparatus in medial canthal reconstruction in patients who have residual canalicular system. Silicone tube intubation with the Crawford method should be used to attempt to align residual canaliculi to promote lacrimal drainage. **A:** Threading of tubing through upper and lower canaliculus into the nasolacrimal area with silicone tubing wedged on lacrimal probes (Crawford). **B:** Final position of silicone tubing fixated intranasally with a single square knot.

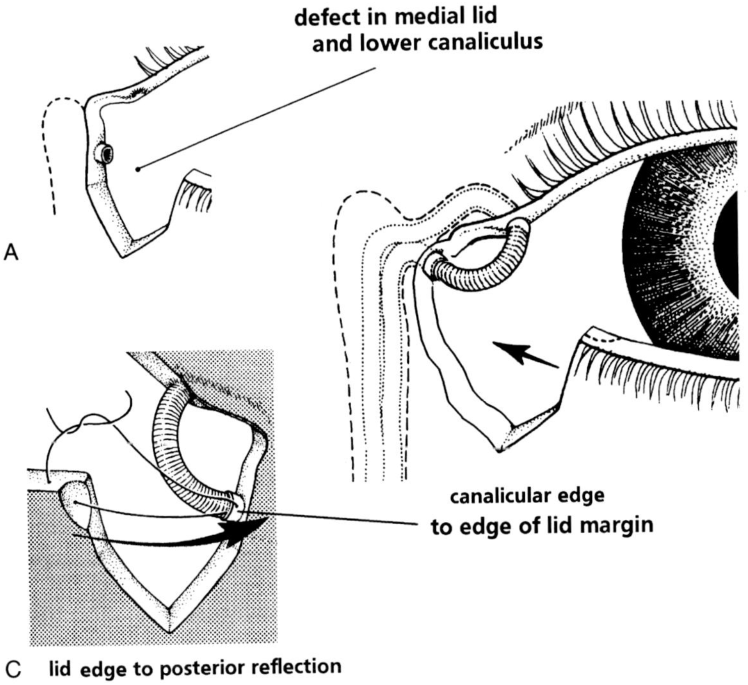

FIG. 16. Reconstruction of medial canthus following lacrimal resection. **A:** Defect in lower lid and medial canthus. **B:** Silicone tubing has been inserted in the residual canalicular system. A resection of the posterior edge of the lid on the outline shown will receive the cut edge of the residual canaliculus. **C:** The lower lid is fixated in the canthus with one of the techniques of medial canthal fixation previously described. The residual cut edge of the canaliculus is brought into the defect created and the edge of the lower lid so that it will assume a position in the lacrimal lake consistent with drainage.

created to reattach the new punctum and lower canaliculus (Fig. 16A–C). The residual canaliculus is then stretched along its axis and sutured to the posterior border of the tarsal notch with 7-0 silk suture. The distal ends of the silicone tubes are recovered through the nasal antrum under the inferior turbinate. The Crawford tube ensures the patency of the newly formed punctum and canaliculus and acts as a supporting splint for the lower lid, ensuring proper direction during the healing process. The ends of the Crawford tube in the nasal antrum are tied with a single square knot; the skin incision is closed with a running vertical mattress suture of 7-0 silk. Sutures are removed in 5 days, but the Crawford tube should be left in position for 5–6 weeks.

REFERENCES

1. McCord CD, Wesley R. Reconstruction of the upper lid and medial canthus. *Oculoplastic surgery*. New York: Raven Press; 1987:73–91.
2. Leibsohn JM, Hahn F. Medial canthal reconstruction with nasal periosteum. *Ophth Plast Reconstr Surg* 1992;8:35–40.
3. Shore JW, Rubin PAD, Bilyk JR. Repair of telecanthus by anterior fixation of cantilevered miniplates. *Ophthalmology* 1992;99: 1133–1138.
4. Beyer CK, Fabian RL, Smith B. Naso-orbital fractures: complications and treatment. *Ophthalmology* 1982;89:457–463.
5. McCord CD. The correction of telecanthus and epicanthal fold. *Ophthal Surg* 1980;11:446–454.
6. Johnson CC. Epicanthus. *Am J Ophthalmol* 1968;66:939–946.
7. Blair V, Brown JB, Hamm WG. Correction of ptosis and epicanthus. *Arch Ophthalmol* 1932;7:832–846.
8. Wilkins RB, et al. Lacrimal drainage system disorders: diagnosis and treatment. *Oculoplastic surgery*. New York: Raven Press; 1987:377–405.

CHAPTER 23

Lateral Canthal Reconstruction

Lateral canthal defects usually involve portions of the upper lid as well as the lower lid, and reconstruction of this area can be challenging. The important priorities in connection with lateral canthal reconstruction are to provide upper lid function, lower lid support, reformation of the outer and internal lamella, and to shape the fissure with canthal fixation.

DIRECT CLOSURE

Smaller defects, particularly in older individuals with stretchable tissue, can be repaired with advancing adjacent tissue.

When at least 70% of both the upper lid and lower lid margins remains, each tarsal plate can be pulled laterally to close the lateral canthal defect. If possible, it is best to convert the defect to a diamond shape; this allows the greatest ease in alignment of skin edges (Fig. 1A) (1). A single 4-0 prolene suture is placed through the lateral cut edge of both the upper and lower tarsal plates and sutured to the superior, inner aspect of the lateral orbital rim periosteum. The proper technique of canthal fixation is seen in Fig. 2.

If periosteum is not available for placement of the lateral canthal suture, other techniques of lateral canthal fixation must be used.

The skin-muscle layer lateral to the canthus is then rotated inwardly via development of two semicircular musculocutaneous flaps and advancement of one each for the upper lid and lower skin (Fig. 1B, C).

TARSAL (TARSOCONJUNCTIVAL) FLAP WITH ROTATIONAL FLAP, GRAFT

If as little as 30% of the upper lid tarsal plate is available medially, the residual tarsus can be used to provide the supporting framework for the upper lid (1). The residual upper lid is everted over a Desmarres retractor or Erhardt clamp. A tarsoconjunctival flap is outlined on the tarsal conjunctiva. This flap is similar to the one described in the chapter on upper lid reconstruction. It is important to leave intact at least 4 mm of the upper lid tarsal margin to prevent instability of the margin (Fig. 3A, B). A careful dissection between the levator aponeurosis and Müller's muscle layer is performed superiorly to the level of the superior fornix. The lateral margin of the tarsal flap is then sutured to the lateral canthus. If the periosteum of the lateral orbital rim is intact, the flap can be anchored to the periosteum in the manner illustrated in Fig. 2. If the periosteum is absent, two 1-mm burr holes are placed through the lateral canthal wall immediately posterior to point D (Fig. 3C, D). The tarsal flap is then anchored to the holes in the orbital wall with nonabsorbable suture. The medial margin of the tarsal flap is then sutured to the lateral cut edge of the original tarsus. The upper lid conjunctival surface now has the configuration shown in Fig. 3D; the anterior aspect of the upper lid is shown in Fig. 3E. The lower lid and lateral canthus are next reconstructed in the manner described as the lateral rotational flap (Fig. 3F). Augmentation of the rotational flap for the lower lid may require a periosteal cartilage flap. If less than 50% of the lower lid tarsus is available, advancement of the tarsal flap from the upper lid may be angled downward in the manner of a modified Hughes procedure (see chapter on lower lid reconstruction) to provide more posterior lamellar support for the lower lid (Fig. 4A–C). With a vertically advanced tarsoconjunctival flap that is shared with the upper and lower lid, fixation with a periosteal flap laterally can provide stronger support for the canthal angle than simple fixation (2,3).

TEMPORAL FOREHEAD FLAP

A transposition flap from the temporal forehead can be used to replace the external lamella if local skin flaps or grafts are not available (Fig. 5A, B). It can be

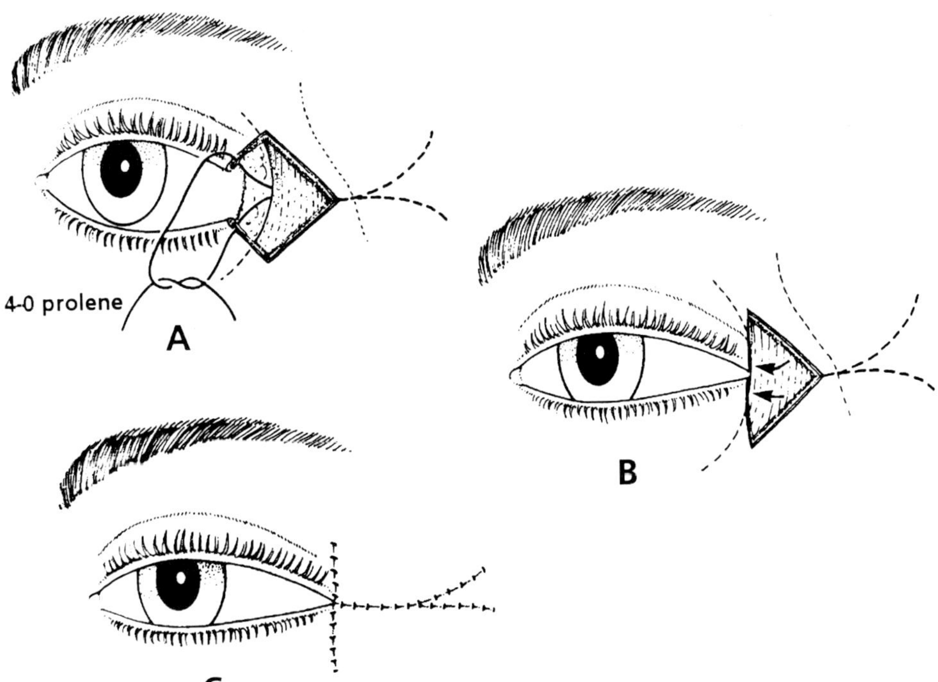

FIG. 1. Reconstruction of the lateral canthus with advancement flaps. **A:** Lateral canthoplasty with attachment of tarsal edges to periosteum and outline of rotational flaps. **B:** Undermining of lateral rotational flaps. **C:** Advancement and closure of lateral myocutaneous advancement flaps.

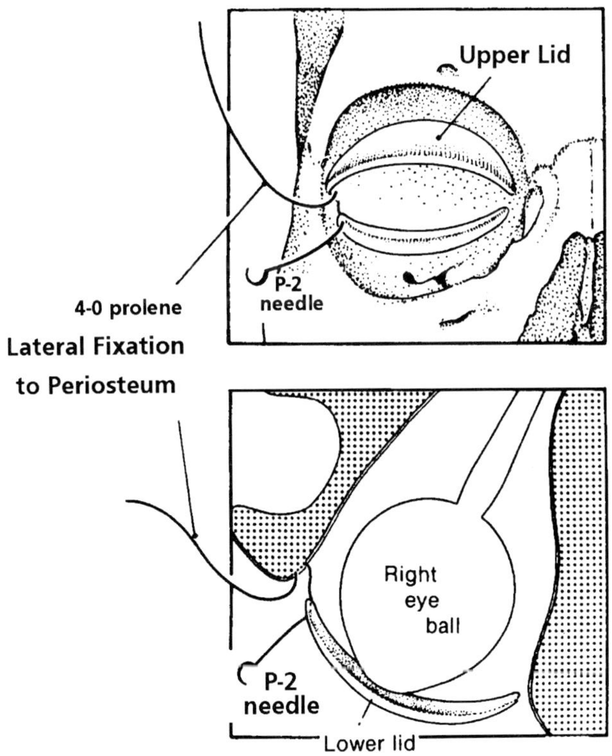

FIG. 2. Lateral canthal reconstruction, canthal fixation. Diagrams emphasizing the fact that for the lower lid curvature to be flush with the globe, the edge of the lower lid should be directed inside the lateral orbital rim. Fixation of tarsus or flaps in this area is best accomplished with the use of a small half-circle needle.

used in conjunction with a tarsal flap or a posterior lamellar graft if it extends to the surface of the globe. This can replace only the external lamella of the lid. The skin in the flap is thicker than is normally found in the area but can be used if local tissue and grafts are not available.

LATERAL CANTHAL FIXATION METHODS

Suture Fixation to the Periosteum

Fixation of the lateral edge of the tarsal plate to the periosteum at the lateral rim can be accomplished with sutures. A small sturdy half-circle needle (P2) is required for taking the periosteal bite inside the rim; 4-0- prolene suture material provides enough support and is nonreactive. After tying, it is important that the ends be kept flat to avoid postoperative irritation of the skin (Fig. 2).

Periosteal Flaps

A rim-based periosteal flap can be used for lateral support to form a pseudocanthal tendon in cases of tissue deficiency (4,5).

The periosteum of the lateral rim is exposed as well as the edge of the temporalis fascia. Two parallel cuts are made 1.5 cm apart beginning at the temporalis fas-

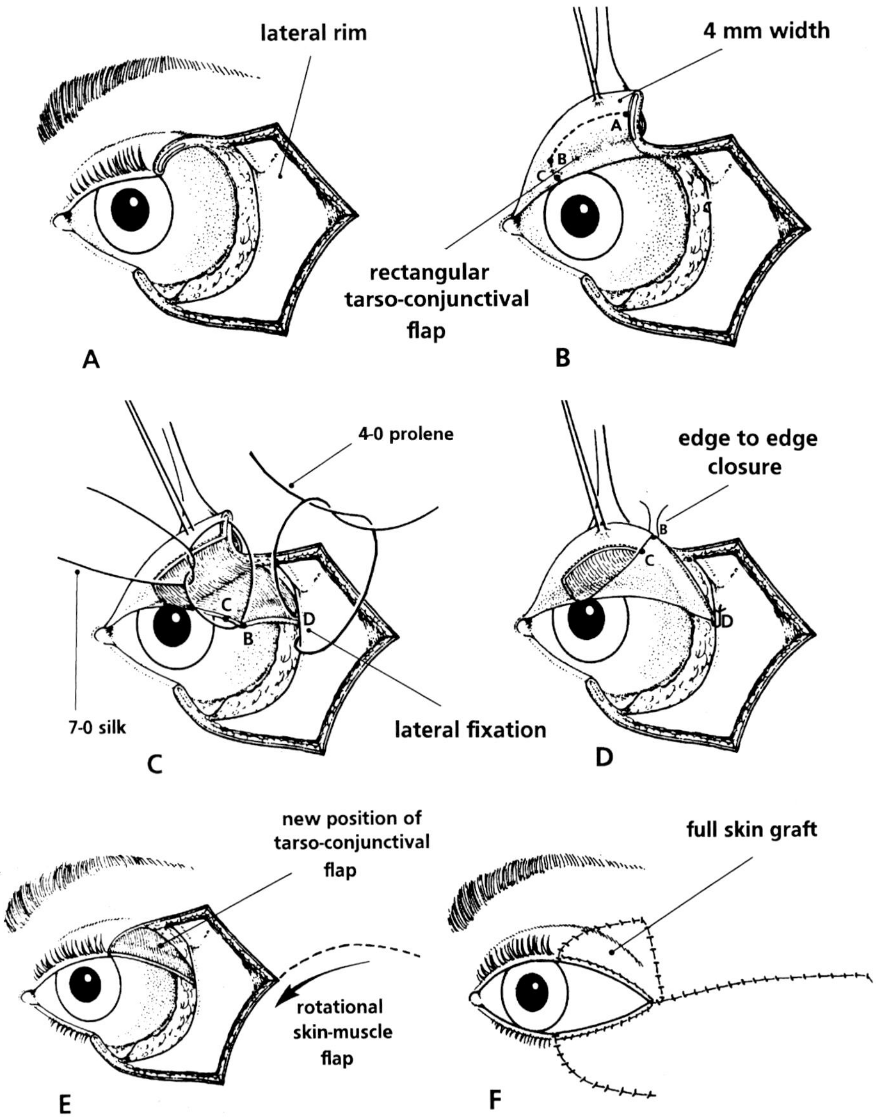

FIG. 3. Reconstruction of lateral canthus with sliding tarsoconjunctival flaps. **A:** Defect shown encompassing temporal portion of upper lower lid and canthal area. **B:** Eversion of the residual upper lid showing design of tarsoconjunctival flap for advancement. **C:** The tarsoconjunctival flap has been developed from the upper lid, advanced to the lateral canthus, and fixated. **D:** The edge of the tarsoconjunctival flap that had been advanced is attached to the lateral edge of the residual upper lid. **E:** New position of tarsoconjunctival flap with outline of rotational myocutaneous flap laterally. **F:** The canthal and lower lid defect has been repaired with a rotational myocutaneous flap in the usual manner. The skin-muscle defect and the upper lid canthal area has been repaired with a full-thickness skin graft.

cia, through the periosteum to the inner edge of the lateral rim (Fig. 6A). The periosteal flap is hinged at the inner edge of the lateral rim, and is raised and split horizontally (Fig. 6B). The flaps are crossed to form an angle that will correspond to the lateral canthal angle. The periosteal edges are sutured to the tarsal-conjunctival layers with 6-0 polygalactin (Fig. 6C). The remaining conjunctiva from the inferior and superior fornices is also mobilized to join the periosteal flaps. There should be a moderate amount of tension in the lids; if they are too loose, the flaps should be shortened. If the periosteum is deficient and there is only enough for a single flap, it should be brought to the lower lid (as in lower lid reconstruction) and the upper lid stretched to the flap base and attached.

Drill Holes

In the absence of periosteum at the lateral rim, the fixation of the edge of the eyelids to the desired rim position must be done with suture fixation to the bone.

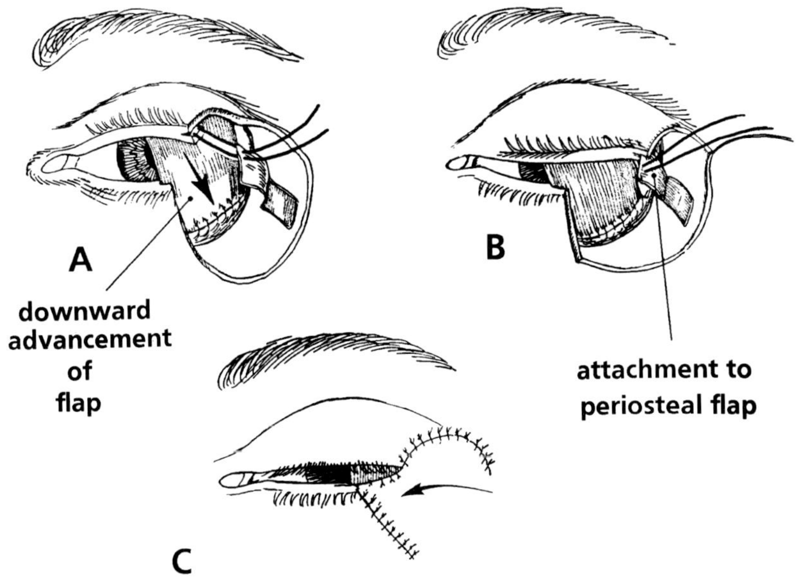

FIG. 4. Tarsoconjunctival flap for repair of lateral canthus, modification for large lower lid defect, and reinforcement with periosteal flap. **A:** The tarsoconjunctival flap has been advanced inferiorly and laterally and a periosteal flap has been elevated laterally to recreate the canthal tendon. **B:** The upper lid has been stretched across and attached to the periosteum. **C:** The lower lid defect has been reconstructed in the outer lamella with a rotational myocutaneous flap.

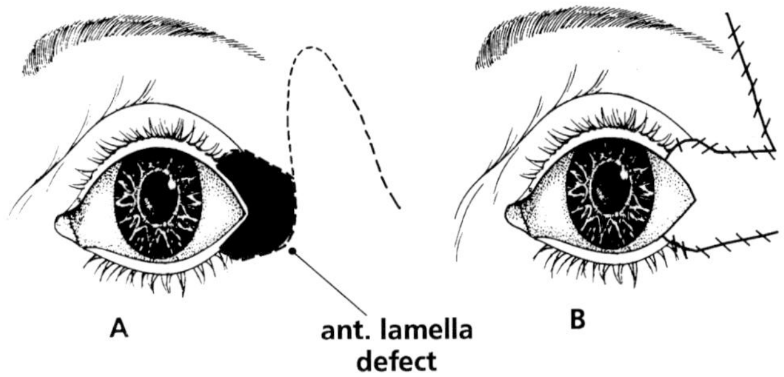

FIG. 5. Repair of canthal defect (anterior lamella) with transpositional temporal flap. **A:** Lateral canthal defect and outline of temporal forehead flap in the thicker skin, lateral and superior to the brow. **B:** Rotation of the flap to the defect and closure of the flap donor site.

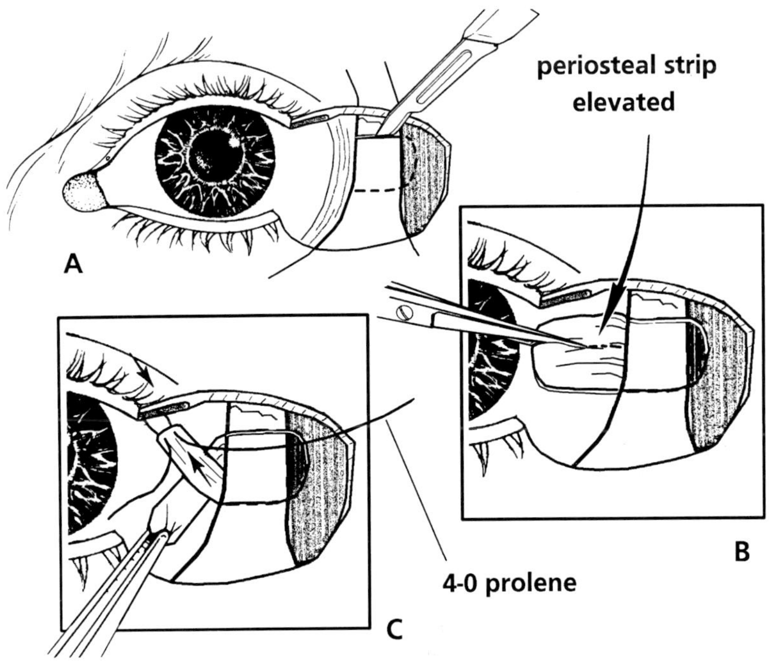

FIG. 6. Lateral canthal reconstruction with crossing periosteal flaps (modified from Leone, ref. 4). **A:** Lateral canthal defect with outline of periosteal flap. **B:** Periosteal flap has been developed, rotated inward, and bisected. **C:** Periosteal flaps have been crossed to provide the proper direction of pull for the upper and lower lid.

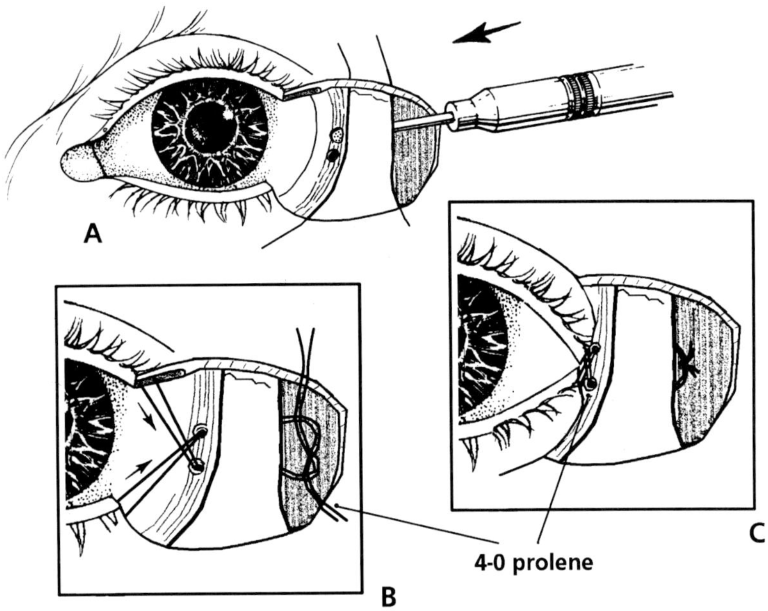

FIG. 7. Lateral canthal reconstruction with direct attachment to the bone. A: Lateral canthal defect. Drill holes are made in the lateral orbital rim to provide entrance for fixating suture at the level of the normal attachment at the lateral tubercle. B: Nonabsorbable sutures have been attached to the lid and threaded through the drill holes in a crossing manner, the lower lid to the upper hole, upper lid to the lower hole. C: Tightening of the sutures pulling the edge of the lid reforming the lateral canthus. Sutures can be loosened or tightened according to the configuration needed and the defect covered with a skin-muscle flap or skin graft.

Two drill holes are made at the appropriate level 3 mm inside the rim (Fig. 7A) and 4-0 prolene sutures from the edges of the upper and lower tarsal plates are crisscrossed through the holes to the outside of the rim and tied permanently. The suture from the lower lid goes through the upper hole, and the suture from the upper lid goes through the lower hole, to provide the proper direction of pull (Fig. 7B, C).

Miniplate

Sometimes because of bony defects in cases of trauma, tumor resection, or after surgery, no support may be available for canthal fixation. A new point of purchase for fixation can be created with a miniplate spanning the bony defect (6). A titanium miniplate of proper length is selected, taking into consideration the need for fixation with two screws at each bony margin (Fig. 8). A seven- to eight-hole miniplate is usually appropriate. A miniplate cutter is used to remove excess length and sharp edges. The plate is molded to the desired contour with the miniplate benders and placed into optimal position at the lateral orbital rim. Two holes are drilled above the frontozygomatic suture and two below the zygomatic arch. These correspond to the holes in the miniplate as it overlaps the bony margins. A 1.5-mm drill bit and guide ensure perpendicularity of the drill holes and avoid oversized hole diameters. A depth gage determines the length of each 2.0-mm diameter screw; 6- to 8-mm screws are used most often. On occasion, 2.4-mm diameter emergency screws are necessary if oversized holes result. After the plate has been cut to length, contoured, and positioned, it is secured with the screws.

The lateral canthal angle is reformed by means of a permanent monofilament suture (4-0 prolene) that is passed through the superior and inferior tarsus independently in a vertical fashion at the lateral, exposed edge of the lateral canthal tendons. The suture is se-

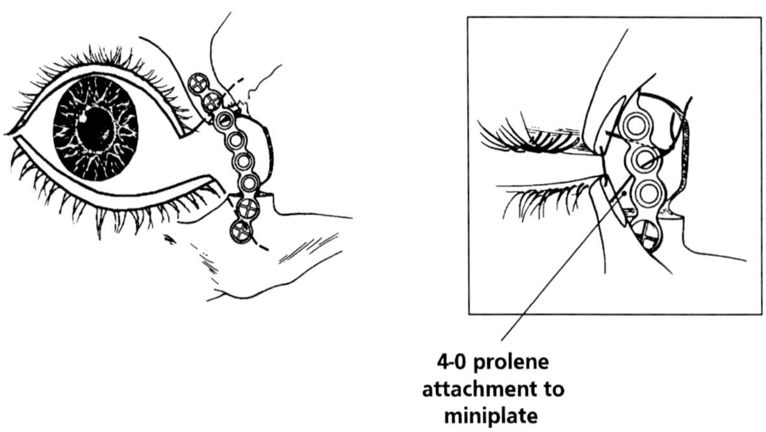

FIG. 8. Reconstruction of the lateral canthus with miniplate fixation. In patients who have loss of bone in the area fixation of the lateral edge of the lids cannot be accomplished normally. A spanning miniplate is used for fixation with suture material. Modified from Shore (6).

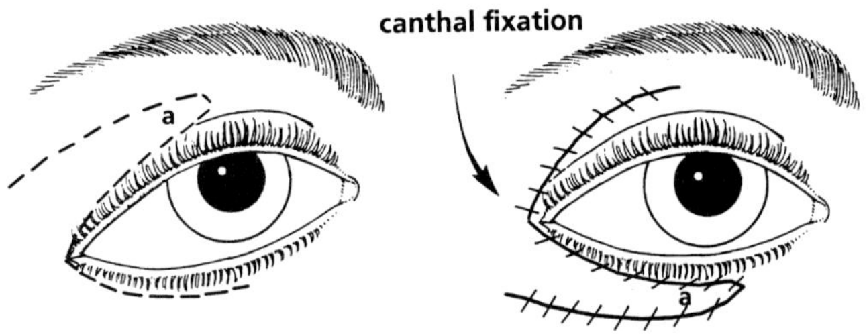

FIG. 9. Vertical displacement of lateral canthus and repair with transposition Z-plasty flap from upper to lower lid (underlying periosteal fixation needed).

cured laterally to the miniplate (Fig. 8) at the proper level for orientation of the lateral canthal angle. Appropriate eyelid tension and apposition to the globe is obtained before securing the knot. Subcutaneous tissue is closed with interrupted absorbable sutures and the skin closed in a standard fashion.

VERTICAL DISPLACEMENT

Transposition Z-plasty

If the canthus is vertically displaced, the position of the canthus can be moved up or down with a vertical movement of canthal fixation with one of the previously described techniques. The fixation techniques involve the tarsoligamentous sling (posterior lamella). The skin availability or laxity may not be adequate to allow the canthus to be moved; consequently, supplemental skin grafts of flaps may be needed. A transposition flap of skin from the lid opposite the direction of displacement can provide local tissue that may have a better appearance than a skin graft (Fig. 9).

LATERAL CANTHAL PHIMOSIS (INWARD DISPLACEMENT)

Canthotomy

In cases in which there is a mild shortening of the lateral canthal soft tissue, in which the underlying structural attachments are generally sound, a lengthening of the fissure can be obtained with excision of the tissue between the upper and lower lid and attachment

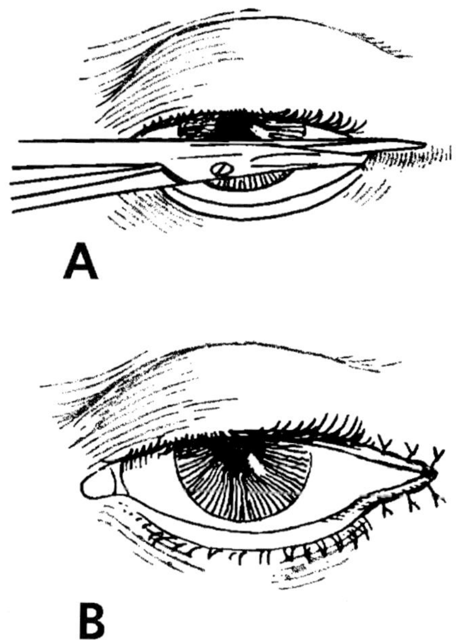

FIG. 10. Lateral canthal phimosis—canthotomy. **A:** Canthotomy is performed. **B:** The conjunctiva has been everted to form a new eyelid margin. Firm fixation of the lids to the lateral rim should be present.

of the skin-muscle conjunctival edges (Fig. 10A, B). This should only be done in cases in which there is firm support of lid position.

Canthoplasty with Flaps

In slightly more severe cases of soft tissue phimosis in which there is good underlying lid support, soft tissue rearrangement can be performed.

The amount of fissure lengthening desired (4–6 mm) is marked off from the lateral canthal angle (Fig. 11A). The lateral quarters of the upper and lower lids are split close to the posterior edge. The conjunctiva is grasped at its lateral point and carefully undermined medially as much as necessary. It is drawn laterally as far as its elasticity will allow and sutured to the upper and lower edges of the cut skin and at B. A double-armed suture is passed through the conjunctiva at the canthal angle and brought out on the skin surface beyond the canthus (Fig. 11B). This will help deepen the new canthal angle and keep it from flattening out and gapping.

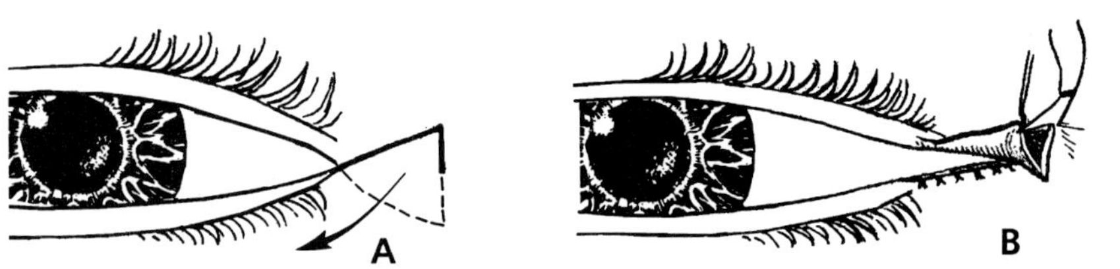

FIG. 11. Lateral canthal phimosis—canthoplasty. **A:** A skin-muscle flap is outlined in the lower lid and allowed to advance forward. Lower lid tension should be firm to prevent retraction. **B:** The conjunctiva is everted and sutured externally to prevent rehealing of the canthal angle.

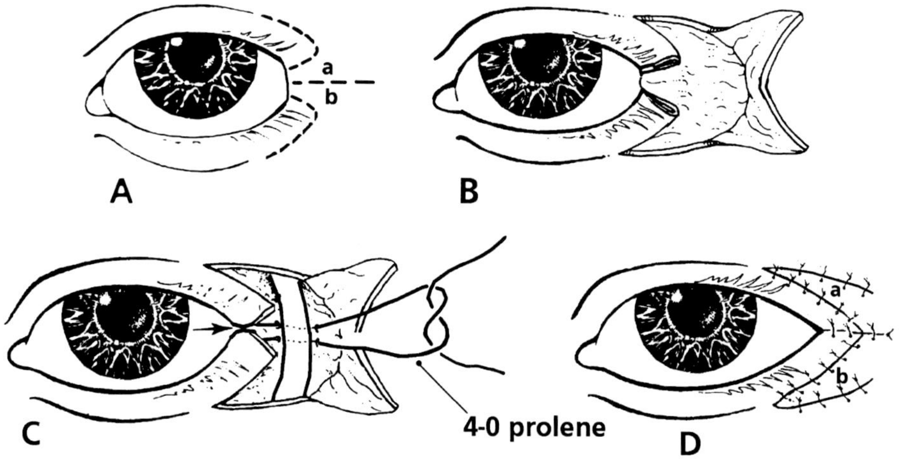

FIG. 12. Lateral canthal rounding and phimosis (cicatricial)—canthoplasty (after Del Campo). **A:** Outline of transposition flaps in area of incision to recreate canthal angle. **B:** Elevation of skin-muscle flaps. **C:** Canthal angle is brought outward to the periosteum laterally, lengthening the fissure. **D:** The flaps have been transposed and sutured into position elongating the lid fissure and correcting the rounding.

Canthoplasty with Drill Holes, Flaps (Del Campo)

Cases of canthal deformity from cicatricial forces and skin shortage may cause rounding and narrowing of the canthal angle. Local transposition flaps combined with canthal fixation can offer improvement without grafts in some cases (7).

The canthal area is divided by a line into two symmetric, laterally based flaps. The length of this line is determined by taking into consideration the distance required to properly position the canthus and to restore normal width to the palpebral fissure (Fig. 12A, B).

Four flaps are developed: an upper and a lower medially based palpebral flap and two laterally based flaps. Underlying fibrous tissue is gathered and pulled laterally and fixated to drill holes in the lateral orbital rim. Conjunctiva and skin are sutured (Fig. 12C, D).

Outfracture Lateral Wall

Narrowing of the lateral fissure can result from inward displacement of the lateral wall and is usually the result of trauma. The normal length of the lateral fissure cannot be obtained with soft tissue surgery alone, and osteotomies and outfracture of the lateral rim to its normal position is needed to allow lengthening of the fissure (Fig. 13).

Exposure of the rim is obtained with a horizontal incision made from the lateral canthal angle. A lateral canthotomy and inferior and superior limb cantholysis are performed. A skin-muscle flap is raised posterior to the orbital rim both superiorly and inferiorly to expose the lateral rim periosteum and the temporalis fascia. Wide undermining is necessary to obtain good exposure of the superior and inferior portion of the lateral orbital wall. The periosteum is incised 3 mm lateral to the outside edge of the rim from above the frontozygomatic suture to the level of the zygomatic arch. Two 2.5-cm relaxing incisions are made in the periosteum, one horizontally along the superior border of the zygomatic arch and the other at the junction of the temporalis fascia and the epicranium at the superior temporal crest. The temporalis muscle is reflected from its insertion at the crest and out of the temporalis fossa using a periosteal elevator. Bone wax may be necessary to control bleeding through venous diploe. The elevator is then used to reflect periorbita from the lateral wall of the orbit and for approximately 1 cm along the roof

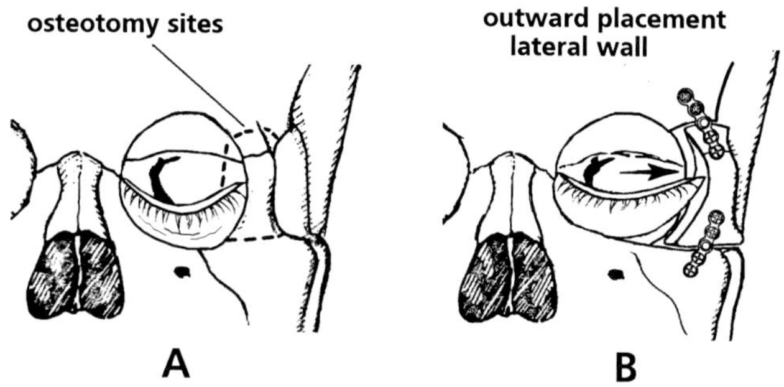

FIG. 13. Lateral canthal phimosis (bony narrowing)—lateral canthoplasty with outfracture of the orbital rim. **A:** Osteotomy sites are shown for lateral orbitotomy, just above the frontal zygomatic suture, and inferiorly just above the zygomatic arch. **B:** The osteotomy has been completed with the bone fractured and fragment moved outward to the desired position to reform the fissure width and fixated with miniplates. Temporalis muscle may have to be detached.

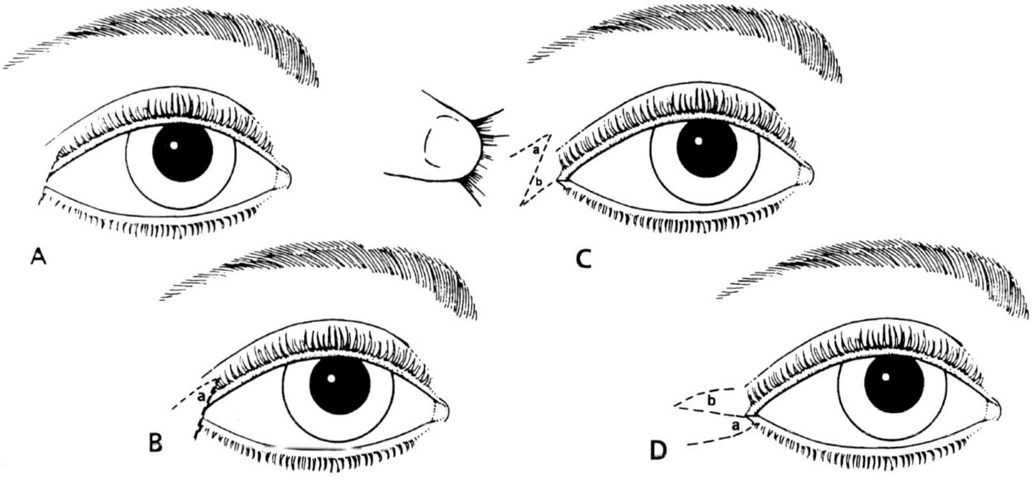

FIG. 14. Canthoplasty for vertical epicanthal folds. **A:** Lateral vertical epicanthal fold. **B:** The marking of the external incision to form transposition Z flaps. **C:** The fold has been retracted for completion of marking of the Z-plasty transposition flaps. **D:** The flaps have been elevated, subcutaneous scarring excised, and the flaps transposed to eliminate the fold.

and floor. Horizontal osteotomies with an oscillating saw are made in the lateral wall, at the level of the superior border of the zygomatic arch, and just above the frontozygomatic suture within the lacrimal fossa. Rongeurs or a saw may be used to completely detach the lateral orbital rim.

The lateral wall bone is now advanced approximately 4–5 mm (or the required amount) laterally and is then rigidly fixated with two 4-hole orbital reconstruction miniplates. This is done by bending soft metallic templates to conform to the osteotomy, followed by bending the titanium miniplates to match the templates. Drill holes are placed in the frontal bone and the zygomatic bone followed by drill holes in the free bone. This free bone is fixated in the lateral position with a bone-holding clamp. Then 1.5-mm self-tapping titanium screws are passed and the bone is rigidly fixated in the lateral position.

The temporalis fascia is reattached with a 4-0 chromic suture to the epicranium at the superior temporal crest.

If the lateral canthal tendon is attached to the lateral periosteum in a normal manner, closure of the periosteum laterally to the rim in its new position will allow the fissure to lengthen normally. If the periosteum is deficient, then an extra step of canthal fixation with drill holes may be necessary.

EPICANTHUS

Transposition Flaps

Vertical epicanthal folds at the lateral canthus may occur posttrauma or following blepharoplasty in which the upper and lower incisions are connected. Skin transposition flaps at the lateral canthus are useful to correct this type of epicanthus palpebralis (Fig. 14A–D). The transfer of the skin flaps should always be accompanied by removal of subcutaneous scarring and adhesions and by debulking of the fold.

REFERENCES

1. McCord CD, Nunery WR. Reconstruction of the lower eyelid and outer canthus. *Oculoplastic surgery*. 2nd ed. New York: Raven Press; 1987: 93–115.
2. Smith B. Eyelid surgery. *Surg Clin North Am* 1959;39:1–12.
3. Smith B. Technique for extirpation and replacement of the lateral canthus. *Trans Am Acad Oph Oto* Sept–Oct 1953:738–742.
4. Leone CR. Lateral canthal reconstruction. *Ophthalmology* 1987; 94:238–241.
5. Meltzer M. Lateral canthal reconstruction with periosteal flaps. In: Wesley R, ed. *Techniques in ophthalmic plastic surgery*. New York: John Wiley and Sons; 1986:368–370.
6. Shore JW, Carvajal J, Westfall CT. Miniplate reconstruction of the lateral orbital rim after orbital decompression for Grave's disease. *Ophthalmology* 1992;99:1433–1438.
7. Del Campo AF, et al. A procedure for reconstruction of the lateral palpebral canthus. *Ophth Plast Reconstr Surg* 1994;10:6–10.

CHAPTER 24

Decision Making in Eyelid Reconstruction

The previous chapters described in detail the specific surgical techniques for repair of eyelid defects. It is helpful when planning the reconstruction of full-thickness defects to group the surgical techniques in terms of their components. Commonly, in the repair of the more complex defects, modifications of these techniques, combining parts or components of one technique with parts of another, must be utilized to successfully repair a particular defect. Grouping the techniques in a functional manner and understanding the anatomic elements of each technique allows the surgeon to undertake this approach more readily. Table 1 groups the techniques in a manner that reflects the source of reconstructive tissue. Table 2 lists the sources of free graft tissue available for reconstructing the layers of the eyelid. For the anterior lamella a split-skin graft may be used if full skin is not available, but the match and flexibility is usually less that ideal. Conjunctival advancement, although not a graft, is listed with methods of posterior lamella lining from the standpoint of convenience. Tissue used to construct or reline the posterior lamella should ideally have a mucous membrane lining and have some rigidity.

It is important for the surgeon to become "defect-oriented" rather than "technique-oriented." With Mohs' surgery (microscopic controlled tumor excision) being performed commonly for removal of eyelid neoplastic disease, all that the reconstructive surgeon may ever see is the eyelid defect. The ability to analyze the eyelid defects created and to apply the proper reparative surgical techniques either singly or in combination will ensure the best possible result for the patient. The surgeon should not learn one or two repair techniques and try to fit them to all defects.

Before applying these techniques to specific defects there are other aspects of the reconstructive process that must be emphasized because of their key role in obtaining a successful result, regardless of the type of flap or technique used.

CANTHAL FIXATION

The newly constructed eyelid must conform to the curvature of the globe particularly in the canthal areas. Methods of attachment of flaps to the canthal areas are summarized in Table 3.

Medial Canthal Fixation

Special attention was given to the canthal areas emphasizing that in repair of the inner canthus fixation of any flap used must be performed by directing the flap toward the posterior lacrimal crest, which is located posterior to the lacrimal sac. Direct inspection of normal people who have visible medial canthal tendons will show that the anterior reflection of the medial canthal tendon angulates about 30° more anteriorly than the normal direction of the lid contour, which travels toward the posterior reflection of the tendon. A common error is to attach the edge of the tarsus of the lower lid to the anterior reflection of the medial canthal tendon, which causes the lid to be pulled away from the globe. Proper fixation to the posterior canthal tendon area may be done with suture fixation if elements of the deep reflection are present. A small but sturdy half-circle P2 needle is invaluable for this fixation. A periosteal flap may be used for fixation. Miniplates and transnasal wiring can be used if an increasing amount of tissue or bone has been removed. In cases of loss of support tissue in the posterior canthal area, compromises are sometimes made if required by the priorities of the situation.

Lateral Canthal Fixation

With lateral canthal defects and with lower lid reconstruction, emphasis was placed on proper fixation of any flap used in this area inside the lateral orbital rim

TABLE 1. *Flap source for eyelid reconstruction*

Use of Adjacent Tissue
Direct closure
Semicircular flap (Tenzel)
Local myocutaneous flap with postlamellar graft
Rotational cheek flap (Mustarde)
Sliding tarsoconjunctival flap (tarsal flap)
Periosteal flap
Use of Opposing Eyelid Tissue
Tarsoconjunctival advancement flap (Hughes)
Tarsoconjunctival transposition flap (Hewes)
Bridge flap (Cutler–Beard)
Pedicle lid margin transposition (Mustarde)
Periorbital Tissue Flap (lined with postlamellar graft)
Glabellar flap
Median forehead flap
Temporal forehead flap (Fricke)
Cheek flap (Imre)
Nasolabial flap (Blasius)

at the lateral tubercle where the normal insertion of the lateral canthal tendon occurs. Lateral canthal fixation is the keystone of lower lid and lateral canthal reconstructive procedures. Fixation can be performed by suturing to the periosteum or to a periosteal flap, or, if the periosteum is absent, by suturing through drill holes placed in the lateral orbital rim at the location of the lateral orbital turbercle. At the lateral canthus the attachment of the eyelid must be inside the lateral orbital rim to assure that the lower lid will be properly curved with the globe in the proper contour, and not separated from the globe. Firm fixation also prevents "lower lid sag" and downward retraction at the lateral canthal area, which in the past has been seen so commonly with many lower lid reconstructive techniques.

REPAIR OF LACRIMAL DRAINAGE APPARATUS

If only a small part of the canalicular system is resected in the inner canthal area, the residual canaliculus may be intubated with a silicone intubation set and a canaliculostomy performed. This technique can be used in conjunction with any of the eyelid reconstructive procedures in that area and may spare the patient the need for a secondary Jones tube placement. If the lacrimal drainage apparatus must be excised completely, then a secondary Jones tube procedure can be performed. This is best done after healing has occurred and the canthal angle has assumed a more normal configuration. It is difficult to satisfy the requirement of a normal-shaped canthal angle for Jones tube placement until healing occurs. The attitude and position of Jones tube placement in the canthal angle is critical for tear drainage to occur. Because of these considerations, the Jones tube procedure is usually performed at a date later than that of the initial eyelid reconstructive procedure.

TABLE 2. *Free grafts for eyelid reconstruction*

Anterior Lamella Eyelid
Full-thickness graft
Skin-muscle flap
Split skin graft
Posterior Lamella Eyelid (ideally mucous membrane lining, some rigidity)
Free tarsoconjunctival graft
Palatal mucoperichondrium
Nasal mucoperichondrium
Buccal mucous membrane
Composite eyelid including margin (including lashes)
Conjunctival advancement from fornix
Conjunctival advancement from opposing eyelid
Ear cartilage graft

TABLE 3. *Methods of canthal fixation*

Medial
Direct suturing to posterior lacrimal crest (posterior reflection)
Direct wiring
Transnasal wiring
Miniplate fixation
Periosteal flap
Lateral
Direct suturing to periosteum (lateral tubercle)
Periostal flap
Wire or suture with drill holes in bone
Miniplate fixation

LID STRETCHABILITY

Eyelid tissue behaves differently in different individuals. Certain individuals, usually those in the older age group, have much more "stretchability" of the eyelid and the defect created may be reduced to a smaller size by simple stretching. In other individuals, especially young people, the eyelid is not as lax and the defect cannot be reduced as much in size by stretching. Particularly severe examples of stiff eyelids are those eyelids that have been damaged by irradiation, actinic changes, previous surgery, scars, burns, or any cicatrizing process such as scleroderma. Table 4 gives a rule of thumb for classifying defects as small, medium, or large, although each case must be individualized. In general, the rule of thumb would indicate that the de-

TABLE 4. *Size classification of eyelid full-thickness defects according to laxity*

Young person/tight lid	Older person/lax lid
Small: up to 20%	Small: up to 30%
Medium: 30%	Medium: 40%
Large: 40% to total	Large: 50% to total

fect can be reduced by stretching 10–15% more in an older person with laxity of tissue than in younger persons with tighter lids.

FULL-THICKNESS DEFECTS OF UPPER LID

This section discusses a variety of eyelid defects and applies the techniques learned in the previous chapters to these defects.

Central Upper Lid

Small Defects

With small defects in the central portion of the eyelid (Fig. 1), direct closure is accomplished more easily because both sides of the defect have residual tarsal tissue that may be approximated as previously described. Canthotomy and cantholysis of the upper limb of the lateral canthal tendon may be necessary. In older patients with more lid laxity, up to one third of a full-thickness eyelid defect may be closed in this manner without cantholysis.

Moderate to Large Defects

At the lower limits of size in this defect, there may be older patients with marked lid laxity whose lids can be repaired with direct closure with cantholysis. In patients with less lid laxity, young patients, or patients with rigid eyelids, other techniques must be used, particularly with the larger defects. Central upper lid defects have the advantage of residual tarsal plate being present on either side of the defect. This allows for direct tarsal-edge-to-tarsal-edge fixation of any flap or graft that may be placed in this position.

Some moderate defects of a larger size may be closed in selected cases by advancing tissue at the lateral canthus with an inverted semicircular flap; however, one should not try to exceed this flap's capability in the upper lid.

A special case of central eyelid defect in the upper lid is that of congenital coloboma, which may or may not be associated with epibulbar dermolipoma. This type of deformity in many cases can be closed directly after the edges of the coloboma have been "freshened." In most cases the repair of the coloboma is successful because the defect is not as great as it appears. Sometimes this occurs because the tarsus has "curled up" as opposed to being completely deficient. Some colobomas may have more complex elements such as symblepharon formation.

With moderate to large total defects, the surgeon has the choice of repair in patients with redundant upper lid and periorbital skin. A local myocutaneous flap backed with a posterior lamellar graft can be used or a bridge flap procedure can be performed. In patients with tighter skin (younger patients) the bridge flap is usually best. The bridge flap can produce an excellent functional and respectable cosmetic result, but it is a two-stage procedure. An "eyelash" graft may be performed prior to separation of the flap in the desired location with a free graft from the eyebrow-bearing hairs. However, the hairs that may be transplanted from the brow or scalp never assume the characteristics of normal cilia. The use of autogenous ear cartilage in conjunction with the bridge flap procedure seems to add more stability to the new upper lid in these authors' experience.

In the absence of available adjacent or lower lid tissue for reconstruction, a periorbital flap backed with a posterior lamellar graft must be used.

Total Upper Lid

With aggressive neoplastic disease, total lid defects may be encountered involving the entire upper lid and, in many cases, a portion of the fornix. In these cases there are no remnants of the tarsal plate left in the eyelid and no residual tissue to be stretched horizontally. In the bridge flap procedure, an autogenous ear cartilage graft should be used in a sandwich-like manner to add stability to the flap. The use of alloplastic

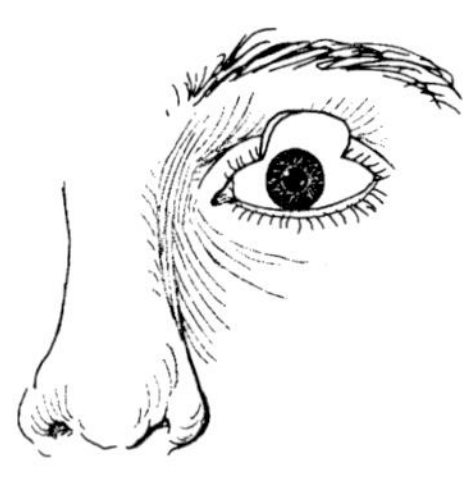

FIG. 1. Techniques for repair of central upper lid defect.

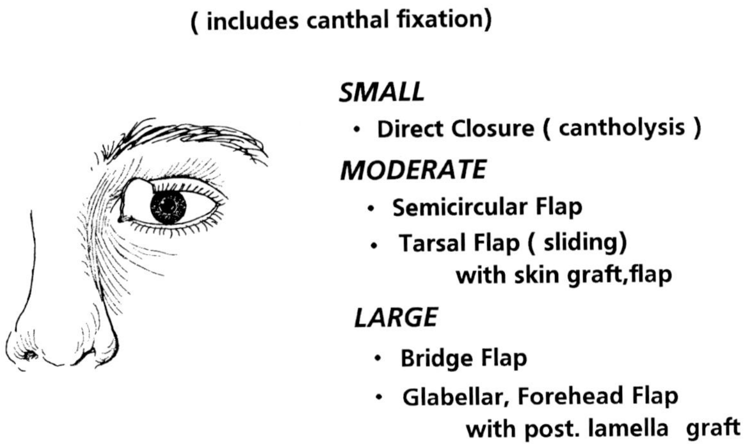

FIG. 2. Techniques for repair of nasal upper lid defect.

material (Gore-tex) in lieu of cartilage to promote stability has been reported as being used successfully in eyelid reconstruction (1). Proper medial and lateral canthal fixation of the flaps and the cartilage grafts must be obtained to ensure proper curvature of new upper lid.

Nasal and Temporal

With smaller defects in these areas (Figs. 2 and 3), direct closure is the procedure of choice combined with the appropriate medial or lateral canthal fixation suture technique. For the moderate-sized nasal and temporal upper lid defects, within the lower range of size, a particularly useful technique is the horizontally sliding tarsal (tarsoconjunctival) flap fixated in the canthus, which is then covered with a full-thickness skin graft or flap (a one-stage procedure). With nasal upper lid defects, the edge of the tarsoconjunctival flap can be attached to the posterior reflection of the medial canthal tendon with a nonabsorbable fixation suture and covered with a full-thickness skin graft. In patients who have an extremely loose upper lid, a sliding myocutaneous flap or skin flap from adjacent upper may be stretched and used to cover this tarsoconjunctival flap, in some cases as an alternative to a skin graft. The method of repair in larger upper nasal eyelid defects should be the bridge flap technique, and it may be the only one that will give an adequate result. Temporal upper lid defects may also be repaired by the sliding tarsoconjunctival flap with a full-thickness skin graft or a myocutaneous flap, and again the tarsoconjunctival flap must be anchored at the proper point laterally with lateral canthal fixation. Larger defects in the upper lid in this area usually require the bridge flap technique. Loss of lashes is much more conspicuous in the nasal portion of the upper lid; in some cases it has seemed beneficial to "convert" a nasal upper lid defect to a temporal defect by performing a lateral cantholysis and canthotomy, sliding the lash-bearing segment of the lid nasally, and then proceeding with the repair of an upper temporal defect.

As a last resort, the transfer of a flap from the forehead area, glabellar-midforehead for nasal defects or temporal forehead for temporal defects, with a posterior lamellar graft can be used.

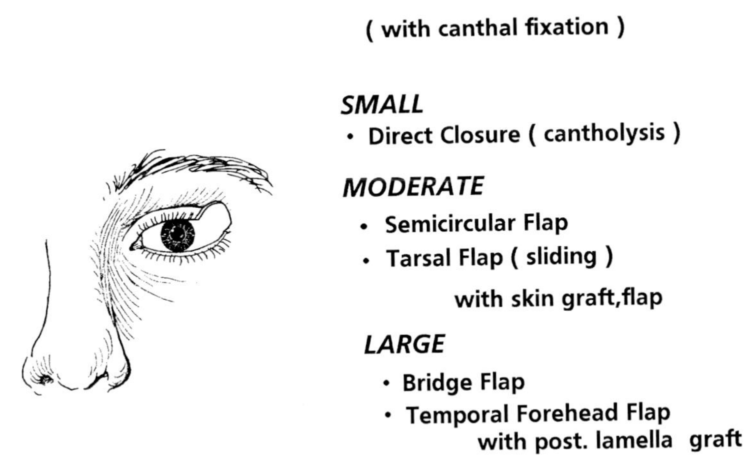

FIG. 3. Techniques for repair of temporal upper lid defect.

NON LID SHARING

- Local myocutaneous advancement flap
  with posterior lamellar graft
  with composite eyelid graft(s)
  (may retain lashes)

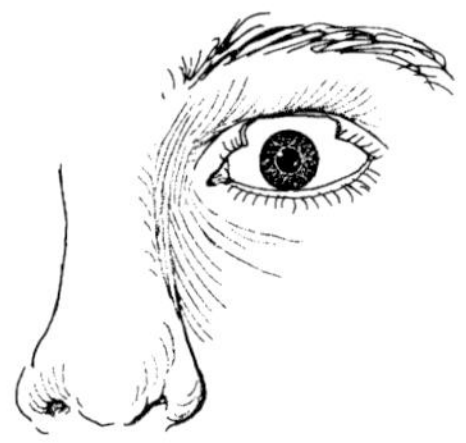

LID SHARING

- Bridge Flap from lower lid
- Pedicle Flap (including margin) from lower lid
  (retains eyelashes)

FIG. 4. Techniques for repair of wide-shallow upper lid defect.

Wide-Shallow Defects

It is not unusual to encounter a lid defect involving mainly the eyelid margin with little vertical involvement of the eyelid (Fig. 4). These shallow defects may occur posttraumatically or in many cases following resection of a superficial or ''sliding'' epithelial neoplastic process. At first glance one tends to minimize the importance of this defect, but one must recognize that the eyelid margin is the most important portion of the eyelid with regards to the preservation of corneal integrity and comfort. The surgeon may be resistant to employing a major reconstructive procedure to repair these shallow defects because in some cases, in order to implement the repair, large amounts of normal tissue may have to be rearranged. If a lesser procedure can be employed to repair the margin, it should be used; however, no shortcuts should be employed that would result in anything less than a completely healthy eyelid margin because of the severe corneal complications that might occur.

In patients with laxity of skin in the upper lid and periorbital area, defects can be repaired in a one-stage procedure with a local myocutaneous graft combined with a posterior lamellar graft. This can only be accomplished if there is skin-muscle laxity in the upper lid (in older patients in most cases). Shallow margin defects can also be repaired by composite grafts or pedicle margin grafts that have a margin containing lashes. Lash follicles remain viable in composite grafts in only 60% of cases. The flaps usually retain close to 100% follicle viability.

In many cases one must resort to a full bridge flap from the lower lid to supply the necessary tissue to reconstruct a healthy lid margin in broad, shallow upper lid defects.

FULL-THICKNESS DEFECTS OF LOWER LID

Central Lower Lid

Small defects are closed by direct closure (Fig. 5). In the lower lid, some defects at the lower range of moderate size may be repaired by direct closure in patients with extremely lax lids. Central lid defects again have the advantage of residual tarsal plate being present on both sides of the defect, allowing for more precise closure. With most moderate-sized defects, the ideal procedure in the lower lid is the semicircular flap, which can produce excellent results. One must not be tempted to stretch its use too far to the upper range of

SMALL

- Direct Closure (cantholysis)

MODERATE

- Semicircular Flap
  (periosteal flap , ear cartilage)
- Local myocutaneous flap (outrotated)
  with tarsal graft

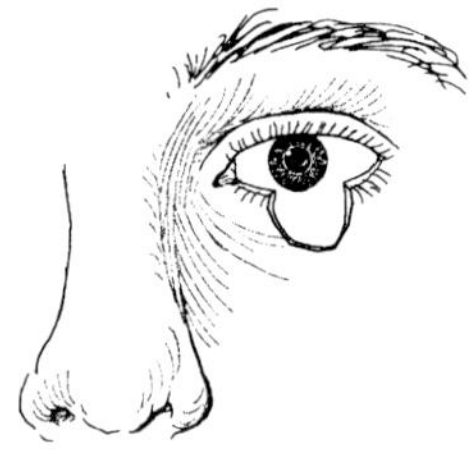

LARGE

- Tarsal Flap from upper lid (Hughes)
  with skin graft, flap
- Rotational Cheek flap (Mustarde)
  with post. lamella graft
- Periorbital flap
  transposition forehead
  nasolabial
  cheek (Imre)
  with post. lamella graft

FIG. 5. Techniques for repair of central lower lid defect.

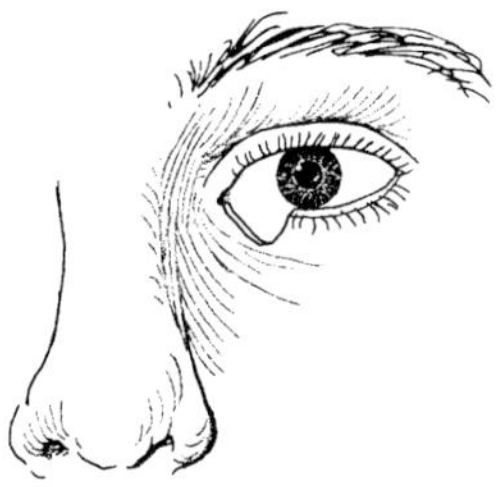

FIG. 6. Techniques for repair of nasal lower lid defect.

this size defect. Its use can be somewhat extended if augmented by a periosteal flap or ear cartilage laterally. In the more shallow defects, a local myocutaneous flap with a posterior lamellar graft can be used. The procedure of choice with the larger defects would be the modified Hughes procedure. The disadvantages of the Hughes procedure (a two-stage procedure, occlusion of the eye) is in most cases negated by the excellent result, which produces a normal-appearing lid with normal movement. However, the Mustarde rotational cheek flap can be used as an alternative for very large lower lid defects in patients who are not willing to tolerate a two-stage procedure or who need to have their eye remain open. Repair of total lower lid defects requires canalicular intubation, if possible, together with canthal fixation of the reconstructive flaps.

In extreme cases that have no adjacent tissue or upper lid tissue available, a periorbital flap—glabellar, cheek, or forehead—with a posterior lamellar graft or lining can be used.

Nasal Lower Lid

In general, the same reconstructive procedures used for central lower lid defects are available for nasal defects (Fig. 6). However, additional consideration is needed in the medial canthal area for proper fixation of the flaps with use of a medial canthal fixation technique. Canalicular intubation, if possible, must also be considered in defects in this area. In some cases inrotated local myocutaneous flaps with posterior lamellar lining can be used.

Temporal Lower Lid

The important aspect of repair of lateral canthal defects in the lower lid is lateral canthal fixation, regardless of whether the defects are small, moderate, or large. Direct closure, the Tenzel semicircular flap, the Hewes procedure, or the modified Hughes procedure is used for defects of a progressively increasing order of magnitude (Fig. 7).

Wide and Shallow

The most effective and efficient method of repair of shallow defects in the lower lid, whether the defects are central, nasal, or temporal, is the outwardly rotated myocutaneous flap (similar to a blepharoplasty)

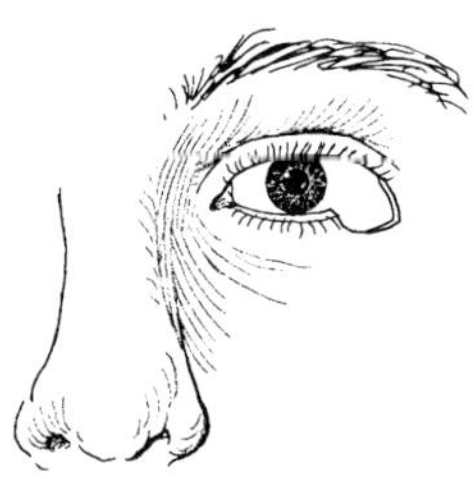

FIG. 7. Techniques for repair of temporal lower lid defect.

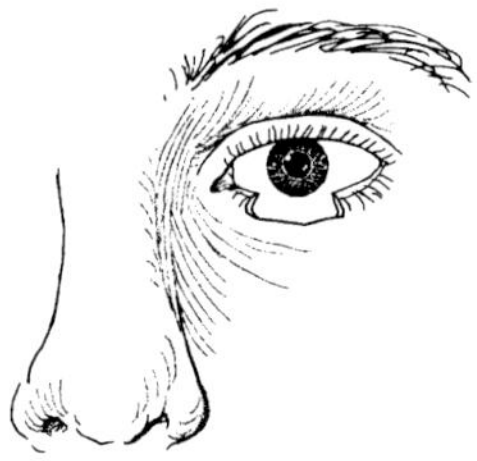

FIG. 8. Techniques for repair of wide-shallow defect in lower lid.

backed by a free tarsoconjunctival graft, a composite eyelid graft, or a palatal mucoperichondrium. Some broad, shallow defects in the lower lid margin can be repaired with a horizontally sliding flap that employs the principle of the Tenzel semicircular flap but also includes an inferior relaxing incision as well (2). This can be used successfully if these shallow defects are not too wide. In the more extensive broad-shallow defects at the lower lid, one may use a Hughes two-stage procedure to adequately repair this area (see Fig. 8). It does not seem justifiable to excise the large amounts of normal lid and cheek tissue that would be necessary to utilize a Mustarde rotational cheek flap for this type of defect. The Hewes procedure can be used if the shallow defect is laterally located.

TOTAL CANTHAL DEFECTS

Total canthal defects in most cases can be considered as a combination of upper and lower lid defects. In the canthal angles the importance of proper fixation of the flaps to the inner canthal area has been previously emphasized. In larger resections with removal of bone for neoplastic disease, fixation of the canthal tendon medially or laterally may be impossible because of the absence of soft tissue and bone. In the medial canthal area, in these cases, one may use microplates or transnasal wires nasally to facilitate fixation of the flap in the proper position. Fixation at the lateral canthus may be obtained with drill holes in the bone or, if the bony wall is absent, a spanning microplate may be used.

COMBINED DEFECTS

In many clinical situations a large canthal defect may occur in conjunction with a large defect of the upper and/or lower lid. Combinations of the previously described techniques must be employed to repair these large defects satisfactorily.

Inner Canthus and Upper Lid

In this difficult defect (Fig. 9), the lower lid canthal defect is first closed by advancement of the lower lid with medial canthal fixation together with canaliculostomy if indicated. A bridge flap procedure is then used as if the lower lid were intact. A flap from the lower lid is brought into the upper lid defect, with implanted ear cartilage between the conjunctiva and the musculocutaneous layer of the flap from the lower lid. In this special situation, adequate vertical bridge of lower lid

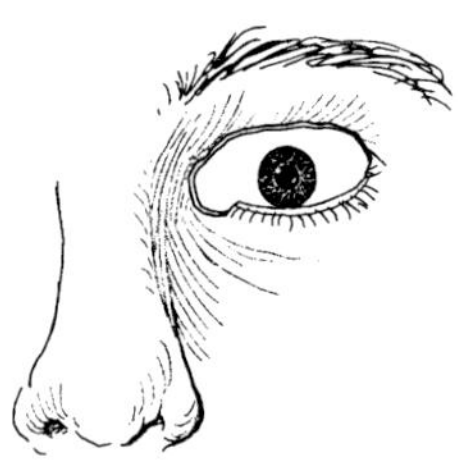

FIG. 9. Techniques for repair of combined defect of upper lid and inner canthus.

(with canthal fixation)

LID SHARING

Repair lower Lid defect
(direct closure , semicircular flap)
then
Bridge Flap to upper lid

NON LID SHARING

Repair lower Lid defect
(direct closure , semicircular flap)

and

Repair Upper Lid
periorbital Flap with
post. lamella graft

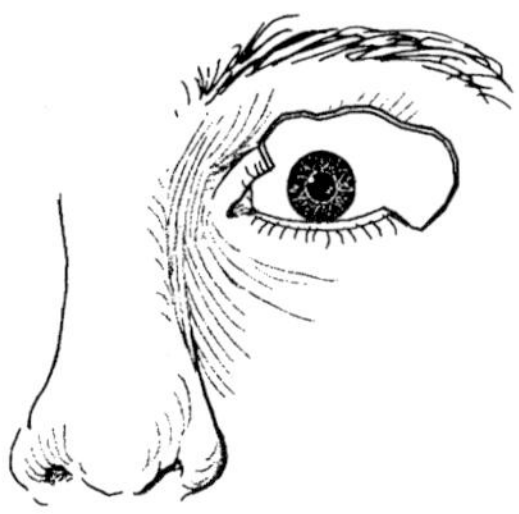

FIG. 10. Techniques for repair of combined defect of upper lid and outer canthus.

margin must be left intact to preserve its integrity because the lid has already been compromised. The lower lid tarsus should not be included in the flap. This is accomplished by making the horizontal incision across the lower lid below the inferior border of the tarsus (5 mm from the margin). The implanted cartilage graft within the flap to the upper lid must be fixed nasally with canthal fixation. Any residual canthal skin defect may be covered with a small full-thickness skin graft, a small glabellar flap, or be allowed to granulate.

In cases in which the eye cannot be closed or a second-stage procedure is not desired, separate non–lid-sharing techniques can be used for the upper and lower lids.

Outer Canthus and Upper Lid

For the upper lid part of the defect (Fig. 10), a bridge flap procedure is used as if the lower lid were intact and lateral canthal fixation of the cartilage graft within the flap were necessary. Great care must be taken to leave the lower lid bridge as vertically "wide" as possible in this situation. A semicircular flap can then be rotated into the lower lateral canthal defect and attached to the lower eyelid "bridge" containing the lower eyelid margin. Proper lateral canthal fixation of this semicircular flap repairing the lower lid and canthal must be obtained. In smaller defects, the temporal edge of the lower eyelid bridge may be attached directly with lateral canthal fixation.

Separate non–lid-sharing techniques can be used if the eyelids cannot be fused until the second stage.

Inner Canthus and Lower Lid

Large lower lid and inner canthal defects (Fig. 11) can be repaired with the modified Hughes procedure in which the tarsoconjunctival flap is brought into the lower lid defect and then stretched nasally and attached to the inner canthal area with medial canthal fixation. A full-thickness skin graft or flap can then be used to cover the flap to the lower lid as well as to cover defects in the inner canthal area. A very acceptable alternative for large lower lid defects involving particularly the inner canthal area is the Mustarde rotational cheek flap with a mucous membrane–bearing graft. The situation

(canthal fixation ,lacrimal intubation)

LID SHARING

tarsoconjunctival flap from upper lid (Hughes)
advance to lower lid and canthus with fixation
cover with skin graft,flap

and

direct upper nasal closure

NON LID SHARING

lower lid repair with periorbital flap
and post. lamellar graft
plus

direct upper nasal closure

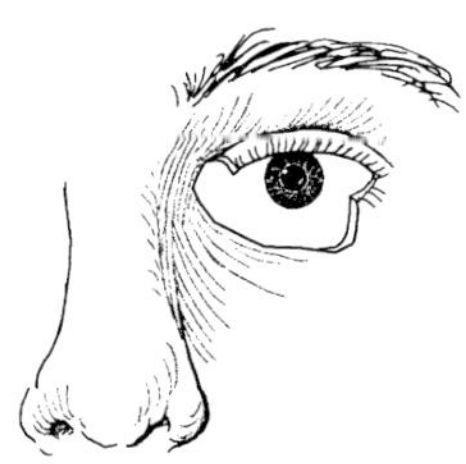

FIG. 11. Techniques for repair of combined defect of lower lid and inner canthus.

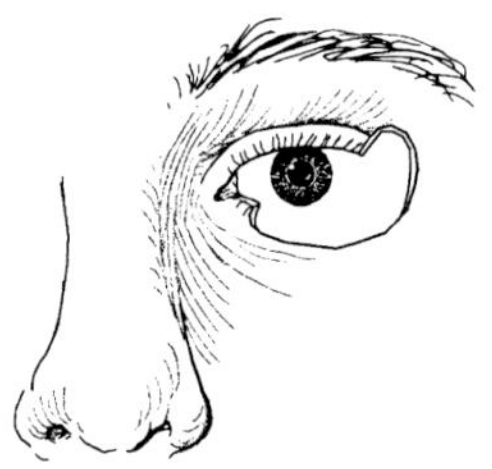

FIG. 12. Techniques for repair of combined defect of lower lid and outer canthus.

in which the Mustarde rotational cheek flap seems to be best used is when lower lid defects are confined mainly to the nasal lower lid or are in combination with inner canthal defects. The vertical suture line that extends downward in the facial area following this type of rotational flap is more appropriate when the defects are located in this area. The portion of this defect that extends to the upper lid may be repaired by a direct advancement of the upper lid or, in larger defects, a sliding tarsoconjunctival flap covered by a full-thickness skin graft. In some cases, a small glabellar flap could be rotated into the upper canthal defect area or simple granulation may provide filling of the defect over a period of time.

Outer Canthus and Lower Lid

For large defects in the lower lid including the outer canthus, the authors have had their best results with the modified Hughes tarsoconjunctival flap, which is brought into the lower lid defect, slid laterally, and fixed inside the lateral orbital rim. A full-thickness skin graft is then applied over the flap and the defect at the lateral canthus and lower lid. A small semicircular flap at the lateral canthus may be used to supplement closure in that area (Fig. 12).

PROBLEM CASES

Repair of eyelid defects is challenging even in the presence of healthy and available tissue. Complicating conditions can occur in which the source of reconstructive tissue is not ideal or the patient's general condition presents problems in management (Table 5).

From time to time the reconstructive surgeon will encounter a total eyelid defect with an inability to share the opposing eyelid tissue because it has been previously reconstructed or damaged by trauma or irradiation, and is therefore unsuitable to use in a lid sharing procedure. In some rare injuries or defects, both eyelids may be absent. Another problem situation is the absence of adjacent tissue that the surgeon may need for advancement or rotation; this can be particularly problematic in the lower lid. In these problem cases, one's priority must be to protect the eye and then secondarily to introduce appropriate tissue into the area to prepare the foundation for formation of a new eyelid. Any tissue that will cover the surface of the globe must be lined with mucous membrane whose epithelial layer faces the cornea. This mucous membrane must be covered in most cases with a flap of thicker skin or muscle that can be brought in from a peripheral area. For the upper lid, the most readily available vascularized skin flap is the median forehead flap or temporal forehead flap, as described in previous chapters. If upper and lower forniceal conjunctiva is present, it can be dissected free from the upper or lower or both forniceal areas and advanced to form the lining for the flap because the forehead skin is stiff. If conjunctival remnants are not present, then one must utilize a free graft of buccal mucous membrane, nasal chondromucosa, buccal mucous membrane, or palatal mucous membrane to line the inner surface of the flap. In this case one must accept the tenuous nature of a free graft lining the inner surface of a primary flap. In a similar situation in the lower lid, a forehead-based flap can also be used. Other periorbital flaps available for lower lid recon-

TABLE 5. *Problem patients eyelid reconstruction*

Irradiated tissue
Reduced stretchability
Actinic shrinkage
Scarring, dermatologic conditions
Young tense lids
Reduced healing (e.g., diabetes)
Bleeding tendencies (coagulation, blood pressure)
Loss of available local tissue
Loss of available remote tissue
Loss of available tissue for free grafts
Inability to seal eyelids with lid sharing technique
Poor patient compliance

TABLE 6. *Prioritization of eyelid reconstruction procedures*

Urgency of corneal exposure
Age of patient—skin elasticity
Expectations
Ability to close eyelids with lid sharing
Convenience and efficiency

struction are those from the nasolabial and cheek area, which may be rotated upward to the lower lid. In some cases, skin grafts may be needed to cover the donor site from where these large flaps originate if it cannot be closed easily. One may rarely encounter the need for this type of procedure; however, knowledge of the techniques may be useful in certain extreme situations.

FINAL CHOICE OF PROCEDURE

When considering the eyelid defect in the patient, the surgeon usually arrives at the choice of procedure that seems the most anatomically correct and promises the most accurate final result. Certain considerations should be given to other factors that may override the most anatomically accurate in choice of reconstructive procedures (Table 6).

REFERENCES

1. Steinkogler FJ, Moser E. A sandwich technique for full thickness reconstruction of the lower lid. *Orbit* 1988;8:37–43.
2. Reese AB. Epithelial tumors of the lid, conjunctiva, cornea, and lacrimal sac. In: *Tumors of the eye*. 3rd ed. New York: Harper & Row; 1936:50.

CHAPTER 25

Management of Eyelid Neoplastic Disease

Much of eyelid surgery is connected with the treatment of eyelid neoplastic disease and can involve diagnosis as well as management. A general knowledge of the common lesions and their behavior is important.

The large majority of all eyelid tumors are benign and more than three quarters of them are keratoses nevi or inflammatory lesions such as chalazions (1). Basal cell carcinoma is the most common eyelid malignancy, composing more than 90% of all eyelid malignancies and nearly 20% of eyelid tumors in general.

In most cases, eyelid lesions that have been present for many years and have not changed in appearance are usually benign. However, some "benign" lesions may change in appearance and the possibility of malignant change should be considered. They should be biopsied.

Clinical features that suggest the presence of a malignancy include *loss of eyelashes, ulceration, changes in size, changes in contour,* and *changes in color.* Recurrence of a lesion after previous treatment should raise the suspicion that a malignancy is present. Neoplastic lesions may increase in size by growing in tissue planes not readily visible to the human eye. The "masquerade syndromes" will be discussed at the end of this chapter (2,3).

BIOPSY AND TISSUE-PROCESSING TECHNIQUES

If an eyelid tumor is suspected of being a malignancy, it should be removed or biopsied for histologic examination. Preliminary photographs should be made to document the appearance and location of the lesion. If the tumor is relatively small, excisional biopsy of the entire lesion may be performed. A shave biopsy is a convenient method for small lesions for which there is a low index of suspicion for malignancy (Fig. 1). In most cases a wedge or plug of the tumor may be excised as a biopsy specimen (Fig. 2). For optimal evaluation, the specimen should be representative of the clinically abnormal lesion, ideally should incorporate adjacent normal tissue, should be sufficiently large for histologic processing, and should not be crushed or excessively traumatized.

Superficial biopsies of epithelium can yield information if the specimen is taken from the lesion itself. Special staining techniques can help to differentiate intraepithelial lesions such as sebaceous carcinomas, squamous carcinomas, and superficial basal cell carcinomas. Of course one must make the assumption that an adequate specimen is obtained and that one has not missed the tumor by biopsying in the wrong place. Many times epithelial biopsies can be misinterpreted as to the exact type of tumor. For example, squamous cell carcinoma can be diagnosed when the lesion is a sebaceous gland carcinoma with pagetoid skin change. The clinician must be aware of this fact and be prepared to perform a *full-thickness eyelid biopsy* to rule out a neoplasm lurking within the lid that has produced only equivocal surface changes (Fig. 3). Tissue should undergo fat staining with permanent sections to be sure that one is not dealing with an occult sebaceous gland carcinoma in these instances (4). Most tumors can be

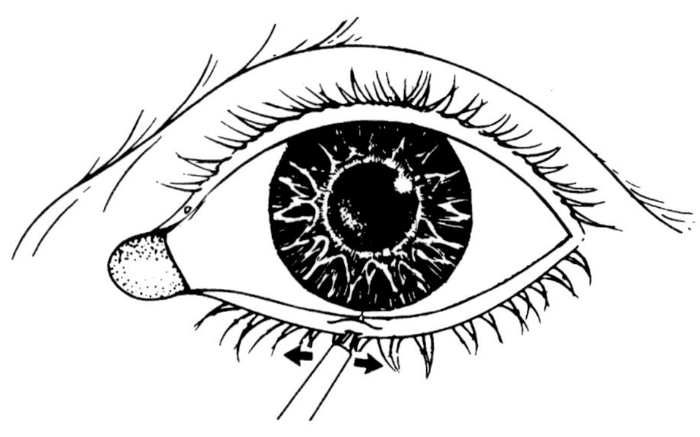

FIG. 1. Shave biopsy. This is the most common convenient way of biopsying small lesions. If malignant neoplastic disease is present, the original location of the lesion may be obscured. It also may be inadequate for diagnosis in some patients.

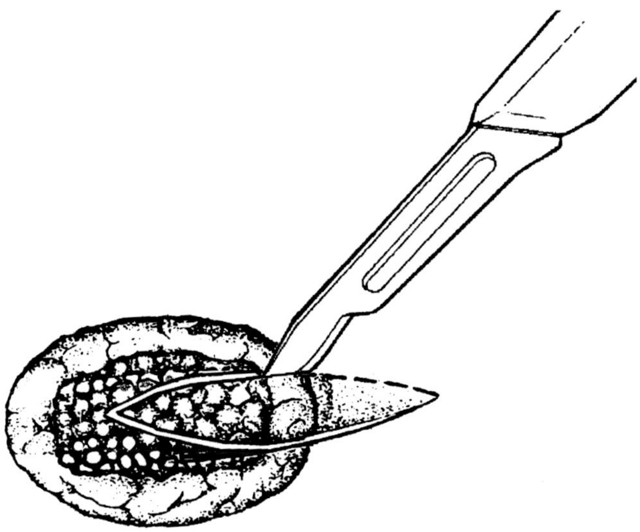

FIG. 2. Ellipse biopsy of visible lesion encompassing normal tissue and lesion. This spectrum of histology will give the pathologist a better opportunity to characterize the true cellular nature of the lesion.

adequately evaluated by conventional formalin fixation and histologic staining with hematoxylin and eosin (H&E). However, lipids are removed from tissues during H&E staining because of alcohol immersion. Therefore, if sebaceous cell carcinoma is suspected, the pathologist should be alerted at the time that the specimen is submitted so that fat stains can be performed. In cases of suspected melanoma, it is usually appropriate to request a review of the slides by a pathologist with wide experience in the examination of pigmented tumors.

A histologic diagnosis should always precede radical or extensive tumor resection.

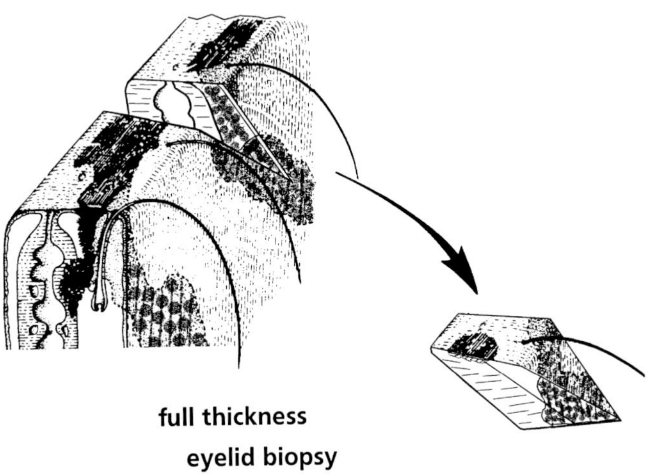

FIG. 3. Full-thickness eyelid biopsy. This type of biopsy is necessary in patients who have diffuse noncircumscribed neoplastic disease, particularly in patients whose malignant process may have an epithelial component but whose primary lesion is deep within the lid. It is mandatory in cases of suspected sebaceous cell carcinoma.

SYSTEMIC WORKUP

Physical examination of a patient with an eyelid tumor should include evaluation of the subcutaneous tissues to determine the clinical depth of the lesion and possible extension to the orbital bones or the globe. The entire conjunctival surface, including the palpebral conjunctiva and the fornices, should be examined when multicentric tumors such as sebaceous cell carcinomas and malignant melanomas are present. Except for basal cell carcinomas, most eyelid malignancies have the potential to spread by regional metastasis. Therefore the preauricular, submandibular, and cervical lymph nodes should be examined and palpated. If possible, photographs and sketches of tumors should be made before initial biopsy or treatment.

In patients with large tumors, extensive recurrent tumors, or tumors that appear to extend to the deep subcutaneous tissues, it is useful to obtain computed tomography (CT) scans. Clinical fixation of a tumor to the underlying periosteum indicates that the adjacent bone may be involved by the malignancy. In such cases bony invasion may be histologically present even though destruction is not seen on X rays or CT scans.

Systemic examinations other than chest X rays, regional node evaluation, and a complete physical examination are usually not required in patients with a basal cell, relatively small squamous cell, or sebaceous cell carcinomas. In patients with malignant melanomas, liver scans and liver function tests should also be performed because even small melanomas may sometimes metastasize rapidly.

TREATMENT OF MALIGNANT EYELID TUMORS

Adequate surgical excision provides the highest cure rate for most malignant eyelid tumors. The adequacy of excision is best determined by histologic examination of the margins around the resected tissue. Such microscopic evaluation can be performed either by examining frozen sections at the time of surgery or by examining tissues that are permanently fixed following surgery.

Frozen section examination of the margins around a resected area allows the surgeon to immediately remove additional tissue if the tumor is histologically found at the edge of the incision (Fig. 4). In the case of tumors such as basal cell carcinomas, which usually grow from a single focus, a very high cure rate can be achieved if the extent of resection is controlled by frozen section examination of the margins (5–8). Surgical excision with histologic control of all margins is usually the most effective treatment for most lesions, particularly basal cell carcinomas and squamous cell carcinomas.

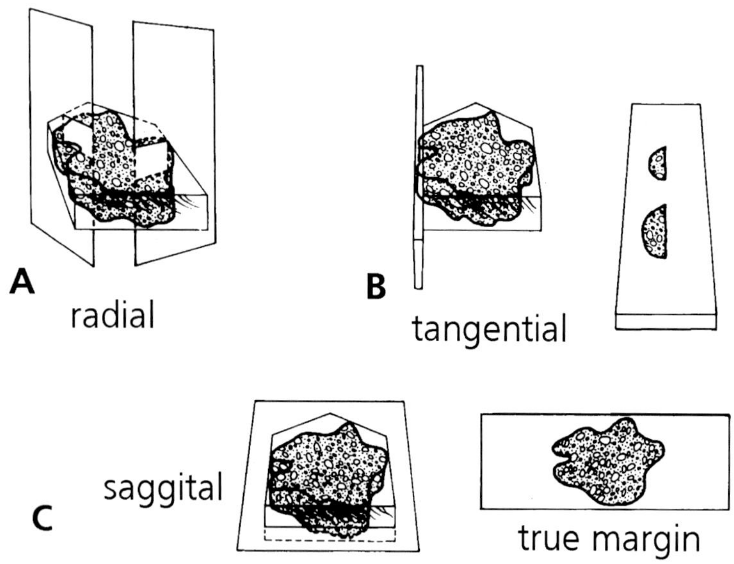

FIG. 4. Orientation of margin sections for eyelid tumors. **A:** The radial sectioning that sometimes is used by hospital pathologists gives the least accurate view of the extent of the lesion. **B:** The tangential view is the one most available for frozen sections in the hospital operating room setting. Its drawbacks are that it may sacrifice more tissue than is necessary for complete excision. In the presence of "positive margins" it may be difficult for the pathologist to determine whether the tumor actually extends through the section taken. A series of additional margins may be necessary to "clear" the excision. **C:** The dimension of the sections that gives the most accurate view of the extent of the margins at that particular level is the sagittal view. This, of course, determines the margin only at that particular level of the lesion and additional levels may be taken further until the sections are clear. This is the basis of the Mohs' microscopic controlled excision.

Histologic examination of the margins is particularly important in the case of morpheaform basal cell tumors because of their irregular edges and microscopic extensions. Frozen section control of the margins at the time of surgery provides an opportunity to assure complete tumor removal before eyelid reconstruction is completed. Orbital exenteration may be required in patients with tumors that invade the eye, the sinuses, or the deep orbit.

In the case of lesions that are usually multicentric in origin (sebaceous carcinomas), it may not be possible to completely rely on examination of resection margins if only one focus of the lesion is removed. In those tumors that may have distant metastases early (nodular melanoma), "clear margins" offer no guarantee of eradication of the process.

Histologically Controlled Methods (of Excision)

The two common venues of tumor excision with immediate frozen section histologic confirmation of margins are the operating room and the micrographic surgeon's (dermatologist's) office. The methods of sectioning and examining the margins generally differ between the two.

Operating Room Frozen Sections

At the time of surgery the initial resection of the lesion (with estimated clear margins of 1–2 mm) is submitted (in saline) as specimen 1 to the pathology lab for examination (Fig. 5). This allows the pathologist to establish the characteristics of the specific lesion. Additional edges of the initial defect created are submitted in a numbered, orderly manner, in separate containers. If a positive margin is encountered, additional edges must be taken until clear. This method will produce a high cure rate; however, if the lesion is very large and irregular it can be taxing on the surgeon and pathologist, possibly resulting in the sacrifice of large amounts of uninvolved tissue.

Mohs' Microscopically Controlled Excision

Mohs' excision is a form of surgical resection in which the tumor is excised in small lamellar tissue blocks, each of which is 5–10 mm^2 and 2–4 mm thick (8–10). The undersurface of each lamellar block is then histologically examined. If tumor is present, additional

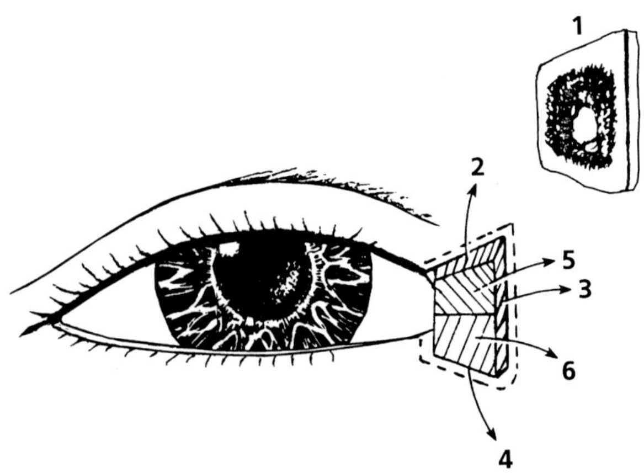

FIG. 5. Microscopic controlled excision of a lesion using operating room frozen sections. This shows the usual sequence of specimens submitted to the pathologist, which should be adequately labeled. These are tangential sections.

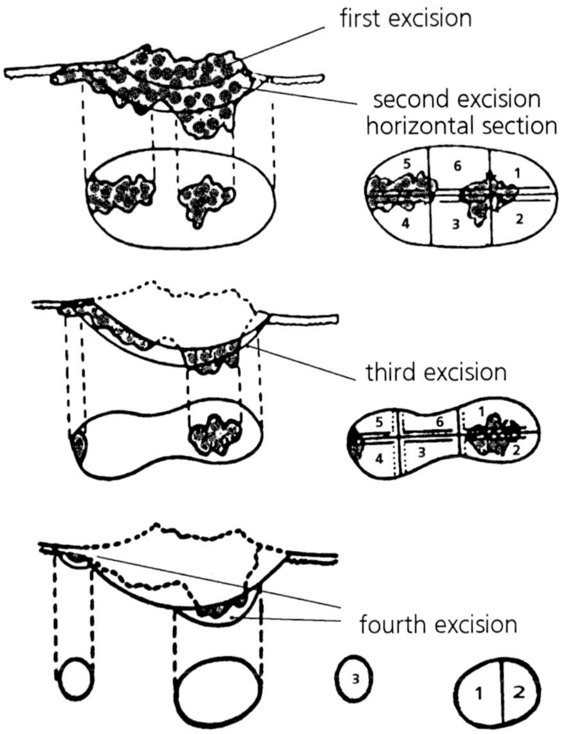

FIG. 6. Mohs' microscopic controlled excision. Current methods uses the "fresh tissue Mohs'" in which layers of tissue are frozen in the dermatologist's office and examined. The undersurface of the layer is examined because it represents the deep most peripheral extent of the lesion vertically. This is the most precise method of tumor excision.

lamellar blocks are excised from the adjacent tissues until all of the malignancy is removed (Fig. 6). This procedure has in the past been termed chemosurgery if the tissues are fixed in vivo with chemicals. More commonly frozen sections are used to examine the tissue and then the procedure is called fresh tissue Mohs' technique. Mohs' excision is time consuming, but it is the most precise of all procedures both to assure complete tumor removal and to preserve normal uninvolved tissues.

This procedure is particularly useful in treating deeply invasive tumors, recurrent (persistent) tumors, and extensive facial-orbital tumors.

Nonhistologic Controlled Treatment

Radiation Therapy

Radiation therapy can destroy many basal cell carcinomas, but it is not as effective as adequate surgical excision because the peripheral margins cannot be histologically examined to assure complete eradication of the tumor. Tumors that recur (persist) after ineffective radiation therapy are usually more difficult to control by subsequent surgery than similar tumors that were untreated. Basal cell carcinomas involving bone are more resistant to radiation than lesions localized to soft tissue (11–13).

Complications of radiation therapy include stenosis of the lacrimal drainage system, loss of eyelashes, skin atrophy with entropion or ectropion, and mucosal drying with conjunctival leukoplakia. Surgical excision and eyelid reconstruction in previously irradiated areas is difficult because of the presence of radiation-induced scarring and atrophy, poor blood supply and difficulty with free grafting.

Cryotherapy

Cryotherapy can be used to treat basal cell carcinoma but, as with radiation therapy, it is not possible to histologically confirm complete eradication of the tumor. Recurrence (persistence) is more frequent than with surgical excision. The main advantage is convenience because most patients can be treated by cryotherapy without hospitalization (14).

If cryotherapy is used to treat eyelid malignancies, the lesion should be carefully chosen and the cryotherapist should be skilled in the technique of treatment. Superficial basal cell carcinomas and tumors arising as part of the basal cell nevus syndrome are particularly suitable to treatment by cryotherapy. It is important to follow patients treated by cryotherapy carefully and to biopsy areas suspected of being persistent tumor.

Complications of cryotherapy include skin depigmentation, loss of eyelashes, and notching of the lid margin. Stenosis of the lacrimal drainage system is relatively uncommon, and subsequent surgery in an area previously treated by cryotherapy is usually not difficult.

TUMOR TYPES

There are a wide variety of rare malignancies that can occur in the eyelids, many of which have been seen by the authors (Table 1). The most common lesions are discussed.

TABLE 1. *Rare malignant eyelid tumors*

Mucoepidermoid carcinoma
Lymphoma
Metastatic
Fibrosarcoma
Merkle cell tumor
Sweat gland carcinoma
Malignant trichoepithelioma
Kaposi's sarcoma
Aberrant lacrimal gland carcinoma

TABLE 2. *Basal cell carcinoma*

Most common eyelid malignancy (80–90%)
Common in sun-damaged skin
More common lower lid, inner canthus
Types
- *Ulceronodular*—"rodent ulcer"—papule progressing to a central depression—rolled edge, may remain fairly demarcated. In many cases can determine clinical extent visually or with low magnification
- *Morpheaform* ("scleroderma-like")—skin thickening with roughness, contracture, ulceration
- Presentation may be insidious
- Infiltrates tissue widely in areas not visible clinically
- Suitable for Mohs' microscopically controlled excision
- *Superficial*—localized plaques of roughness, most commonly from sun-damaged skin and predisposing lesions (i.e., keratosis). Not very invasive but usually multicentric

Spread
- Ulceronodular enlarges microscopically but demarcated by palisading of cells.
- Morpheaform infiltrates tissue in strands and is not well demarcated microscopically
- Basosquamous variant behaves similarly
- Under normal circumstances there is no metastatic activity, only local invasion
- In eyelids, microscopic controlled excision is necessary, particularly with the morpheaform variety

Basal Cell Carcinoma

Basal cell carcinoma is the most common eyelid cancer, arising over 25 times more frequently than any other malignancy in this location. Most of these tumors arise on the sun-exposed lower eyelids in middle-aged persons with light complexion (Table 2). Although basal cell carcinomas often invade local tissues, they seldom metastasize. When these tumors arise near the canthi, they tend to become deeply infiltrative and may involve the eye or the lacrimal drainage system (15–17).

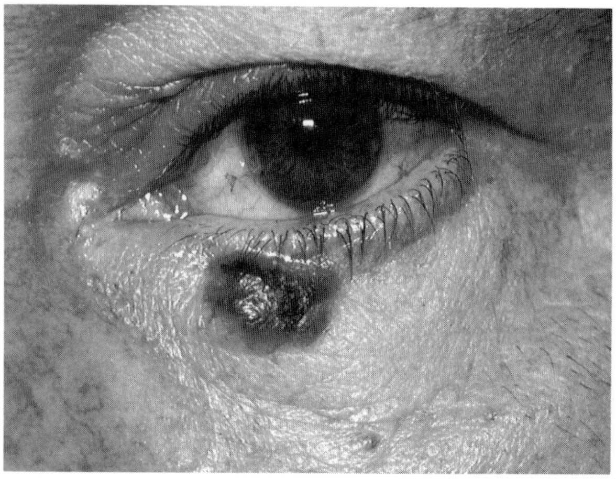

FIG. 7. Nodular basal cell of a pigmented variety. Central umbilication and ulceration has not occurred at this stage.

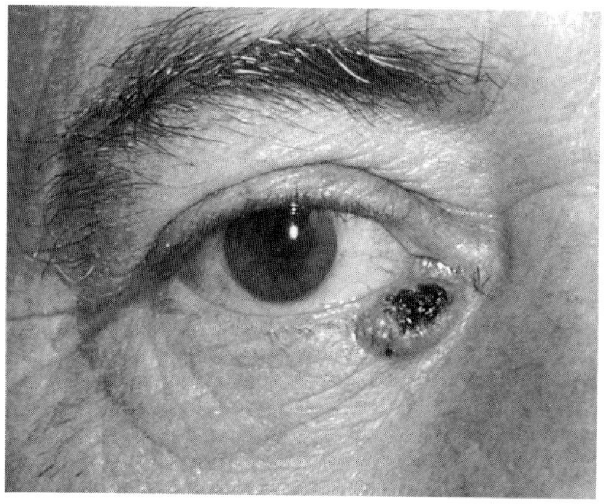

FIG. 8. Ulceronodular basal cell of the lower lid. This is the most common location for basal cells to occur on the eyelid.

Most basal cell carcinomas of the eyelids grow in one of three types: (a) nodular-ulcerative, (b) morpheaform, and (c) superficial. Occasionally these tumors can be pigmented (Fig. 7) and resemble nevi or melanomas. An unusual variant is found in the basal cell nevus syndrome (Gorlin's syndrome).

The margins of nodular-ulcerative tumors are usually pale, elevated, and nodular with telangiectatic vessels. The central area is often necrotic and ulcerated (Figs. 8 and 9). Morpheaform tumors are characterized by indistinct margins and a smooth, leathery surface, and often extend for a considerable distance beyond their clinical margins. They frequently produce cicatrization of the surrounding tissues (Fig. 10A, B). Superficial basal cell carcinomas are relatively rare on the face and usually consist only of slightly elevated, erythematous scaling patches.

Histologically, basal cell carcinomas are composed of small, oval cells containing dark nuclei and relatively little cytoplasm. The nuclei are usually rather uniform in size with little anaplasia. Groups or clusters of cells

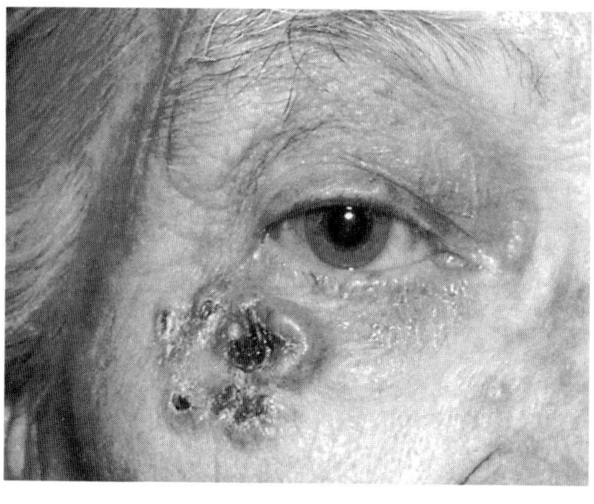

FIG. 9. Ulceronodular basal cell in a patient with neglected disease showing method of progression.

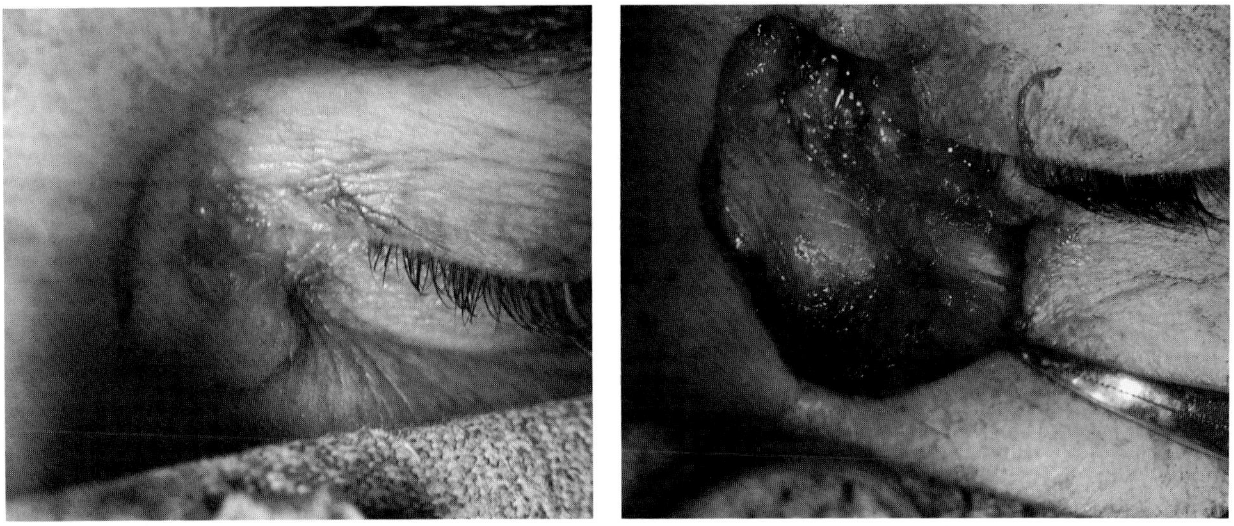

A B

FIG. 10. Morpheaform basal cell. **A:** Patient with a superficial ulcerative, scaly plaque of the inner canthus. The clinical evaluation of the extent of the lesion is marked. **B:** Using operating room frozen section control, the lesion was excised. The resulting defect indicates that the tumor had a much greater extent than that shown by clinical inspection.

are often surrounded by palisading columnar cells that are arranged in rows. During histologic fixation, the peripheral cells often separate from the surrounding stroma to leave empty spaces or clefts, which are a useful diagnostic feature. Morpheaform tumors have abundant, fibrous connective tissue that produces clinical cicatrization and a smooth, leathery surface.

Squamous Cell Carcinoma

Squamous cell carcinoma, of epidermoid carcinoma, is the second most common malignant skin tumor and can arise de novo or from a preexisting lesion (e.g., sun-induced keratosis). It may demonstrate intraepithelial spread only or advance with vertical invasion of the dermis with the risk of regional lymph node metastasis and ultimately distant metastasis. Understanding of the biological behavior of squamous cell carcinoma in the clinical settings in which it occurs is a requisite to proper management (Table 3) (18–21).

Squamous cell carcinomas frequently arise from previously sun-damaged skin, typically solar keratoses or actinic keratoses. These lesions affect an older population, the greatest risk factor being history of sun exposure and a fair complexion. The typical location of these lesions is on the face, forearm, and dorsa of the hands. Squamous cell carcinoma commonly occurs on the eyelid margin and may appear as an erythematous lesion, usually elevated and sometimes scaly (Fig. 11A, B). It may also be primarily in the eyelid skin and remain intraepithelial for a long period (Fig. 12). Squamous cell carcinomas arising in sun-damaged skin have a low propensity to metastasize (approximately 0.5%). With sun exposure a significant risk factor, it is not surprising that squamous cell carcinoma is more common on lower eyelids than the upper eyelids. Squamous cell carcinoma can commonly occur on the conjunctival surface and is not related to sun exposure (Fig. 13). Although squamous cell carcinoma is the second most common malignant eyelid tumor, it is esti-

TABLE 3. *Squamous cell carcinoma*

2nd most common eyelid malignancy (9%)
In Skin
Occurs commonly in fair-complexioned individuals with history of sun exposure, may arise from keratosis, can occur in old scars or areas of chronic irritation. More common in upper than lower lid, has predilection for the margin and canthus. Regional metastasis as high as 15–20%
Appearance
1—Rough scaly patch with erosion or ulceration
2—Nodular, plaque-like growth on lid margin
3—Chronic dermatitis (i.e., fungus), Bowen's disease
In Conjunctiva
Presents as *chronic conjunctivitis (blepharo conjunctivitis)*
Unrelated to sun exposure or pigmentation
Higher incidence of metastasis if occurs in fornix or palpebral conjunctiva
May present as pingueculum-pterygium
Epibulbar lesions generally remain intraepithelial but may invade globe
Spread
Infiltrative deep and subepithelial, intraepithelial, regional metastasis in aggressive cases
Excise with histologic controlled technique (regional node dissection in aggressive cases, if indicated)
Exenteration necessary with many cases of fornix involvement or orbital invasion

A 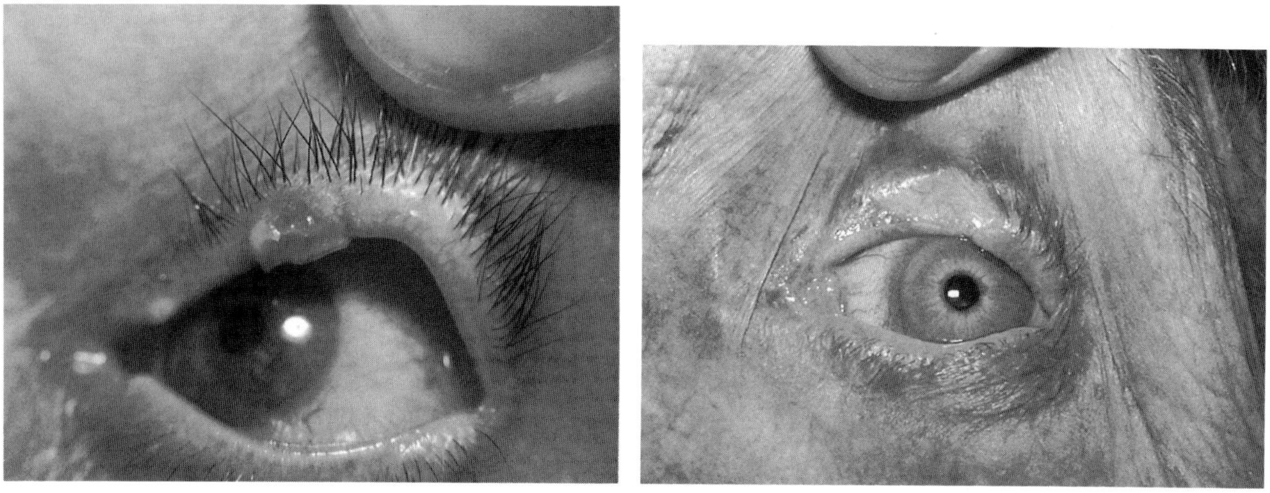 B

FIG. 11. Squamous cell carcinoma of the upper lid margin. **A:** A small, pearly hyperkeratotic plaque of the eyelid margin. Loss of lashes has not yet occurred. **B:** Another patient with a more advanced lesion with thickening and shiny induration. Loss of lashes has occurred.

mated that basal cell carcinoma is more frequent, at a rare of 40:1.

Squamous cell carcinoma can also arise from radiation-damaged skin, chronic ulcers, burn scars, and osteomyelitic sinuses. Squamous cell carcinomas arising from these lesions metastasize at a rate of 20–40%. Squamous cell carcinomas arising from non–sun-exposed normal skin (e.g., the mucocutaneous junction of the lip, glans penis, or vulva) have a high rate of metastatic disease.

Bowen's disease is usually a solitary lesion, commonly in non–sun-exposed skin, that slowly enlarges as a flat, erythematous encrusted patch (Fig. 12). Because metastasis can occur from this superficial-looking lesion, this carcinoma in situ should be differentiated from the similar-looking but benign solar or actinic keratosis.

Squamous cell carcinoma can be suspected clinically but must be biopsied for definitive diagnosis. Intraoperatively, frozen section control is necessary to ensure adequate margins of excision. Histologically, squamous cell carcinomas are composed of large, pale cells with abundant cytoplasm. Cellular atypia, dyskeratoses, and loss of normal dermal cell polarity are important features. Areas of keratin pearls are seen within the masses of invading cells.

Local spread of squamous cell carcinoma is often by narrow cellular strands rather than by uniform advancement of the entire border of the tumor. Because of this propensity and the potential to metastasize, a wider resection margin is removed from around a squamous cell carcinoma than in the case of most basal cell carcinomas. Frozen section control is mandatory when undertaking surgical excision. Radiation therapy offers

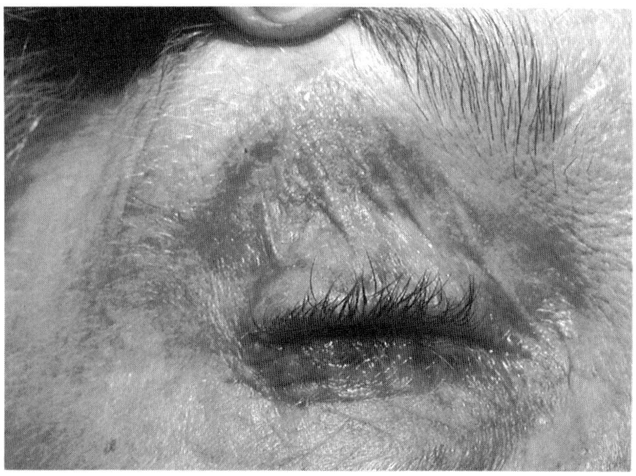

FIG. 12. Squamous cell carcinoma of upper lid skin. Intraepithelial with early deep invasive squamous cell carcinoma (Bowen's disease) of the upper lid.

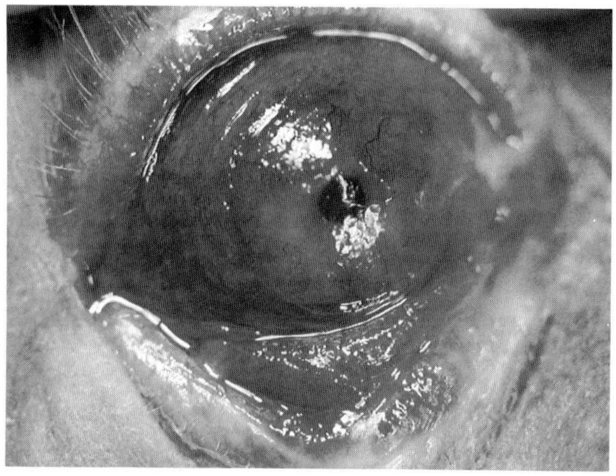

FIG. 13. Squamous cell carcinoma of the conjunctiva, which initially started in the fornices progressing over the surface of the cornea. The patient required exenteration for cure.

TABLE 4. *Sebaceous carcinoma*

Arises from sebaceous glands (Zeis, meibomian, hair follicle, brow, caruncle)
Onset usually in 60s
Commonly in fair-complexioned individuals
Presents as *chalazion, chronic blepharoconjunctivitis*
More common in upper lid (both upper and lower approx 20%)
"Masquerade" presentation common
Spread
Local infiltration
Intraepithelial spread (pagetoid) in 50–70% (higher incidence of regional metastasis in these cases)
Regional lymphatic metastasis (20–30%) significant mortality risk
Multicentric origin common, recurrence rate high, close follow-up mandatory
High percentage of patients require exenteration for cure
High incidence of secondary (other) malignancies
High incidence in irradiated tissue, radioresistant tumor
Diagnosis
Full-thickness lid biopsy with fat stains

less control and may be contraindicated in skin previously damaged by X rays. The role of local chemotherapy is not well defined. Exenteration of the orbit may be necessary if the tumor is extensive or deeply invasive. Lymph node removal may be appropriate if the tumor has undergone regional metastases.

Sebaceous Cell Carcinoma

Sebaceous cell carcinoma is the third most common eyelid malignancy, accounting for approximately 1–2% of all eyelid malignancies. Sebaceous cell carcinoma most commonly arises from the meibomian gland but it can arise from the glands of Zeis, hair follicle glands, and sebaceous glands of the caruncle and of the brow. Most of these tumors are slow-growing neoplasms, occurring in patients greater than 60 years of age. They occur in the upper eyelid with twice the frequency of occurrence in the lower eyelid, presumably because of the greater number of meibomian glands in the superior tarsus (Table 4). The rarity of the lesion and its presentation as a benign eyelid condition requires a high index of suspicion on the part of the clinician in order to diagnose this condition (2–4,18,22–26).

It is well recognized that sebaceous cell carcinoma may mimic symptoms of a chronic chalazion (Fig. 14A), chronic unilateral blepharoconjunctivitis (Fig. 14B), keratitis, or superior limbic keratoconjunctivitis and commonly "masquerades" as an inflammatory process. It can also present as localized eyelid or conjunctival inflammation, caruncular tumor, conjunctival mass, cutaneous horn, or lacrimal fossa tumor (26–28). In its more recognizable form, sebaceous cell carcinoma will cause a nodular induration and thickening of the eyelids, with a yellowish, erythematous coloration. Loss of cilia and distortion of the meibomian gland orifices of the eyelid margin is typical (Fig. 14B).

In many cases it requires a high index of suspicion and a knowledgeable clinician to diagnose this condition. Surgeons not only must perform the correct type of biopsy but must submit the specimen for the proper type of pathologic exam. Simple shave biopsies are often inadequate. Pagetoid spread (intraepithelial sebaceous cell carcinoma) may be indistinguishable on a shave biopsy from squamous cell carcinoma in situ, superficial spreading malignant melanoma, or other lesions. It should be emphasized that a *full-thickness eyelid biopsy* with adequate tarsus is the definitive biopsy for diagnosing sebaceous cell carcinoma. Because of

A

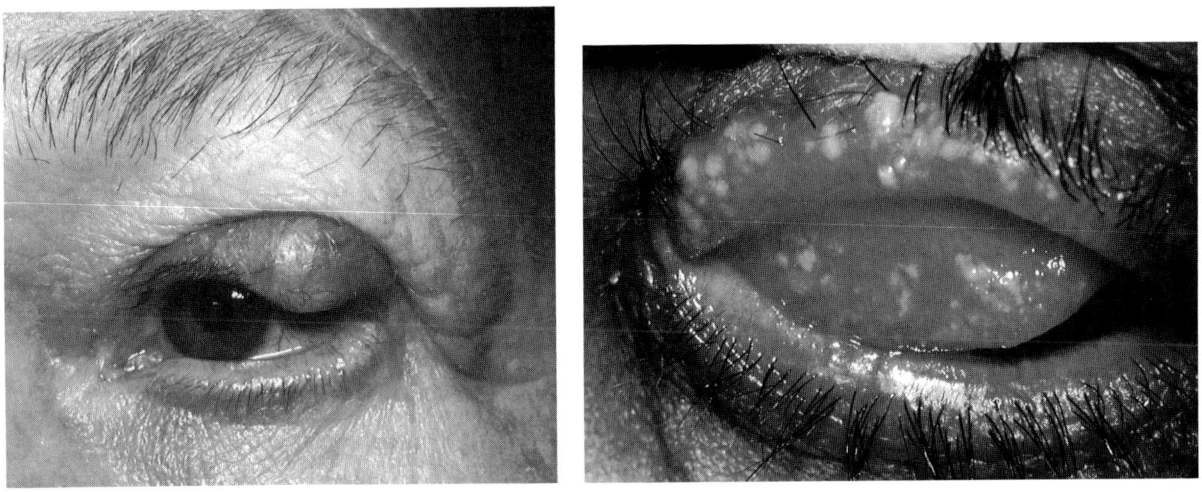

B

FIG. 14. Sebaceous carcinoma of the eyelid. **A:** A localized, well-differentiated lesion presenting as a chalazion. **B:** The diffuse infiltrative lesion presenting as blepharoconjunctivitis in the upper lid.

the frequently multicentric origin of these tumors, multiple biopsies are often necessary.

Histologically, most sebaceous cell carcinomas are composed of large anaplastic cells with a foamy cytoplasm. Lipid vacuoles within the cytoplasm are usually positive for fat stains. Because routine histologic processing with alcohol will dissolve the lipid vacuoles, frozen sections on fresh tissues stained with oil red O stain must be performed (28). Foci of lipid in this cytoplasm and evidence of sebaceous differentiation are histopathologic hallmarks of this tumor. Electron microscopy or immunoperoxidase studies can serve as useful adjuncts. Poorly differentiated tumors, with scanty cytoplasm and prominent nucleoli, have a relatively poor prognosis.

The delay in diagnosing sebaceous cell carcinoma may be attributed to a number of factors: relative rarity of the lesion, resemblance to other more common benign conditions, and inexperience of both the clinician and the pathologist. It should be remembered that sebaceous cell carcinoma is rare in other parts of the body and that the general pathologist may have little experience in diagnosing this malignancy of predominantly the eyelids. There seems to be a significant correlation between the duration of symptoms of sebaceous cell carcinoma prior to excision and prognosis (28). If the duration of symptoms is between 1 and 6 months, the mortality was found to be 14%. If the duration of symptoms was greater than 6 months, the mortality was 38% (24). A delay in diagnosis typically correlated with larger-sized tumors, intraepithelial spread, and orbital invasion. Once the diagnosis is established, the preferred management is wide surgical excision with frozen section monitoring. Excision may include 5- to 6-mm margins of normal tissue. Even wide excisions with frozen section control may not be curative because the presence of multiple, unconnected lesions is a well-known characteristic of sebaceous cell carcinoma (25). Close clinical follow-up of every patient treated for sebaceous cell carcinoma is mandatory. Ultimately, many patients require orbital exenteration, as recurrence or multicentricity of the lesion becomes apparent during follow-up. Initial tumor metastases usually occur in the ipsilateral parotid gland and anterior cervical lymph nodes. Radical neck dissection is the treatment of choice for local lymph node metastatic disease. Enlarged lymph nodes must always be biopsied prior to radical neck surgery because localized lymphadenitis without tumor metastases may occur with sebaceous cell carcinoma. Distant metastasis to the lungs, liver, and brain may occur as a later sequela. The role of radiation therapy in the treatment of sebaceous cell carcinoma remains controversial (29). Although not a primary choice of therapy, radiation treatment has been used in selected patients who are not surgical candidates. Sebaceous cell carcinoma is somewhat radiosensitive and may regress initially, although recurrence is typical. Radiation therapy must also be questioned in that irradiation has been implicated as one of the causes of sebaceous cell carcinoma.

Malignant Melanoma

Malignant melanoma rarely involves the eyelids. Melanomas of the cheek may spread onto the eyelids, and conjunctival melanomas may extend over the lid margin on the eyelid skin (Table 5). Cutaneous melanomas are usually classified into one of three types: (a) lentigo maligna melanoma (malignant melanoma arising in Hutchinson's freckle), (b) superficial spreading melanoma, and (c) nodular melanoma. Lentigo maligna is an acquired pigmentation that usually appears after the fifth decade of life on the face or on other body surfaces that have been exposed to the sun (Fig. 15A) (30). Malignant melanoma may arise within the lesion and produce an elevated nodule (Fig. 15B). Acquired melanosis is a conjunctival abnormality that is sometimes considered analogous to lentigo maligna, and malignant melanoma may similarly arise in this lesion (Fig. 16) (33,34). Nodular melanoma is a tumor with a predominantly vertical or invasive growth phase and usually has a relatively poor prognosis, whether it arises within the skin or the conjunctiva.

Histologically, malignant melanomas are composed of atypical melanocytes that demonstrate varying de-

TABLE 5. *Melanoma*

In Skin
Nodular with vertical growth pattern (dermal invasion)
Lentigo maligna
Superficial spread (lentigo maligna is precursor)
More radial growth phase
Most common lower lid
No sex predilection
Most common clinical characteristics: growth, pigmentation, ulceration/hemmorrhage
Also irregular borders, variegated shades or color
In Conjunctiva
Behaves like lentigo maligna, superficial spreading, may go into vertical growth phase, may be amelanotic
Spread
Direct invasion, regional nodes, blood borne
May have systemic (blood borne) metastasis early from vertical growth
Treatment is wide local excision followed by incontinuity regional node resection if indicated
Wide local excision biased toward the regional lymph drainage
"Premalignant lesion" may become malignant and matastasize early—dilemma in management because wide local excision may involve globe
Clarke levels of vertical invasion or estimate of tumor volume allow prognostication

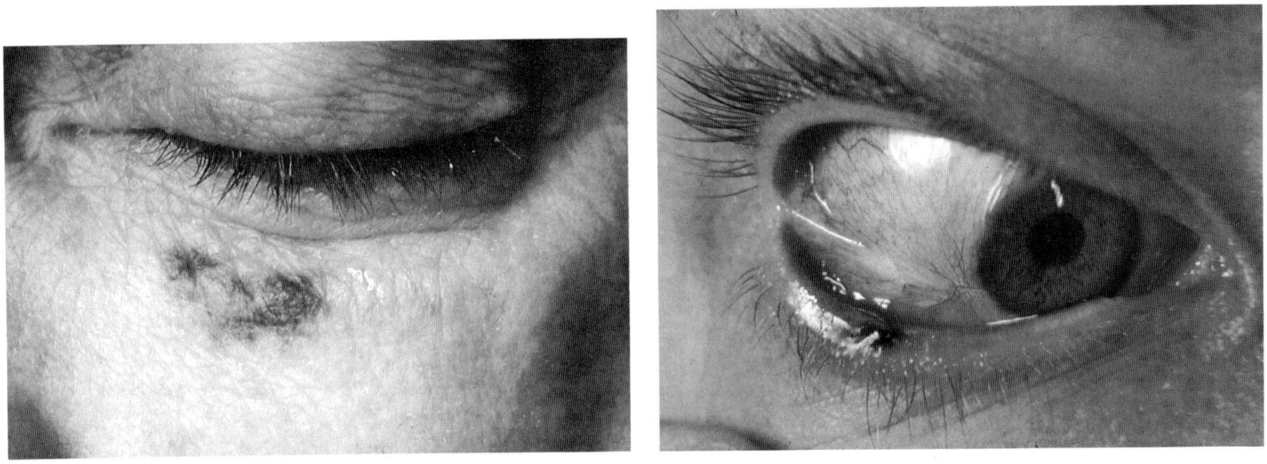

A B

FIG. 15. Malignant melanoma. **A:** An example of lentigo maligna which may progress to superficial spreading or nodular melanoma. There is an irregular outline, variegation in pigmentation, and history of growth. **B:** Nodular melanoma of the eyelid margin. This lesion occurred 8 months following excision of conjunctival melanoma.

grees of differentiation and tissue invasion. In both skin and conjunctiva, melanomas that measure less than 0.75 mm in thickness have a very high cure rate. In all tissues, melanomas confined to the epithelium can usually be completely removed by wide local excision (33,34).

Wide local excision (excisional biopsy) of lesions that are suspected of being a melanoma should be performed. Before more aggressive therapy is instituted, histologic confirmation and, if possible, histologic staging should be performed. Systemic evaluation should include not only examination of the regional lymph nodes and chest X rays but liver scans and liver function tests as well. The commonly accepted treatment for localized melanomas is surgical excision of the malignant tissue alone. Exenteration should be considered in patients with extensive or invasive tumors. The exact role of prophylactic regional lymph node dissection has not been established for patients with eyelid melanomas; however, the Clark levels now serve as a guide (33,34). Similarly, adjunctive chemotherapy, immunotherapy, and hormone therapy are of unknown value in the management of eyelid melanomas that have no evidence of metastatic spread.

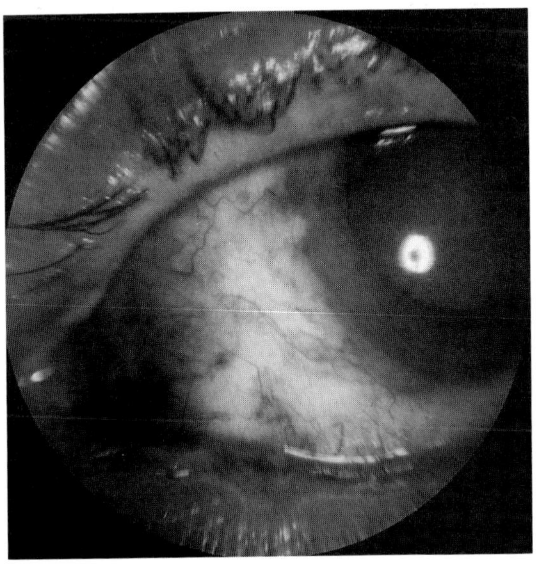

FIG. 16. Malignant melanoma. Conjunctival melanoma initially appearing as lentigo maligna of the conjunctiva. It progressed to a nodular change in the fornix and progressed to the eyelid margin.

Metastatic Eyelid Carcinoma

Metastatic carcinoma is a very rare form of malignant eyelid tumor (16,35–37). Because it may be the presenting sign of lethal disease, its diagnosis is critical and it is discussed here for this reason. Forty-six cases have been reported in the medical literature, with eight of the cases also showing orbital involvement. Without doubt there are patients with known metastatic carcinoma who never have suspicious eyelid lesions biopsied and are never reported. In 38% of the cases in the literature, the eyelid lesion was the presenting sign of carcinoma. Thus, the oculoplastic surgeon should certainly be familiar with this condition.

Metastatic eyelid carcinoma will typically present in one of three ways (37). Approximately two thirds of patients will present with a *solitary eyelid nodule*. This nodule may be a painless growth or may be acutely inflamed and tender. Approximately one third of the patients with metastatic eyelid carcinoma will present with *diffuse eyelid induration*. Less than 10% of the patients will present with a ulcerative lesion. Metastatic eyelid carcinoma may be accompanied by orbital disease in patients who have proptosis or motility dysfunction. Metastatic eyelid disease should be readily differentiated from eyelid melanomas and lymphoid tumors or lymphomas, which have a different coloration and general appearance.

Metastatic eyelid disease is most commonly due to carcinoma of the breast (65%), lung (15%), and stomach (10%). Although the eyelid lesion is the presenting sign of carcinoma in approximately one third of cases, two thirds of patients will already have known carcinoma, which stresses the importance of a thorough history. The mean time interval between the diagnosis of carcinoma and the occurrence of metastatic eyelid disease is 4 years. The late occurrence of metastatic disease is most typical of slow-growing breast carcinoma; at the time at which metastatic eyelid carcinoma is diagnosed, over two thirds of patients have metastatic disease elsewhere, most commonly in the liver, spleen, lymph nodes, or bones.

If feasible, the treatment of choice is excisional biopsy with eyelid reconstruction. Palliative local radiation therapy can induce significant tumor regression, especially in metastatic breast carcinoma. The mean survival in all patients with metastatic eyelid disease is less than 10 months. The prognosis is better with slow-growing metastatic breast carcinoma, which, when presenting as a solitary eyelid nodule, has a mean survival of greater than 20 months.

MICROSCOPIC GROWTH PATTERNS AND MASQUERADE PRESENTATIONS OF EYELID NEOPLASTIC DISEASE

If all neoplastic disease in the eyelid were confined to visible mass lesions and the extent of tissue involvement could be readily seen with the naked eye, the diagnosis and treatment of these lesions would be less formidable. Ordinarily, one would expect the growth of skin cancer, regardless of the histologic type, to be uniform in all directions producing an enlarging, protruding mass that could be easily identified. Many eyelid tumors, however, expand involving different tissue planes at a microscopic level, so that the process does not present as a discrete lesion that is a round bump or ulcerated lesion that can be readily diagnosed as skin cancer (18).

Intraepithelial Spread

Some neoplastic disease may progress primarily within the epithelial layer of the skin or mucous membrane in a radially spreading manner as shown in Fig. 17. This occurs commonly in cases of squamous cell carcinoma of the conjunctiva or Bowen's disease of the skin. It can also occur in some cases of malignant

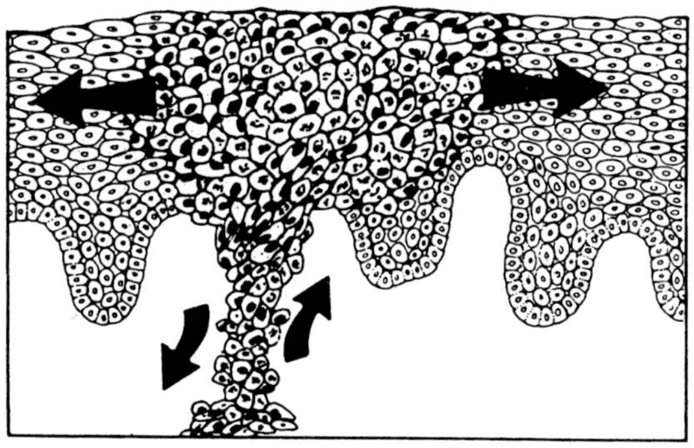

FIG. 17. Diagrammatic representation of the intraepithelial spread of eyelid neoplastic disease. This type of microscopic behavior can mimic an inflammatory process.

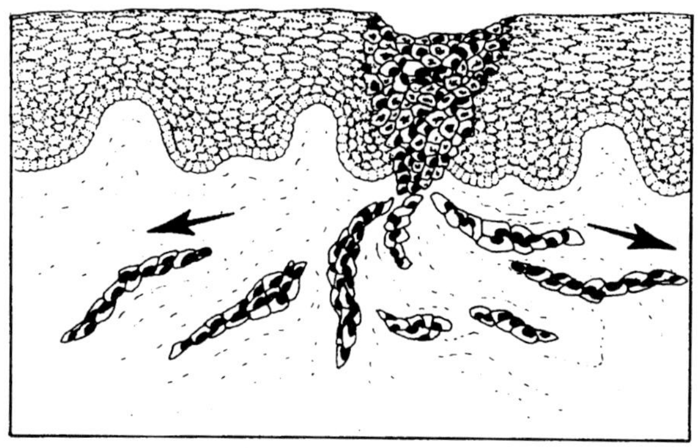

FIG. 18. Diagrammatic representation of subepithelial spread of neoplastic disease. This process allows aggressive tumors to invade surrounding tissue without clinical evidence of involvement.

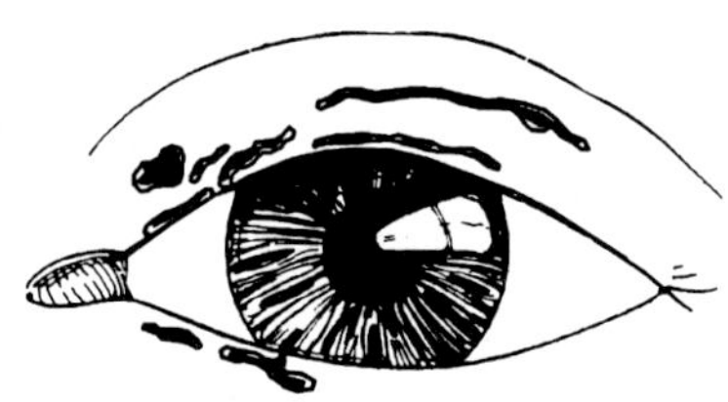

FIG. 19. Multicentric origin of sebaceous carcinoma. The sebaceous carcinoma is notorious for arising in multiple areas in the eyelid and can in many cases arise in both the upper and lower lids in the same patient.

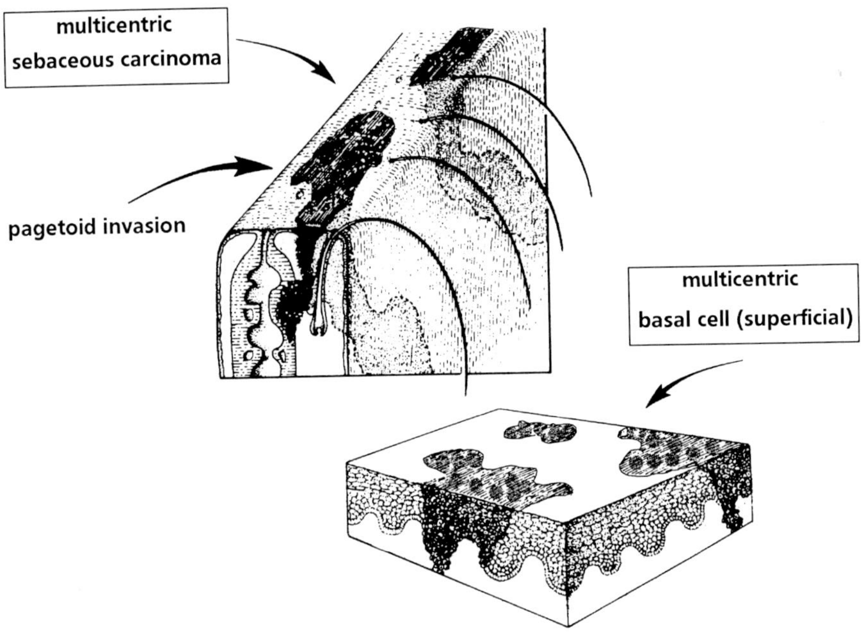

FIG. 20. Diagrammatic representation of types of multicentric origination of tumors. This characteristic does limit the value of microscopic controlled excision in patients with this process.

melanoma. Other lesions, such as sebaceous carcinoma, show "epidermotropic" characteristics with epithelial or pagetoid skin or conjunctival involvement.

Subepithelial Spread

Many neoplasms that originate in the epidermal layer may invade the dermis and exhibit a radial growth spread beneath normal overlying cutaneous epithelium. The most common lesion behaving in this manner is the "sclerosing," "fibrosing," or "morphea"-like basal cell carcinoma or that with squamoid differentiation, which is depicted in Fig. 18.

Multicentric Origination

Multicentric origination is a particularly distressing type of microscopic behavior. Patchy areas can certainly occur with squamous cell carcinomas or basal cells; however, the most troublesome lesion that shows multicentricity is the ominous sebaceous carcinoma (Fig. 19). This relegates the use of frozen sections for margin confirmation to a very minor role. When the lesion is excised one may get clear margins and still have multiple foci of neoplasm remaining in the tissue. This characteristic, as well as pagetoid intraepithelial spread, is demonstrated in Fig. 20.

Vertical Invasion

Invasive cutaneous tumors, as many melanomas, are classified (Clark–McGovern) according to the invasion level into the dermis and subcutaneous tissues to which they vertically extend beneath the epidermal surface: level I—in situ; level II—papillary dermis; level III—uppper reticular dermis; level IV—reticular dermis; and level V—subcutaneous fat (Fig. 21). In gen-

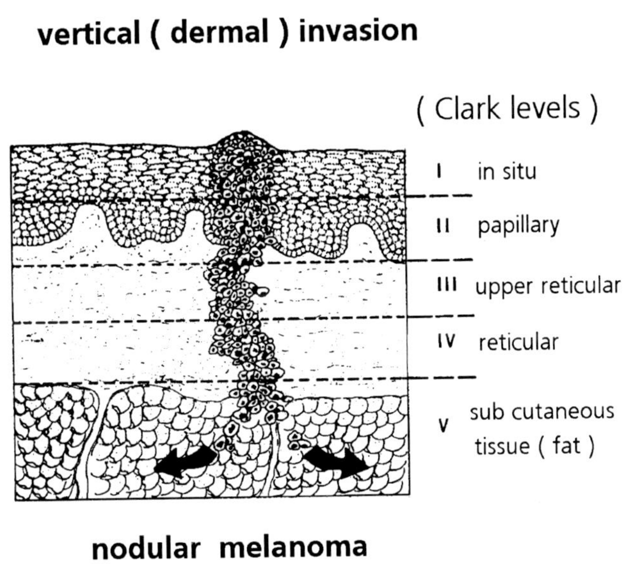

FIG. 21. Diagrammatic representation of the vertical growth phase of certain tumors. This is particularly important in determining a prognosis in patients with nodular melanoma in that the chance of regional or systemic metastasis is greater the further into the dermis or deep tissue the lesion penetrates. This has also been correlated with the mass of the tumor, particularly in the vertical direction. Once the tumor cells reach the subcutaneous and fat tissue they may more readily invade the body through the bloodstream, lymphatics, or specific tissue plains such as the peripheral nerve sheaths. Histologic evaluation of this behavior also imparts prognostic value in patients with lesions other than nodular melanoma.

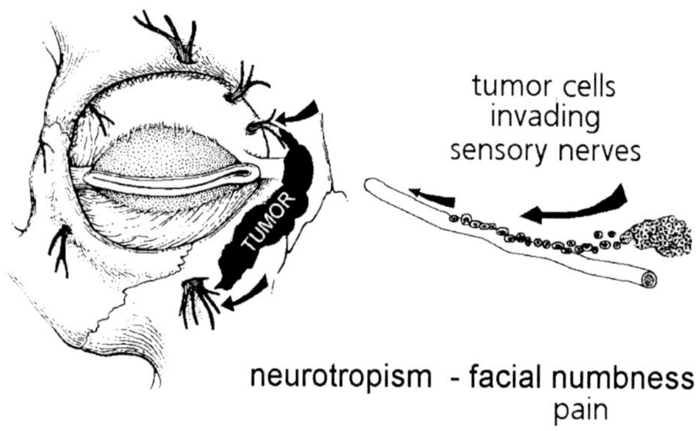

FIG. 22. Neurotropism of eyelid neoplastic disease. Facial numbness or pain can be a presenting sign or a sign of recurrence in patients with invasive squamous cell or malignant melanoma (less commonly basal cell) if the tumor involves the branch of the fifth cranial nerve producing a loss of sensation or pain.

eral, it is felt that Clark level I is an in situ lesion with almost no metastatic potential. Clark level II has a 2.5% potential for regional metastasis. Clark level III has a 20% metastasizing potential and IV and V a 40% and 70% potential, respectively. Consideration for regional node dissection occurs at level III (33,34). Although the Clark–McGovern invasion levels were originally described in connection with melanomas, they are also applicable to other invasive cutaneous tumors such as squamous cell and sebaceous cell carcinomas. In general, metastasis occurs more often when tumors extend more deeply into the dermis or the subcutaneous fat. These invasion levels are not generally used to describe conjunctival tumors because the conjunctival epithelium is relatively thin as compared to the epidermis of the skin and because the conjunctival substantia propria is similarly much thinner than the cutaneous dermis.

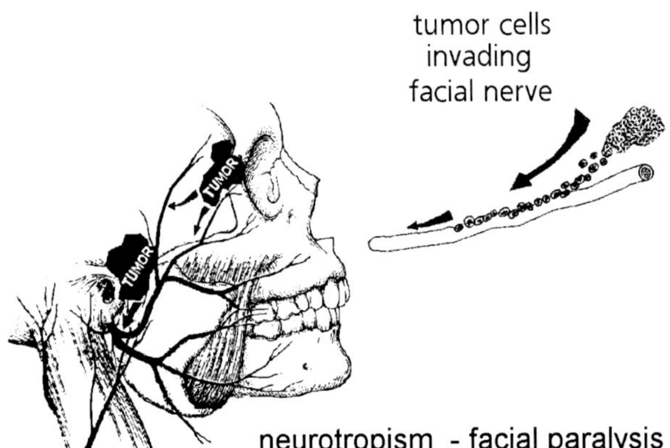

FIG. 23. Neurotropism of eyelid neoplastic disease. A complete or partial facial paralysis may be the initial presenting sign or sign of recurrence in a patient with eyelid neoplastic disease if the nerve sheath has been invaded by the tumor. This is common in squamous cell carcinoma and malignant melanoma.

Neurotropism

Poorly differentiated neoplasms can invade peripheral nerve sheaths and is a poor prognostic sign. This behavior occurs most commonly with squamous cell carcinoma and malignant melanoma (desmoplastic variant). The resulting effect on the nerve can be a presenting sign of the neoplasm or the first sign of a recurrence. Nerve invasion can produce facial numbness, facial pain, or partial or complete facial paralysis (Figs. 22 and 23) (38–43).

MASQUERADE PRESENTATIONS

The following presenting clinical situations have occurred in which an eyelid neoplasm has been misdiagnosed as an inflammatory lesion or nonneoplastic disease because of disguise of involvement of the eyelid by the mechanisms described above.

Chronic Conjunctivitis (Squamous Cell Carcinoma, Sebaceous Cell Carcinoma)

Lesions can present insidiously with a chronic reddening of the conjunctiva in the conjunctival fomix or the bulbar conjunctiva, and may persist over a long period of time despite treatment with antibiotics or antiinflammatory agents. Many times the process will seem to improve slightly with the antibiotic agents and the doctor may feel encouraged to try more agents. The doctor may feel that the patient is noncompliant or that the doctor has not found the "right drop yet." The doctor may feel that the problem is explained by

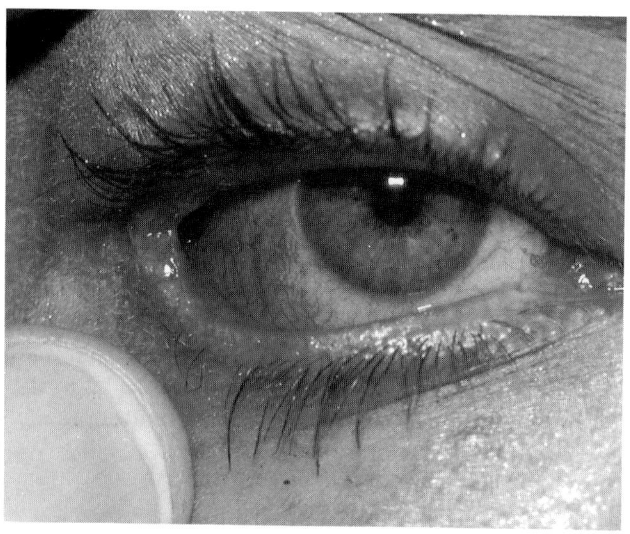

FIG. 24. Squamous cell carcinoma of the eyelid margin and conjunctiva. This patient had been treated for 6 months or more for a fungal blepharoconjunctivitis with intermittent response. A full-thickness lid biopsy was taken showing it to be a squamous cell carcinoma.

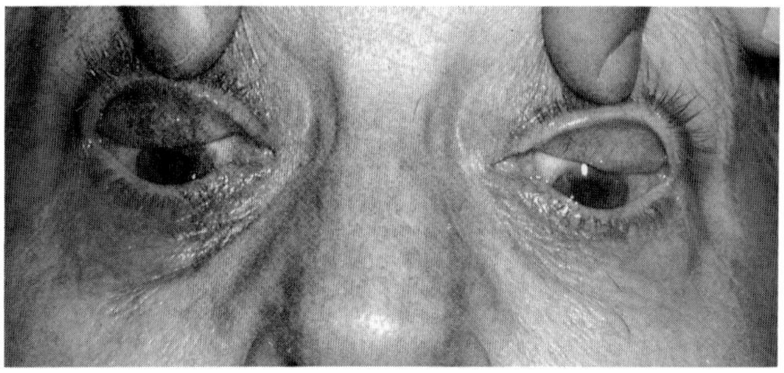

A

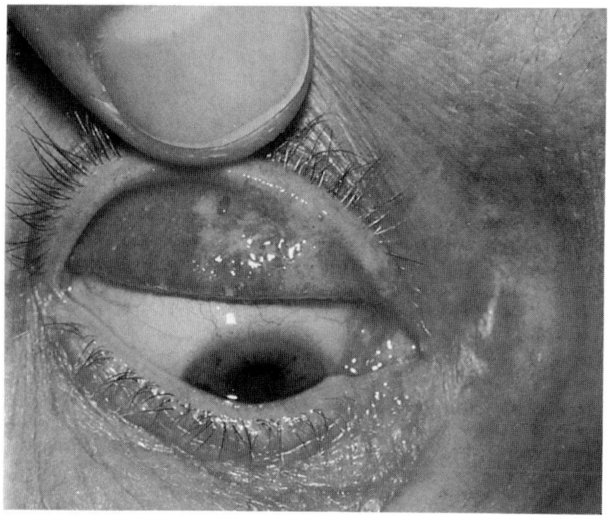

B

FIG. 25. A: Squamous cell carcinoma. This patient was treated for a chronic conjunctivitis of her right upper lid. **B:** Closer view showing the thickening and induration of the lid. A biopsy was taken showing it to be a squamous cell carcinoma. The lesion was treated with lid resection and repair.

an unusual condition such as a fungus conjunctivitis and indeed many times these pathogens can be cultured from patients with these longstanding chronic red eyes (Fig. 24). It may be misdiagnosed as a process such as unilateral pemphigoid or unilateral Stevens–Johnson syndrome. Unfortunately, many of these cases will turn out to be squamous cell carcinoma of the conjunctiva as seen in Fig. 25A and B, or a sebaceous carcinoma as seen in Fig. 14B. In any longstanding case of chronic conjunctivitis that is not responding to reasonable medical care, a biopsy (full eyelid thickness) should be performed to rule out these processes.

Chronic Chalazion (Sebaceous Cell Carcinoma, Trichoepithelioma)

Through the past years, the most common masquerade syndrome proposed has been a sebaceous carcinoma masquerading as a chalazion (Fig. 14). In fact, sebaceous cell carcinoma's most common presentation is that of a chronic blepharoconjunctivitis; however, very localized sebaceous carcinomas can present as a chalazion, which is why it is very important to submit suspicious chalazion tissue to pathology. A very rare situation occurs with metastatic eyelid carcinoma in which approximately two thirds of lesions metastatic to the eyelid present as metastatic nodules. Characteristically these lesions are painless but in 38% of the cases in the literature the eyelid lesion was a presenting sign of a carcinoma elsewhere, most commonly that of breast or lung. Other neoplastic processes that may present as a chalazion are lymphoid lesions or extranodal lymphomas.

Dermatitis

Intraepithelial involvement of the skin by a squamous cell carcinoma (Bowen's disease) can produce a reddened, roughened appearance to the skin of the eyelid not unlike that of a benign dermatologic process (Fig. 26). Treatment for allergies and a variety of exzemoid problems may be undertaken before a neoplastic process is considered. The pagetoid (intraepithelial) component of sebaceous carcinomas produce a dermatitis-like picture. Morpheaform basal cell carcinoma produces a stiffness, thickening, and scaliness to the skin mimicking scleroderma.

Cicatricial Ectropion (Morpheaform Basal Cell; Usually Lower Lid)

A large number of patients with sun-damaged skin will have a tightening of the skin from the actinic

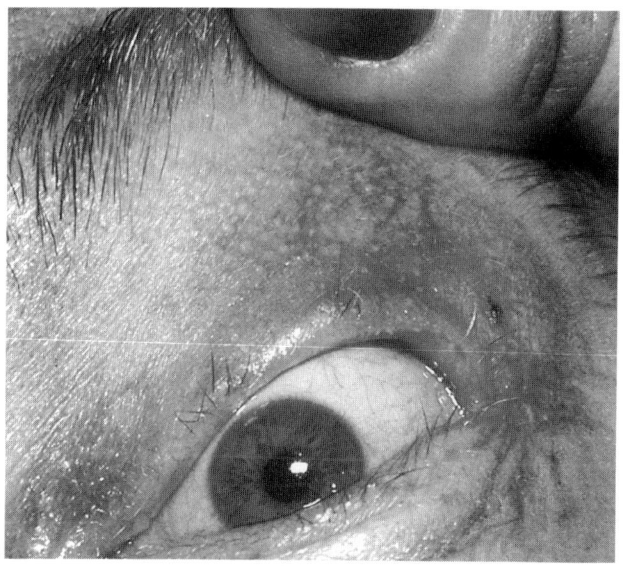

FIG. 26. Squamous cell carcinoma of the upper lid presenting as dermatitis. This patient was treated for chronic dermatitis of the skin and eyelid margin. Was subsequently biopsied and diagnosed as Bowen's disease with intraepithelial and invasive areas.

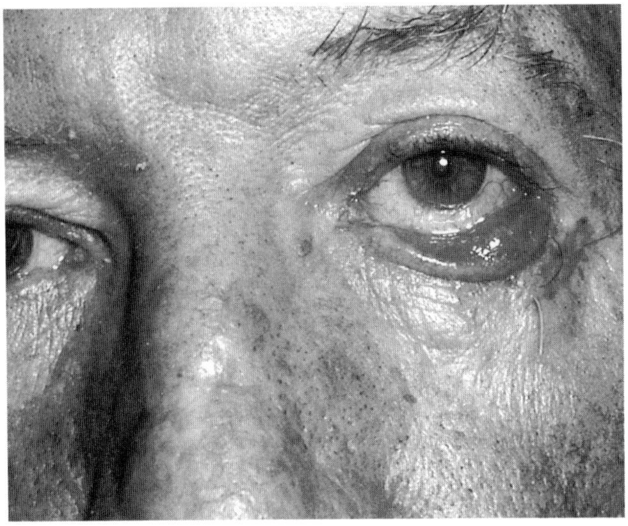

FIG. 27. Morpheaform basal cell carcinoma of the left lower lid and lateral canthus presenting as a cicatricial ectropion. This patient was diagnosed with cicatricial ectropion from actinic skin shrinkage and referred for treatment. The biopsy did show it to be a morpheaform basal cell carcinoma requiring Mohs' excision and reconstruction.

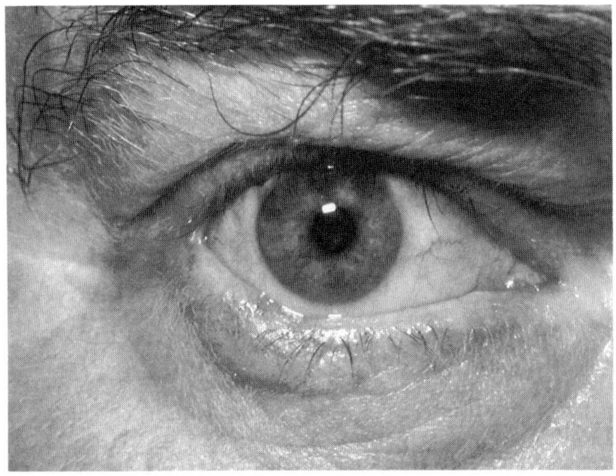

FIG. 28. Basal cell carcinoma of the eyelid margin presenting as recurrent trichiasis. This patient was treated for localized blepharitis and styles, and underwent epilation for a year. The biopsy taken in the area of the lid notch proved it to be a basal cell carcinoma.

changes, which in many cases will cause lid retraction and ectropion in the lower lid. Although most of these people truly have only actinic shrinkage, morpheaform basal cell carcinoma can produce a skin shrinkage. Patients have been treated for simple cicatricial ectropion when indeed they have invasive morpheaform basal cell carcinoma (Fig. 27), in which the skin may be indurated and thickened. This change can also occur with Bowen's disease or squamous cell carcinoma in situ. When repairing any cicatricial ectropion with sun-damaged skin, tissue should be submitted to rule out this process.

Cicatricial Entropion—Trichiasis (Sebaceous Cell Carcinoma, Usually Upper Lid)

A small epithelioma on the eyelid margin may at first cause only distortion of the cilia before there is actual loss of cilia. Trichiasis is not an uncommon early presentation of an eyelid margin lesion (Fig. 28).

Most patients are assumed to have entropion of the upper lid on the basis of a scarring inflammatory process or a mucocutaneous disease because they are the most common causes. These conditions are notoriously difficult because recurrence is common and in most cases will not arouse suspicion of a neoplastic process. Patients who have refractory, progressive disease, particularly with thickening of the eyelid, should

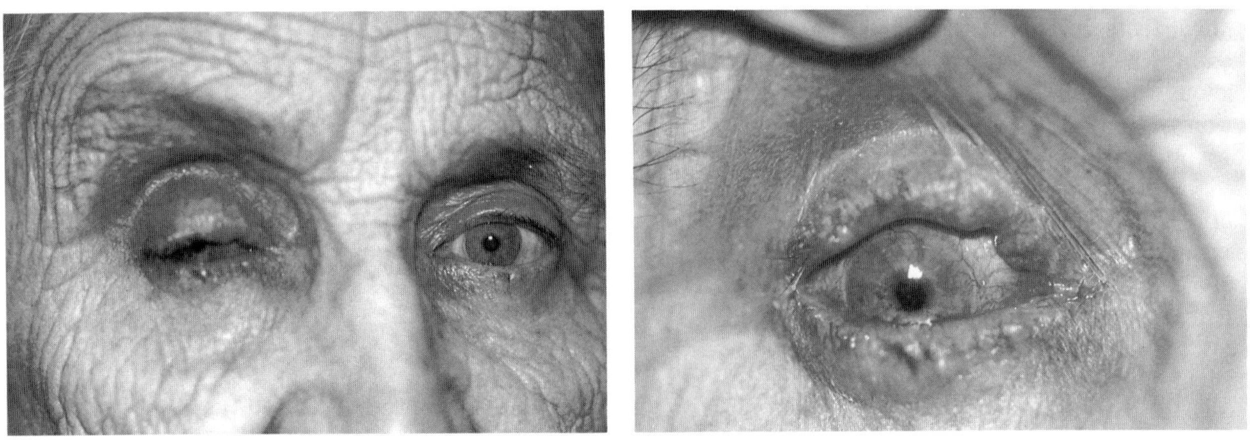

FIG. 29. A: Patient who is treated for inflammatory eyelid disease and a cicatricial entropion of her upper lid. The changes were initially felt to be pseudopemphigoid secondary to glaucoma drops. After a number of entropion procedures, a biopsy was taken and the lid was shown to contain a sebaceous cell carcinoma. **B:** Close-up view of the eyelid of the same patient.

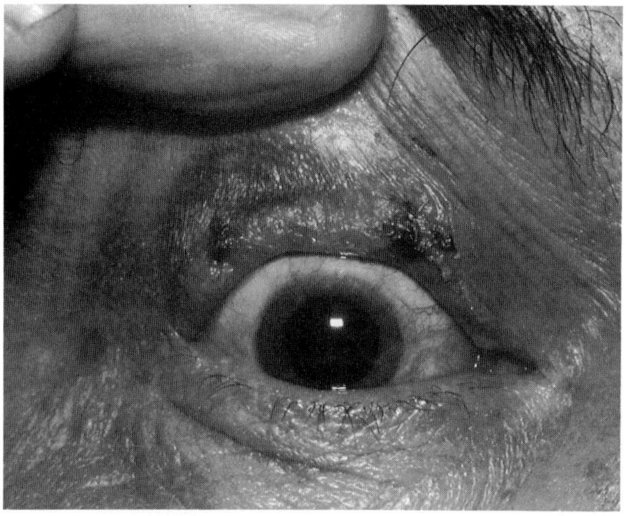
A

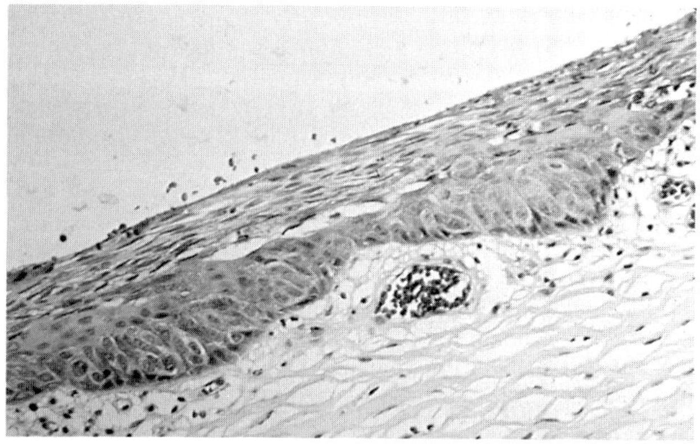
B

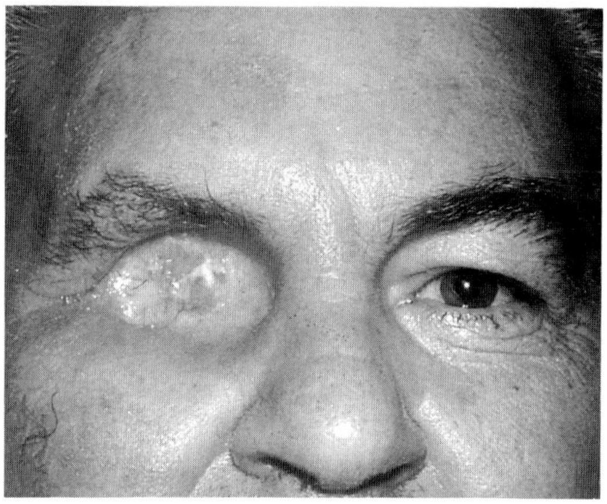
C

FIG. 30. **A:** Sebaceous cell carcinoma of the right upper lid that had undergone a year and a half of treatment for recurrent blepharitis. A biopsy was taken and it was determined that the lesion was a sebaceous cell carcinoma. The patient underwent 6000 rads of irradiation to the upper lid alone. Recurrent thickening occurred at 8 months. An additional biopsy showed recurrence of sebaceous carcinoma. Multiple biopsies were taken of the upper and lower lids and conjunctiva, which were positive for neoplastic invasion. The patient required exenteration for cure. **B:** Section of the cornea from the globe of the exenterated patient showing pagetoid invasion of the corneal epithelium. **C:** Patient postexenteration.

be suspected of having neoplastic disease and biopsied (Fig. 29A, B).

Blepharitis—Entropion

Chronic blepharitis is a common presentation of an eyelid neoplastic process that in most cases will ultimately be diagnosed by biopsy. The patient will have recurrent redness and a thickening of the lid that will not clear up with lid hygiene and cortisone-antibiotics. Any of the neoplasms can present in this way and when loss of lashes becomes evident one must be very suspicious of a neoplastic process. Purely dermatologic conditions such as rosacea can of course mimic this, but one should be aware that neoplastic disease may need to be ruled out in some cases. The most insidious process that can present in this manner is sebaceous cell carcinoma (Fig. 30A) of the eyelid in which the main focus of neoplasm is deeper than the surface changes on the lid margin, which are the pagetoid changes common to this lesion (Fig. 30B, C). It is imperative to biopsy the patients in these categories to rule out an underlying neoplastic process, which can be treated best if diagnosed early.

Facial Numbness–Pain—Paralysis

Neurotropic invasion is most commonly seen with squamous cell carcinoma and desmoplastic malignant

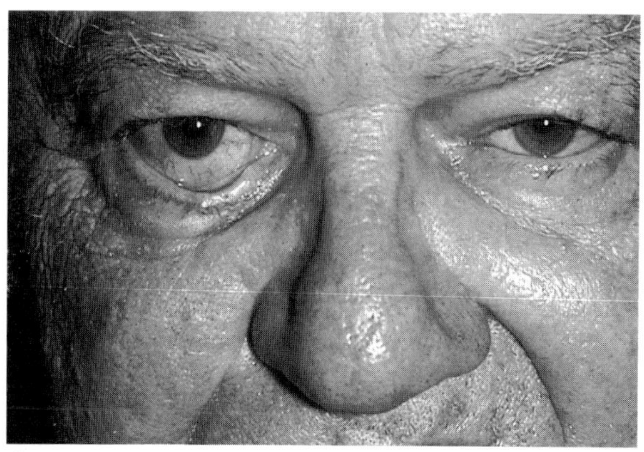

FIG. 31. Facial numbness and ectropion as a presenting sign in a patient with recurrent squamous cell carcinoma. The patient had a squamous cell carcinoma excised from the lip a year and a half previously. The initial symptom was facial numbness in the area, which progressed to a cicatricial ectropion in the right lower lid. There was deep involvement of the infraorbital nerve and the tumor extended into the orbit.

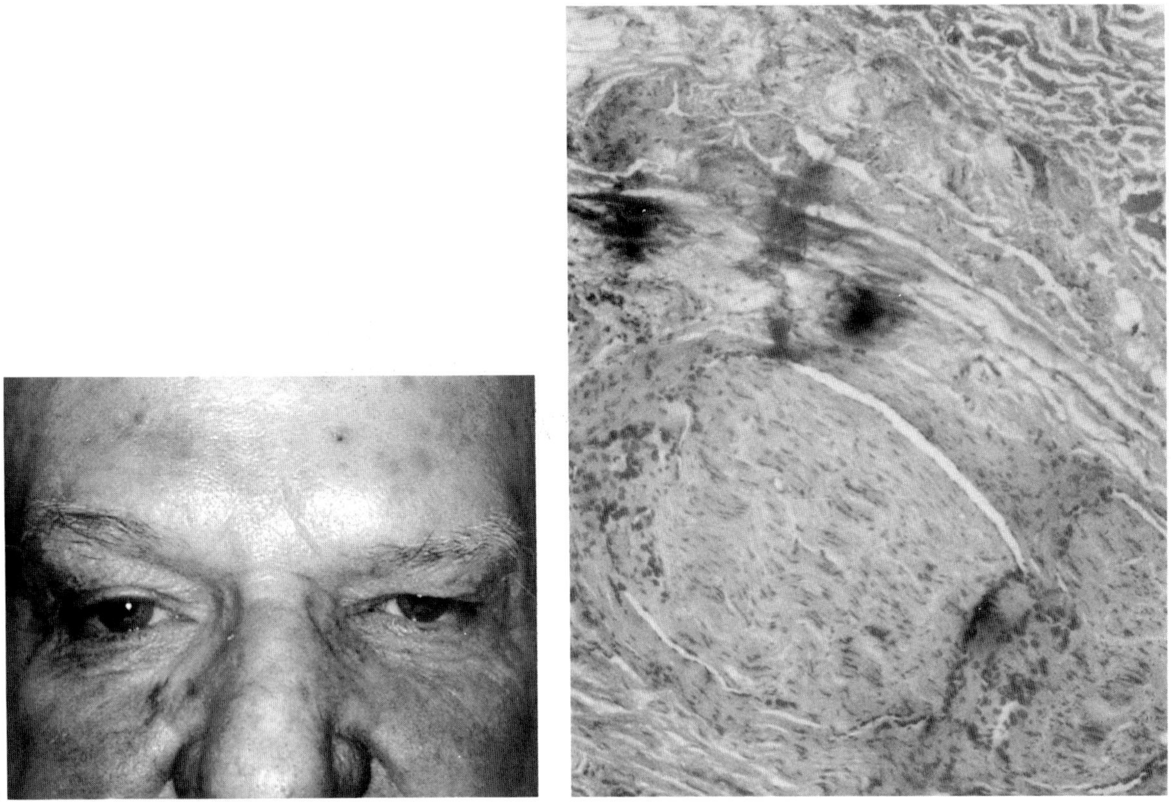

A B

FIG. 32. A: Patient with neoplastic disease presenting with eyebrow forehead numbness and paresis of the superficial temporal branch of the facial nerve. The patient had a previous history of squamous cell carcinoma of the eyelid. Computerized tomography and magnetic resonance imaging were negative in this patient. **B:** Histologic section of a biopsy of the frontal nerve in the midsuperior orbit showing invasion of the nerve with a neoplastic process. The patient died before further workup could be performed. At postmortem it was felt that the neoplastic process had arisen from the parotid gland.

melanoma (Fig. 31). A neoplastic process adjacent to the eyelids that has neurotropic tendencies is carcinoma of the lacrimal gland. In the authors' experience there have been 14 patients in which neurotropic invasion was the presenting sign or the first sign of recurrence (Fig. 32A, B). Most were squamous cell carcinomas and most were considered surgically unresectable and treated with radiation.

The infiltrative lesions previously described can escape the lid and fornices and invade the orbit to the point where the only method of cure is radical surgery. With systemic metastatic disease there may be no cure. Because of microscopic behavior of these lesions, the phrase "what you see is what you get" may not apply to many instances of eyelid neoplastic disease because of its ability to spread through tissue planes in an insidious manner.

REFERENCES

1. Friedman AH, Henkind P. Clinical and pathological features of eyelid and conjunctival tumors. In: Fox SA, ed. *Ophthalmic plastic surgery*. 5th ed. New York: Grune and Stratton; 1976: 24–63.
2. Brownstein S, Codere F, Jackson WB. Masquerade syndrome. *Ophthalmology* 1980;87:259–262.
3. Condon CP, Brownstein S, Codere F. Sebaceous carcinoma of the eyelid masquerading as superior limbic keratoconjunctivitis. *Arch Ophthalmol* 1985;103:1525–1529.
4. Yeatts RP, Waller RR. Sebaceous carcinoma of the eyelid: pitfalls in diagnosis. *Ophth Plast Reconstr Surg* 1985;1:35–42.
5. Older JJ, Quickert MH, Beard C. Surgical removal of basal cell carcinoma of the eyelids utilizing frozen section control. *Trans Am Acad Ophthalmol Otolaryngol* 1975;79:658–663.
6. Dahlin DC. Seventy-five years' experience with frozen sections at the Mayo Clinic. *Mayo Clin Proc* 1980;55:721–723.
7. Grove AS Jr. Staged excision and reconstruction of extensive facial-orbital tumors. *Ophth Surg* 1977;8:91–109.
8. Mohs FE. Chemosurgical treatment of cancer of the eyelid. A microscopically controlled method of excision. *Arch Ophthalmol* 1948;39:43–59.
9. Mohs FE. Chemosurgery for facial neoplasms. *Arch Otolaryngol* 1972;95:62–67.
10. Mohs FE. Chemosurgery for skin cancer. *Arch Dermatol* 1976; 112:211–215.
11. Levene MB. Radiotherapeutic management of carcinoma of the eyelid. In: Brockhurst RJ, Boruchoff SA, Hutchinson BT, Lessell S, eds. *Controversy in ophthalmology*. Philadelphia: WB Saunders; 1977:390–397.
12. Cladstein AH. Radiotherapy of eyelid tumors. In: Jacobiec FA, ed. *Ocular and adnexal tumors*. Birmingham, AL: Aesculapius; 1978:508–516.
13. Hirshowitz B, Mahler D. Incurable recurrences of basal cell carcinoma of the mid-face following radiation therapy. *Br J Plast Surg* 1971;24:205–211.

14. Fraunfelder FT, Zacarian SA, Limmer BL, Wingfield D. Cryosurgery for malignancies of the eyelid. *Ophthalmology* 1980;87: 461–465.
15. Payne JW, Duke JR, Butner R, et al. Basal cell carcinoma of the eyelids. *Arch Ophthalmol* 1969;81:553–558.
16. Aurora AL, Blodi FC. Lesions of the eyelids: a clinicopathological study. *Surv Ophthalmol* 1970;15:94–104.
17. Ferry A. The eyelids. In: Sorsby A, ed. *Modern ophthalmology*. vol 4. Philadelphia: JB Lippincott; 1972:833–853.
18. McCord CD Jr, Cavanagh HD. Microscopic features and biologic behavior of eyelid tumors. *Ophth Surg* 1980;11:671–681.
19. Doxanas MT, Iliff WJ, Iliff NT, Green RW. Squamous cell carcinoma of the eyelids. *Ophthalmology* 1987;94:538–541.
20. Reifler DM, Hornblass A. Squamous cell carcinoma of the eyelids. *Surv Ophthalmol* 1986;30:349–365.
21. Stroll HL. Squamous cell carcinoma. In: Fitzpatrick TB, Eiser AZ, Wolff K, et al, eds. *Dermatology in general medicine*. New York: McGraw-Hill; 1979;362–377.
22. Brauniger CE, Hood L, Worthcrn DM. Sebaceous carcinoma of the lid masquerading as a cutaneous horn. *Arch Ophthalmol* 1974;90:380–381.
23. Shields JA, Font RL. Meibomian gland carcinoma presenting as a lacrimal gland tumor. *Arch Ophthalmol* 1974;92:304–306.
24. Rao NA, Hidayat AA, McLean LW, Zimmerman LE. Sebaceous carcinomas of the ocular adnexa: a clinicopathologic study of 104 cases, with five-year follow-up data. *Human Pathol* 1982;13:113–122.
25. Cavanagh HD, Green WR, Goldberg HK. Multicentric sebaceous adenocarcinoma of the meibomian gland. *Am J Ophthalmol* 1974;77:326–332.
26. Margo CC, Lessner A, Stern GA. Intraepithelial sebaceous carcinoma of the conjunctiva and skin of the eyelid. *Ophthalmology* 1992;99:227–231.
27. Lisman RD, Jakobiac FA, Small P. Sebaceous carcinoma of the eyelids. *Ophthalmology* 1989;96:1021–1026.
28. Doxanas MT, Green RW. Sebaceous gland carcinoma. *Arch Ophthalmol* 1984;102:245–249.
29. Hendley RL, Rieser JC, Cavanagh HD, et al. Primary radiation therapy the meibomian gland carcinoma. *Am J Ophthalmol* 1979;87:206–209.
30. Grossniklaus H, McLean IW. Cutaneous melanoma of the eyelid. *Ophthalmology* 1991;98:1867–1873.
31. Grove AS Jr. Melanomas of the conjunctiva. *Int Ophthalmol Clin* 1980;20(2):161–175.
32. Jakobiec FA. Conjunctival melanoma. Unfinished business. *Arch Ophthalmol* 1980;98:1378–1384.
33. McGovern VJ, Mihm MC Jr, Bailly C, et al. The classification of malignant melanoma and its histologic reporting. *Cancer* 1973; 32:1446–1457.
34. Breslow A. Thickness, crossectional areas and depth of invasion in prognosis of cutaneous melanoma. *Ann Surg* 1970;172: 902.
35. Arnold AC, Bullock JD, Foos RY. Metastatic eyelid carcinoma. *Ophthalmology* 1985;92:114–119.
36. Hood CL, Font RL, Zimmerman LE. Metastatic mammary carcinoma in the eyelid with histiocytoid appearance. *Cancer* 1973; 31:793–800.
37. Riley FS. Metastatic tumors of the eyelids. *Am J Ophthalmol* 1970;69:259–264.
38. Conley J, et al. Metastatic melanoma to the facial nerve. *Plast Reconstr Surg* 1991;87:341–345.
39. Hufnagel TJ, Savino PJ, et al. Painful ophthalmoplegia caused by neurotropic malignant melanoma. *Can J Ophthalmol* 1990; 25:38–41.
40. Shields JA, Elder D, et al. Orbital involvement with desmoplastic melanoma. *Br J Ophthalmol* 1987;71:279.
41. Khalil MK, Duguid WP. Neurotropic malignant melanoma of right temple with orbital metastasis: a clinicopathologic case report. *Br J Ophthalmol* 1987;71:41–46.
42. Howard GR, Nerad JA, et al. Clinical characteristics associated with orbital invasion of cutaneous basal cell and squamous cell tumors of the eyelid. *Am J Ophthalmol* 1992;113:123–133.
43. Trobe JD, Hood CI, et al. Intracranial spread of squamous carcinoma along the trigeminal nerve. *Arch Ophthalmol* 1982;100: 608–611.

CHAPTER 26

Upper Lid Crease: Sulcus Problem Solving

The surgeon will find that even if a good functional result is obtained with one of the various upper eyelid surgical procedures, if the eyelid crease and upper lid fold are not in the desired location, the surgery may be considered unsuccessful by the patient. Examples of this problem are shown in the chapters on ptosis, blepharoplasty, and trauma. Although upper lid crease formation is discussed to some degree in those chapters, it is felt that its importance warrants a more in-depth discussion.

The overall appearance of upper lid contour in the skin above the lash line depends largely on the shape and amount of visible skin exposed in the pretarsal area (the "eyeshadow area"). The amount of visible skin is an interplay between the upper lid crease position and the overhanging skin fold. The upper lid crease, which is formed by a firm attachment of the levator aponeurosis, is the uppermost limit of the pretarsal area. The pretarsal skin is held firm by its own attachments to the pretarsal connective tissue. The vertical amount of pretarsal skin exposed is a function of the height of crease fixation and the amount of loose skin above the crease that overhangs the crease, i.e., the crease–fold interplay. In some patients the overhanging fold will obscure the crease and a portion of the pretarsal skin, whereas in other patients the skin above the crease will be taut and not overhang at all, with all of the pretarsal skin and the crease being visible (see Fig. 1).

Upper lid crease positioning and the amount of visible pretarsal skin is very important in cosmetic blepharoplasty, ptosis surgery, and reconstructive procedures following trauma or tumor resection.

Crease abnormalities that can occur postoperatively are *asymmetry* of the crease-fold with the opposite side. The eyelid crease may be attached at a different level than the contralateral side. In some cases crease attachments may be symmetric but there is a difference in the amount of overhanging fold (loose skin) above the crease producing a different amount of visible pretarsal skin. If the crease is attached too high or there is less overhanging skin, the effect is a *wider visible space of skin above the lashes*. If the crease is attached too low or if there is more overhanging fold than on the opposite side, there is a *more narrow visible space of skin above the lashes*. There may be a complete *loss of crease* with dehiscence of the skin attachments from the levator and the pretarsal area. In many patients this degree of dehiscence of skin attachments will produce ptosis or entropion of the lashes. The crease may be *irregular* from scarring, as the result of surgery or trauma, in which the normal attachments of the skin have been disrupted.

NORMAL SOFT TISSUE ATTACHMENTS

The pretarsal skin is normally attached to the tarsal plate with small fibrous strands interdigitating through the orbicularis fibers to the tarsal plate that are probably extensions of levator aponeurotic connective tissue. This flat pretarsal area of skin extends to the upper lid crease. This firm upper crease attachment is the result of extensions of the levator aponeurosis proper to the eyelid skin. The orbital septum normally inserts at the superior tarsal edge so that the preaponeurotic fat is held above the pretarsal skin area. The skin above the crease forms the lid fold; with redundancy of skin or protrusion of the preaponeurotic fat it can extend downward covering the crease and reducing the amount of visible skin between the lashes and the crease. The fold of skin above the crease is supported by the brow and the amount of overhanging fold can be a function of the amount of brow laxity or position (Fig. 2).

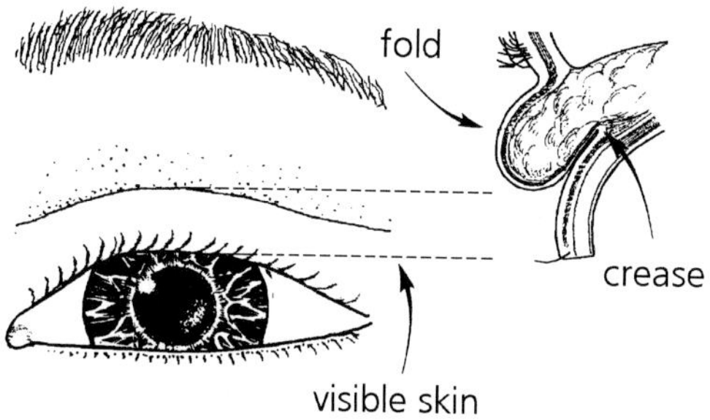

FIG. 1. Interaction of eyelid crease–upper lid fold–visible skin in the upper lid. In addition to the level of the upper lid margin, the overall impression of upper lid contour and appearance is the result of the amount of visible skin seen above the lashes—the "eye shadow space." In cases in which there is no fold overhanging the upper lid crease, the amount of visible skin is the same as the distance between the lashes and the crease. As the overhanging fold increases, the amount of visible skin is reduced. For definition purposes, the crease is the highest position of the attached pretarsal skin, and the upper lid fold is the skin above the crease that overhangs the crease area.

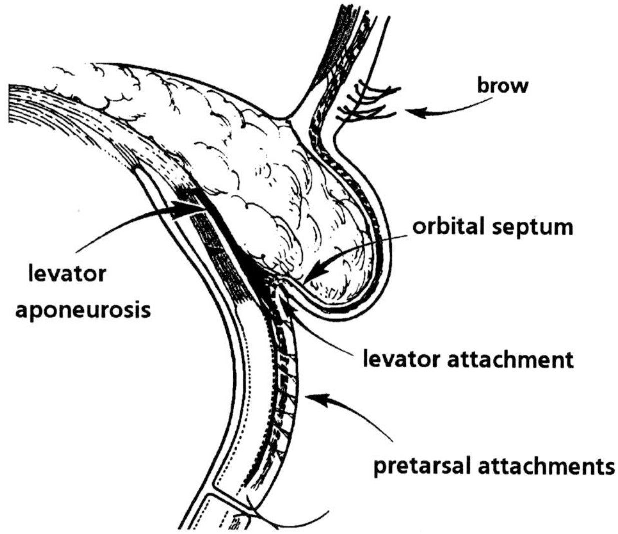

FIG. 2. Sagittal view showing the soft tissue attachments and structures that influence the eyelid crease–fold–visible skin complex in the upper lid. The pretarsal skin is attached to the tarsal plate with fibrous strands and connects at a higher level with extensions of the levator aponeurosis. The superiormost attachment of the pretarsal skin is a very firm attachment designated as the eyelid crease that is the result of a direct insertion of fibers of the levator aponeurosis. The tissue above the crease is the lid fold, which consists of the outermost layer of skin and muscle and the orbital septum, which confines the preaponeurotic fat. Varying degrees of laxity of these tissues and protrusion of fat can cause varying degrees of overhanging fold. Normally the orbital septum inserts on the levator aponeurosis at the level of the superior tarsal edge but can insert further down in different ethnic groups. The eyebrow is the "curtain rod" of the upper lid fold and its elevation or lowering can influence the amount of fold that overhangs the pretarsal skin area.

FACTORS ALTERING THE CREASE–FOLD–VISIBLE SKIN INTERPLAY

Attachments to Levator Aponeurosis

The effect of loss of levator attachments, pretarsal attachments, and change of position of the insertion of the orbital septum can be seen in the Asian eyelid. Many Asians will have no crease because of their normal anatomic variation from the Western upper lid (Fig. 3). A common situation that can occur in the Western eyelid producing ptosis is dehiscence of the levator aponeurosis. In these patients the upper lid crease can migrate higher as the levator retracts from dehiscence of its lower insertions (Figs. 4A,B).

In routine blepharoplasty and ptosis surgery the surgeon may be operating in the area of the crease attachments and, as recommended in preceding chapters, specific measures can be taken to ensure that crease formation forms at the desired location. The usual method is the use of transcutaneous crease sutures that attach the pretarsal skin to the levator. In frontalis suspension ptosis surgery, crease sutures are also used but in some cases they are also attached to the superior tarsal edge for more stable fixation.

Pretarsal Attachments

In patients who have had previous upper lid surgery, commonly ptosis procedures, there can be a dehiscence of the attachments of the crease and pretarsal skin causing loss of crease and, in some cases, lash

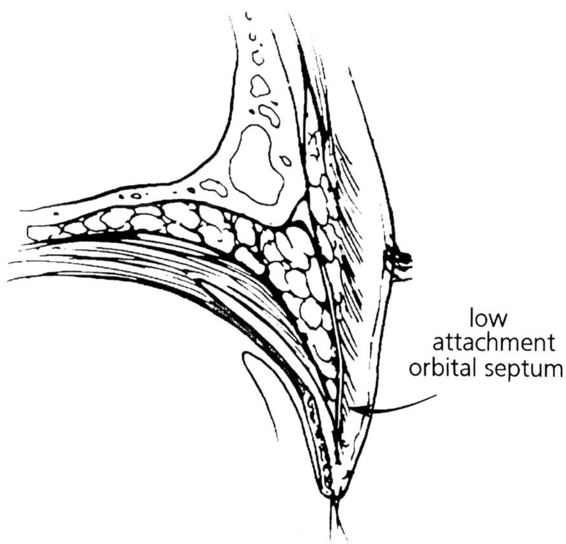

FIG. 3. Asian eyelid showing an absence of insertion of the levator aponeurosis in the skin and a low insertion of the orbital septum causing a creaseless eyelid.

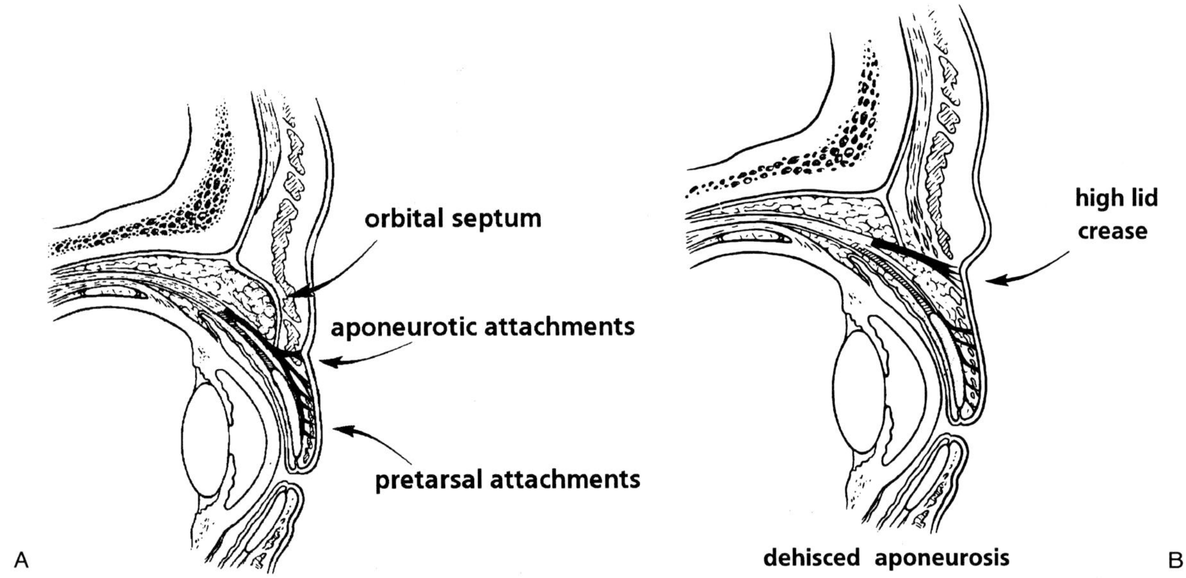

FIG. 4. A: Sagittal view of the upper lid showing the normal attachments emphasizing the upper lid crease formation by the insertion of the levator aponeurosis. **B:** High lid crease with dehiscence of the levator aponeurosis causing ptosis. The upper lid crease is pulled upward because of residual levator attachments to the skin. This high lid crease in some patients with severe dermatochalasis or eyebrow ptosis may be obscured by an overhanging fold that covers some of the pretarsal skin.

ptosis or entropion (Fig. 5). A secondary crease procedure can restore the normal attachments with reformation of the crease (Figs. 6 and 7). In these cases, not only should transcutaneous sutures be placed from the skin to the levator aponeurosis but quilting sutures in the pretarsal area should be used to reattach the pretarsal skin to the tarsal plate. Reoperated ptosis patients in particular will have a tendency for contracture of the pretarsal skin area postoperatively causing loss of the upper lid crease.

Orbital Septum Attachments

The influence of the orbital septum insertion on the position of the upper lid crease is most conspicuous in Asian patients (Fig. 3). Many Asian patients will have no attachments of the levator to the skin and have an orbital septum that inserts in the pretarsal area close to the lash line on the tarsal plate. This allows the preaponeurotic fat to prolapse forward into this area without formation of the crease and little if any visible pretarsal space. The surgical formation of the crease in the Asian patient has been discussed in the chapter on blepharoplasty.

Globe Prominence

The position of the globe can influence the formation and position of the upper lid crease and sulcus.

Exophthalmos

Exophthalmos is most commonly seen in Graves' patients who have a forward position of the globe, sometimes asymmetric in nature (Fig. 8). When performing upper lid surgery in the Graves' patient who has residual proptosis, if significant amounts of fat are removed from the preaponeurotic area the indentation of the globe on the upper lid will be seen and the indentation will produce an abnormally high lid crease. This may accentuate the prominence of the eye. It can be difficult in patients with asymmetric globe position in

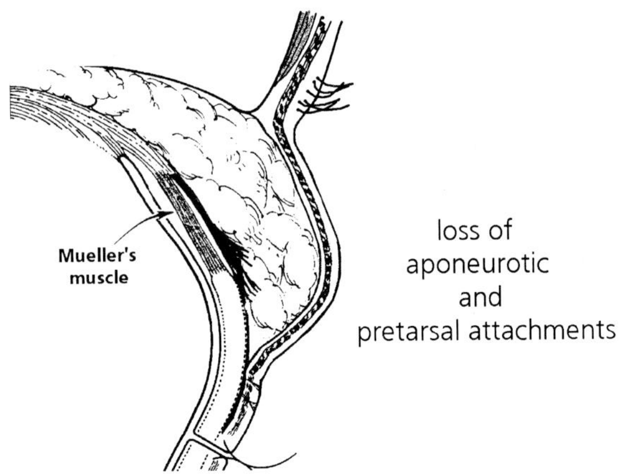

FIG. 5. Loss of upper lid crease from loss of levator and pretarsal attachments. This can occur postsurgically or posttraumatically.

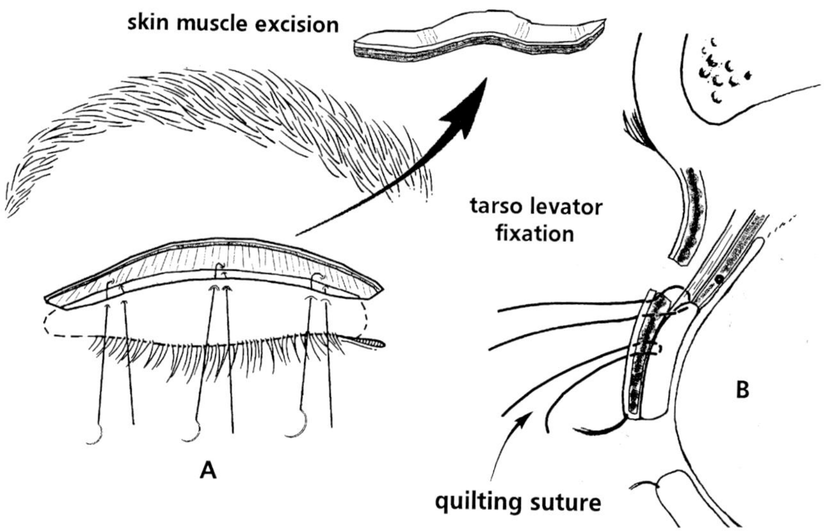

FIG. 6. Eyelid crease procedure. **A:** A strip of skin-muscle and subcutaneous tissue (and sometimes a small degree of preaponeurotic fat) is excised. **B:** The skin edges are then reattached to the edge of the levator aponeurosis with transcutaneous sutures. Additional quilting sutures can be placed in the pretarsal skin if needed.

Graves' disease to obtain a completely symmetric crease because of the indenting effect and other reasons. Upper lid surgery should be modified in these patients by marking the incision for the crease lower in the patients with more exophthalmos and leaving more preaponeurotic fat in position. In some cases, no crease formation sutures are used because of the already present tendency to form a high crease by the indenting globe. If the skin edges are attached for crease formation, they should be attached to the superior tarsal border, which remains relatively symmetric between the two sides.

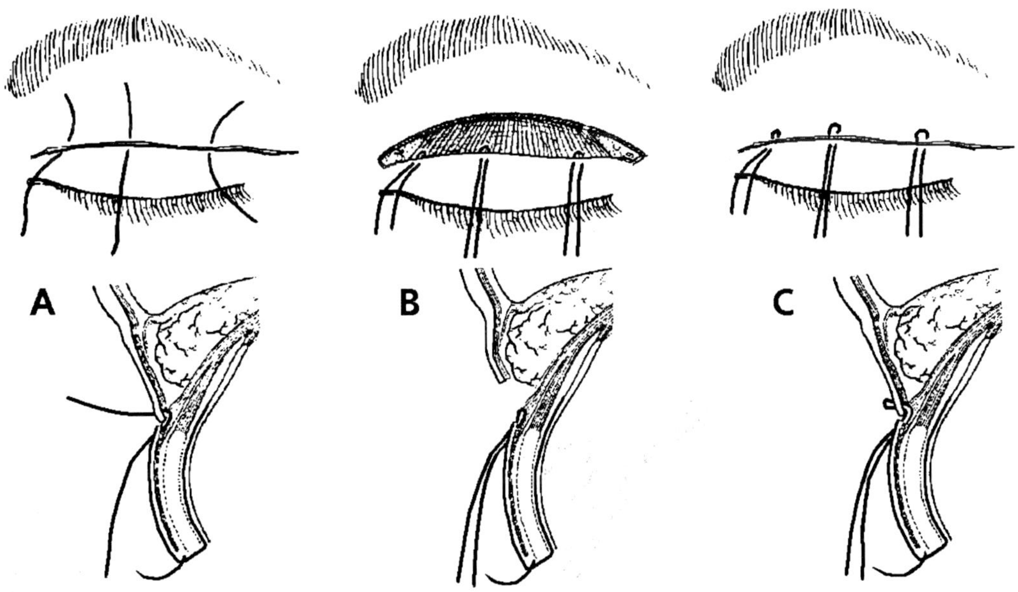

FIG. 7. Crease suturing. **A:** Edge-to-edge attachment of skin edges with interrupted sutures. This produces a moderately indented crease. **B:** Eyelid crease procedure with mattress sutures. This reattaches the pretarsal skin to the levator aponeurosis with transcutaneous sutures. The upper lid fold skin is closed passively to the incision. This technique produces a softer eyelid crease and is most commonly used with the blepharoplasty patient. **C:** Through-and-through skin mattress sutures for crease formation. This produces the most indented crease and is used for refractory cases.

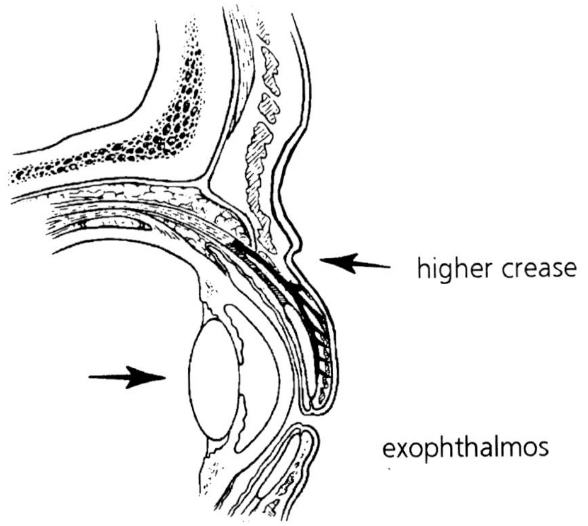

FIG. 8. Sagittal view of a patient with exophthalmos showing how the forward-placed globe produced a higher lid crease because of indenting the lid. This effect is particularly true in patients with Graves' disease and is the reason that conservative removal of skin and fat is performed in these patients so as to avoid producing an abnormally high crease.

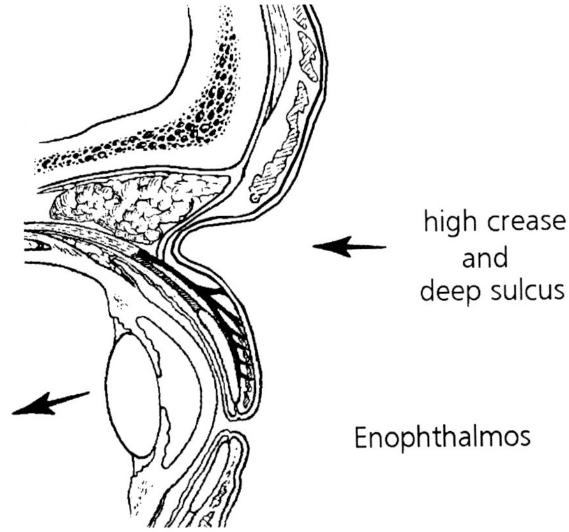

FIG. 9. Sagittal view showing patient with enophthalmos causing a deep superior sulcus and a higher lid crease. This situation occurs because of the lack of indention of the globe on the upper lid and superior orbit.

Enophthalmos

Inward and downward settling of the globe can occur in patients who have had trauma with orbital fractures and can also be seen from settling of a prosthetic eye. A deep sulcus and a very high lid crease may be present in these patients (Fig. 9). If there is severe volume deficiency, then in some cases it may be appropriate to restore orbital volume with an orbital volume implant. If orbital augmentation is inappropriate in the patient because of medical problems or the patient's wishes, then correction of the deep sulcus and high lid crease can be obtained with grafting of dermis-fat to the superior sulcus or sliding existing superior orbital fat forward into the preaponeurotic space (Fig. 10).

Skin Stiffness

Skin stiffness in the eyelid with scarring following trauma or skin grafting can cause distortion of the upper eyelid crease–fold–visible skin area. In most cases the problem is a loss of floppiness of the skin above the eyelid crease increasing the visibility of the pretarsal skin and giving the appearance of a very high lid crease on the involved side (Fig. 11). In some patients the high-appearing lid crease can be compensated for by a blepharoplasty crease procedure on the opposite (normal) side.

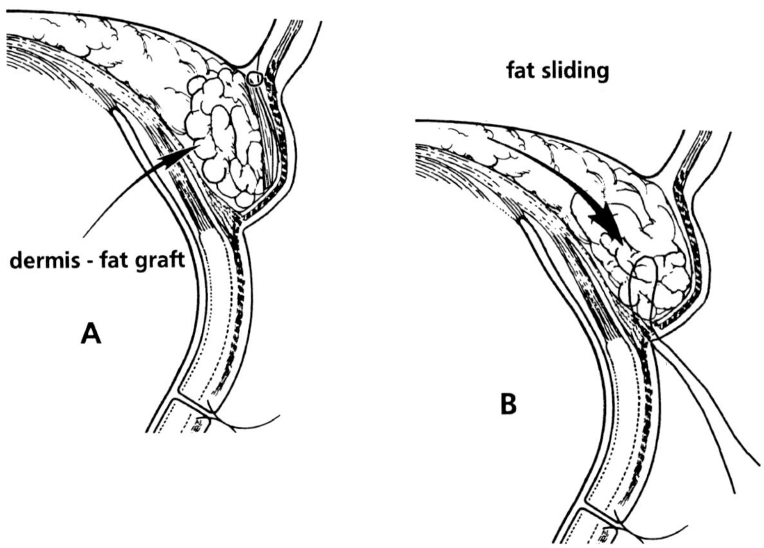

FIG. 10. Sulcus augmentation. **A:** Correction of an upper lid crease deep sulcus deformity with dermis-fat grafting. Through a lid crease incision, tissue plane is created into the preaponeurotic space exposing the superior orbital rim. A dermis fat graft can be taken from the iliac crest area and the edge of the dermis sutured to the arcus marginalis at the superior orbital rim, leaving the fat graft, "hanging" over the levator. No suturing of the graft to the inferior structures is performed to avoid tethering levator movement. Simultaneous plication of the levator can also be performed if necessary. There is usually an absorption of 30% of the fat. **B:** Fat sliding. If adequate residual orbital fat is present superiorly, it can be brought forward into the preaponeurotic space by traction. It is then fixated in the forward position (preaponeurotic space) with quilting sutures, which fills out the upper fold.

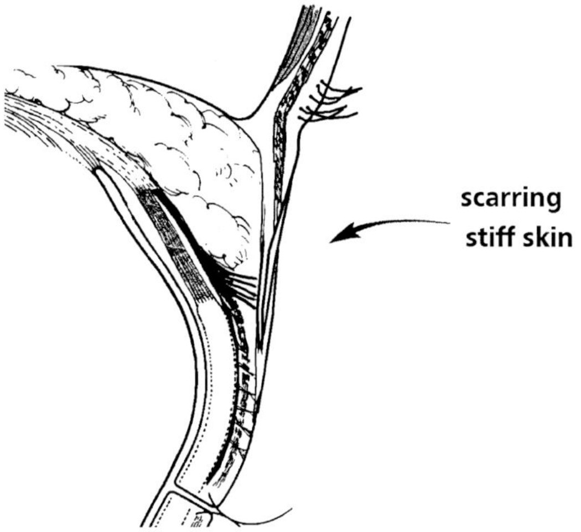

FIG. 11. Flattening of upper lid fold from scarring or stiffness of skin following trauma or skin grafting. Stiffness of the skin of the upper lid fold can impair its flexibility and "floppiness" and its ability to overhang the upper lid crease. When this occurs, it produces a very asymmetric appearance compared to the opposite (normal) side, which will have retained its "floppy" upper lid fold. This effect also creates the illusion of a higher lid crease on the "stiff side" even though the actual crease position is in some cases the same.

Surgery to the involved, stiff side can compensate for this problem by placing the crease incision at a lower level than the normal side. To fill out the upper fold, fat sliding or grafting techniques, which can cause a protrusion of the skin above the crease, may recreate the floppy skin fold to match the opposite side. In many cases fat grafts are not needed because fat already present in the superior orbit can be mobilized and brought forward to fill out the fold above the supratarsal crease in these patients (Fig. 10).

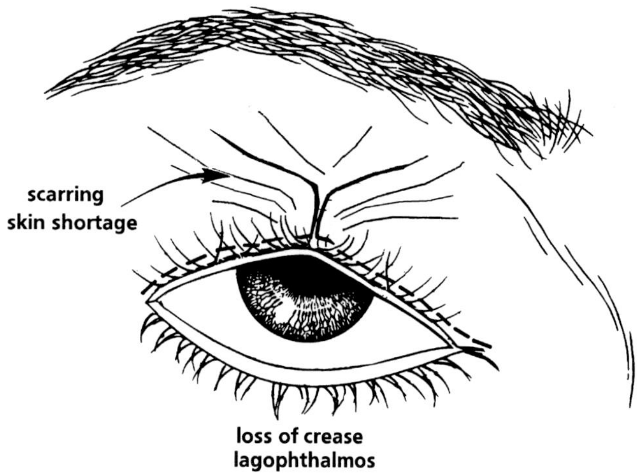

FIG. 12. Lagophthalmos, notching, and skin shortage with loss of lid crease in the upper lid usually from trauma.

Skin Grafting

Frequently patients who have skin shortage and scarring from trauma or previous surgery require grafting of full-thickness skin to the upper lid. It is important to avoid placing a full-thickness skin graft in the upper lid in a position that crosses over the lid crease from the pretarsal area to the fold area or vice versa because it will impair crease formation as a result of graft stiffness. For grafting purposes the upper lid should be divided into two separate units: the pretarsal area from the lash line to the crease, and the fold area from the crease to the brow skin. If at all possible, grafts should first be placed in the pretarsal area (Figs. 12 and 13). If skin grafting is required above this area (the fold area), then it should be placed as a separate graft and,

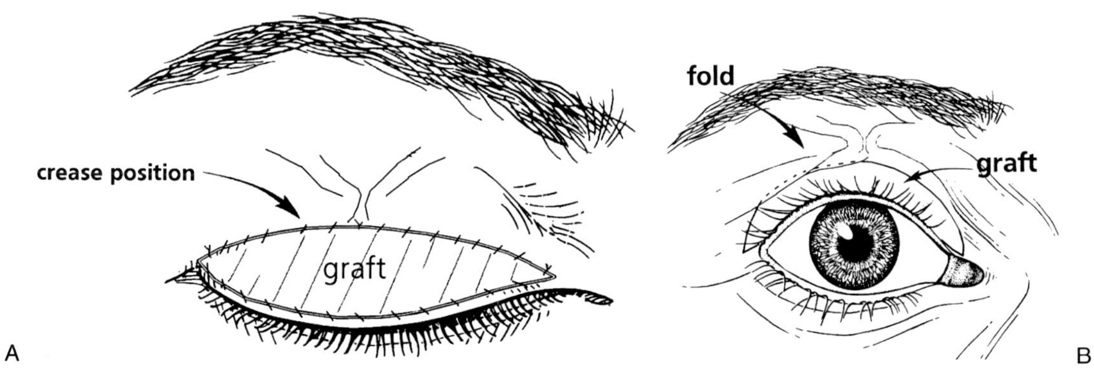

FIG. 13. Full-thickness graft to upper lid. **A:** Proper placement of the full-thickness skin graft to the upper lid. The inferior edge of the graft is placed just above the lash line and the superior edge of the graft is placed at the desired position of the crease. This restores the pretarsal area shape and form. In many cases the skin that is allowed to retract to the upper lid fold area will become looser, form a more folding appearance, and retain the position of the eyelid crease. Fat sliding can also be used at this time to enhance this effect. **B:** Postoperative view of position of the full-thickness skin grafting. Additional skin grafting can be performed in the fold (supracrease) area, but if performed should not extend below the crease level to avoid loss of crease line.

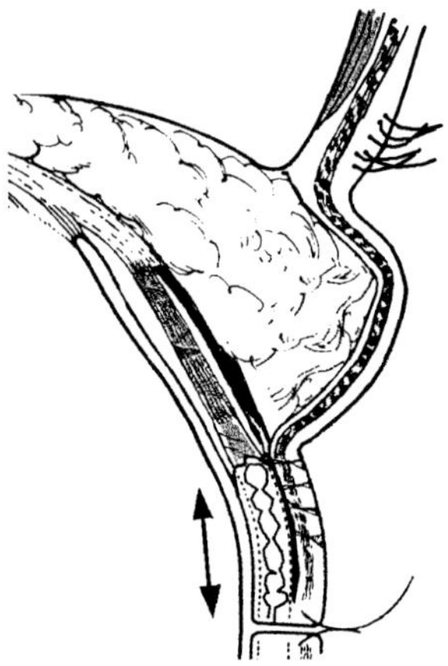

FIG. 14. Loss of lid crease complicated by attenuation of the tarsal plate and loss of crease pretarsal attachments of skin. This can occur following trauma or prior ptosis surgery.

if possible, billowed out with fat sliding underneath the graft to recreate the fold. Skin grafts placed in the pretarsal area can be flattened for smooth healing in the postoperative period either with splints or with multiple quilting sutures.

Height of the Tarsal Plate

Disruption of the tarsal plate either from trauma, eyelid reconstruction, or ptosis surgery (Fasanella procedure) can cause abnormalities in the upper lid crease. The abnormalities can be the result of a "dragging down" of the normal attachments of the lid crease to the levator if it has been lowered and if some of the pretarsal skin attachments to the tarsus have been disrupted. In many of these patients lash ptosis and entropion can also occur because of instability of the tarsal plate. The tarsal plate is the skeleton of the eyelid and it is difficult to produce desired surgical results in the presence of its instability. In cases of tarsal attenuation, restoration of tarsal stability can be accomplished by augmenting the tarsus with autogenous ear cartilage. Flat, thin, cartilage grafts taken from the scaphoid portion of the ear can add stability to the upper lid and allow formation of the crease (Figs. 14 and 15).

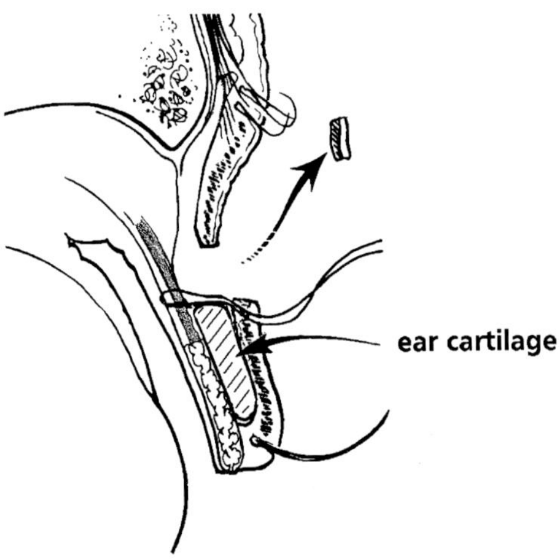

FIG. 15. Ear cartilage grafting to the upper lid in patients with deficient tarsus to restore stability to the lid and allow crease formation.

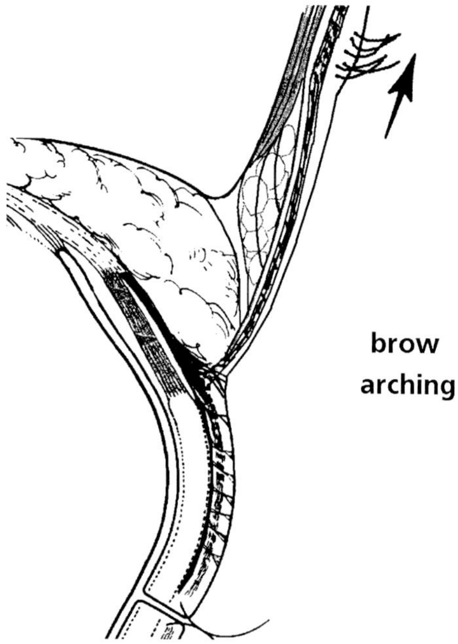

FIG. 16. Brow arching causing retraction of fold simulating a "higher lid crease" (more visible skin on the affected side). This effect occurs in patients who have unilateral brow arching. Techniques of brow surgery for lowering or elevating the brow have been described.

Brow Position

The eyelid crease–fold–visible skin complex is greatly altered by animation of the eyebrow. In patients whose eyebrow has become loose or ptotic it will allow the fold to overhang the lid crease and may obscure the visible skin area. In patients who chronically arch their brow or who have the brow elevated from scarring, the lid fold will be pulled upward exposing more pretarsal skin and crease (Fig. 16). If brow movement is not symmetric with the opposite side, then there will be a perceived asymmetry of the crease position because of assymetry of the amount of visible pretarsal skin exposed. Many patients, due either to habit or to compensation from a weighing down of the upper lid, will unconsciously arch their brows. This habit can persist even following corrective surgery and will cause asymmetry of appearance. Eyebrow position can be altered surgically and the techniques for elevating the brow were described in the chapter on blepharoplasty. Eyebrows that are chronically arched upward or scarred upward can also be remedied. The internal brow pexy procedure can be used in a reversed manner to stitch the eyebrow down to the orbital rim and fixate it in a more symmetric position that, in many cases, can eliminate chronic arching.

CHAPTER 27

Facial Paralysis

Seventh nerve disorders, with weakness or paralysis of the facial and eyelid muscles, always invoke concern for the health of the eye because denervation of the eyelid closure muscles (orbicularis oculi) takes away an important eye protective mechanism. The eye protects itself by movement from intact extraocular muscles, with moisture from lacrimation, with sensation from fifth nerve innervation, and with closure of the eyelids from the seventh nerve innervation. It is quite possible for the patient to "get by" with a deficiency in one of these mechanisms; however, in many cases, extra effort on the patient's part or some restorative surgical procedure must be undertaken if one of the protective mechanisms is permanently damaged.

FINDINGS WITH FACIAL PARALYSIS

The loss of muscular tone and contraction of the upper and lower lid orbicularis muscles and the frontalis muscle are the underlying cause of most of the problems associated with facial paralysis.

Upper Lid

Lagophthalmus or poor closure of the upper lid can lead to corneal exposure with drying, pain, possible scarring, and visual loss. Over a period of time, contracture of the antagonist levator muscle can also result in upper eyelid retraction intensifying the lagophthalmos and corneal exposure problem.

Brow

Denervation of the frontalis muscle in the forehead can cause a ptosis of the eyebrow, particularly in the older patient. Paralysis of the frontalis muscle will also produce a loss of forehead creases (flattening) in addition to brow ptosis. The brow ptosis and the bulk of the upper lid skin produce a mechanical eyelid ptosis on the affected side (Fig. 1A, B). Contralateral upper eyelid retraction is commonly observed due to Hering's law of equal innervation. This eyebrow ptosis can weigh down the upper lid and impair vision in upgaze. (An exception occurs in the central supranuclear seventh involvement in which the bilateral forehead innervation spares the frontalis muscle.)

Lower Lid

Loss of muscular tone in the lower lid in patients who already have some lid laxity can cause sagging or an ectropion of the lower lid. In younger patients who still have elasticity and tone in their lid, the lid position may only be displaced downward with some "scleral show" as opposed to a frank ectropion; however, increased exposure of the eye and keratopathy can be encountered in some patients with only minimal displacement (Fig. 1C, D). The loss of contracture of the orbicularis fibers also interferes with the "pumping" effect of the lids, which promotes tear drainage. Excessive tearing is encountered in patients with facial palsy because of the loss of the "eyelid pump," which eliminates tears from the eye. Tearing in these patients is intensified by increased tears that are produced by the eye in an attempt to protect itself from exposure. The combination of these two disturbances can be a great annoyance to the patient because of the "watery eye" produced.

Ocular

The cornea of the eye may become damaged from exposure keratitis depending on the adequacy of the other eye protective mechanisms. Faulty eyelid closure due to orbicularis oculi involvement will produce varying degrees of exposure conjunctivitis and keratitis. In its mildest form, the exposure can be tolerated.

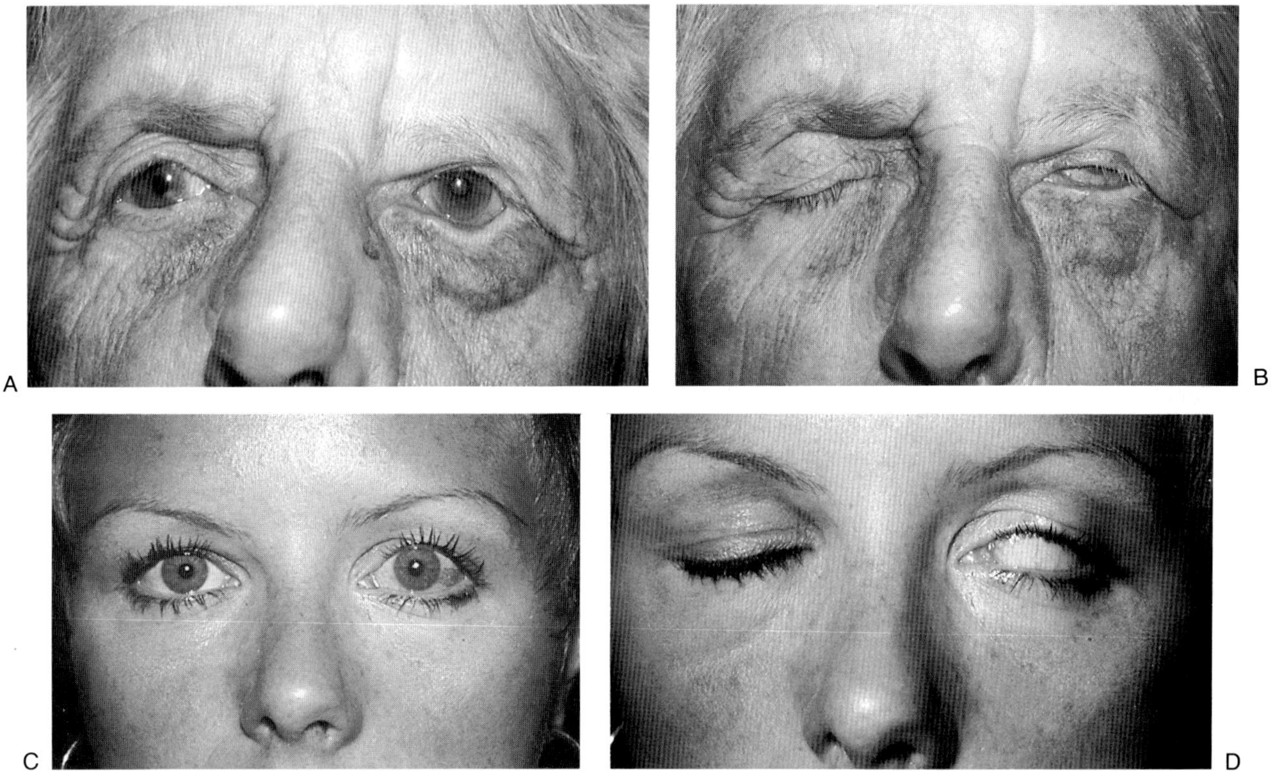

FIG. 1. Characteristic appearance of eyelids and eye in patient with facial paralysis. **A:** Older patient after Bell's palsy with eyebrow ptosis and severe ectropion. The ptotic brow masks upper lid retraction. **B:** Same patient as in A showing lagophthalmos with attempted eyelid closure. **C:** Younger patient following seventh nerve paralysis from trauma. There is less of a tendency for ectropion and eyebrow ptosis. However, significant exposure is present. **D:** Same patient as in C showing lagophthalmos with attempted eyelid closure.

However, depending on the degree of lagophthalmos and underlying integrity of the corneal tear film, varying degrees of corneal breakdown will result. Inferior punctate epithelial staining may progress to corneal ulceration. Clinical and surgical treatments should minimize or control progressive corneal breakdown. Decreased corneal sensation can be encountered if the pathologic process affecting the seventh nerve also affects the fifth nerve, which can occur with tumors in proximity to the cerebellopontine angle. This has also been reported in cases of Bell's palsy and zoster in cases involving inflammation of the fifth nerve. May and Hardin reported the polyneuronal nature of Bell's palsy (the most common cause of facial paralysis), citing as evidence decreased corneal sensation, hearing, and taste discrimination and numbness of the face, shoulder, and neck (1). Neurotropic corneal ulceration may aggravate the exposure difficulties. The combination of fifth nerve paresis combined with a seventh nerve paresis may preclude maintaining a "normal" fissure width even with compensatory eyelid surgery because of the problem of cornea protection with the loss of eye protective mechanisms. Other ocular changes are due to other cranial nerve involvement. Miosis and reduced intraocular pressure have been reported. An increased incidence of cataracts has also been reported in patients with longstanding Bell's palsy or in patients with acoustic neuroma.

Lacrimal

Epiphora is frequently an annoying sequel of facial palsy. This may result from the eversion of the puncta from the lacus lacrimalis (punctal ectropion) or from ectropion of the eyelid. Epiphora also results from a nonfunctioning lacrimal pump that requires orbicularis muscle contractures. The closing of the eyelids expands the lacrimal sac and creates a negative pressure within the sac. The tears are drawn into the lacrimal sac and then drain into the nose by gravity. The lack of orbicularis function paralyzes eyelid movement (the lacrimal pump) and causes epiphora. Epiphora may be partially relieved by managing the exposure or correcting eyelid malposition. If the lacrimal system is patent to irrigation with an open, well-positioned puncta but still is nonfunctioning as confirmed by dye tests, a Jones tube may be required to bypass the inadequate pump. However, a Jones tube may function poorly with paralyzed lids because of the absence of the palpebral movement also necessary for tear elimination.

As previously mentioned, there may be an excess of tears because of compensation by the eye to protect itself and a reduction of flow through the draining ducts because of loss of pumping. If the pathologic process involving the seventh nerve affects the parasympathetic fibers accompanying the nerve at the level of the greater superficial protrosal nerve intracranially, the lacrimal gland will be denervated from its secretory fibers. The orbital and palpebral lobes of the lacrimal gland function as "emergency tear glands" and their function can be impaired with a lesion involving the nerve at this level. A Schirmer test comparing tear function with that of the opposite side would give an indication of this level of involvement. This involvement usually occurs when the nerve lesion is at the level of the geniculate ganglion.

LOCALIZATION OF PATHOLOGY

Understanding of the anatomy and the course of the facial nerve helps in the comprehension of the signs and symptoms that occur with facial paralysis (2) (Fig. 2). The facial nucleus is in the pons and the genu of the facial nerve arches over the abducens nucleus and exits the brainstem. The nerve passes the cerebellopontine angle and enters the internal auditory meatus and a rigid bony canal, which is the longest bony canal in the body. The facial nerve has four anatomic portions prior to exiting from the stylomastoid foramen: the meatal, labyrinthine, tympanic, and mastoid. Involvement of each of these segments will produce specific features. It should be noted that the more proximal the involvement of the facial nerve in Bell's palsy, the more profound and permanent the sequelae of involvement. Involvement of taste and salivary flow reflects compression of the mastoid segment. Diminished tear production and disturbances of balance and hearing are associated with involvement of the proximal portion of the fallopian canal, i.e., the labyrinthine segment. A diminished stapes reflex is associated with involvement of the tympanic segment. Loss of taste on the anterior tip of the tongue and decreased salivation in the sublingual and submandibular glands occur when lesions occur further down in parasympathetic secretory fibers accompanying the facial nerve (chorda tympani) in the tympanomastoid area of the cranial bone. Because of the proximity of the eighth nerve to the seventh nerve in the internal auditory canal and because of the branch nerve to the stapes, audiologic testing and a test of the stapedial reflex can be of localiz-

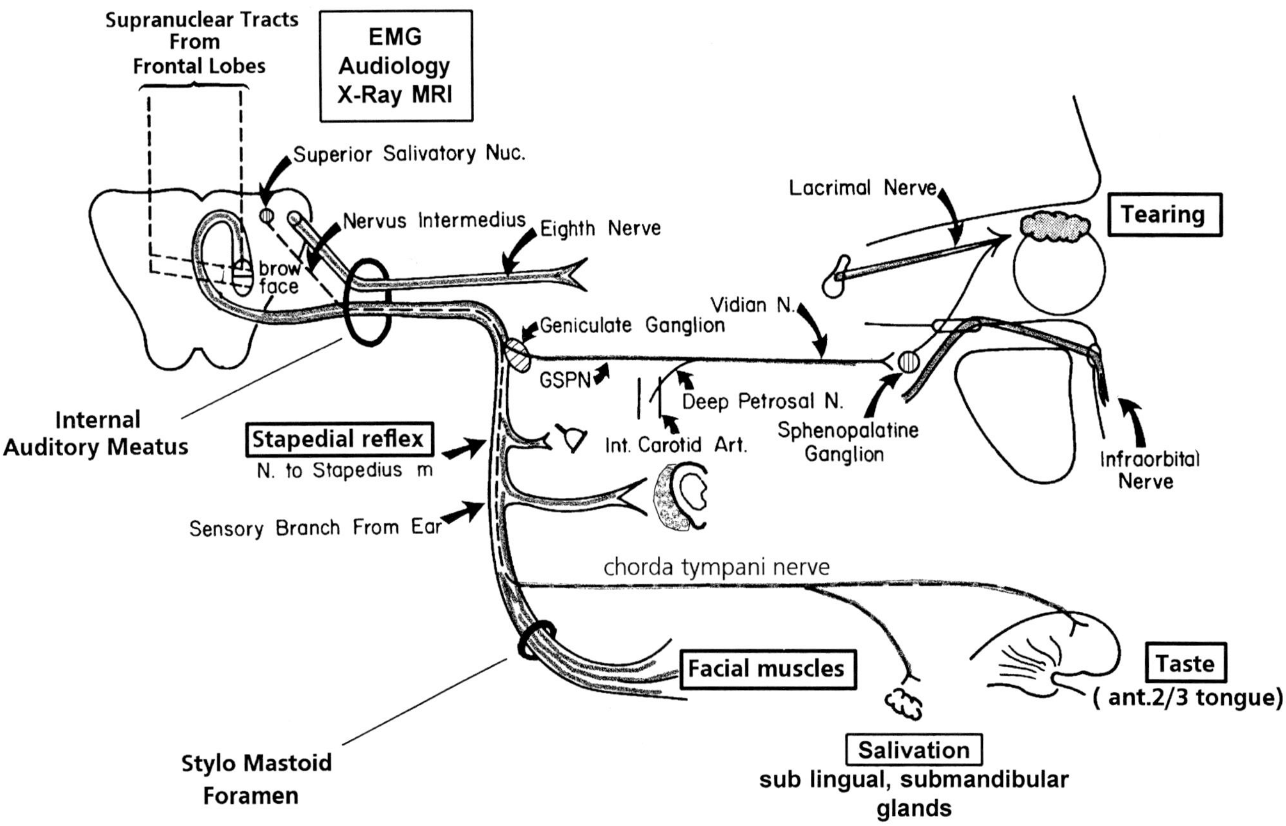

FIG. 2. Pathways of facial nerves showing areas of localizing neurologic signs (after Bajandas, ref. 2).

ing value. The recognition of the sites of involvement and electromyographic analysis allow identification of the location of the compression of the facial nerve.

CAUSES OF FACIAL PARALYSIS

Seventh nerve paralysis may result from injury, tumors, or inflammatory conditions (3). Facial nerve paralysis from tumors, surgery, or trauma is usually a severe and total paralysis. The facial nerve is in close apposition to the auditory nerve. Surgical resection of acoustic neuromas may produce a facial paralysis postoperatively. Lesions affecting the facial nerve may be central and include other cranial nerves, and may occur as a nuclear or intrapontine lesion. Lesions between the pons and the internal auditory meatus (cerebellar pontine angle lesions) are frequently caused by acoustic neuroma, meningioma, basal meningitis, and meningocarcinomatosis. Lower motor neuron damage occurring in the intracanalicular portion of the nerve and causing paralysis of the facial nerve can result from otitis media and chronic mastoiditis, cholesteatoma middle ear surgery, hemorrhage of the facial nerve, and inflammatory processes such as Guillain–Barré, sarcoidosis, mumps, porphyria, and idiopathic facial palsy (Bell's palsy). As the nerve exits from the stylomastoid foramen, paralysis can be caused by trauma of various kinds, including surgical involvement with tumors, parotid tumors, and neuritis (3). With one exception, peripheral branches of the facial nerve, if damaged, usually do not cause paralysis because of numerous interconnections; the exception is the temporal branch of the facial nerve to the frontalis muscle (important for eyebrow position), which is vulnerable because of its length.

Fortunately, the most common causes of facial palsy can be temporary. In a series of 1575 patients with facial paralysis seen consecutively (3), Bell's palsy (57%) and herpes zoster cephalicus (7%) comprised the largest segment of patients. Trauma (17%), tumor (6%), infection (4%), birth (3%), and others (6%) constituted the remainder of etiologic categories (Table 1).

TABLE 1. *Causes of facial nerve disorders*

Cause	Patients (%)
Bell's palsy	57
Herpes zoster cephalicus	7
Trauma	17
Tumors	6
Birth (congenital and acquired)	4
Hemifacial spasm	2
Central nervous system (axial) disease	1
Questionable	1

After May (ref. 3).

TABLE 2. *Diagnosed Bell's palsy*

True cause of facial palsy	No. patients
Tumor	47 (4.8%)
Herpes zoster cephalicus	19 (1.95%)
Infection	12 (1.2%)
Birth	4 (0.4%)
Trauma	2 (0.25%)
Other	12 (1.25%)
Bell's palsy	878 (90%)

After May (ref. 3).

Bell's Idiopathic Facial Palsy

Bell's palsy, the most frequent cause of acute facial palsy, is idiopathic and is confirmed after all other diagnoses have been excluded. The acute onset may occur overnight and often resolves within a few weeks. The most dangerous aspect of Bell's palsy consists of the ophthalmologic sequelae. The maximum progression of the facial paralysis in Bell's palsy usually occurs within 2 weeks (4). Remission is usually spontaneous, often occurring within 3 weeks. The earlier the recovery, the better the function results. The extent of facial function recovery is usually complete in 6 months (5). Because of the preponderance of the cases caused by Bell's palsy, other causes may receive the diagnosis erroneously (Table 2) (3,5). Clinical features that preclude a diagnosis of Bell's palsy or suggest tumor or other lesions include the following (5):

Facial paralysis, which is slowly progressive beyond 3 weeks
No return of facial function beyond 6 months
Simultaneous bilateral facial palsy
Recurrence of facial palsy unilaterally (30% will have tumor)
Facial hyperkinesis or dyskinesis

The etiology of Bell's palsy, or idiopathic facial paralysis, remains obscure. Viral, inflammatory, and immune factors have been implicated as offenders in this disorder. In adult facial paralysis an etiology other than Bell's palsy can be determined in roughly 20% of cases, whereas in children an etiology can be established in more than 50% of cases. Approximately 70–80% of patients with Bell's palsy have a complete or satisfactory return of function. Patients who have an incomplete facial paralysis are most likely to have a complete return of function. Approximately 50% of patients who have a complete paralysis at the onset of affliction will have a satisfactory return of function. If the paralysis is incomplete at the time of onset but progresses to complete, approximately 25% of patients will have a satisfactory return of function. An aggressive approach to Bell's palsy, which has been recommended, is to recognize and treat patients with poor prognostic indicators for functional return (3). Early identification of patients who are likely to proceed to irreversible facial paralysis can be recognized based on clinical features.

The diagnostic workup for facial paralysis differs between adults and children. Adults generally undergo electrophysiologic testing emphasizing nerve excitability. Imaging studies are not required uniformly but ordered on an individualized basis. Children undergo electrophysiology, magnetic resonance imaging (MRI) and computed tomographic (CT) imaging, and serologic and neurologic evaluations. Patients with other neurologic symptoms such as chronic headaches or diminished hearing, or an atypical clinical course, should be evaluated for a structural lesion with a CT scan of the head (3,4,6). The physician must direct special attention to the base of the skull and cerebellopontine angle when requesting the CT scan.

Common causes of facial nerve dysfunction in children include trauma, congenital malformation, immune disorders, hematopoietic derangement, and neoplasms. Traumatic neonatal facial palsy usually comes from uncomplicated forceps delivery because the nerve is most vulnerable at the lateral stylomastoid foramen and may be compressed against the sacrum during prolonged and difficult labor. Mobius syndrome is a congenital facial nerve paralysis combined with a sixth nerve palsy due to hypoplasia of the facial motor nucleus and of abducens nucleus. Lyme disease should be considered in the differential diagnosis of acquired facial palsy in pediatric patients.

Electrophysiologic testing includes Hilger nerve stimulation, electroneurography, and electromyography (6). The Hilger nerve stimulator is used most often to predict prognosis. Percutaneous electrical stimulation of the facial nerve trunk or peripheral nerve branches can be employed. Patients have less pain with peripheral nerve stimulation.

Electroneurography evokes a myogenic response to evaluate facial nerve paralysis, providing a reliable prognosis for acute facial nerve paralysis. Bipolar surface electrodes are used for both stimulating and recording. Test results are used to calculate the percentage of conduction-blocked fibers as well as degenerated fibers. Injury leading to Wallerian degeneration has a worse prognosis than that seen with conduction blockage (neuropraxia). Bell's palsy patients with a maximal degeneration of 90% could be considered for surgical decompression within the first 3 weeks. Degeneration of 90% or less should be treated with steroids. High-dose steroid therapy is thought to be efficacious during the first 2 weeks after onset of Bell's palsy (5,6).

Tumors

Facial palsy with slow progression, fluctuation, or facial hyperkinesis raises the suspicion of neoplasm. The most common tumor is the acoustic neuroma of the adjacent eighth nerve, which occurs insidiously. The acoustic neuroma affects the facial nerve indirectly by pressure, whereas neuromas of the facial nerve occur frequently near the geniculate ganglion as part of the facial nerve. The smaller tumor size correlates with a better prognosis for return of facial function. Facial nerve paralysis due to parotid tumors is a reflection of the aggressive behavior of the tumor (3,5–7).

Intraoperative electromonitoring of the facial nerve during removal of cerebropontine angle tumors has resulted in improved preservation of the facial nerve function. Neuromuscular blockade or local anesthetics, however, render the nerve unresponsive to stimulation (6).

Malignant tumors of the ear, external auditory canal, and temporal bone, such as squamous cell carcinoma and adenoid cystic carcinoma, can extend into the temporal bone to produce facial palsy. Metastatic lesions are uncommon.

Ramsey–Hunt Syndrome

Herpes zoster can cause a painful facial palsy called Ramsey–Hunt syndrome. Herpetic lesions at the external ear canal provide the specific diagnosis. Acyclovir has been used with dramatic pain relief (3,5).

Lyme Disease

The sole manifestation of Lyme disease can be facial palsy from *Borrellia burgdorferia* transmitted by the bite of the deer tick. Lyme disease frequently occurs in the early summer and one third of the patients have bilateral facial palsy. The facial palsy can begin acutely, as with Bell's palsy, and partial paralysis is common. Serologic testing provides the diagnosis of Lyme disease. Patients with neurologic disease should be treated with currently recommended antibiotics such as tetracycline or ciprofloxcin (3,5).

Immunocompromised Patients

Patients with immunodeficiency virus (HIV) infection can present with facial palsy, but the palsy frequently resolves without treatment after 2–10 weeks. Facial palsy may be associated with other cranial neuropathies or peripheral neuropathies, although the isolated facial palsy constitutes the most frequent presentation (3,5).

Leprosy

Leprosy can produce lagophthalmos through a facial palsy affecting the zygomatic and temporal branches of the facial nerve. The lepromatous type of leprosy is responsible for the majority of ocular and facial nerve complications. Facial palsy may be complicated by trigeminal nerve involvement with loss of corneal sensation (3,5).

Sarcoidosis

A common neurologic manifestation of sarcoidosis is facial palsy, occurring in 22–50% of patients. Early in the course of the disease, one third of the patients have facial palsy as the only sign of neurologic involvement. The onset is usually acute followed by a spontaneous recovery (3,5).

Bacterial Infection

Prior to antibiotic therapy, acute otitis media was a common cause of facial palsy but now chronic otitis is a more common cause of facial palsy.

Cholesteatoma

Bone destruction from cholesteotoma, an epidermal type cyst, can affect the facial nerve by infiltration, compression, and infection, and necessitates surgical treatment (3,5).

Trauma

Fractures of the temporal bone or the peripheral face can cause injuries to the facial nerve. Exploration of the nerve for primary repair may be necessary either from a neurosurgical approach to the temporal bone or in the face (3,5).

Cerebrovascular Accidents

Facial nuclear and supranuclear paralysis arise most often from cerebrovascular accidents, although neoplasms and trauma can sometimes produce similar changes. Most strokes in the corticobulbar tracts present with sparing of the nerve fibers to the upper face due to bilateral innervation. The lower face seventh nerve fibers have only contralateral innervation from the facial motor nuclei (3,5).

REGENERATION SYNDROMES

Fortunately for many, patients some regeneration of nerve fibers or restoration of nerve function may occur. This is always an improvement over paralysis; however, in some patients, the nerves regenerate aberrantly. Misdirection syndromes and anomalous innervations occur that can create a nuisance to the patient. Presently, there is no remedy for these regeneration syndromes.

Marin–Amat Syndrome

The most commonly encountered regeneration syndrome causes the synchronous contracture of the eyelid orbicularis fibers with contracture of the lower facial fibers. Patients with this syndrome will have a spasm of eyelid closure when they smile or move their lower facial muscles. "Eyelid closure with smiling" has been described in the past as the "syndrome of Marin–Amat" (8). This condition must be differentiated from patients who have hemifacial spasm or benign essential blepharospasm. Smaller variations and localized tics can occur as a result of misdirection of these peripheral nerve fibers.

Gustatory Syndromes

When the facial nerve regenerates the parasympathetic innervational fibers to the nose, lacrimal and sweating apparatus becomes aberrantly regenerate and becomes associated with the chorda tympani, which supplies sensation to the anterior tip of the tongue. With gustatory rhinorrhea, the nose produces secretions and "runs" when the tongue is stimulated with spicy food. With gustatory lacrimation, the eye will produce tears when the tongue is stimulated with spicy food ("crocodile tears"). With gustatory sweating (Frey's syndrome), facial and retroauricular hyperemia and sweating can occur with stimulation of the tongue. These regeneration syndromes are frustrating to the patient and to the doctor because of lack of remedy. However, they are important to recognize.

TREATMENT OF THE EYE CHANGES IN FACIAL PARALYSIS

Temporizing

Fortunately for most patients the most common causes of facial palsy have a high recovery rate, i.e., 84% in Bell's palsy and 60% in herpes zoster. Both tend to resolve in a 3- to 4-week period and during

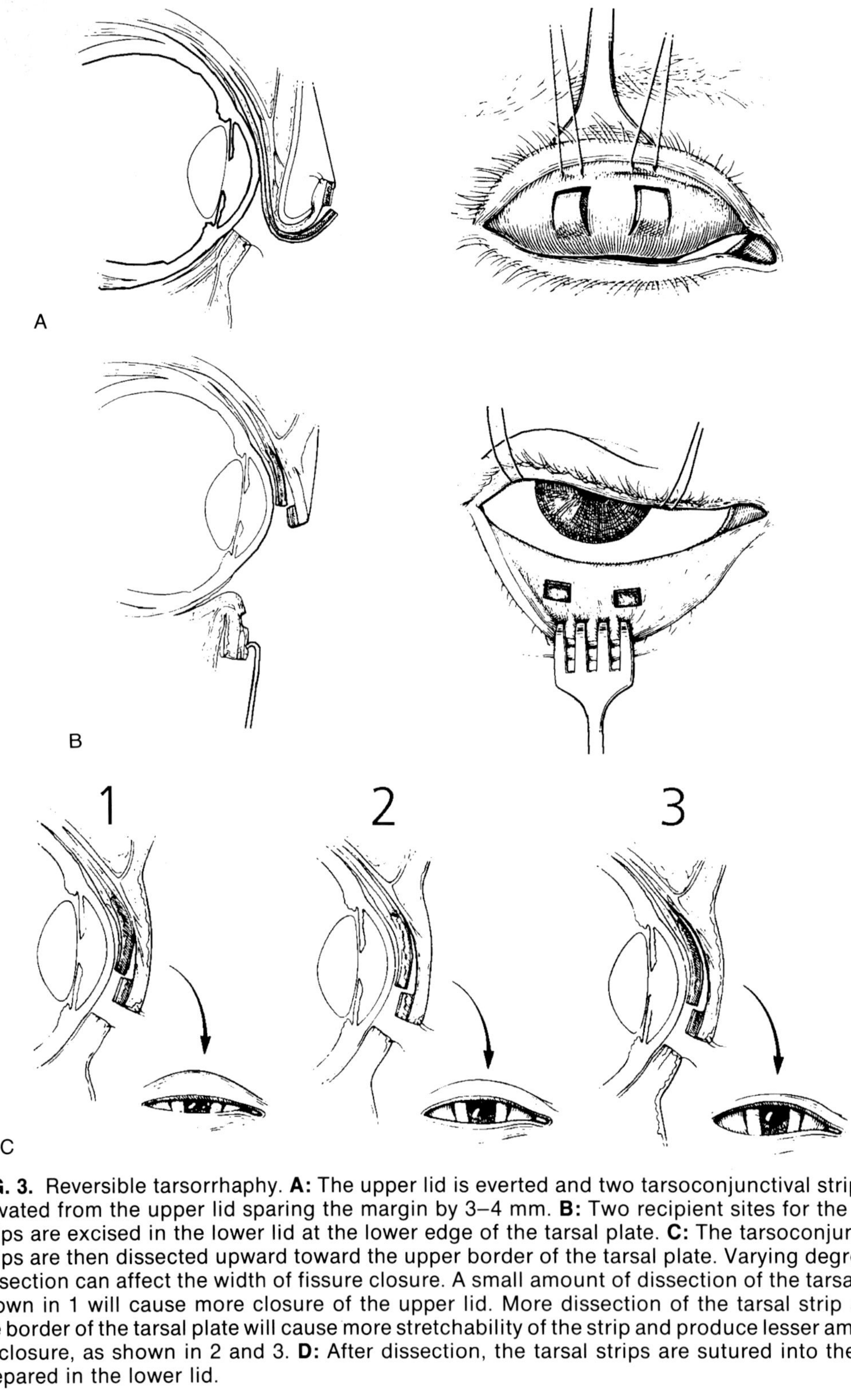

FIG. 3. Reversible tarsorrhaphy. **A:** The upper lid is everted and two tarsoconjunctival strips are elevated from the upper lid sparing the margin by 3–4 mm. **B:** Two recipient sites for the tarsal strips are excised in the lower lid at the lower edge of the tarsal plate. **C:** The tarsoconjunctival strips are then dissected upward toward the upper border of the tarsal plate. Varying degrees of dissection can affect the width of fissure closure. A small amount of dissection of the tarsal strip shown in 1 will cause more closure of the upper lid. More dissection of the tarsal strip above the border of the tarsal plate will cause more stretchability of the strip and produce lesser amounts of closure, as shown in 2 and 3. **D:** After dissection, the tarsal strips are sutured into the sites prepared in the lower lid.

this period of time, if necessary, a monofilament nylon suture can be used to perform a temporary tarsorrhaphy for the eyelids. The suture can be tolerated for as long as 3 weeks if polysporin ointment is applied with it. Many patients will not require even this and may get by with only lubricants.

Tarsorrhaphy

"Reversible" Tarsorrhaphy

Some patients require a more prolonged closure of the eyelids than can be provided by a suture tarsorrha-

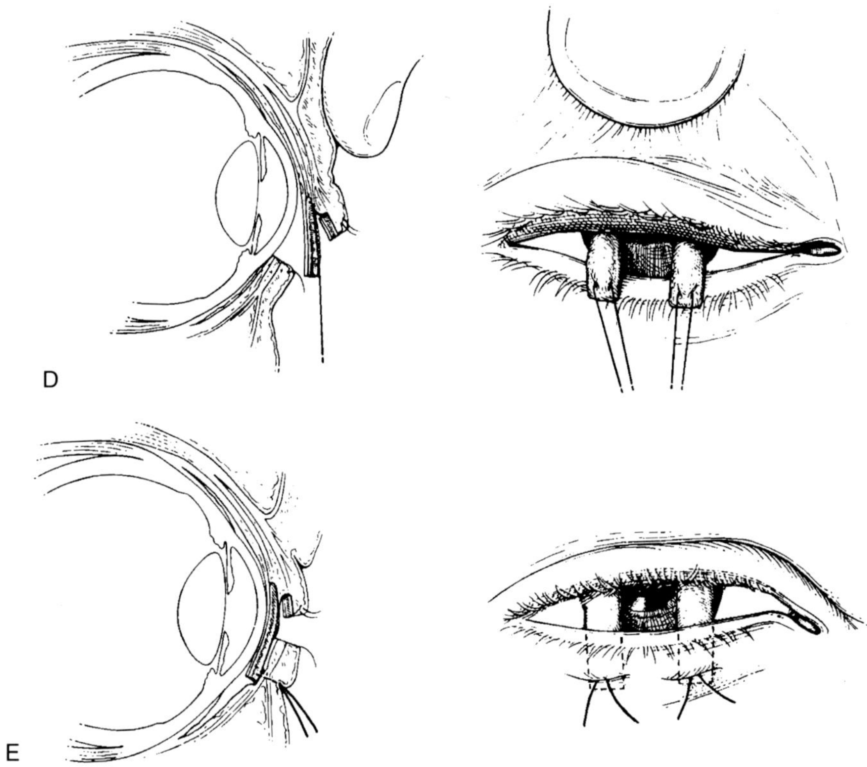

FIG. 3. *Continued.*

phy. In patients who expect a more prolonged or even permanent loss of function of the nerve to the eyelids, a tethering of the eyelids together will be necessary in some cases for protection, particularly if there is decreased corneal sensation accompanying the seventh nerve paresis. There are numerous ways to perform a tarsorrhaphy; however, it should be emphasized that the proper technique is the one that damages the eyelid margin the least. This is important because eyelid margin adhesions very commonly cause inturning eyelashes. If the patient is fortunate enough to have a "takedown" of the tarsorrhaphy at a later time, the intact healthy eyelid margin is a very important commodity. Surgical separation of these "permanent" adhesion tarsorrhaphy procedures, as may sometimes be desired at a later date, often result in localized lid notching and trichiasis.

Very adequate closure of the eyelids can be obtained by strips of tarsoconjunctiva brought from behind the upper lid margin to the lower eyelid, sparing the margins and closing the eye without damage to the eyelid margin. This surgical tarsorrhaphy is easy to perform, offers prolonged protection of the globe from exposure, and is readily undone.

For this procedure, the upper and lower lids are infiltrated with lidocaine 2% with epinephrine 1:100,000 and hyaluronidase (Wydase). The upper lid is everted over a cotton-tipped applicator and held under tension traction suture. A thin strip of tarsoconjunctiva is elevated. The upper lid margin is spared by at least 4 mm. A single tongue of tarsoconjunctival tissue may be elevated for a lateral tarsorrhaphy, or two strips may be used for a combined medial and lateral tarsorrhaphy (Fig. 3A). The upper lid tarsoconjunctival strips are dissected a variable amount depending on the degree of eyelid closure desired (Fig. 3C). Extensive dissection of the strip above the superior border of the upper lid tarsus will allow for minimal eyelid closure with the tarsorrhaphy. Minimal dissection of the elevated tissue strip will allow for greater narrowing of the palpebral fissure with the tarsorrhaphy.

Divets of tarsoconjunctiva from the lower lid that corresponds to the tongue of tarsoconjunctiva from the upper lid are excised (Fig. 3B). A double-armed 4-0 prolene mattress suture is installed through the upper lid strip of tarsoconjunctiva, into the lower lid recipient bed, and out the skin of the lower eyelid (Fig. 4D). The suture is tied and cut, and polysporin ophthalmic ointment is applied for the first postoperative week. This tarsorrhaphy may be left in place indefinitely. It is easily undone by simple excising of the tarsoconjunctival strip(s) flush with the inner eyelid surfaces.

"Permanent" Tarsorrhaphy

A permanent tarsorrhaphy can be used when permanent closure of the medial and lateral canthal angles is

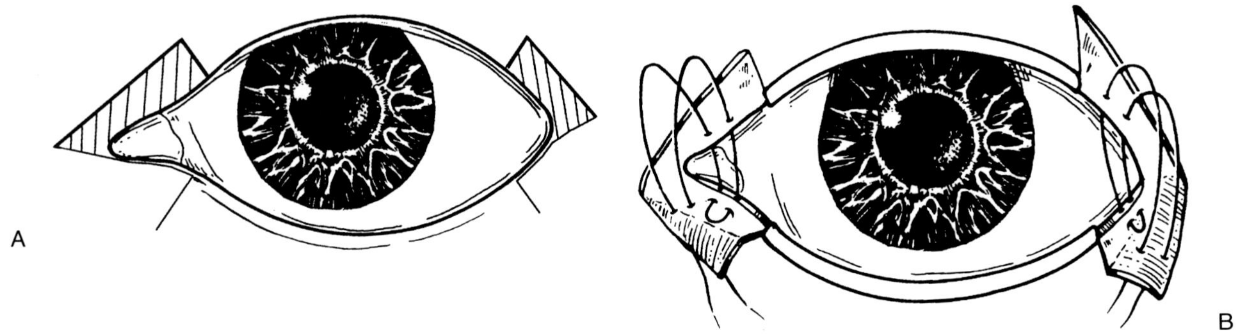

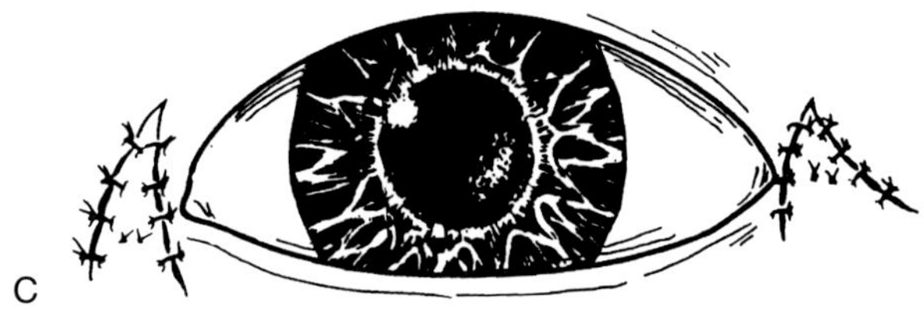

FIG. 4. Permanent tarsorrhaphy. **A:** The skin-muscle flap is undermined in the areas marked in the lower lid and excised in the marked areas in the upper lid. **B:** The edge of the tarsal plate margin is deepithelialized. Mattress sutures are inserted closing the canthal angles and the skin-muscle flap from the lower lid is sutured to the upper lid. **C:** Shows position of the flap sutured to the upper lid and closure of the fissure.

desired. A combined medial and lateral tarsorrhaphy gives more protection than either alone. The lateral canthoplasty is the most effective and is preferred if used singly. The lateral lid margins are denuded in the areas to be approximated. The freshened edges of the lid margin are approximated with a mattress suture that is brought through the musculocutaneous flap from the lower eyelid. A triangle of skin is excised from the upper eyelid to create a bed for the triangle of skin to be rotated in from the lower lid (Fig. 4A–C).

A medial canthoplasty is performed in the same manner as a lateral canthoplasty. Canalicular probes can be placed during the procedure to protect the canaliculi.

Reinnervation Procedures

If the patient has had paralysis for less than a year with minimal facial muscle atrophy, or if the patient demonstrates residual muscle function by electrical testing, reestablishment of a nerve supply to the facial muscles can in some patients restore tone and movement.

Myoneurotinization

Flaps of adjacent muscles of mastication (temporalis) can reinnervate the facial muscles; however, the innervation is anomalous and contracture only takes place with chewing actions (9). Attachment of the temporalis muscle to the eyelids with facial strips to the eyelids and lower face has been performed. The most common transfer is the temporalis transfer to the eyelids and lower facial area. Theoretically this has some advantage of animation, but the muscular movement of the face is not mimetic with the contralateral side and most surgeons who have performed this procedure over the years have noticed that these attachments become static with time. These procedures do have some value in severe cases. Even a purely static facial sling with fascia lata can be helpful for the lower face in severe cases.

Cross-Facial Grafting

A Sural nerve graft anastomosing the nonparalytic facial nerve to the paretic nerve in some cases has given reasonable reinnervation. If the facial muscles have atrophied, muscle transplantation (extensor digitorum brevis) in conjunction with a Sural nerve cross-facial graft can restore some innervation or tone. These procedures are unpredictable and may take as long as 3–4 years to produce any results (10).

Cranial Nerve Anastomosis to the Facial Nerve

Hypoglossal to Facial (12 to 7)

Anastomosis of the ipsilateral twelfth nerve to the paretic seventh can restore lower facial tone. However, it has a much lesser effect on the eyelids and does cause a deficit in the use of the tongue with hemiglossal atrophy (11).

Spinal Accessory to Facial (11 to 7)

Anastomosis of the spinal accessory nerve to the facial nerve can restore tone to the paralyzed face and contracture of facial muscles occurs with contracture of the trapezius muscle (shrugging of the shoulder).

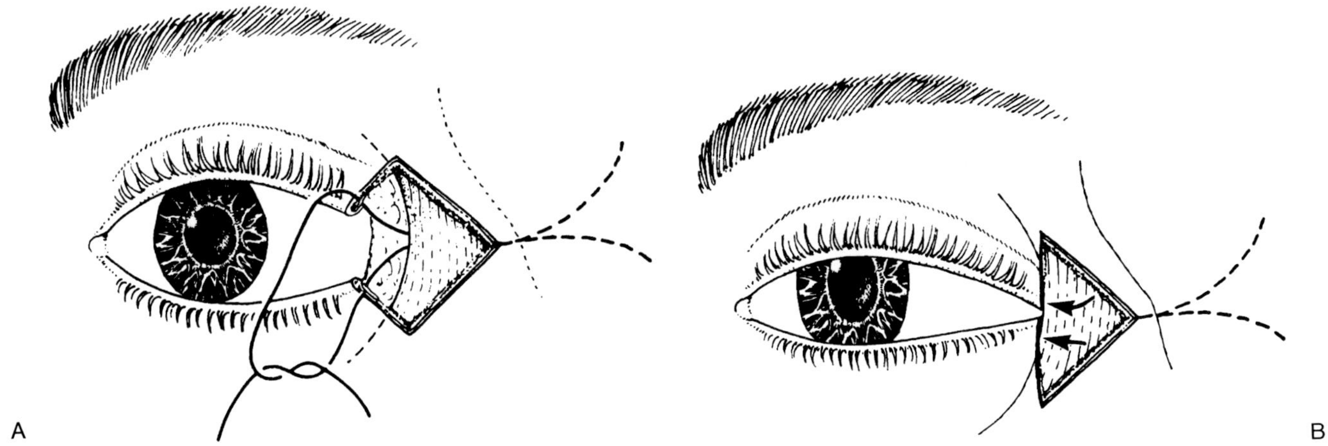

FIG. 5. Lateral canthoplasty with eyelid tightening. **A:** Full-thickness resection of the edge of the upper and lower lids has been performed in a triangular manner. Rotational advancement flaps have been marked. A 4-0 prolene suture is used to tighten the lower lid and the upper lid toward a point inside the periosteal rim. **B:** The lateral edges of the lids have been tightened to the periosteum, tensing the upper and lower lids. The lateral flaps will be advanced to cover the periosteum.

Compensatory Eyelid Surgery

Reinnervation procedures give hope for the future in the rehabilitation of the patient with facial paralysis. As a practical matter, however, the eyelids seem particularly unresponsive and most patients usually end up with eyelid procedures to help improve eyelid closure or position. Compensatory eyelid surgery involves three areas: lower lid, upper lid, and eyebrow.

Lower Lid Surgery

The normal position of the lower lid margin is at the lower limbal area, so that the tear film of the eye flows at the proper level across the cornea. Normally both lower and upper lids move up and down vertically, although the lower not as much as the upper lid. The main importance of the lower lid movement is its contribution to the tear pump. In some younger people who have not lost elasticity, a horizontal tightening of the lid via plication of the lateral tendon can restore the lower lid to its normal position and appearance. Unfortunately, this does not restore normal movement to the tear pump and a degree of tearing may persist.

In our experience with the the lower lid tightening procedure it has been helpful to perform a tightening resection of the upper lid along with the lower lid tightening at the lateral canthus in order to tighten the tarsoligamentous sling of the upper lid; this combination seems to at least temporarily help upper lid closure if a specific upper lid closure device is not used (Fig. 5A, B).

In more severe cases, such as in individuals with frank ectropion, the horizontal tightening procedure must be supplemented with a strip of facia lata (donor homologous or autogenous) to serve as a hammock support to the lower lid. This was described in the chapter on ectopion. This repositioning of the lower lid flush against the globe, at a level to reinstate the tear film, is quite helpful to the protection of the eye and to the person's appearance (Fig. 6A–D).

Upper Lid Surgery

Over the years a number of implant devices have been used to replace the contraction of the orbicularis fibers lost with paralysis to improve closure of the upper lid. All of these devices are intended to simulate the protractor closure effect of the eyelid muscle and, in some cases, reposition the eyelid. Lid "loading" with gold weights has been used in the upper lids with varying degrees of success (12). However, the gravitational effect only works if the patient is in the upright position and moves only the upper lid. Morel et al. (13) introduced a palpebral spring, which mainly affected upper lid closure and has been used on and off for many years; however, in most cases it has not been effective, and most have extruded. Arion (14) introduced an encircling elastic silicone rod to simulate the squeezing of the protractor muscle. This seems to be effective, although it has its inherent problems of erosion and in many cases must be considered a temporary procedure.

Morel-Fatio Palpebral Spring

The palpebral spring seems to be the least successful of the devices. There is a tendency for erosion and

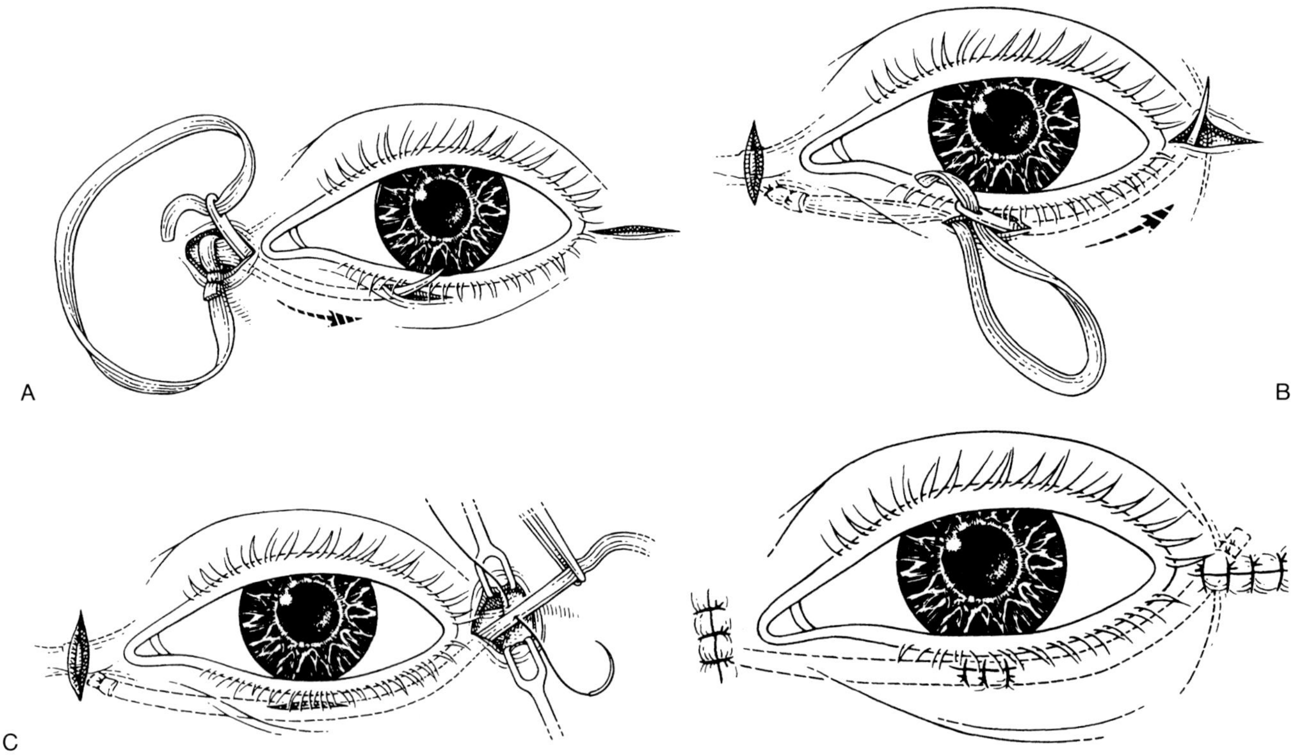

FIG. 6. Fascia sling to the lower lid (autogenous or donor fascia). **A:** A fascia strip 3–4 mm in width has been threaded underneath the anterior reflection of the medial canthal tendon and threaded in the submuscular plain to a central incision. **B:** The fascia is then threaded from the central incision to the incision at the lateral orbital rim. **C:** Horizontal tightening of the lid has been performed and a suturing of the fascia to the rim periosteum with a permanent suture tenses the lid. **D:** The fascia in position with tightening and elevation of the lower lid.

extrusion with time and it is very difficult to fine-tune the amount of closure desired. Very commonly ptosis of the upper lid is created.

Arion Silicone Rod (Cerclage)

The technique described here is similar to Arion's original technique, but modifications have been introduced. The most recent modification, which will be described in detail here, is using the elastic portion of the rod for the upper lid only. It is usually combined with a fascia graft to the lower lids. Incisions in the medial canthus exposing the anterior reflection of the medial canthal tendon and in the lateral canthal area exposing the bony lateral rim are made. A 1-mm silicone rod is threaded from the lateral canthal area in the suborbicularis plane in the pretarsal area to the inner canthus. It is attached to the undersurface of the medial canthal tendon. It is then brought through a drill hole at the lateral canthal area through the orbital rim and fixated in those two areas. A Watzke sleeve threaded over the rod is helpful as a bolster for fixation in the medial canthal tendon and the lateral orbital rim area to prevent sutures cutting through the silicone rod. The tensile strength of the silicone is excellent; however, it is not elastic enough to allow the lid to open to its normal width and then snap shut completely. To get more closure one must sacrifice opening of the upper lid when the person is awake in primary gaze. There can be a tendency for erosion of the silicone through the tarsal plate with time; however, many patients have had the silicone implant in position for a number of years without mishap. The 1-mm silicone rod can be obtained from specialty companies as described in the chapter on ptosis.

The lateral orbital rim is exposed about 3 mm below the lateral palpebral tendon. The 0.8- to 1.0-mm-thick silicone rod is passed behind the anterior limb of the medial palpebral tendon. The curved Keith needle is passed as close to the lid margin as possible (2–3 mm ideally). A 1.5-mm hole is then drilled in the lateral orbital rim about 3 mm below the lateral canthal angle (Fig. 7A). The silicone from the upper eyelid is pulled through the hole created in the lateral orbital wall from the inside to the outside of the orbit and fixated with a Watzke sleeve (Fig. 7B). The tension is adjusted, preferably in the awake patient. A slight to moderate ptosis should be created because 1–2 mm of ptosis is needed in the final result to give adequate protection

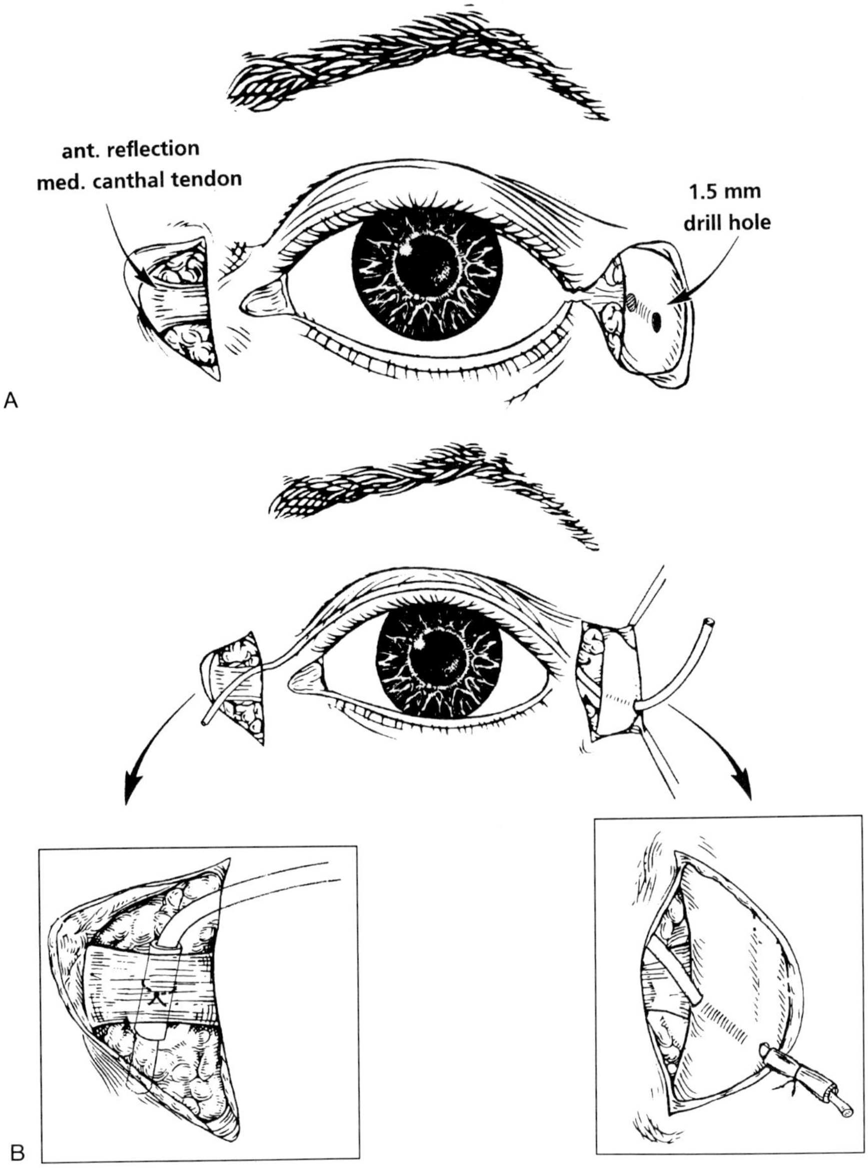

FIG. 7. Arion silicone filament to upper lid. **A:** The anterior reflection of the medial canthal tendon has been exposed through a medial incision. The lateral orbital rim has been exposed with a lateral incision and a through-and-through drill hole is placed slanting upward from the outside to the inside. It is placed in a location to create a downward pull on the upper lid. **B:** A 1-mm silicone rod has been threaded in the submuscular (pretarsal plain) in the upper lid exiting in the medial canthus and in the lateral canthus. The 1-mm silicone rod is then sutured to the undersurface of the medial canthal tendon, bolstering it with a Watzke (polyethelene) sleeve. Laterally, the rod is inserted through the drill holes and fixated externally with a Watzke sleeve. In the absence of voluntary cooperation by the patient, the proper tension can be determined by hanging a small mosquito hemostat on the silicone rod to produce tension.

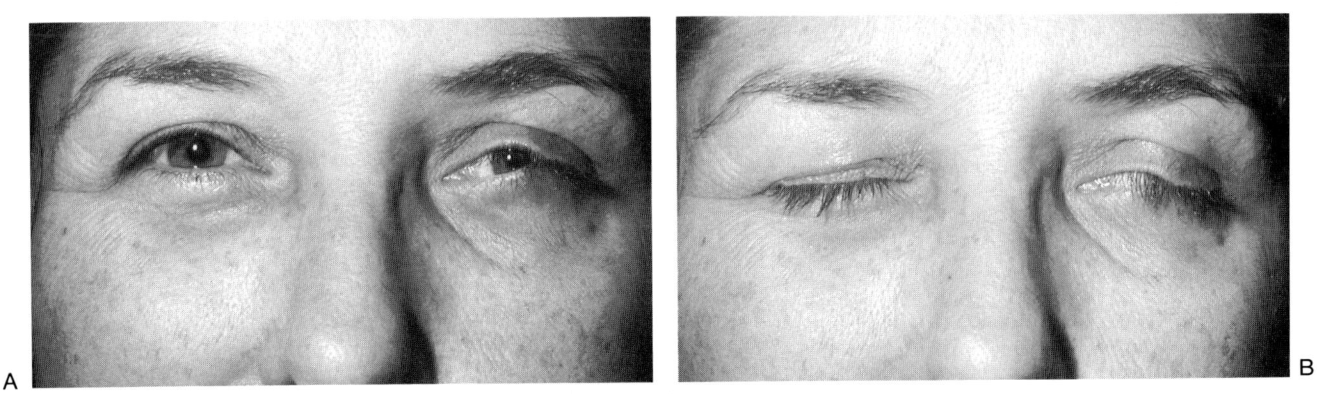

FIG. 8. A: Patient with a seventh nerve palsy following the removal of an acoustic neuroma requiring a wide, visually obstructing tarsorrhaphy for protection of the cornea. **B:** Patient in A with attempted closure of the eye with tarsorrhaphy in position.

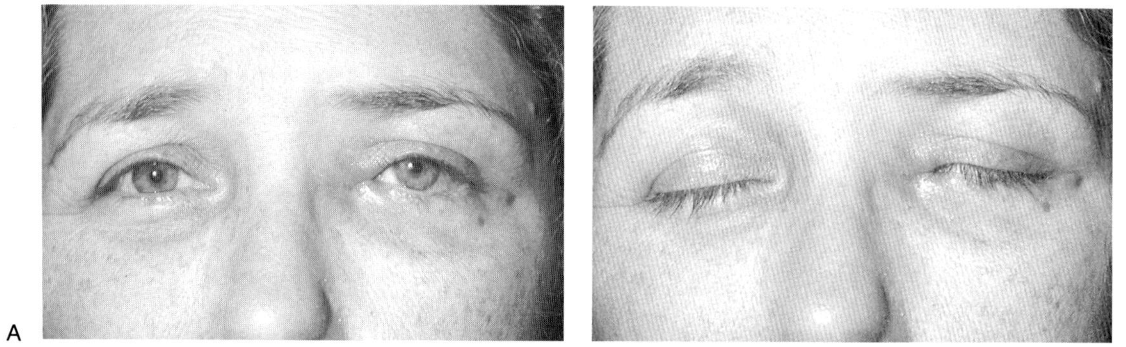

FIG. 9. **A:** Same patient as in Fig. 8 following implantation of the Arion silicone rod to the upper lid together with lower lid tightening showing the patient's ability to have almost full opening of the eye with good corneal protection. **B:** Same patient showing closure of the eye with the aid of the silicone rod in the upper lid.

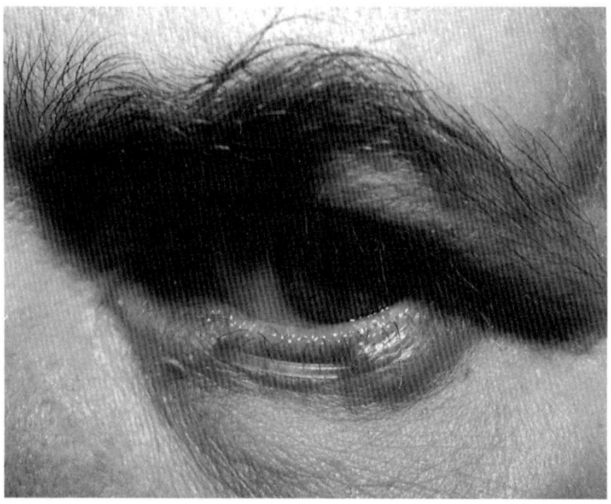

FIG. 10. Patient showing erosion of a silicone rod that has been placed in the Cerclage manner through the upper and lower lid.

to the globe. An overcorrection at this stage allows for loosening with time. If the patient is asleep, the pressure achieved with a hanging standard hemostat is a fair approximation of the tension required. Closure is made in layers to keep the silicone deep to orbicularis and subcutaneous tissue. If adjustments are needed later, these ends may be reexposed, untied, and readjusted. Prophylactic antibiotics should be considered postoperatively to reduce the chance of infection (Figs. 8A, B; 9A, B).

Problems encountered with the Arion filament are several. A rod that is not passed through the bone laterally may tear free. Subcutaneous migration of the rod can occur in the medial area if the rod is too superficial nasally or not well behind the medial limb of the medial palpebral tendon. Infection requires removal and replacement of the silicone rod. Undercorrection is most common and occurs from a reluctance to initially create enough tension on the silicone rod. Finally, erosion of the silicone through the medial canthal tendon or the eyelid proper will occur with time in many cases (Fig. 10).

Gold Weight Implant (Lid Loading)

More popular than the silicone implant because of ease of implantation is the eyelid load prosthesis, a gold weight that can be obtained from the Meddev Cor-

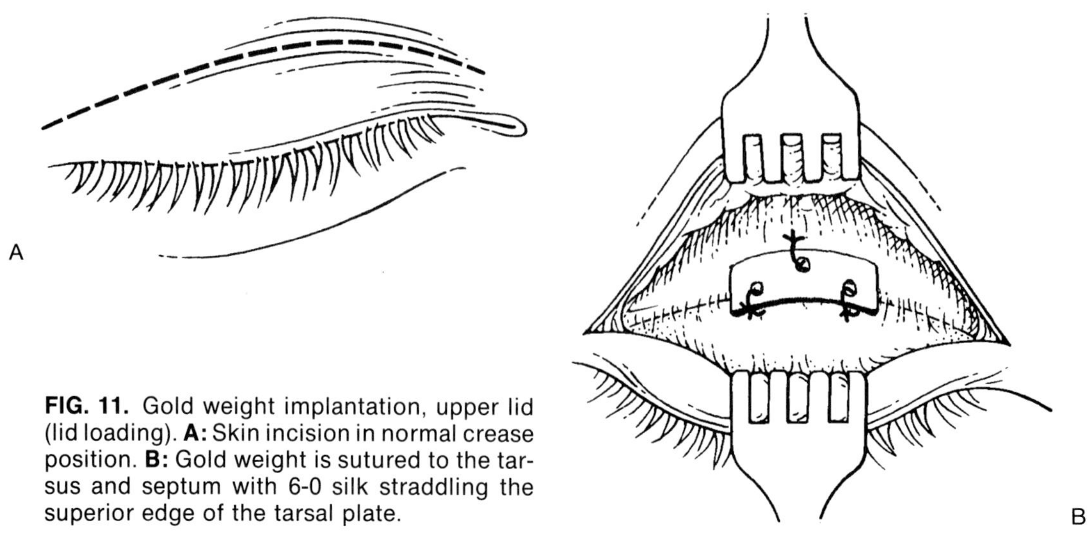

FIG. 11. Gold weight implantation, upper lid (lid loading). **A:** Skin incision in normal crease position. **B:** Gold weight is sutured to the tarsus and septum with 6-0 silk straddling the superior edge of the tarsal plate.

poration (Los Altos, California). The weights vary from $^{6}/_{10}$ g to $^{16}/_{10}$ g; however, the most commonly used weight is a 1- to 1-$^{4}/_{10}$-g weight. In the upright position, gravity acts on the gold implant in the upper lid and assists upper lid closure when the levator muscles relaxes.

The technique that is preferred by these authors is to use a midrange weight (1.2–1.4 g) placed at the superior tarsal border (Fig. 11A–D). The weight is placed in the upper lid under local anesthesia maintaining lid kinesia and patient cooperation. It has not been the authors' experience that pretaping a weight to the upper lid and

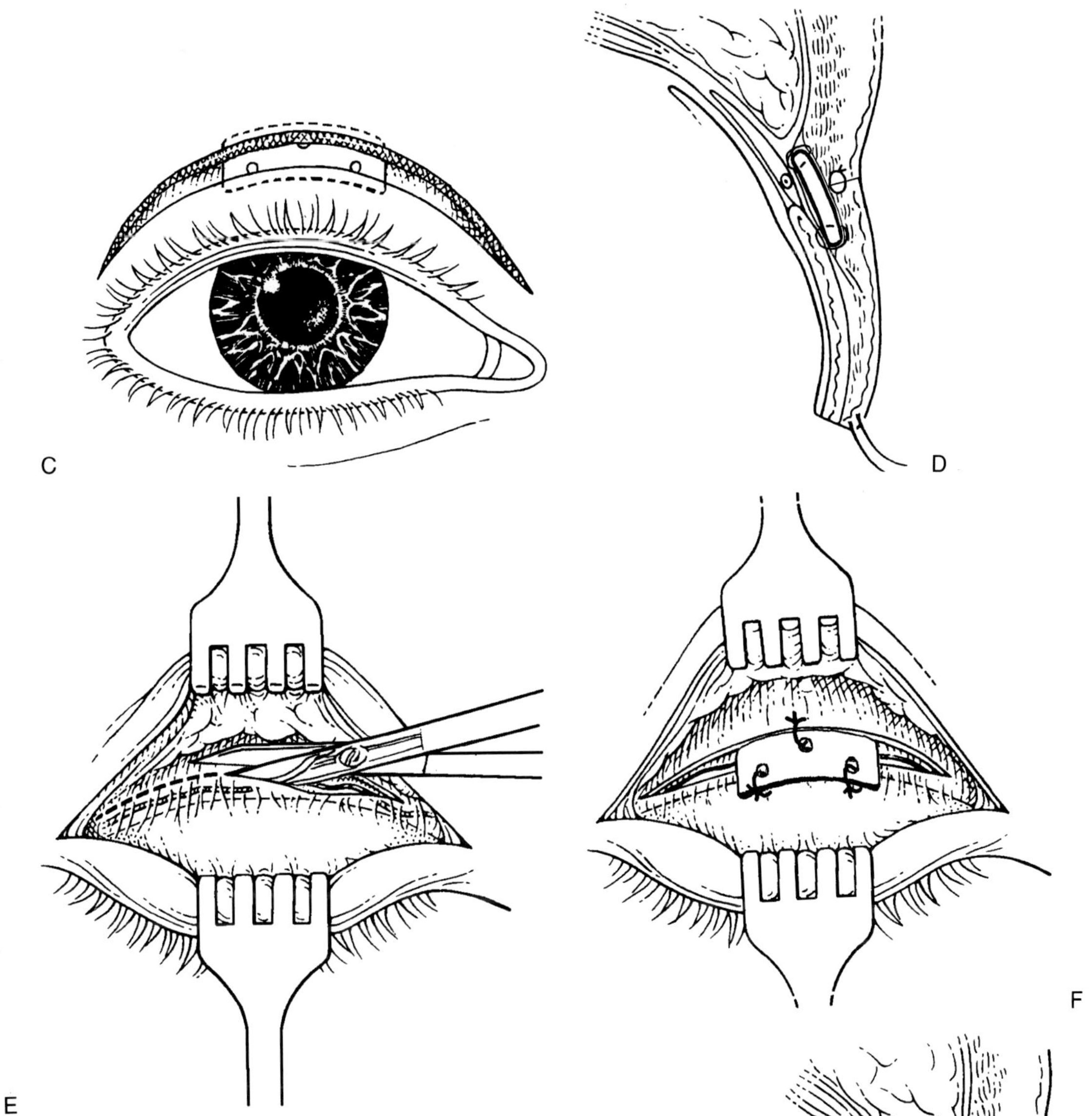

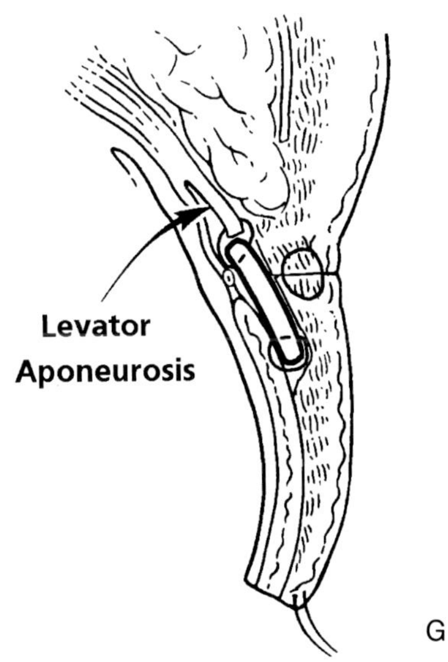

FIG. 11. *Continued.* **C:** Position of the gold weight at the superior tarsal edge. **D:** Saggital view showing position of the gold weight. The orbicularis fibers and skin are closed separately. **E:** Dissection of levator aponeurosis for recession of the upper lid. **F:** Suturing of gold weight to the tarsus and recessed levator. **G:** Sagittal view showing position of gold weight with the recessed levator. The orbicularis fibers are closed separately.

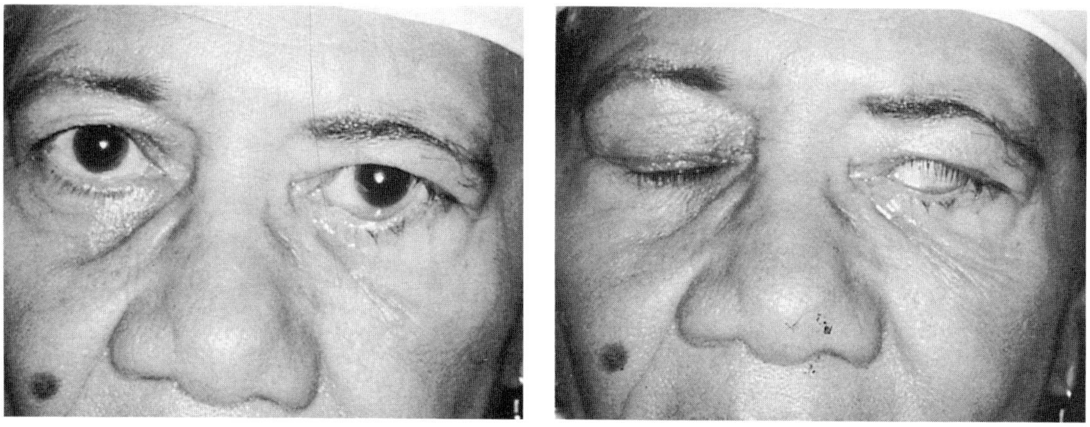

FIG. 12. **A:** Patient with unresolved Bell's palsy on the left side with ectropion and eyebrow ptosis. **B:** Same patient showing lagophthalmos and poor lid closure.

observing closure in the office always correlates with the effective weight used.

In most facial paralysis cases of long standing (a year or more), there is contracture of the antagonist levator muscle causing retraction of the upper lid. This is almost invariably present but in some cases may be masked by brow ptosis or by a previously placed tarsorraphy. A common procedure used is placement of the gold weight at the superior tarsal border in combination with recession of the levator aponeurosis (Fig. 11E–G) and has given optimum closure with fewer side effects from heavier weights (Figs. 12A, B; 13A, B).

There are other variations in the method of implantation in the upper lid. One technique involves the placement of the weight just above the lashes to reduce the amount of weight needed and to increase the leverage of closure. Side effects of this method, which can occur in some cases, are an erosion of the upper lid, entropion of the lashes, and an unsightly appearance (Figs. 14A, B; 15).

Eyebrow Surgery

The loss of innervation of frontalis muscle causes a downward displacement of the eyebrow. In patients who do have some preexisting laxity, the brow will slide down on the upper lid causing tethering of movement and ptosis, which can be quite frustrating to the patient. The direct supra brow pexy with excision of a strip of skin is the most common way of correcting this problem (15). This is a variation of technique used for brow pexy in cosmetic patients with the difference that the brow is sutured to the galea as opposed to the

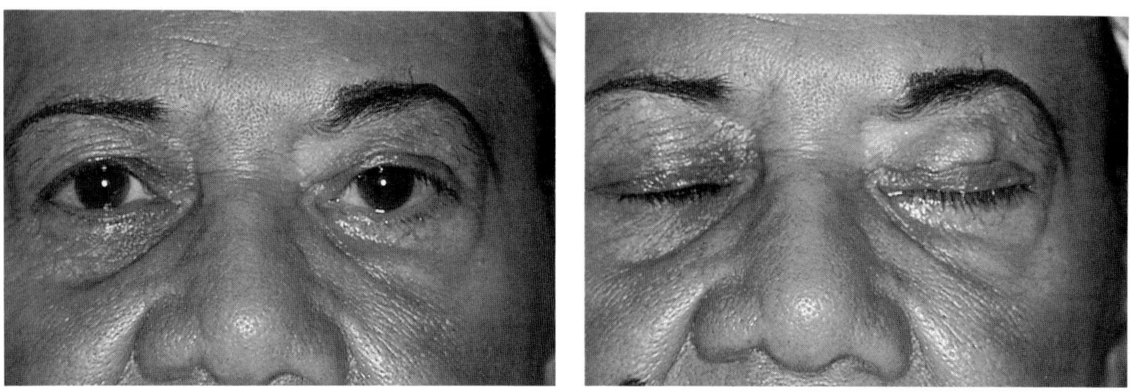

FIG. 13. **A:** Same patient as shown in Fig. 12 following levator recession and a 1.4-g gold weight in the upper lid, a direct supra brow pexy, and a fascia sling to the lower lid. **B:** Same patient in A showing eyelid closure with the gold weight visible at the superior tarsal edge.

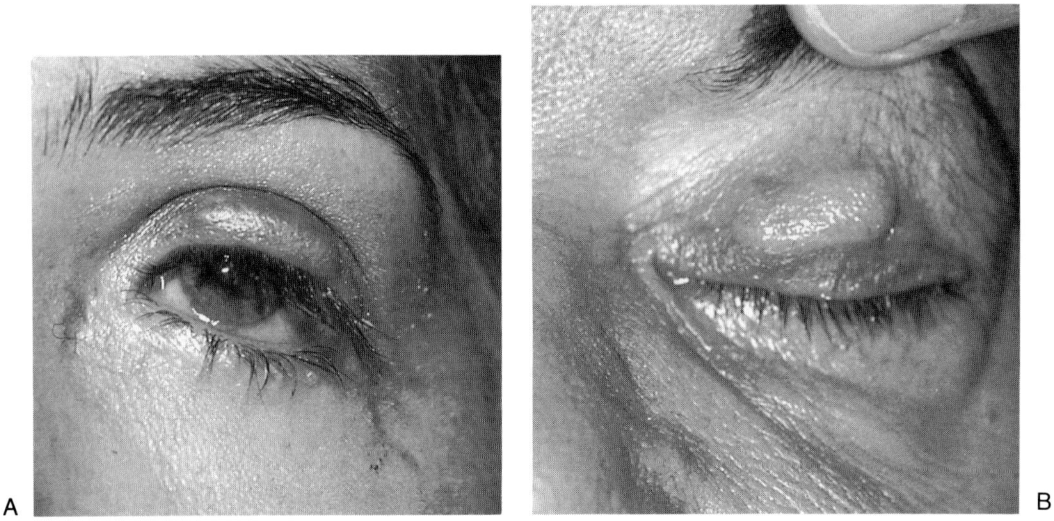

FIG. 14. A: Patient showing gold weight that was placed lower down on anterior tarsal surface causing entropion of the lashes and visual blockage. **B:** A more desirable position of the gold weight higher above the lash line.

frontalis muscle (Fig. 16). In most patients this is quite satisfactory. An alternative brow forehead lift (open coronal or endoscopic) may be used in younger patients.

Reanimation of the Eyelids and Face with Temporalis Muscle Attachment

Eyelid closure synchronous with contracture of the temporalis muscle can be obtained in the paralyzed eyelid with fascial attachments to the lid which are in turn attached to a flap of temporalis muscle. The movement is anomalous in that it is not synkinetic with the opposite eyelid movement, but the procedure can be used in patients with exposure not correctable by other methods. The technique also has the advantage of using the same temporalis muscle segment to attach the fascial strip to the lower face to improve mouth and facial sagging, which is unsightly and can interfere with eating and talking (15–17).

The original procedure was thought to restore movement to the eyelids and lower face with mechanical effect of temporalis contracture transmitted through the fascial strips. It is very probable, however, that some of the eyelid animation actually comes from myoneuritonization of the eyelid muscles from the temporalis muscle itself. Even though attached to the temporalis muscle, the fascia strips to the lower face tend to become static in time. The procedure can, however, be

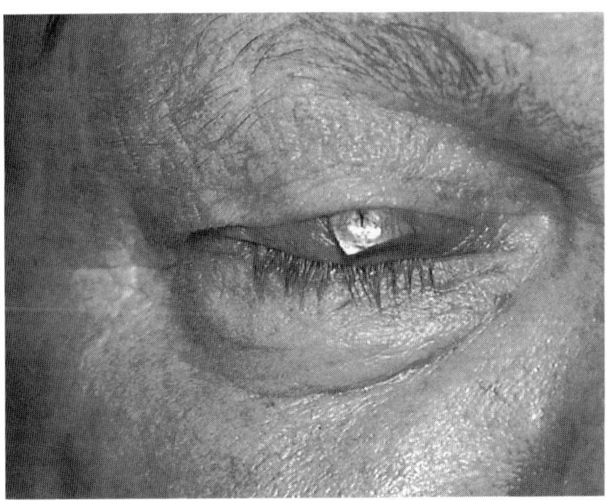

FIG. 15. Patient with extrusion of a Job weight through skin dehiscence possibly from poor closure of orbicularis and skin.

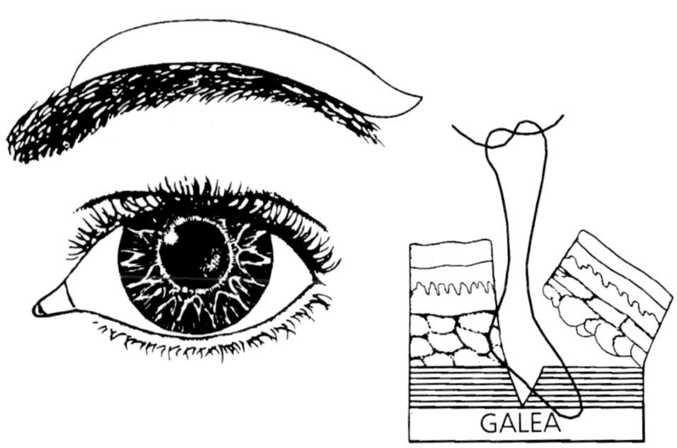

FIG. 16. Direct supra brow pexy used in patients with facial paralysis showing suturing of the brow to the deep tissue and galea for firm fixation.

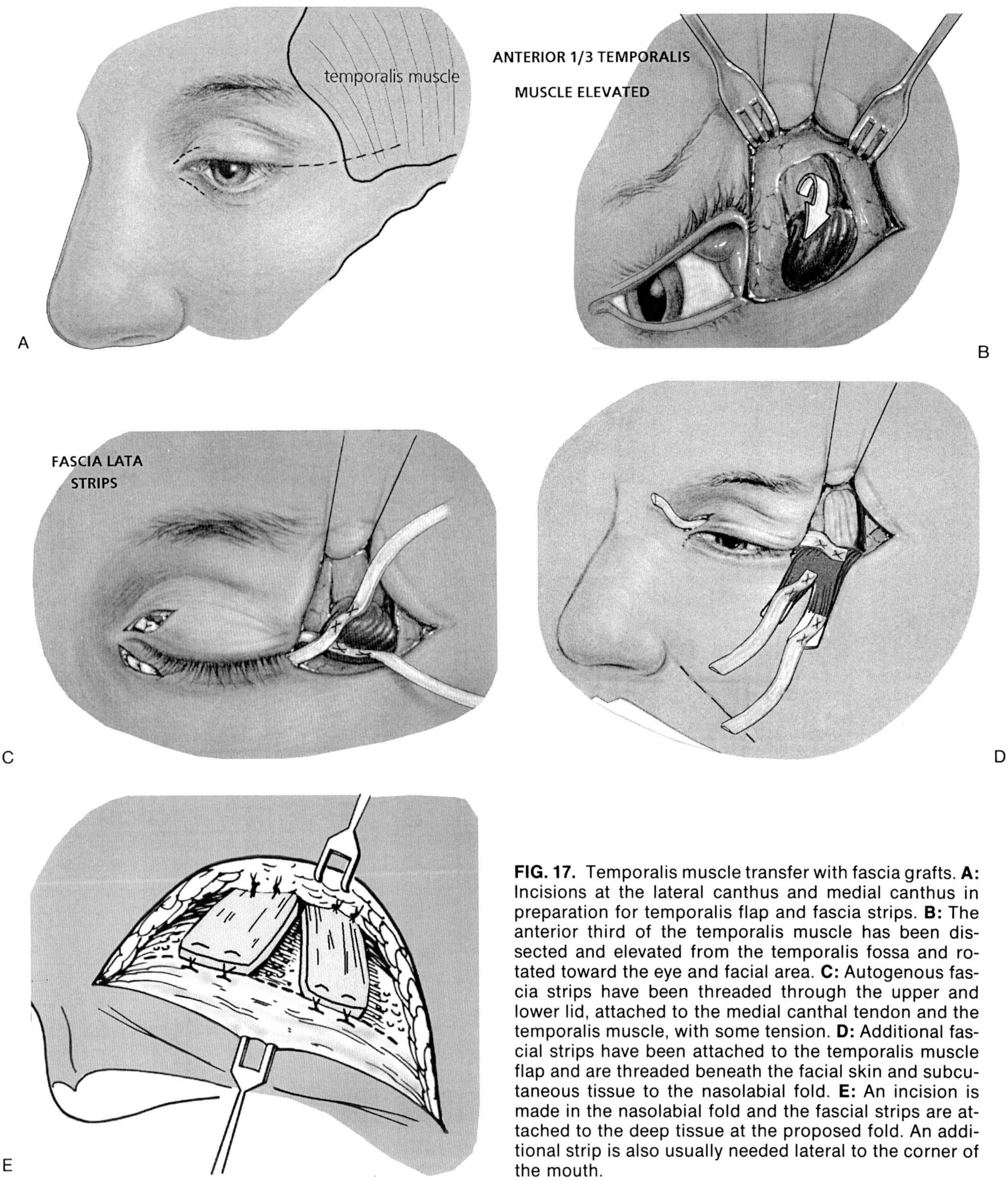

FIG. 17. Temporalis muscle transfer with fascia grafts. **A:** Incisions at the lateral canthus and medial canthus in preparation for temporalis flap and fascia strips. **B:** The anterior third of the temporalis muscle has been dissected and elevated from the temporalis fossa and rotated toward the eye and facial area. **C:** Autogenous fascia strips have been threaded through the upper and lower lid, attached to the medial canthal tendon and the temporalis muscle, with some tension. **D:** Additional fascial strips have been attached to the temporalis muscle flap and are threaded beneath the facial skin and subcutaneous tissue to the nasolabial fold. **E:** An incision is made in the nasolabial fold and the fascial strips are attached to the deep tissue at the proposed fold. An additional strip is also usually needed lateral to the corner of the mouth.

quite beneficial in patients with this severe deformity. Some patients who would benefit greatly from the procedure are those with combined fifth and seventh nerve paralysis. Because the temporalis muscle is innervated by the fifth nerve, it is denervated also and usually cannot be used in these patients.

A lateral canthotomy and horizontal incision exposes the temporalis fascia. Incisions are made in the

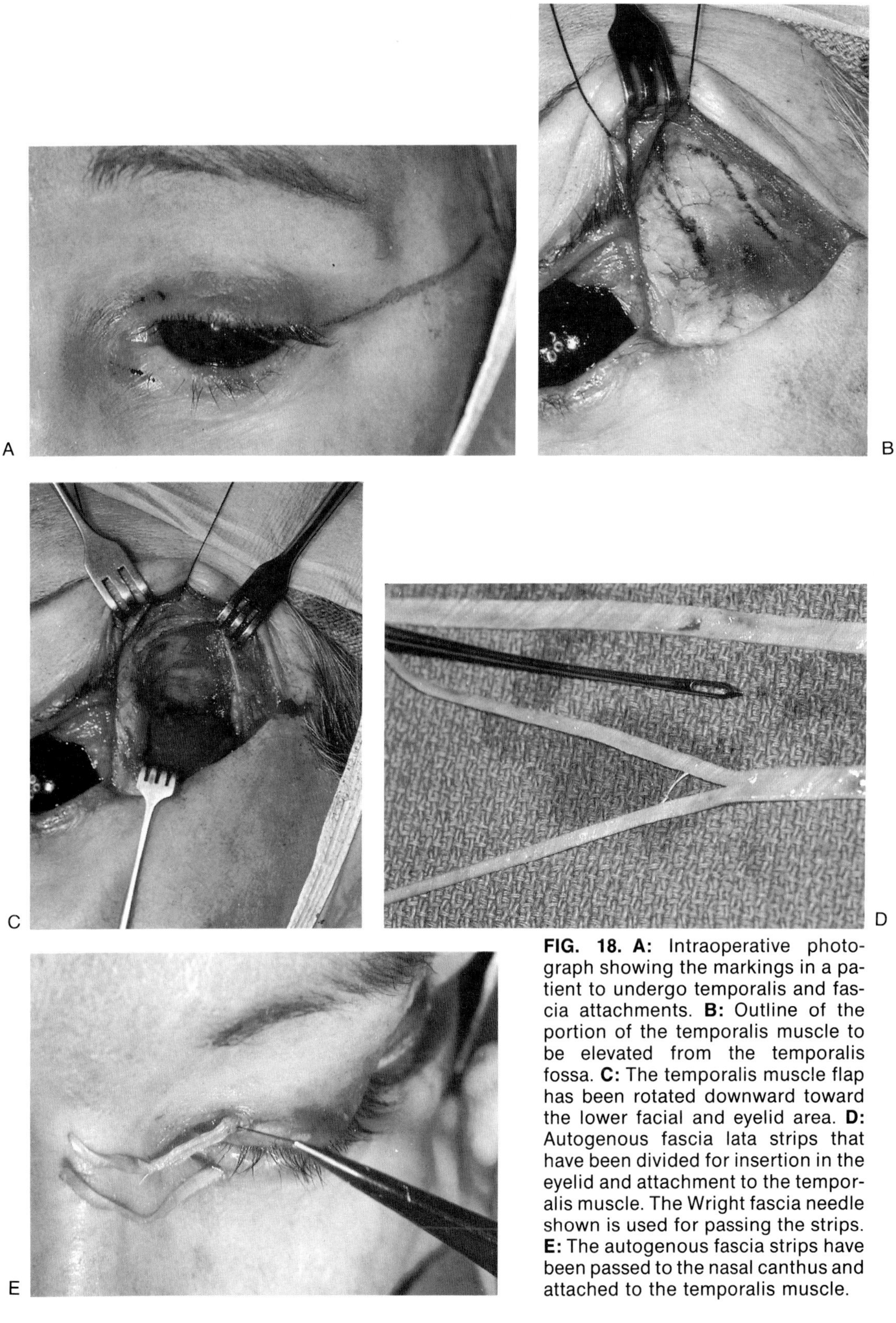

FIG. 18. A: Intraoperative photograph showing the markings in a patient to undergo temporalis and fascia attachments. **B:** Outline of the portion of the temporalis muscle to be elevated from the temporalis fossa. **C:** The temporalis muscle flap has been rotated downward toward the lower facial and eyelid area. **D:** Autogenous fascia lata strips that have been divided for insertion in the eyelid and attachment to the temporalis muscle. The Wright fascia needle shown is used for passing the strips. **E:** The autogenous fascia strips have been passed to the nasal canthus and attached to the temporalis muscle.

medial canthus exposing the anterior reflection of the medial canthal tendon (Figs. 17A, 18A). The flap to be elevated is outlined on the temporalis fascia and is marked and incised with the cutting Bovie and periosteal elevator (Fig. 17B; Fig. 18B, C). It is helpful to thoroughly infiltrate the muscle with xylocaine and adrenalin before incision. Autogenous fascia lata strips are fashioned and threaded in the submuscular plane

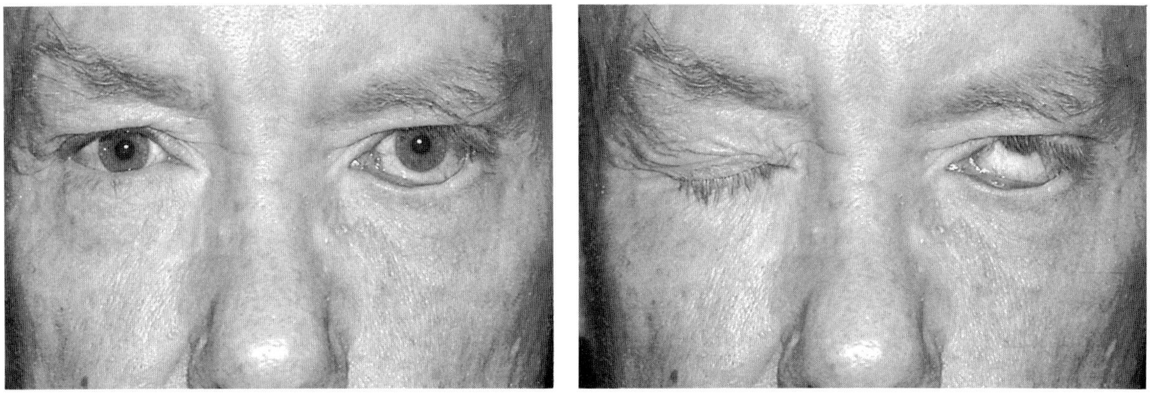

A B

FIG. 19. A: Patient with facial paralysis on the left following tumor resection with poor closure and exposure. **B:** Same patient showing attempted closure of eyelids.

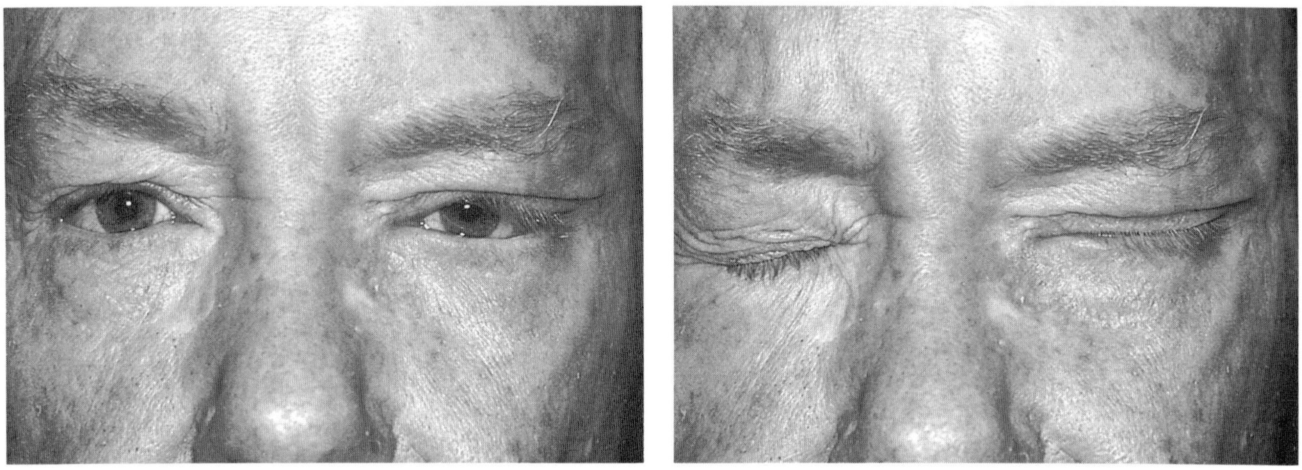

A B

FIG. 20. A: Same patient shown in Fig. 19 following temporalis muscle transfer with fascia strips to the eyelid showing the patient without jaw clenching and open eyelids (a lower facial suspension was also performed). **B:** Same patient in Fig. 19 following temporalis muscle transfer with fascia strips to the eyelid showing the patient with jaw clenching and eyelid closure.

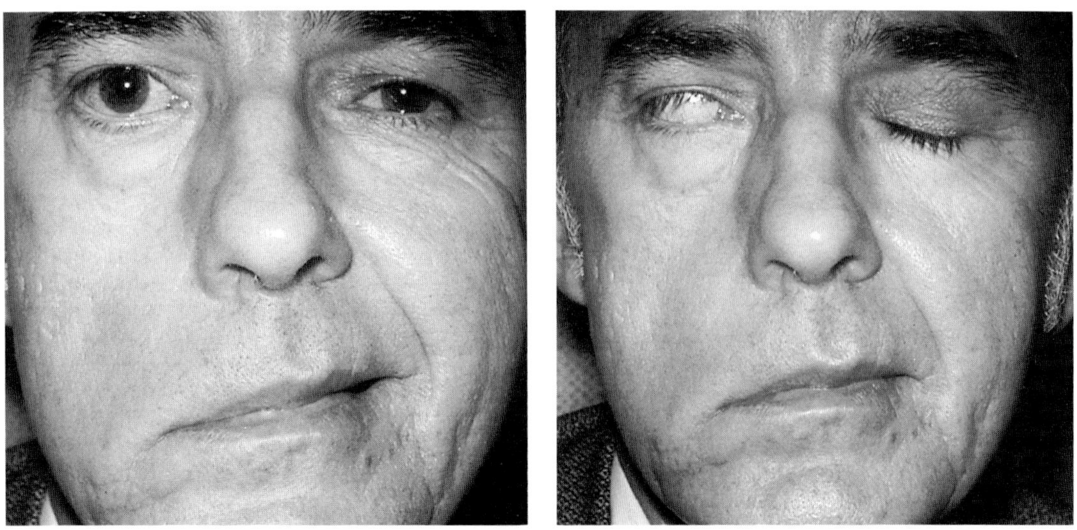

A B

FIG. 21. A: Patient with facial paralysis on the right showing mouth drop and lagophthalmos. **B:** Same patient showing poor eyelid closure and corneal exposure.

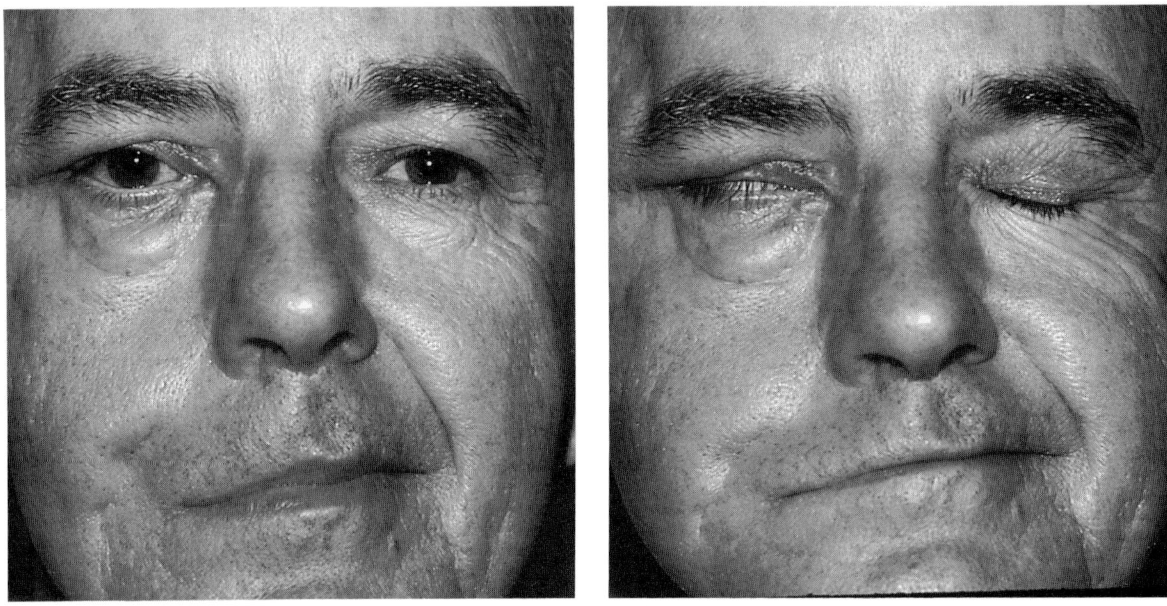

A B

FIG. 22. A: Same patient in Fig. 21 following temporalis transfer with fascia strips attached to the eyelids and to the nasolabial fold area showing support of the midface and improvement of the lip and mouth position. The jaw is unclenched. **B:** Same patient showing closure of the eyelids with jaw clenching and some face movement following the procedure.

from the lateral incision to the medial canthal tendon and fixated to the tendon (Figs. 17C and 18D). They are then sutured to the flap of temporalis muscle under moderately firm tension (Figs. 17C and 18E). Additional strips of fascia lata can be threaded to the nasolabial fold area and then attached to the temporalis muscle flap for movement, or attached to the zygoma as a static sling for the lip and mouth (Fig. 17D, E). The eyelid procedure is usually reserved for patients who have not responded well to other surgical procedures. The procedure, however, can protect and restore the patient to useful vision in many of these cases (Figs. 19A, B; 20A, B). The patient can also be offered an added benefit of improved mouth and lip function with additional fascia strips to the upper lip and mouth area (Figs. 21A, B; 22A, B).

REFERENCES

1. May M, Hardin WB: Facial palsy: interpretation of neurologic findings. *Laryngoscope* 1978;88:1352–1362.
2. Bajandas FJ. The seven syndromes of the facial nerve. In: *Neuro-ophthalmology board review manual*. Thorofare, NJ: Charles B Slack; 1980:139–141.
3. May M. Differential diagnosis by history, physical findings, and laboratory results. In: *The facial nerve*. Vol. 9. New York: Theime; 1986:183–184, 186.
4. Peitersen E. The natural history of Bell's palsy. *Am J Otolaryngol* 1982;4:107.
5. Wesley RE, Jackson CG, Glasscock ME III. Management of facial palsy. *Oculoplastic surgery*. 3rd ed. New York: Raven Press; 1995.
6. Kartush JM. Electroneurography and intraoperative facial monitoring in contemporary neurotology. *Otolaryngol Head Neck Surg* 1989;101(4):496–503.
7. Jackson CG, Glasscock ME, Hughes GB et al. Facial paralysis of neoplastic origin: diagnosis and management. *Laryngoscope* 1980;90:1581.
8. Marin Amat M. Sobre un nuevo caso de Marcus Gunn. *Arch Oftalmol Hisp-Am* 1930;30:530–536.
9. Masters FW, Robinson DW, Simons NJ. Temporalis transfer for lagophthalmos due to seventh nerve palsy. *Am J Surg* 1965; 110:607–611.
10. Jelks GW, Smith B, Bosniak S. The evaluation and management of the eye in facial palsy. *Clin Plast Surg* 1979;6:397–419.
11. Glasscock ME, Jackson CG, Hays JW. Facial hypoglossal anastomosis for treatment of facial paralysis. In: Silverstein H, Norrell H, eds. *Neurologic surgery of the ear*. Vol. 20. Birmingham, AL: Aesculapius; 1979:189.
12. Smellie GD. Restoration of the blinking reflex in facial palsy by a simple lid load operation. *Br J Plast Surg* 1966;19:279–283.
13. Morel J, Fatio D, Lelardrie JP. Paliative surgical treatment of facial paralysis: the palpebral spring. *Plast Reconstr Surg* 1964; 33:447.
14. Arion HG. Dynamic closure of the lids in paralysis of the orbicularis muscle. *Int Surg* 1972;57:48–50.
15. Beard C. Canthoplasty and brow elevation for facial palsy. *Arch Ophthalmol* 1964;71:386.
16. Rubin LR. *Reanimation of the paralyzed face: new approaches*. St. Louis: CV Mosby; 1977:53–80, 125–131.
17. Rubin LR, Lee GW, Simpson RL. Reanimation of the longstanding partial facial paralysis. *Plast Reconstr Surg* 1986;77: 41–49.
18. Rubin LR. Entire temporalis muscle transposition. In: *Reanimation of the paralysed face: new approaches*. St. Louis: CV Mosby; 1977:294–315.

CHAPTER 28

Principles of Management of Eyelid Trauma

Surgical techniques and principles that were described in previous chapters can be utilized in the treatment of eyelid trauma in acute and posttraumatic situations. It is important to recognize, however, that there are special aspects of evaluation and treatment of eyelid tissues unique to the clinical setting of acute eyelid trauma. This chapter will emphasize primarily general principles of management and care of these patients and will refer to surgical techniques previously described when necessary.

Traumatic events that damage the eyelid tissue can also damage other important structures. In some situations this fact may be obscured by the urgency of the visible eyelid injury; however, these other injuries should be recognized so the surgeon can preserve threatened visual function and so medicolegal considerations can be satisfied.

In these situations of acute eyelid trauma, before proceeding to the repair of an eyelid the surgeon should conscientiously search for other possible injuries and evaluate the surrounding tissue with a systematic approach. It is important to rule out any injury to the globe itself because its treatment may take priority over the management of the eyelid. Adequate inspection of the globe to ensure that there is no corneal laceration, measurement of the visual acuity, and fundus examination should allow the surgeon to rule out a direct injury to the globe or any penetration from a foreign object.

Many patients will present with a very small eyelid puncture wound or laceration; however, close questioning of the patient regarding the mechanisms of the injury is necessary and the possibility of retained foreign bodies should be considered. A common situation is the story of a person running through the woods and being hit in the eye with a branch of a tree. The patient may present with a minimal external puncture wound but have a retained wooden foreign body (Fig. 1A, B).

Many very small lacerations of the eyelid skin can be managed without suturing if the edges are well approximated; however, the eyelid margin should be inspected very closely for any damage because uncontrolled healing in that area may lead to notching of the lid and trichiasis.

The eyelid movement should be inspected to determine any facial nerve injury or any damage to the levator muscle. It is possible that ptosis from levator damage may need subsequent surgery regardless of the situation, but it is very important to record this finding.

In the inner corner of the eyelids, lacerations may extend into the lacrimal canaliculus. If the canaliculus is not splinted internally during the healing period, stenosis will occur causing tearing at a later date. Silicone intubation with the use of Crawford intubation is a convenient method for splinting the canalicular system.

REPAIR OF FULL-THICKNESS EYELID LACERATION INCLUDING MARGIN

The most common eyelid problem that the specialty surgeon will be called on to repair in the acute situation is a laceration including the eyelid margin and skin-muscle layer. Many times these full-thickness injuries are a result of a wound from a sharp object or in some cases can be the result of a shearing effect. An important principle involved in the repair of these defects in order to avoid postoperative notching (Fig. 2) is the same principle mentioned in Chapter 24 on full-thickness eyelid reconstruction of upper and lower lids. The edges of the tarsal plate should be parallel when realigned so that the margin of the lid will form a normal contour and not produce a notch. In many cases if the edges of the wound are irregular and the tarsal plate is fragmented, the tarsal edges will not line up in the desired manner. Some judicious trimming of the edges of the tarsal plate to produce parallel sides for closure must be performed (Figs. 3 and 4). The lid should be closed in layers with the most important closure being that of the tarsal plate (Fig. 3).

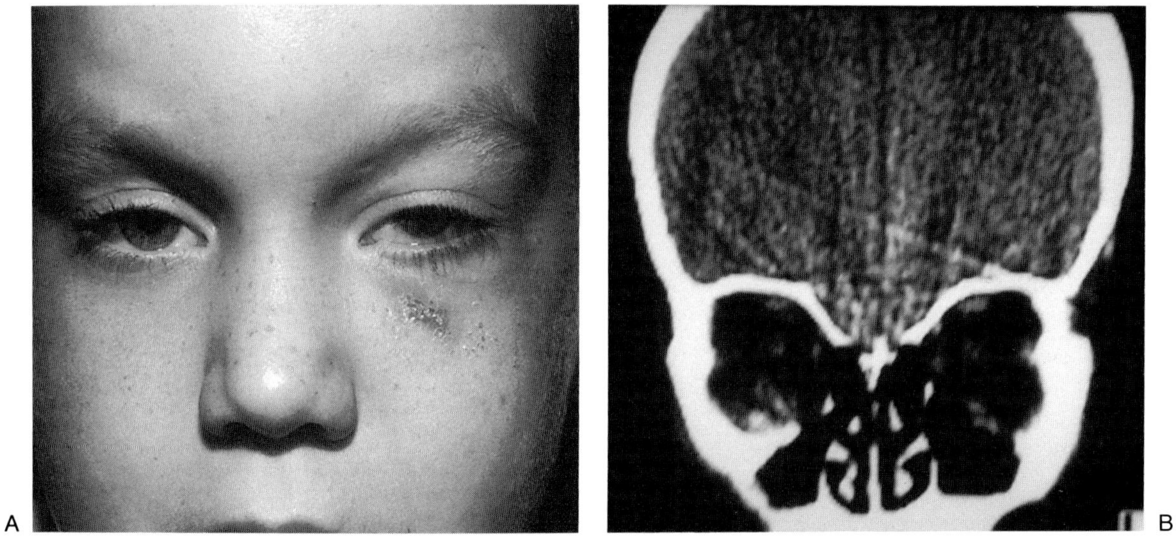

FIG. 1. A: A young patient who was struck by a branch running through the woods, lacerating his eyelid. After further questioning, the possibility of a retained wooden foreign body was entertained. **B:** Coronal CT scan of the patient (with a "narrow window") showing a retained wood fragment in the lower lid, inferior fornix, and inferior orbit.

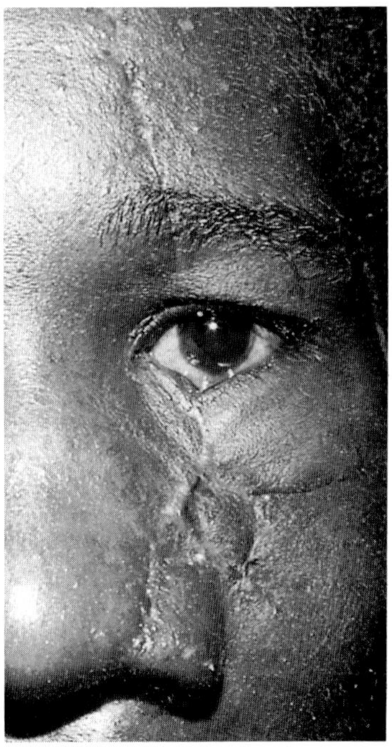

FIG. 2. Patient with notching and depressed scars following vertical laceration of the brow and lower lid and cheek. The notching and retraction is due to adhesions formed between the deep tissue, periosteum, and skin.

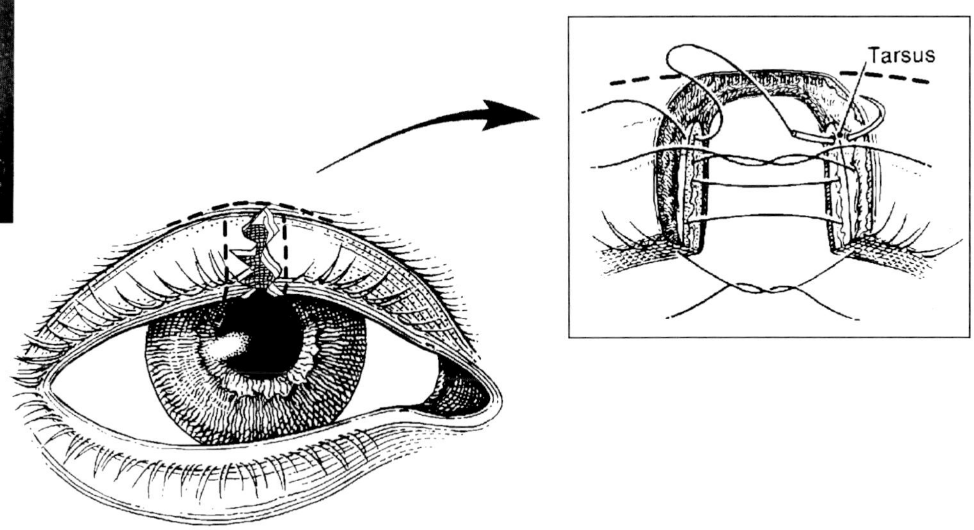

FIG. 3. Diagram showing a full-thickness laceration through the upper lid margin. This type of laceration requires trimming of the edges of the tarsal plate to produce parallel-sided edges to allow closure of the upper lid without notching.

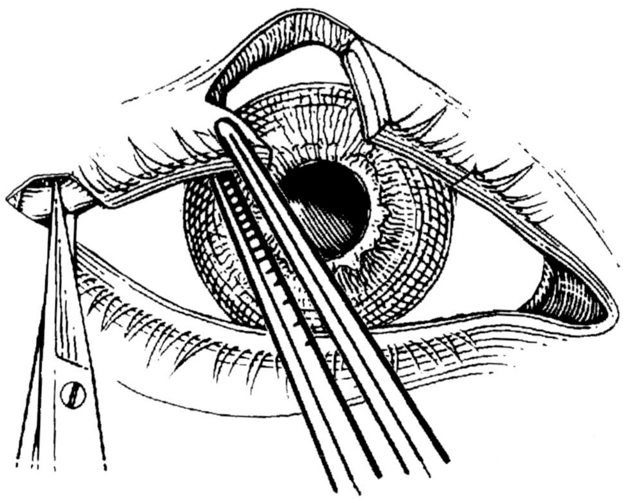

FIG. 4. Canthotomy and cantholysis of the upper canthal tendon. If there has been tissue loss (from the injury or after trimming) there may be more tension on the margins than allows direct closure. To produce laxity for closure, cantholysis is necessary in some cases.

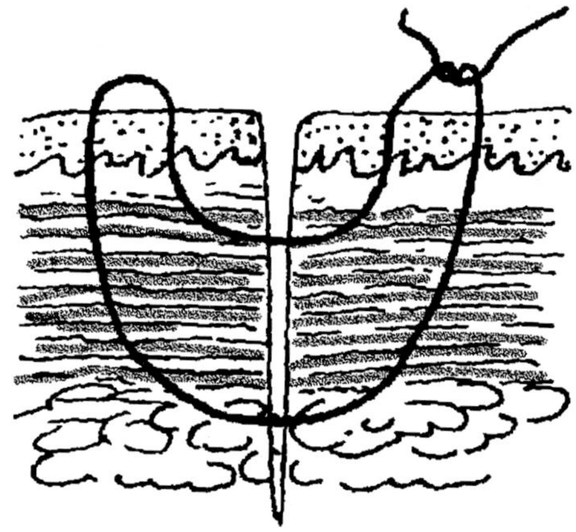

FIG. 6. Preliminary mattress sutures (before skin closure sutures) can aid with deep closure and skin eversion.

REPAIR OF LID–BROW–CHEEK LACERATIONS

Many wounds through the eyelid will extend to the orbital rim and deeper tissue into the facial or brow area. Devices such as chain saws may even penetrate the wall of a sinus. If the tissue is not closed in every layer, there will be a tendency for fibrous bands to form between bony structures and the deep tissue and the external skin layer causing depressed scars. This will cause retraction of the lid and notching. Skin edges should be everted to minimize indentation of the scar with healing (Figs. 5 and 6). When faced with deep wounds, care must be taken to close the tissue in layers and to ensure deep tissue closure of fascia layers, muscular layers, beneath the skin-dermis edges to prevent the formation of vertical adhesions (Figs. 7–9).

Figure 10A shows a patient who suffered a chain saw injury that damaged the orbital rim, penetrating the antrum and frontal sinus. It also lacerated the patient's globe and produced deep lacerations to the face, forehead, and orbit. The injury was closed initially with sealing of the sinuses and closure of deep tissue in layers. The patient required enucleation of the globe and has had one subsequent revision with dermabrasion. Figure 10B shows the results that can be obtained by observing principles of layered closure.

FULL-THICKNESS EYELID DEFECTS

When, in an acute situation, the surgeon is confronted with significant missing full-thickness eyelid tissue creating a defect, the defect must be repaired as described in the chapters on eyelid reconstruction. When faced with these acute full-thickness defects, the surgeon should not temporize but instead should insti-

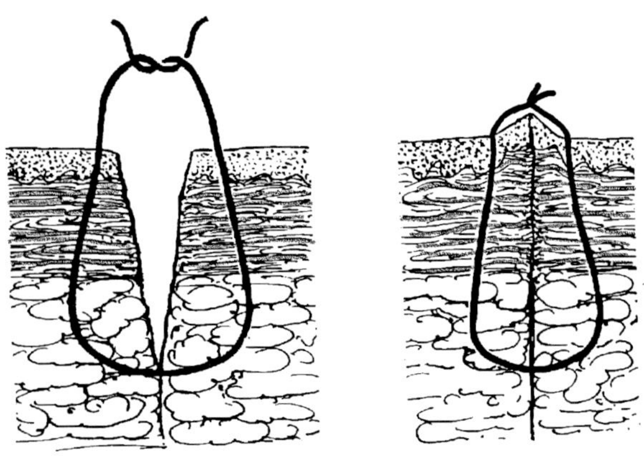

FIG. 5. Eversion of the skin edges reduces indentation of the scar line after healing. Skin closure sutures should encompass a wider amount of tissue deeper than in the skin edges to create eversion.

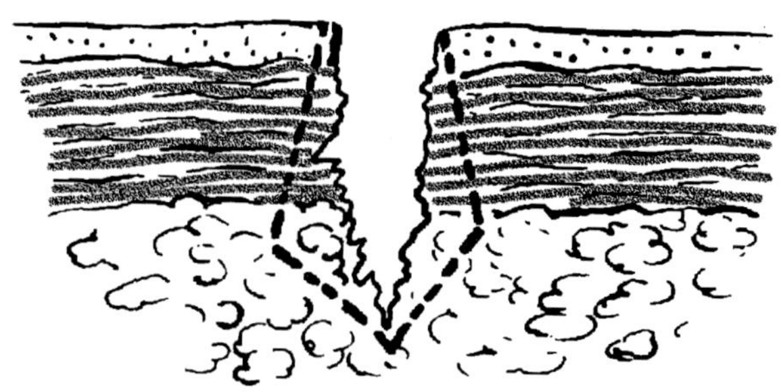

FIG. 7. Debridement for closure of deep layers. Deep muscle and fascia planes must be closed in the cheek and brow areas to prevent a depressed scar. As in the tarsus, some trimming may be necessary to allow even closure.

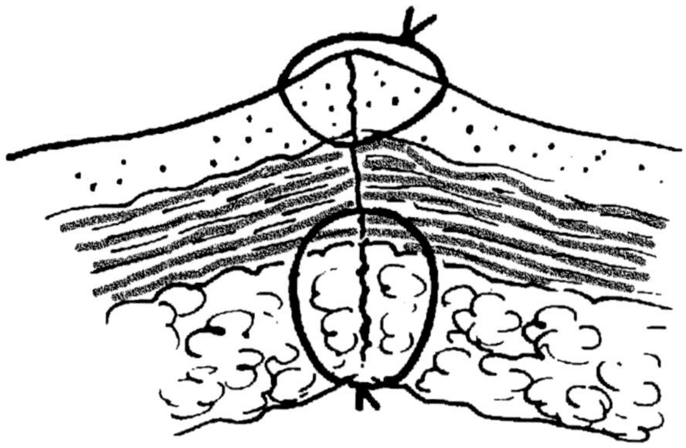

FIG. 8. Deep closure and skin-everting suture.

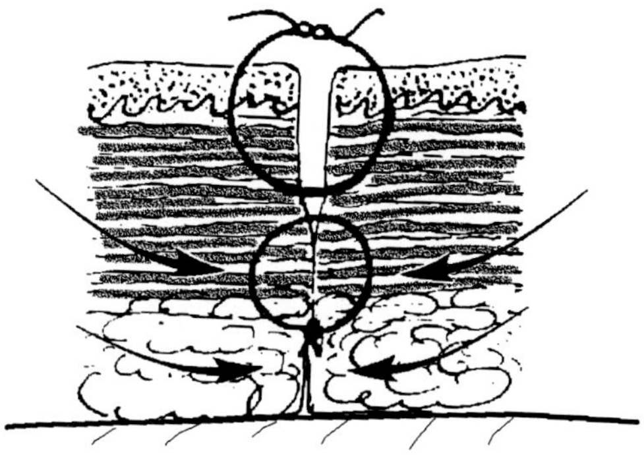

FIG. 9. Prevention of vertical adhesions to bone with deep closure.

tute the needed repair in the acute situation after analyzing the defect as described in the chapter on decision making in eyelid reconstruction.

PRESERVATION OF EYELID TISSUE

Other than the minimal debridement required to square off the tarsal edges or possibly deep tissue, no eyelid tissue should be discarded. Many patients will present with extensive injuries and tissue that seems macerated or disconnected from the eyelid and orbital area. There may be a tendency on the surgeon's part to discard this tissue or to consider it unviable and not use it in the initial repair. Figure 11A shows an extreme example of facial avulsion in which the lids have been totally separated from the orbit in this unusual and severe injury. It was noted that the avulsed facial tissue could be reposited and the eyelid fissure repositioned over the globe and orbital area. The subsequent healing over the next few weeks showed good viability of the eyelid tissue with a much more normal fissure than would occur if the tissue was discarded (Fig. 11B). In some cases, eyelid tissue will be completely detached

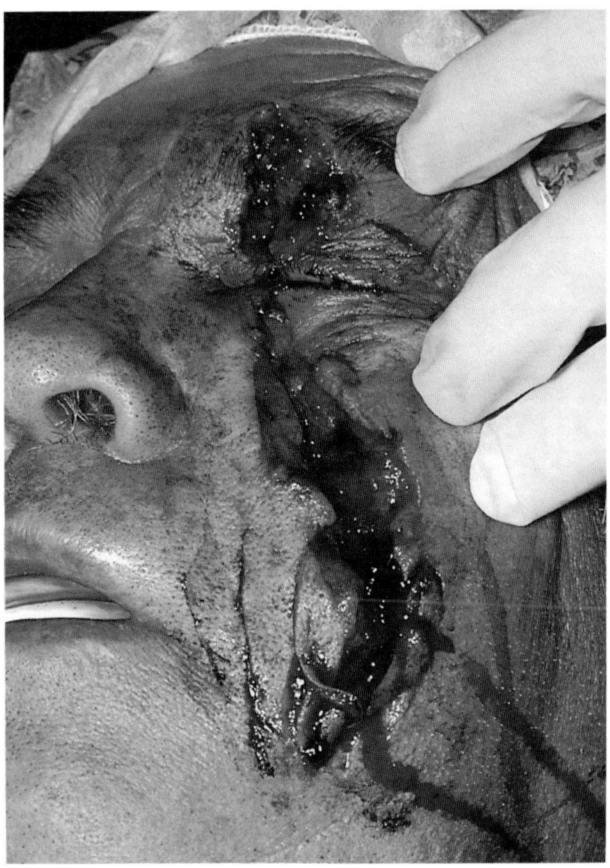

A

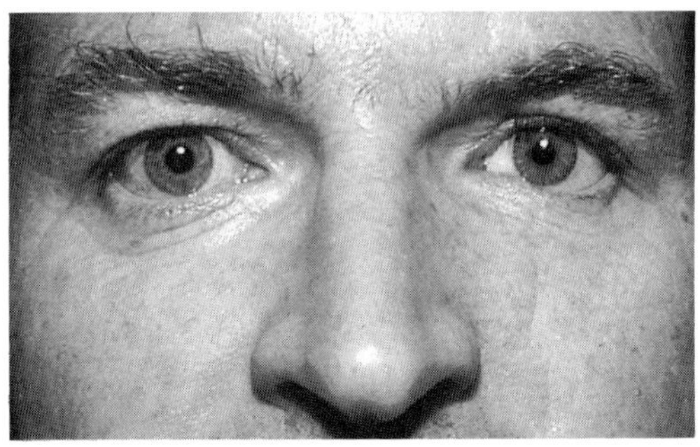

B

FIG. 10. A: Vertical chain saw laceration through the brow, upper lid, frontal sinus, inferior orbital rim, and antrum. B: Same patient postoperatively with good alignment of the tissue. The patient is wearing a prosthetic eye on the left.

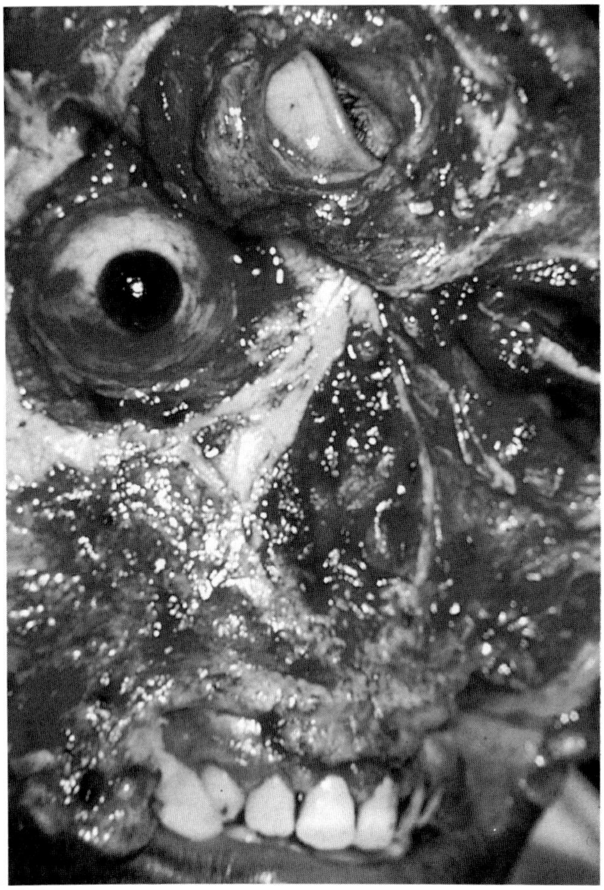
A

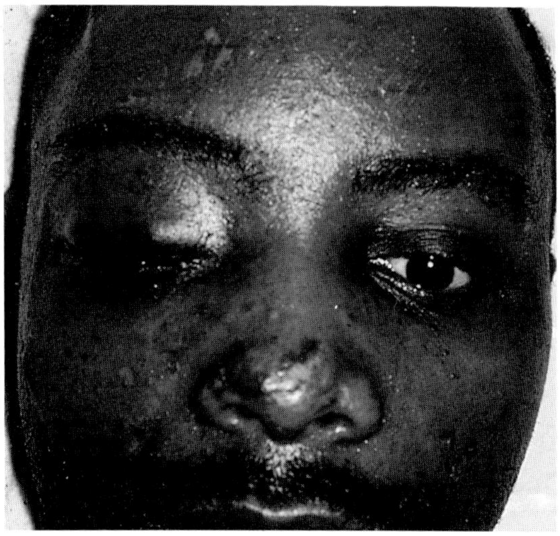
B

FIG. 11. A: Lower facial avulsion with total avulsion of the eyelid, nose, and facial soft tissue. This injury occurred in an automobile accident. **B:** Same patient after suturing of the facial flap with repositioning of the nose and the eyelids. The patient subsequently had normal contour of the lower lid but required ptosis surgery in the upper lid. Facial nerve function was retained.

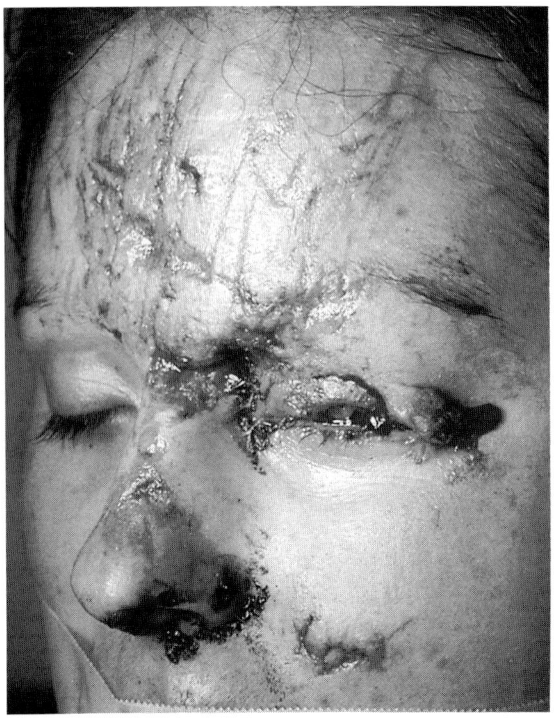
A

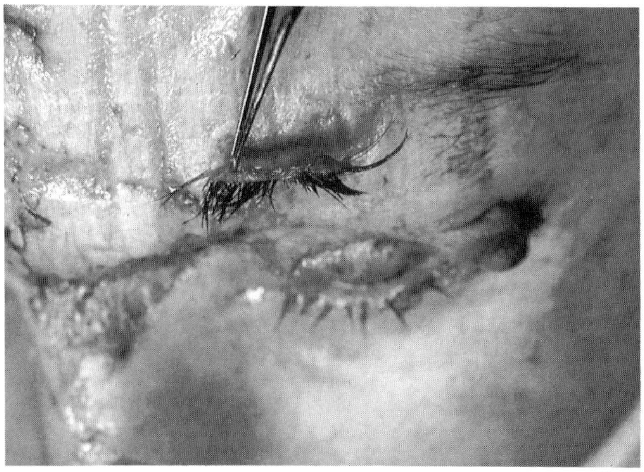
B

FIG. 12. A: Patient in an automobile accident with avulsion of the upper lid and margin. **B:** The avulsed margin of the eyelid that was sent along with the patient. It was placed in iced saline.

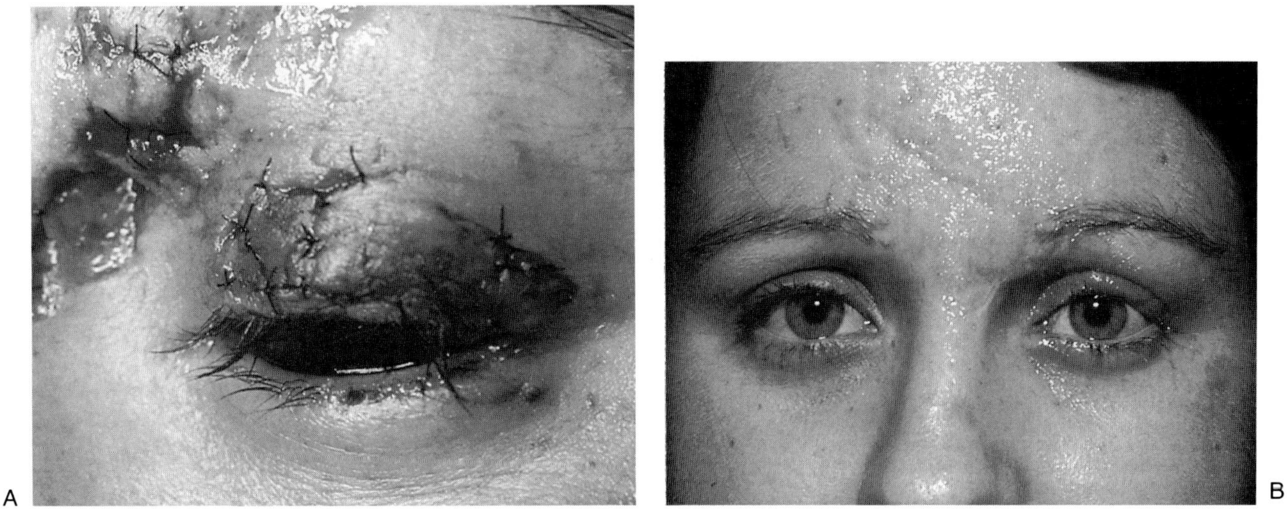

FIG. 13. **A:** The remnant of the lower lid margin has been sutured into position with initial closure. **B:** Same patient at 2 months with good upper lid contour and good margin architecture. The lashes have been only partially retained. It is difficult for the lash follicles to retain viability.

from the body and be discovered somewhere in the geographic vicinity.

Figure 12A shows a patient with an avulsion and detachment of eyelid tissue including most of the upper lid margin and tarsal plate. The detached tissue was discovered by the emergency team, placed in a saline ice bath, and returned with the patient (Fig. 12B). The detached tissue could be sutured in place (Fig. 13A) with good restoration of the contour, but unfortunately eyelash follicles may not survive this devitalization process. The patient had only partial eyelash recovery but good margin restoration (Fig. 13B). This points out that because of the excellent blood supply in the facial and eyelid area, detached tissue, despite being macerated and disconnected from the body, should be preserved because it can be viable and contribute to the substance of the lid.

ACUTE SKIN GRAFTING

In acute situations, many times occurring in the wee hours of the morning, the surgeon is tempted to simply "close what is present" and let the tissue granulate in. In small defects, in thick skin, away from the eyelid

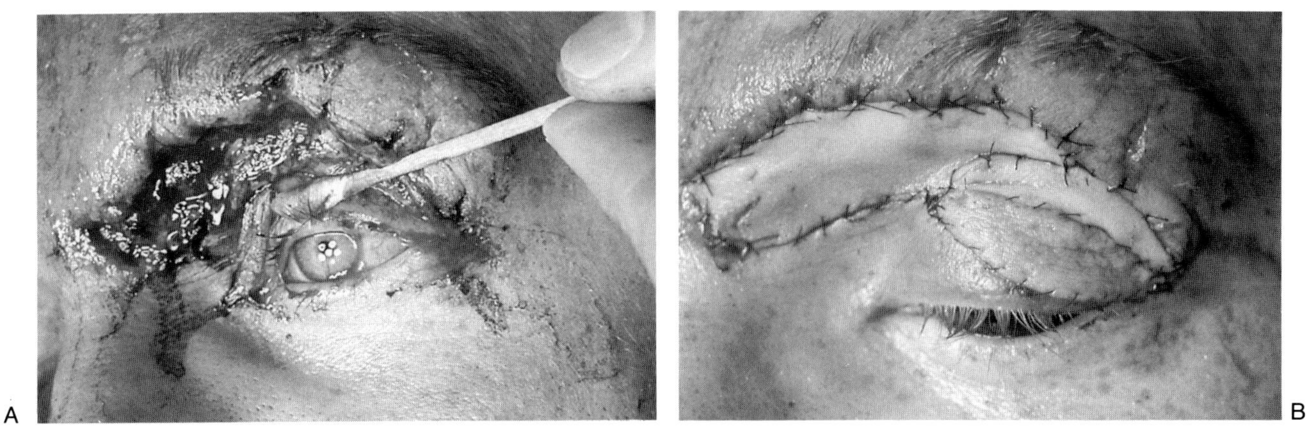

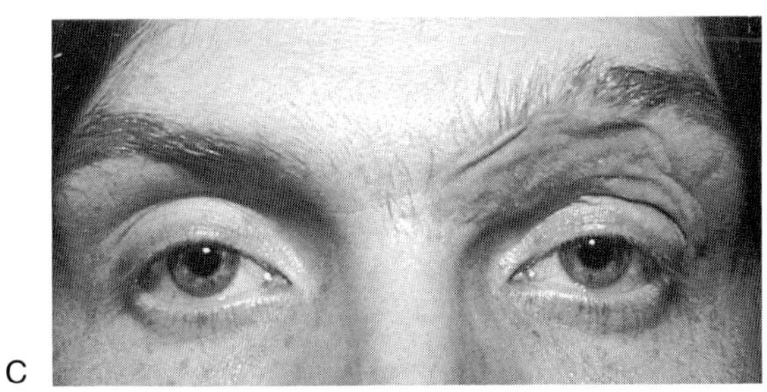

FIG. 14. **A:** Avulsion of the skin-muscle layer of the eyelid in an automobile accident. Defect encompasses brow, glabellar area, and upper lid skin. **B:** Skin grafts from both posterior auricular areas and supraclavicular area are needed to cover the defect. **C:** Same patient at 3 months following take of the grafts. The eyelid functioned normally. The patient did not desire further revisional work.

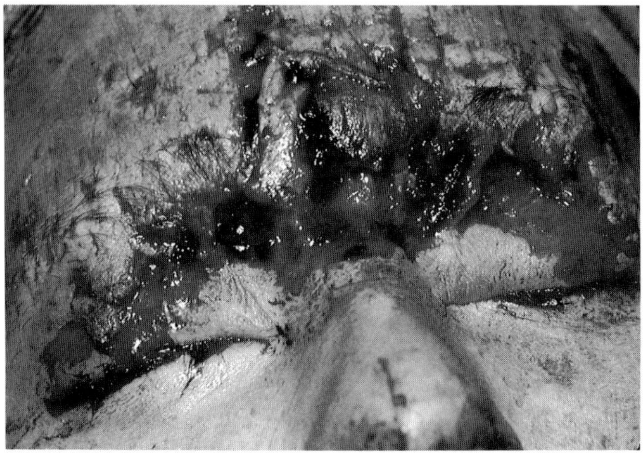

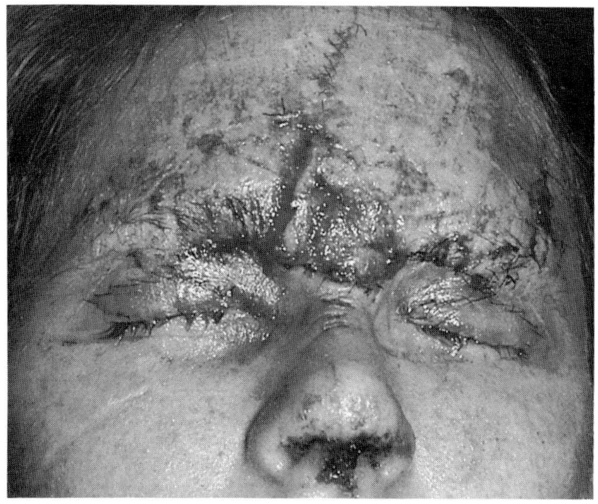

FIG. 15. Patient in an automobile accident with avulsion of the skin from the upper lid, brow, and glabellar area. **A:** Defects of skin are seen in the temporal portion of the lid in the nasal glabellar area with multiple abrasions and flaps in the forehead area. **B:** Same patient following placement of skin grafts in the upper lid from the retroauricular areas. The grafts were placed in the pretarsal eye shadow area and the existing eyelid skin was rotated up to the glabellar area as a flap. Repositioning and suturing of the flaps of forehead tissue was performed.

margin, granulation is effective in filling in defects. If large amounts of tissue are missing from the eyelid, one can be most certain that the tissue will contract postoperatively. If this occurs, the eyelids will be retracted from the globe, producing an exposure problem, and subsequent grafting will surely be necessary. Acute grafting can produce an excellent cosmetic result and can relieve the patient of the need to go through an unnecessary contracting phase with its morbidity over a period of weeks or months. Figure 14A shows a patient with a large area of avulsion of the skin-muscle layer of the upper lid and brow which, if ungrafted, most certainly would produce severe retraction of the upper lid with lagophthalmos and exposure. Full-thickness skin grafting was performed in this patient in the acute situation, with grafts taken from the supraclavicular and retroauricular areas (Fig. 14B). Available skin donor sites are described in the chapter on free grafts. The same patient is shown in Fig. 13C with good eyelid closure and reasonable contours, which, if better cosmetics is desired, can be revised if necessary. Figure 15A shows another patient who had an automobile accident involving driving her car underneath a trailer truck. She had avulsion of skin from the upper lids, multiple smaller areas of avulsed skin, tags of avulsed skin, and irregular abrasions and flaps in the forehead area. This patient was treated with acute skin grafts to the upper lids, suturing of all flaps, and shaving of irregular skin tags (Fig. 15B). Small areas of skin defects were smoothed by abrasion and allowed to granulate. Figure 16A and B shows the same patient and the results obtained.

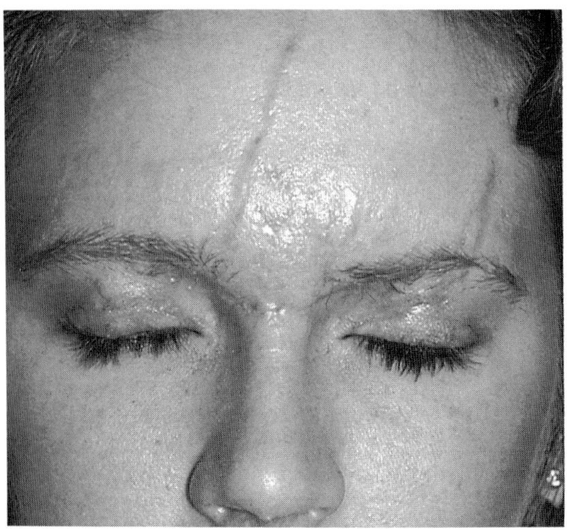

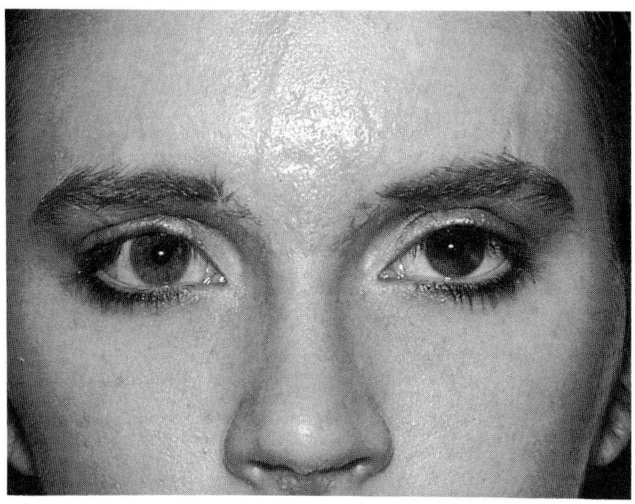

FIG. 16. A: Same patient as in Fig. 15 showing complete lid closure (8 weeks). **B:** Same patient showing symmetric upper lid creases (3 months).

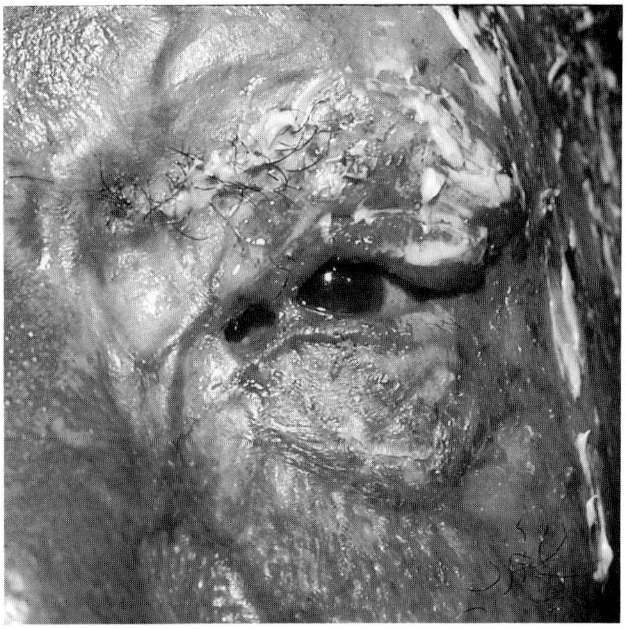

FIG. 17. Chemical burn with loss of skin-muscle layer and lid eversion. Chlorine burn of the face and eyelids with marginal tarsorrhaphy. Despite split-skin grafts and tarsorraphy the lids have retracted with corneal exposure.

ACUTE BURNS OF THE FACE AND EYELID AREA

Severe chemical or thermal burns of the eyelid area can cause a complete contracture of the external layers of the lid and periorbital area resulting in retraction of the lids and exposure of the eye. Corneal damage and ulceration is always a concern in these patients. In many burn cases, swelling and prolapse of the conjunctival fornices provide a temporary protection of the cornea. However, the conjunctiva soon becomes dried and irritated, with infection usually ensuing.

In some cases, because of other severe problems that the patient may have, there is a temptation to simply perform tarsorrhaphies that can, in a very temporary manner, protect the eye. The contracting process over a period of time will overcome the tarsorrhapies and they will prove inadequate in preventing the eyelids from separating. Small grafts to the upper and lower lid (in many cases only split-thickness grafts are available) are usually employed to retard retraction and exposure. Figure 17 shows a patient who suffered a chlorine burn to the facial area. Despite nasal tarsorrhaphy and split-skin grafting, the lids are being retracted apart. The adequate protection in some of these patients can be obtained only by the "masquerade graft" technique (complete overlay graft) as described in the chapters on eyelid reconstruction for total reconstruction of the eyelid. In some patients this procedure is needed to preserve vision for the long term, and these benefits far outweigh the inconvenience of the long period of eyelid closure required.

BITE EVULSIONS OF THE EYELID

A common setting seen with dog bites of the eyelid in young children is that of a child playing with the neighbor's dog, which then nips "at" the child, many times without malice (depending on the personality of the dog). The usual injury, because of the tendency for dogs to bite toward the nose and the eye, is the presence of one laceration in the inner canthus and a second one in the forehead or scalp area corresponding to the opened jaws of the dog (Fig. 18A). If the bite is mild the canthal injury may be superficial, but in many cases

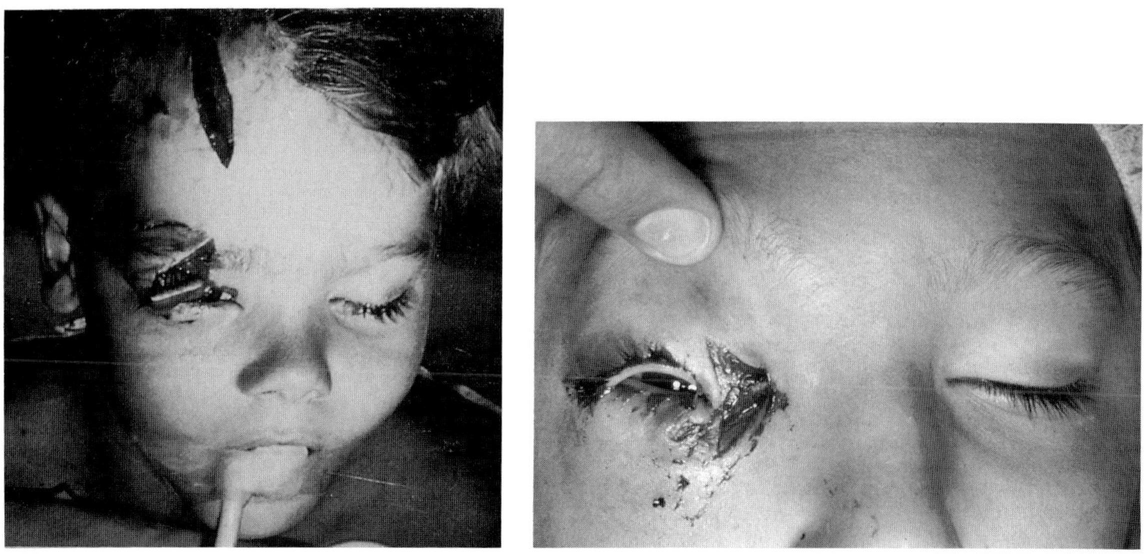

A B

FIG. 18. Dog bite eyelid lacerations. **A:** Patient with dog bite showing the characteristic bite in the eyelid canthal area and scalp corresponding to the lower and upper lid teeth of the animal. **B:** Patient with avulsion of the inner canthus including the upper and lower canaliculus and medial canthal tendon.

it involves damage of deep tissues in the canthus including the superior oblique tendon and lacrimal canalicular system (Fig. 18B). If not repaired adequately, these injuries will create a posttraumatic telecanthus with lacrimal drainage insufficiency.

Repair of these wounds can be difficult but with a knowledge of postoperative sequela the surgeon can direct efforts toward repairing the structures necessary to prevent the known problems. The techniques described in the chapter on medial canthal reconstruction are useful in this situation.

Human bites of the eyelid can occur in unusual settings, usually a passionate encounter. In these cases the lid may be separated from the globe with avulsion of the eyelid from the bite with complete sparing of the globe. The exact mechanism is not clear.

CANALICULAR LACERATION REPAIR WITH SILICONE INTUBATION

If the canalicular system is lacerated and allowed to heal unattended, it will fibrose and cause lacrimal drainage insufficiency with annoying tearing. Figure 18B shows a patient with a severe medial canthal injury from a dog bite including the canthal tendon and upper and lower canaliculus. The eyelid and canthal laceration could be repaired with a reconstructive procedure but the canalicular system must be intubated at the same time for restoration of lacrimal drainage. Some severe avulsing injuries will be unrepairable with intubation because of lost tissue. These patients will acquire a Jones tube intubation at a later date.

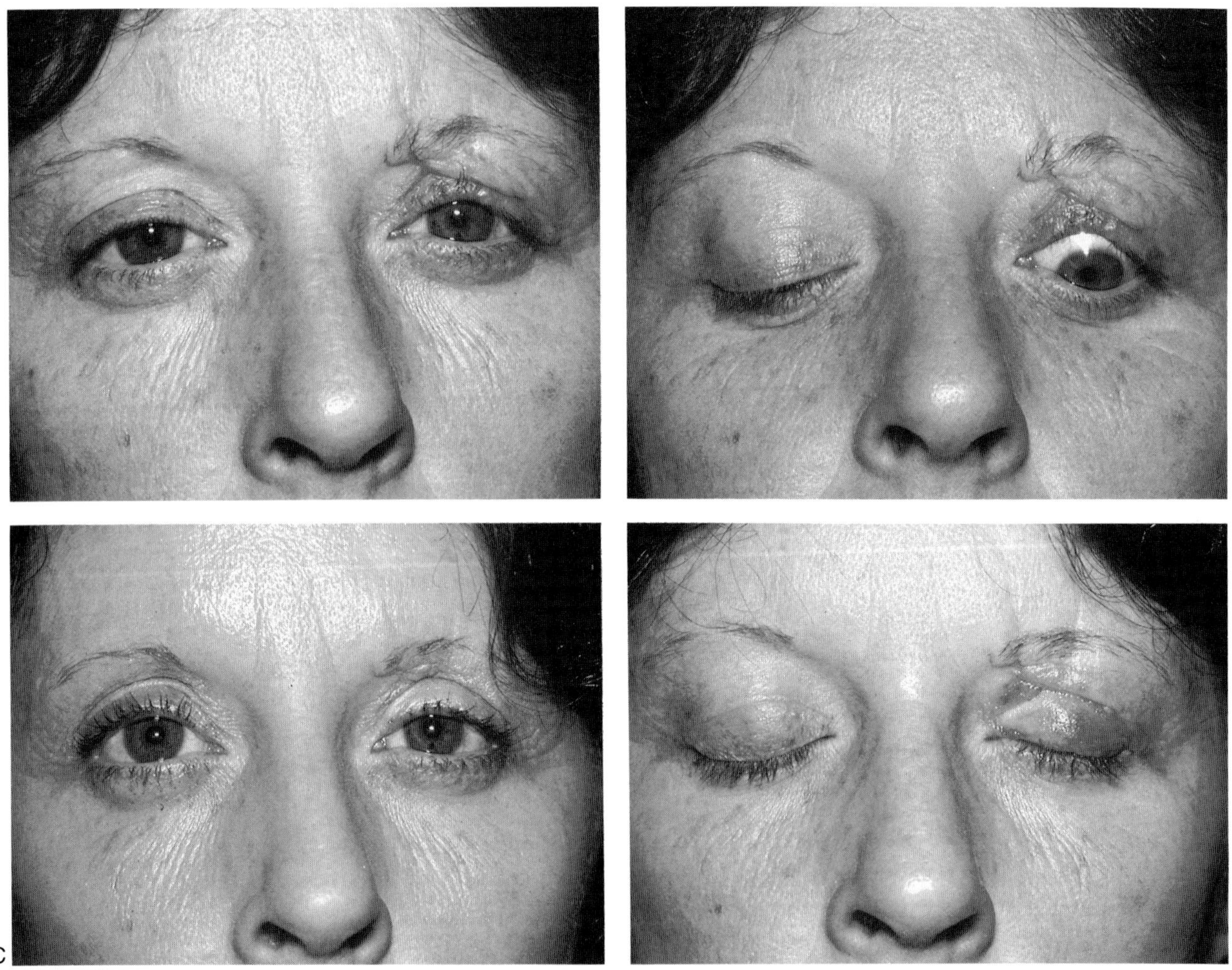

A B C D

FIG. 19. Vertical scar in the upper lid causing lagophthalmos and distortion of the lid crease. This is a very common deformity following eyelid laceration. It is caused by vertical traction bands and deep adhesions. **A:** Patient preoperatively, primary position. **B:** Preoperatively on downgaze showing lagophthalmos and tethering of the upper lid. **C:** Same patient following placement of full-thickness skin graft. Graft has been placed in the area between the lash line and the crease or eyeshadow area. **D:** Same patient showing retention of the eyelid crease and eyeshadow space because of the placement of the graft avoiding distortion of the lid crease.

LATE REPAIR OF EYELID TRAUMA

The surgical techniques for repair and reconstruction of full-thickness defects have been covered in previous chapters. Other chapters, such as that on ectropion, may also contain useful techniques available for correction of posttrauma deformities.

Upper Lid

A recurring situation is seen in patients who have healed upper lid lacerations. In these patients the upper lid will have skin shortage, lagophthalmos, and damage to the eyelid crease. This problem is often associated with a vertical scar that may extend to the eyelid margin causing a notch that may need excision with revised closure. For correction of the skin shortage, it is felt that skin grafting gives better results than transposition flaps. The technique of skin grafting in the upper lid to preserve the upper lid crease position has been covered in the chapter on complications of upper lid blepharoplasty and in the chapter on upper lid crease considerations. This typical injury is shown in a patient in Fig. 19A and B. To preserve crease position, a single graft should not straddle the crease if possible. If two skin grafts are to be used, one should be placed below the crease (from the supralash area to the crease) and a second skin graft, if necessary, above the crease with the interface placed at the desired position of the crease as shown in Fig. 19C and D.

Care should also be taken when removing vertical traction bands and scar tissue to avoid loosening the levator aponeurosis and to prevent a postoperative ptosis. If ptosis does occur, then secondary levator surgery may be needed.

Lower Lid

Posttraumatic cicatricial ectropion or entropion can be treated by methods described in previous chapters. Commonly, tissue must be added back to the lid either in the form of a full-thickness skin graft or an internal lamellar graft from ear cartilage or mucoperichondrium.

Eyelid margin deformities can be treated as described in previous chapters.

CHAPTER 29

Endoscopic Forehead Lift

The evolution of methods to improve the appearance of the forehead and brow region has been recently influenced by the application of endoscopic techniques to conventional surgical procedures. The main disadvantage of the open coronal brow lift has been directly related to the length and location of the incision. The morbidity associated with this approach has included significant scarring, hair loss, and posterior scalp numbness that can often be permanent. The use of minimally invasive endoscopic techniques provides the surgeon with the opportunity to achieve the same surgical results with considerably reduced morbidity.

Advances in minimally invasive surgical procedures have occurred in virtually all specialties including general surgery, gynecology, orthopedic, otolaryngology, urology, thoracic surgery, and plastic surgery. The primary advantage of endoscopic surgery includes a reduction in scar length and scalp numbness associated with the conventional technique. The innervation to the scalp is preserved by avoidance of the coronal incision. This minimally invasive technique has reduced alopecia and posterior hairline displacement. Although patients with thin hair or a high hairline are frequently not considered candidates for the traditional forehead lift, these patients are often good candidates for the endoscopic method. In addition, blood loss is markedly reduced and the overall operating time for the endoscopic-assisted brow lift is shorter. There is a significant reduction in postoperative edema as well as postoperative pain. These advantages have contributed to higher patient acceptance and surgeon satisfaction. In the past, patients have often refused a forehead lift because of the coronal incision. The endoscopic forehead lift has reduced the degree of patient unwillingness resulting in a higher overall acceptance rate.

It should be emphasized that the endoscope is a tool that assists the surgeon in the performance of a standard surgical procedure. Proper training and experience with the open forehead lift is a mandatory prerequisite prior to performing the endoscopic technique. Although improved endoscopic visualization is obtained due to better magnification and lighting, the trade-off for these advantages includes surgery that is highly dependent on new technological equipment and is subject to technical limitations and failures.

Patients undergoing endoscopic surgery should be informed that these limitations may require that the procedure be stopped if proper visualization is not achieved or that an open coronal incision be performed for control of bleeding that cannot be controlled endoscopically. Although there is a distinct learning curve associated with the performance of the endoscopic forehead lift, the surgeon can anticipate good, predictable surgical results with significantly reduced morbidity.

HISTORY

Since the original description of the forehead lift, several surgical modifications for brow elevation have been proposed that include the coronal incision temporal incision, hairline incision, midforehead incision, direct brow lift through a superciliary incision, and the internal brow pexy (1–6). All of these modifications attempt to balance the goal of brow elevation with minimal scar visibility and surgical morbidity. The closer the incision is located to the brow, the more effective the elevation but the more visible the scar. Although the coronal incision has remained the foremost method for brow elevation in the past, the development of endoscopic techniques has rapidly contributed to the gaining popularity of this procedure.

Investigation of minimally invasive procedures in the forehead region was initially performed by the use of endoscopic visualization of the subgaleal anatomy from incisions made posterior to the hairline. Initial surgical procedures performed included ablation of the frontalis and corrugator muscles to improve forehead and glabella wrinkling (7,8). As endoscopic instrumentation and techniques improved, wider subperiosteal dissection and brow fixation methods evolved that allowed effective brow and forehead elevation (9). Considerable clinical experience with the endoscopic-assisted brow lift has demonstrated similar early surgical results when compared to the conventional coronal forehead lift with significantly reduced morbidity (10).

INSTRUMENTATION

Advances in the field of minimally invasive surgery are closely linked to the development and availability of endoscopic instrumentation (Fig. 1). Following the success of endoscopic procedures in other surgical specialties, there has been momentous growth in instru-

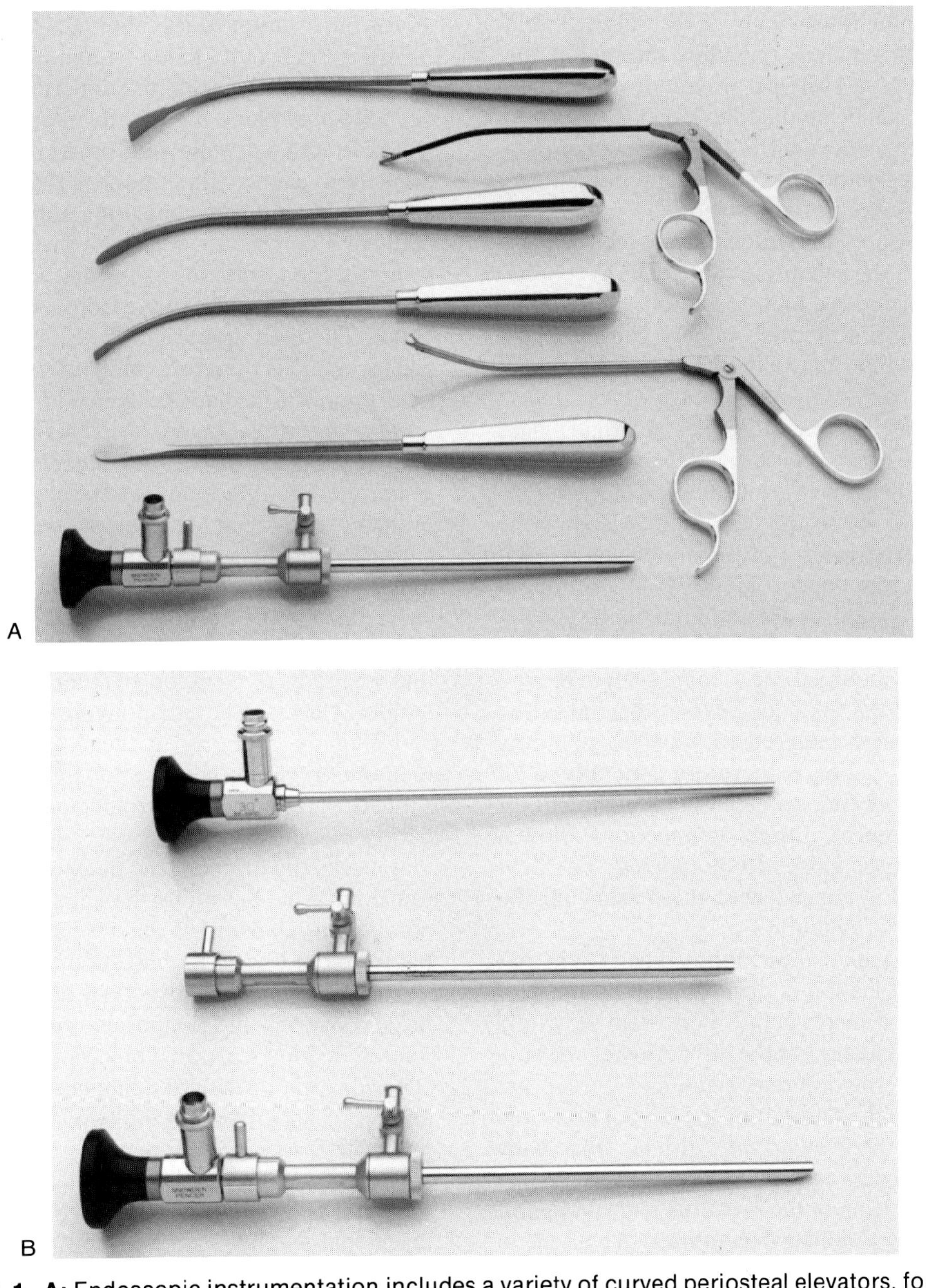

FIG. 1. A: Endoscopic instrumentation includes a variety of curved periosteal elevators, forceps, scissors, and endoscope. **B:** The 4-mm endoscope with retractor sheath is shown. Courtesy of Snowden-Pencer, Inc.

mentation. The main instrumentation requirements include a camera and video equipment, endoscope, light source, retractor, and endoscopic surgical instruments. These instruments are used to create a closed, air-filled working space termed the optical cavity (8). The primary requirement in endoscopic surgery is the development of this cavity, which is maintained by a retractor-mounted endoscopic system (10). This allows the surgeon to maintain the optical cavity with the nondominant hand while performing the procedure with the opposite hand.

The video equipment consists of a camera that attaches to the endoscope and provides output signals to the video monitor for viewing of the surgical field. The camera systems include one-chip, three-chip, and digital formats. These systems provide a high degree of resolution and can be mounted to various size endoscopes. In order to achieve the correct vertical orientation, the camera body has an external alignment marker to indicate the upright position. Video cables connect the camera to the video cart, which is positioned adjacent to the operating table. The video cart setup generally includes a high-resolution video monitor, VCR recorder and printer, camera source, and a light source with fiberoptic attachment to the endoscope.

The currently available endoscopes are rigid, glass Hopkins rod–type endoscopes that are 4, 5, and 10 mm in external diameter. The various angles of visualization are 0, 30, and 70° to the longitudinal axis of the endoscope. Because the size of the optical cavity that can be created during endoscopic brow lift is limited, the smaller endoscope sizes are recommended. The optical cavity is maintained through tissue retraction using the retractor-mounted endoscopic system or with the use of a sleeve that extends beyond the end of the endoscope. The angle required to view the anatomy in the supraorbital region is therefore generally a 30° downward view. The endoscope has an attachment for an external light source. Proper connections allow a variety of light source cables to be utilized. The light source connection is aligned with the marker on the camera for proper orientation.

Once adequate visualization of the optical cavity has been achieved, dissection is begun using a variety of endoscopic surgical instruments. Periosteal elevators can be used for dissection of the subperiosteal or subgaleal space. Several different sizes and curves are used depending on the contour of the frontal bone and the distance from the brow to the hairline. Once wide undermining has been completed, biopsy forceps are used to resect a portion of the procerus and corrugator muscles to correct glabellar frown lines. A variety of biopsy forceps are available. Blunt-tipped Takahashi forceps allow control over the depth of the myotomy. Following subperiosteal release and procerus corrugator resection, brow elevation and fixation are performed. Several methods for brow fixation have been proposed ranging from posterior retraction of the frontogaleal–occipital layer to tissue advancement flaps and screw fixation to the outer calvarial table.

ANATOMY

The anatomy of the forehead, brow, and temporal region has been well defined, and an appreciation of the relationship of the nerves and muscles to the fascial planes is critical for the preservation of sensory and motor innervation to this region (11).

The optical cavity in the frontal region can be developed in the subgaleal or subperiosteal planes. The subperiosteal plane has an advantage of direct periosteal reattachment following brow elevation. Once the dissection reaches the supraorbital rim, the periosteum is divided to allow visualization and access to the procerus and corrugator muscles. There are three fascial layers in the temporal region that are important landmarks for localization of the frontal branch of the facial nerve. The temporoparietal fascia is the most superficial layer and is therefore often referred to as the superficial temporal fascia. The deep temporal fascia is made up of a superficial layer, which is often termed the innominate fascia, and a deep layer.

The temporoparietal fascia contains the frontal branch of the facial nerve on the deep subaponeurotic surface. This layer represents an extension of the submuscular aponeurotic system (SMAS) and is in the same plane as the frontogaleal–occipital layer (12). The subaponeurotic plane consists of loose areolar tissue that separates the temporoparietal fascia from the deep temporal fascia. The subaponeurotic plane is avascular and extends inferiorly to the zygomatic arch. In the temporal region, the subaponeurotic space and the subperiosteal space are connected by division of the periosteal reflection along the superior temporal line that marks the origin of the deep temporal fascia. This transition zone lies along the anterior crest of the temporal bone. Division of this fascial reflection is essential for lateral brow mobilization.

The deep temporal fascia is a dense, double-layered fascia covering the temporalis muscle. The temporal line of fusion is a transverse line at the level of the superior orbital rim extending laterally over the fascia and represents fusion of the two layers superior to this line. The fascia is separated inferior to the line by the superficial temporal fat pad, which is located between the superficial and deep layers of the deep temporal fascia and extends to the level of the zygomatic arch. The deep temporal fat pad lies beneath the deep temporal fascia 2 cm above the zygomatic arch and overlies the temporalis muscle and tendon. The deep temporal fat pad is a cephalic extension of the buccal fat pad through the zygomatic arch. Appreciation of the anatomic relationship of the frontal branch of the facial nerve to the fascial layers is important in order to define the safe level of dissection and protect the nerve when operating in the temporal region.

The frontal branch of the facial nerve provides motor innervation to the upper facial musculature. The course and depth of the nerve has been well defined and extends along a line beginning 0.5 cm below the tragus to 1.5 cm above the lateral aspect of the brow. The frontal branch lies within the temporoparietal fascia as it traverses the zygomatic arch and is at greatest risk for injury at this level. Superior to the zygomatic arch, the nerve is superficial to the superficial layer of the deep temporal fascia and provides innervation to the frontalis and corrugator muscles.

The supratrochlear and supraorbital nerves provide sensory innervation to the forehead region and scalp. The ophthalmic (V1) division of the trigeminal nerve traverses the cavenous sinus and enters the orbit through the superior orbital fissure. The ophthalmic nerve has three divisions: the frontal, nasociliary, lacrimal nerves. The frontal nerve runs along the superior orbital wall and divides into the supratrochlear and supraorbital nerves. The supratrochlear nerve emerges from the medial aspect of the superior orbital rim and provides sensory innervation to the glabella, medial forehead, medial upper eyelid, and conjunctiva. The supraorbital nerve exits the orbit in the central aspect of the superior orbital rim most commonly through a notch. A true supraorbital foramen exists as an anatomic variant in 25% of orbits (Fig. 2) (13). The supraorbital nerve provides sensory innervation to the scalp, lateral forehead, lateral upper eyelid, and conjunctiva.

The musculature in the upper face that contributes to prominent lines in the forehead and glabella region include the frontalis, procerus, and corrugator supercilii muscles. The frontalis muscle is a paired muscle that is an extension of the galea aponeurotica and occipitalis muscle. The vertically oriented fibers insert into the supraorbital dermis and elevate the eyebrow during contraction. Increased frontalis muscle tone, in order to maintain an elevated brow position in response to brow ptosis, causes transverse lines across the forehead. The frontalis is a primary brow elevator and should therefore not be weakened during a procedure aimed at brow elevation. Rather, repositioning of the brow at a higher level will decrease the baseline tone of the frontalis thereby reducing the transverse forehead lines.

The procerus muscle is a paired midline muscle that originates from the nasal bones and upper lateral cartilages. The vertically oriented fibers insert into the dermis of the glabella at the medial border of the frontalis. Contraction of the procerus causes inferior and medial

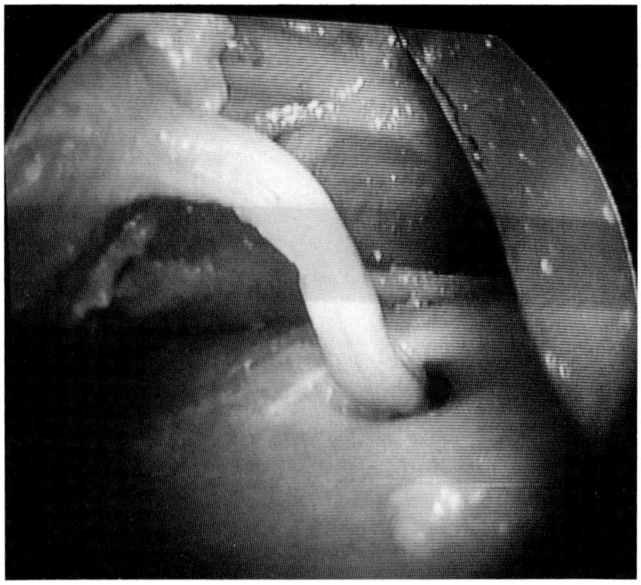

FIG. 2. Endoscopic view of the supraorbital nerve and a supraorbital foramen in a cadaver dissection.

displacement of the medial eyebrow and a transverse line at the nasal radix. The procerus muscle has innervation from the buccal branch of the facial nerve. The procerus is a primary brow depressor and should therefore be weakened in order to achieve medial brow elevation.

The corrugator supercilii muscle is a paired muscle that originates from the periosteum of the medial superior orbital rim. The fibers are oriented in a lateral oblique direction. They insert into the dermis of the medial eyebrow skin and have lateral interdigitations with the medial portion of the orbicularis oculi muscle and depressor supercilii superior to the brow. Contraction of the corrugator muscles cause inferior and medial displacement of the eyebrow and vertical oblique lines of the glabella. Therefore, weakening the medial portion of the corrugator along with fibers of the orbicularis oculi and depressor supercilii will contribute to medial brow elevation and correction of glabellar frown lines. The lateral portion of the corrugator causes slight lateral brow elevation and should be preserved. Motor innervation of the corrugator is from the frontal branch of the facial nerve.

BROW POSITION

In addition to correction of the lines associated with facial aging and increased activity of the forehead musculature, the surgical goals of the endoscopic forehead lift are to elevate the brow to a more youthful position. Fixation of the eyebrow in proper position avoids creating brow ptosis in an unstable brow following upper eyelid blepharoplasty. Brow ptosis is defined as an ab-

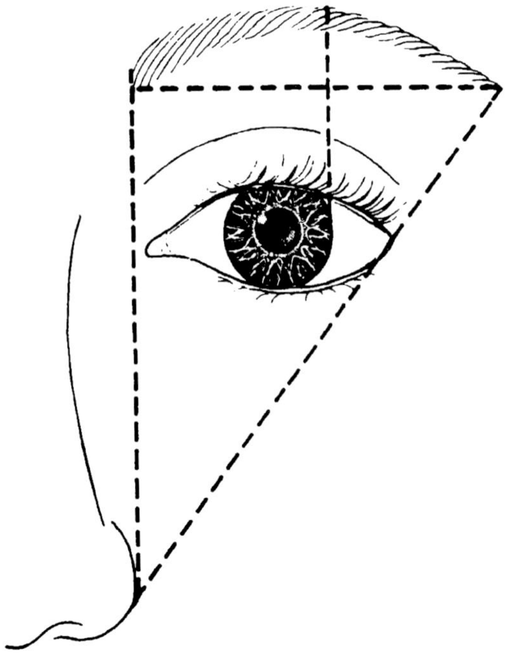

FIG. 3. Vectors demonstrating the basic aesthetic relationship of the female eyebrow to the lateral nasal ala and the eye landmarks.

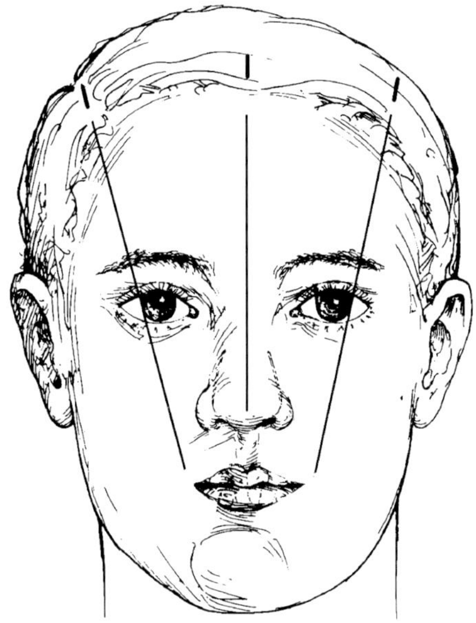

FIG. 4. Location of endoscopic incisions are shown in the midline and along a vector intersecting the lateral oral commissure and the lateral limbus.

normal position of the brow relative to the orbital rim or as a narrowing of the brow–lash distance. Transverse brow position is influenced by partial medial or lateral brow ptosis. Correction of unilateral brow ptosis can also be achieved with the endoscopic forehead lift. In addition, isolated procerus and corrugator resection can be performed if the brow is in proper position to improve the appearance of the glabellar region.

The eyebrow position has a basic aesthetic relationship to the fixed position of eye landmarks and superior orbital rim (Fig. 3) (14). In women, the medial and lateral ends of the brow are at the same approximate horizontal level. The apex of the brow arch lies on a vertical line directly above the lateral limbus and is 1 cm above the superior orbital rim. The medial aspect of the eyebrow begins at a vertical line directly above the lateral nasal ala. The lateral aspect of the eyebrow is positioned on an oblique line intersecting the lateral nasal ala and the lateral canthus. The eyebrow is oriented in a more horizontal position in the male patient at the level of the superior orbital rim.

SURGICAL TECHNIQUE

Once the surgical goals have been determined and individual preferences for brow position have been considered, vector analysis is used to mark the location of the incisions (Fig. 4). A total of three radial incisions are marked within the hairline. One vertical incision 1.5 cm in length is marked in the midline and two lateral along a vector from the lateral oral commissure to the lateral limbus beginning 2 cm posterior to the hairline. The lateral incisions are individualized depending on the degree of lateral brow ptosis. Generally, the lateral incisions are 4 cm from the midline and are located over the periosteum of the superior temporal line (Fig. 5). The central incision is used to approach the pro-

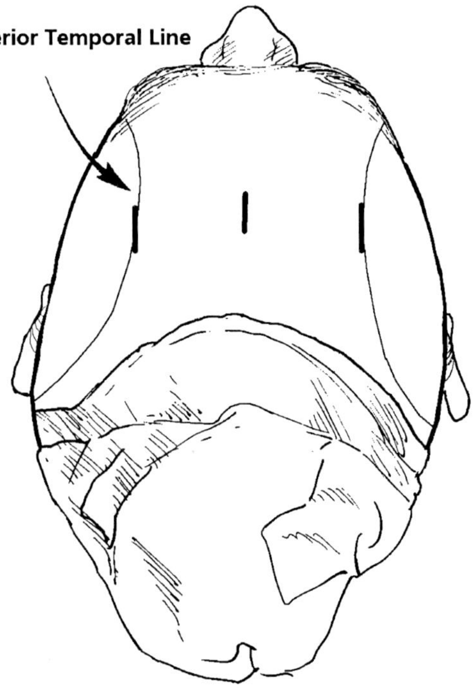

FIG. 5. Three longitudinal incisions are made within the hairline for subperiosteal access to the forehead. The lateral incisions generally cross the superior temporal line.

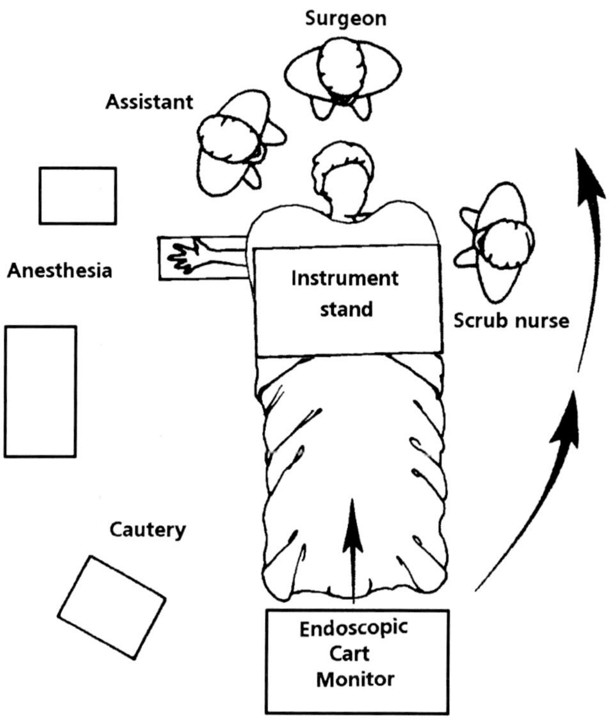

FIG. 6. Schematic diagram demonstrating the operating room setup and patient positioning during endoscopic browlift.

cerus and corrugator muscles and to release and elevate the medial brow. The lateral incisions are used to release and elevate the lateral brow.

The location of the incisions are based on the aesthetic relationship of the eyebrow to the eye. This aesthetic relationship must be maintained in order to avoid the surprised look from overelevation of the brow. In addition, the incisions are placed posteriorly within the hairline to minimize scar visibility. The incisions should avoid the site of maximal hairline recession, which generally occurs along a line from the lateral oral commissure intersecting the lateral canthus. Furthermore, the midline incision can be omitted or placed paramedian if the patient has a hairstyle with a midline part.

The patient is placed on the operating table with the head suspended in a headrest to facilitate clearance for the use of the endoscope and instruments. The endoscopic cart with the monitor is placed at the left side of the operating table and the assistant stands at the right side (Fig. 6). The procedure can be performed effectively under general or local anesthesia with sedation. Generous infiltration with 0.25% xylocaine with epinephrine (1:400,000) aids in hydrodissection of the scalp and forehead region. Subperiosteal dissection is begun anteriorly without using the endoscope through the central incision stopping 1–2 cm above the superior orbital rim (Fig. 7). The 4-mm 30° endoscope with a retraction sleeve or retractor is inserted into the optical cavity at this point to continue dissection of the lower forehead under endoscopic visualization (Fig. 8). The dissection proceeds down to the superior orbital rim and the periosteum is divided transversely with a sharp periosteal elevator. A curved periosteal hook and curved endoscopic scissors can also be used to divide the periosteum (Fig. 9). The procerus and corrugator muscles are clearly visualized once the periosteum is divided. The supratrochlear nerves are seen with the underlying oblique fibers of the corrugator muscle and the transverse supratrochlear vein. The supraorbital nerves are dissected and mark the lateral extent of muscle removal. Periosteal division continues laterally along the orbital rim to the level of the lateral canthus using a narrow, curved elevator. Subperiosteal release of the superior temporal line transition zone and the lateral orbital rim is necessary for effective lateral brow lift.

The remainder of the lateral subgaleal release is performed through the lateral incisions with endoscopic-assisted dissection directly on the superficial layer of the deep temporal fascia. For an effective lateral brow lift, division of the periosteal reflection along the superior temporal line is performed in a lateral-to-medial direction to avoid entering the temporal fossa (Fig. 10). Dissection in the temporal region down to the level of the lateral orbital rim is performed taking precaution to avoid injury to the frontal branch of the facial nerve. Nerve injury is minimized by remaining deep to the

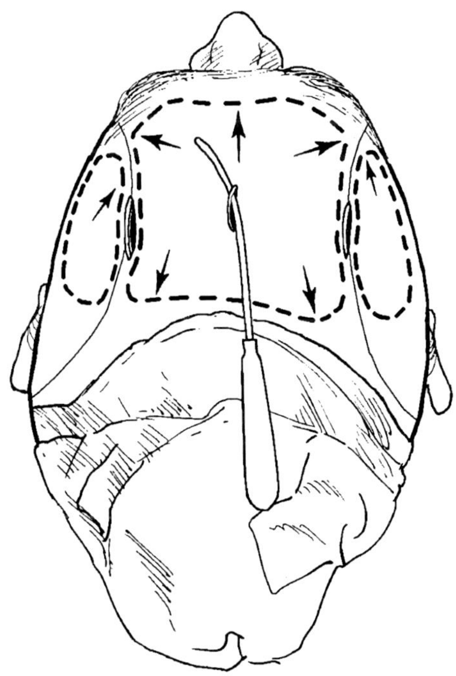

FIG. 7. A periosteal elevator is used to create the central subperiosteal and lateral subgaleal optical cavities through the three access incisions.

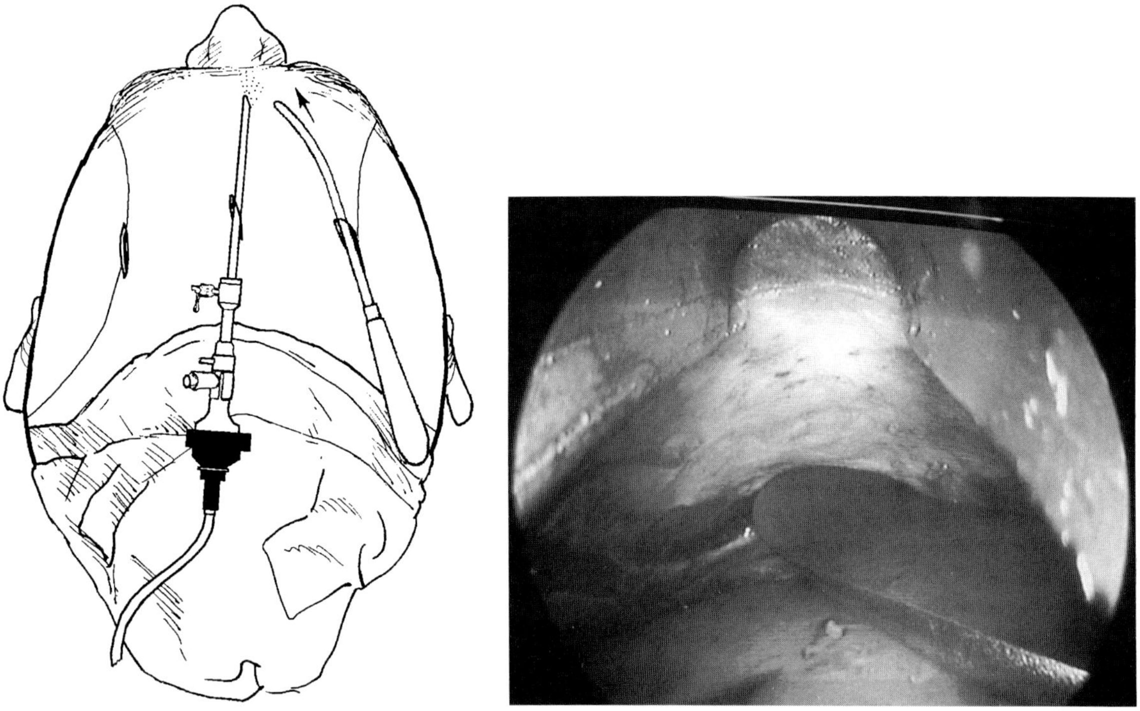

A B

FIG. 8. A: The endoscope is inserted through the central incision and subperiosteal dissection of the glabellar and supraorbital region is performed with endoscopic visualization. **B:** Intraoperative endoscopic view demonstrating division of the periosteum along the supraorbital rim.

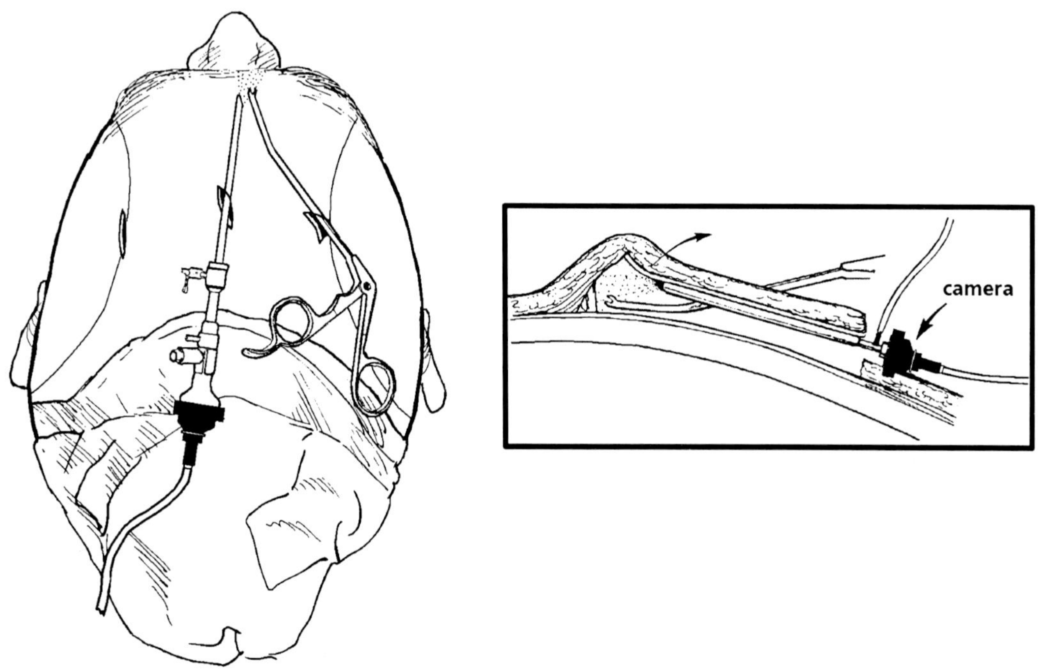

FIG. 9. The periosteum is divided in the glabellar region to provide access to the procerus and corrugator muscles. Upward retraction of the endoscope sheath maintains the optical cavity.

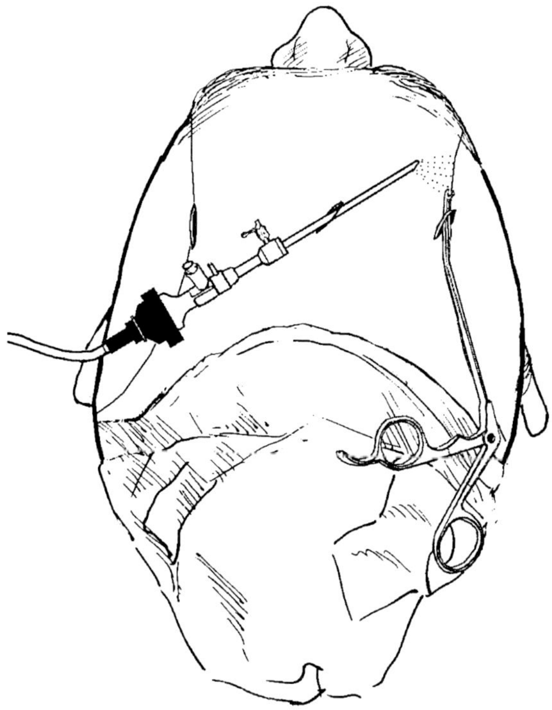

FIG. 10. In order to mobilize the lateral brow, division of the periosteal reflection along the superior temporal line is performed.

nerve and avoiding vigorous upward retraction with the endoscope, which could cause a stretch-induced neuropraxia.

Once adequate undermining of the forehead region has been performed, muscle removal is performed to correct lines in the glabellar region (Fig. 11). Hypertrophy of the procerus or corrugator muscles is treated by myectomy to weaken these muscles. A blunt-tipped Takahashi biopsy forcep allows precise muscle resection and minimizes potential dissection of the underlying subcutaneous tissue and dermis, which could result in a visible deformity in the glabellar region. Removal of procerus is performed in the midline at the level of the superior orbital rim. Dissection proceeds laterally with removal of corrugator on both sides of the supratrochlear nerve. The supratrochlear nerve crosses the corrugator and is deep to the orbicularis oculi fibers. A nerve hook can be used to retract the supratrochlear nerve. Myectomy of the underlying orbicularis oculi and depressor supercilii is performed and dissection continues to the supraorbital nerve, which marks the lateral extent of the muscle removal. It is important that the muscles located between the supratrochlear and supraorbital nerves are resected.

Following procerus and corrugator myectomy, endoscopic inspection for hemostasis is performed. An insulated grasper is used with electrocautery to control any bleeding points. At this point, brow elevation and fixation are performed. Several methods for brow fixation have been used. The central incision located over periosteum can be fixed with tissue advancement flaps or rigid screw fixation methods. Screw fixation methods have included permanent placement of surgical screws that anchor galeal support sutures or temporary percutaneous screws that are removed 1–2 weeks after surgery and rely on periosteal fixation. The lateral incisions are located over the transition zone so that the

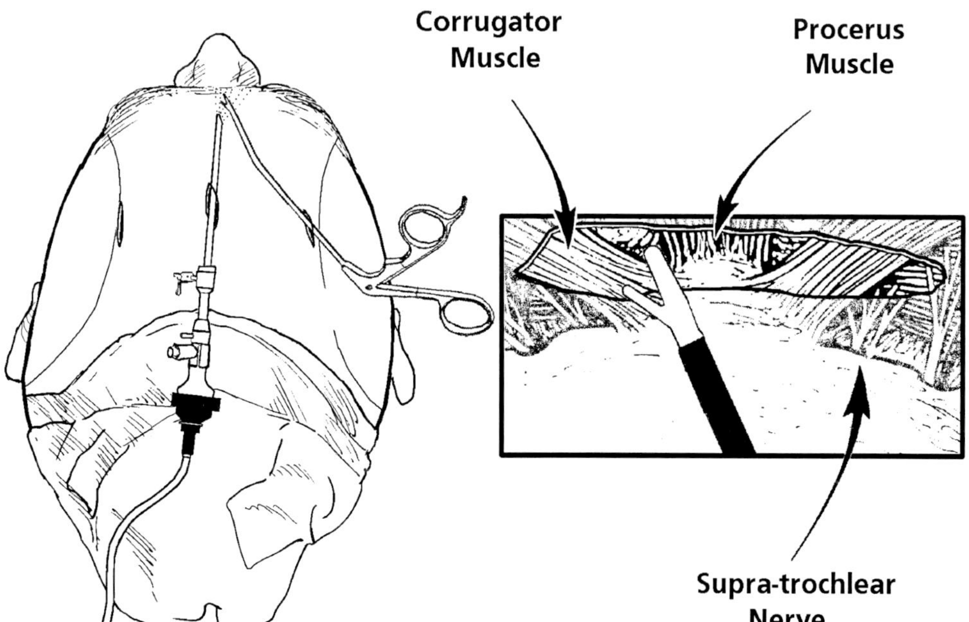

FIG. 11. In order to correct glabellar frown lines, myectomy of the procerus and corrugator muscles is performed using endoscopic forceps.

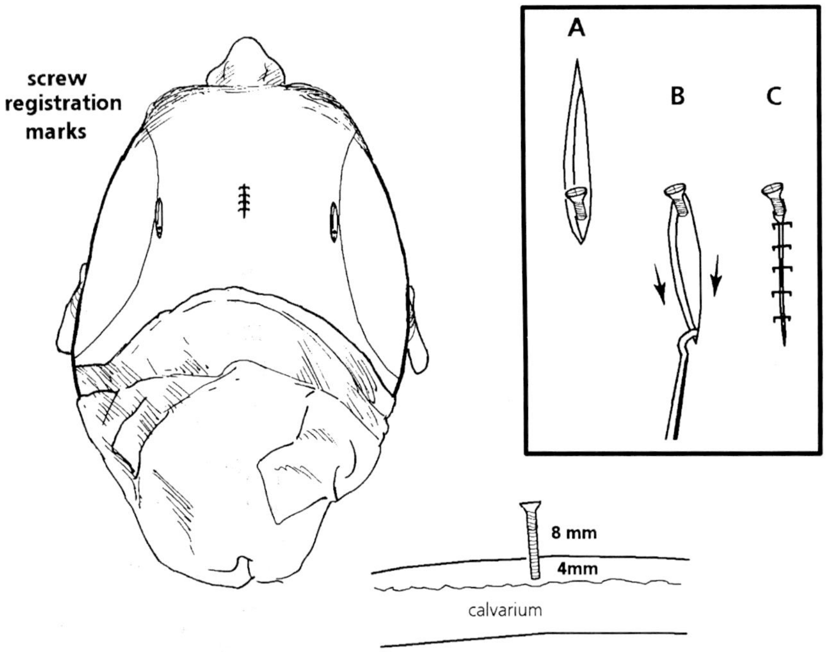

FIG. 12. Lateral forehead elevation is maintained using screw fixation techniques. Bovie electrocautery is used to make screw registration marks. A 12-mm titanium screw is placed into the outer cortex. The scalp is advanced posteriorly and held in place with surgical staples.

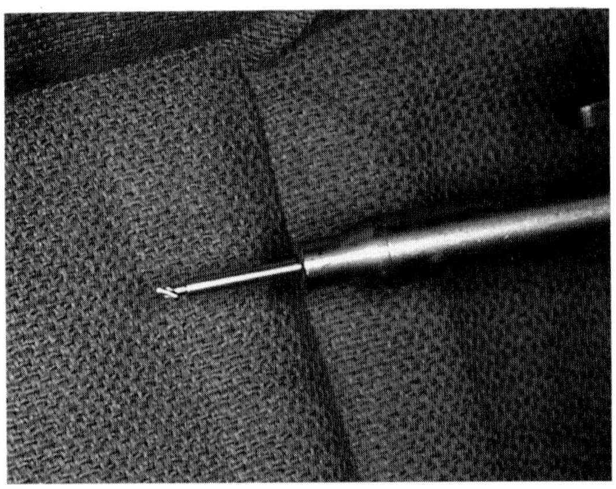

FIG. 13. A guarded 4-mm drill bit is used to control the drill depth used in screw fixation.

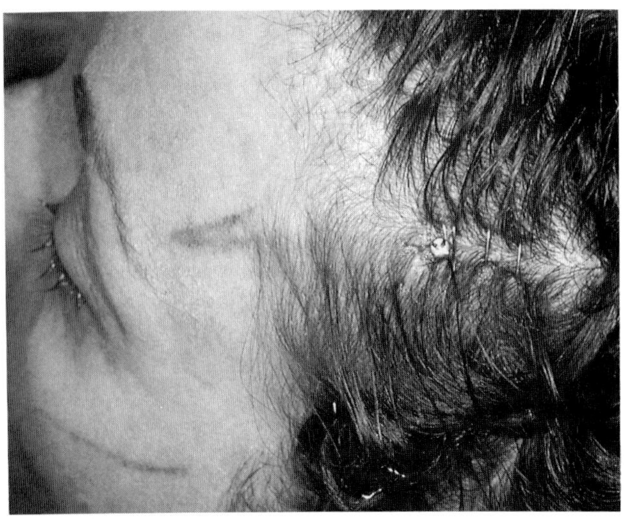

FIG. 14. Posterior scalp advancement and forehead elevation maintained with screw fixation.

deep temporal fascia can be used for suture fixation or screw fixation of the lateral forehead can be performed (Fig. 12). Another method includes the application of a posterior scalp bolster with posterior fixation following complete subgaleal undermining of the posterior scalp.

When temporary percutaneous rigid fixation is used to elevate the lateral brow and set the height of the brow arch, a guarded drill bit 4 mm in depth is used to place a 2-mm diameter titanium screw (Fig. 13). The screw length is 12 mm thereby allowing an 8-mm length to traverse the scalp and allow the screw head to remain external to the scalp. Once the screw is secured at the posterior aspect of the radial incision, the scalp is advanced posteriorly along the vector of the incision with a single-hook retractor. After the scalp has been advanced to achieve proper brow elevation with some consideration for overcorrection, surgical staples are placed posterior to the screw to close the incision and maintain the scalp advancement (Fig. 14). In order to avoid a dog ear type of deformity, 2–3 cm of posterior scalp undermining is performed. The lateral incisions can also be used to elevate the lateral brow with suture fixation. The temporoparietal fascia and galea are advanced posteriorly along the lateral vector and sutured to the deep temporal fascia using a nonabsorbable suture (Fig. 15). The incisions are closed after posterior undermining. If medial brow elevation is not required, the midline incision can be closed primarily. In order to elevate the medial brow, the central incision can be closed with a tissue advancement flap or an additional screw can be placed for fixation.

A pressure head dressing is placed for the first 24–48 h following surgery. Patients are placed on antibiotics with return for screw and staple removal 10–14 days after surgery. No drains are required. The postoperative edema is mild and the incidence of hematoma appears to be markedly reduced compared to the conventional coronal incision. Postoperative results have demonstrated clinical improvement in the glabellar region with satisfactory brow elevation (Fig. 16).

CONCLUSION

The surgical indications and objectives for the endoscopic forehead lift are similar in principle to the conventional coronal approach. Wide subperiosteal undermining in the forehead region is performed, including release of the fascial periosteal reflection along the superior temporal line, in order to redrape and elevate the brow. The periosteum is divided along the orbital rim and the procerus, corrugator, and orbicularis oculi muscles are partially removed in order to correct prominent glabellar lines. Finally, forehead and brow elevation are performed with fixation for the correction of brow ptosis. Reattachment of the periosteum at a higher level combined with soft tissue contraction from pull of the occipitalis muscle likely contribute to further brow elevation.

Although the advantages of the endoscopic-assisted forehead lift are evident, the procedure is not without potential pitfalls. Endoscopic surgery is dependent on technology and therefore subject to video equipment failure. If an adequate video image cannot be produced due to technical difficulty, the procedure must either be discontinued or converted to an open procedure. All patients undergoing endoscopic surgery should be informed that there is a slight risk of conversion to an open approach being necessary.

The endoscopic forehead lift has significantly reduced the morbidity associated with the conventional approach. Early postoperative results have revealed a

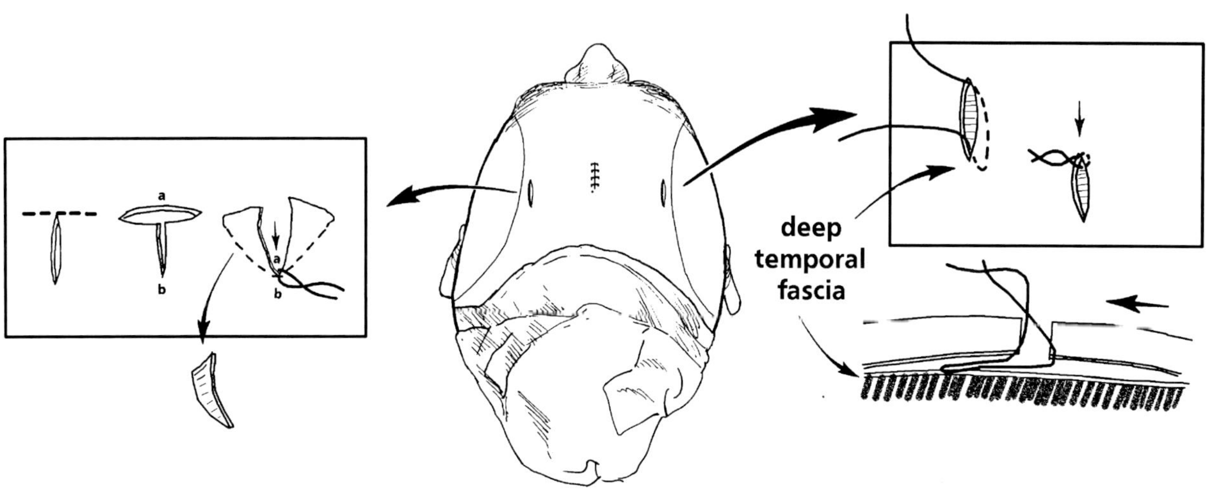

FIG. 15. Alternate fixation methods include tissue advancement flaps and galeal advancement with fixation to the deep temporal fascia.

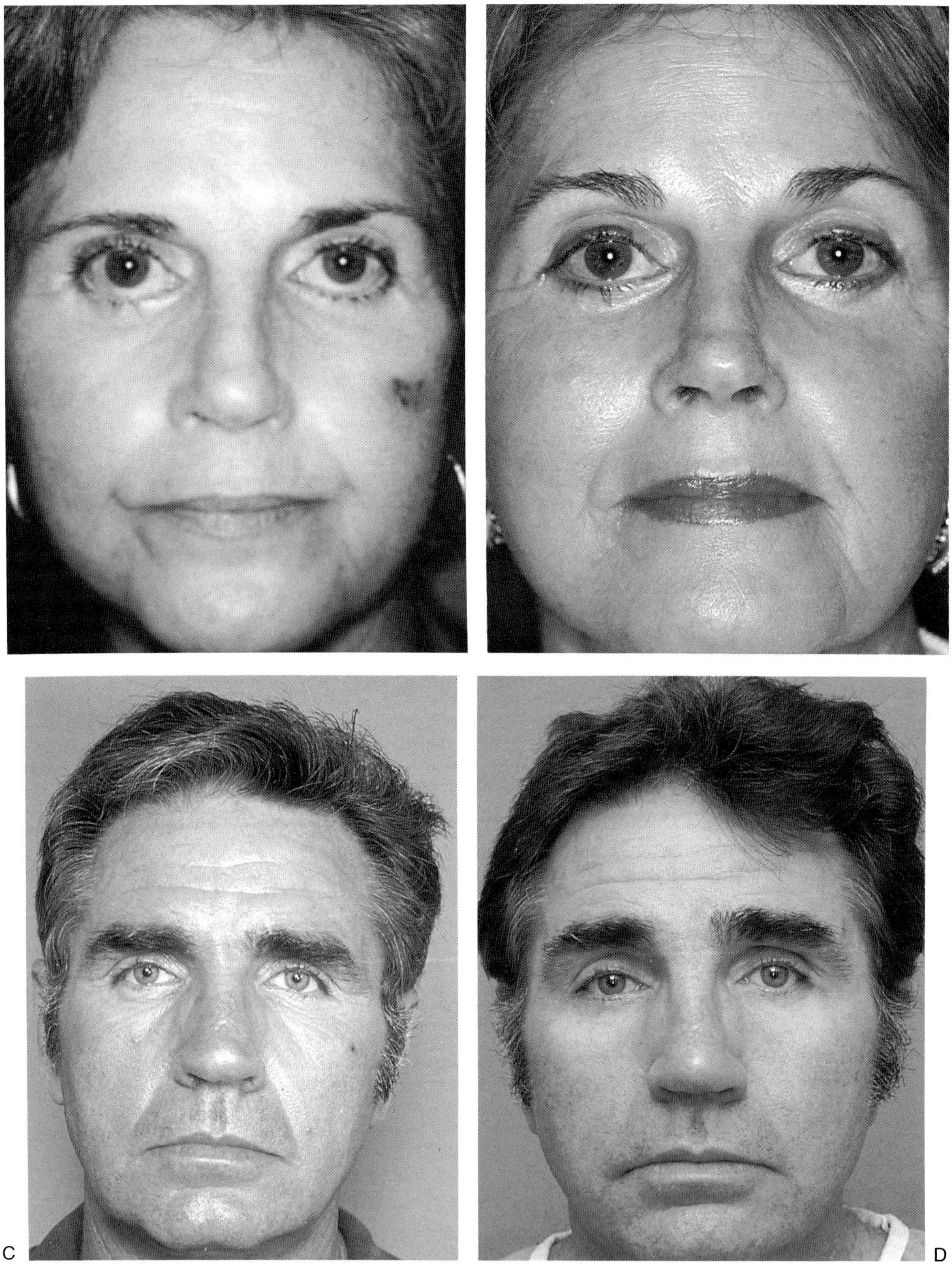

A B C D

FIG. 16. Postoperative results following an endoscopic forehead lift in a female patient before **(A)** and after surgery **(B)**. A male patient with brow ptosis before surgery **(C)** and 6 months after endoscopic forehead lift **(D)**.

marked reduction in facial edema. Furthermore, the surgical correction of the glabellar region with endoscopic procerus and corrugator resection appears excellent when compared to the open approach (15). The ability to adequately mobilize the forehead and lateral orbital region as well as to avoid injury to the frontal branch of the facial nerve is facilitated by the use of the endoscope. The critical aspect of this procedure involves maintaining long-term brow elevation without the removal of a strip of full-thickness scalp. Although early results suggest adequate brow elevation, long-term results remain to be evaluated.

REFERENCES

1. Hunt HL. *Plastic surgery of the head, face, and neck*. Philadelphia: Lea and Febiger; 1926.
2. Gonzalez-Ulloa M. Facial wrinkles: integral elimination. *Plast Reconstr Surg* 1962;29:659.
3. Passot RL. *Chirurgie esthetique pure: techniques et resutats*. Paris: Gaston Doin et Cie; 1930.
4. Gurdin MD, Carlin GA. Aging defects in the male: a regional approach to treatment. In: Master FW, Lewis JR, eds. *Symposium on aesthetic surgery of the face, eyelid, and breast*. St. Louis: CV Mosby; 1972.
5. Passot RL. La chirurgie esthetque des rides du visage. *Presse Med* 1919;27:258.
6. Sokol AB, Sokol TP. Transblepharoplasty brow suspension. *Plast Reconstr Surg* 1982;69:940–944.
7. Liang M, Narayanan K. Endoscopic ablation of the frontalis and corrugator muscles: a clinical study. *Plast Surg Forum* 1992;15: 54.
8. Vasconez LO. Coronal facelift with endoscopic techniques. *Plast Surg Forum* 1992;15:227.
9. Isse NG. Endoscopic facial rejuvenation: endoforehead, the functional lift, case reports. *Aesth Plast Surg* 1994;18:21–29.
10. Eaves EF, Price CI, Bostwick J, Nahai F, Jones G, Carlson GW, Culbertson J. Subcutaneous endoscopic plastic surgery using a retractor-mounted endoscopic system. *Persp Plast Surg* 1993; 7(2):1–27.
11. Stuzin JM, Wagstrom L, Kawamoto HK, Wolfe SA. Anatomy of the frontal branch of the facial nerve: the significance of the temporal fat pad. *Plast Reconstr Surg* 1989;83(2):265 271.
12. Mitz V, Peyronie M. The superficial muscloaponeurotic system in the parotid and cheek area. *Plast Reconstr Surg* 1976;58: 80–88.
13. McCord CD, Tanenbaum M. *Oculoplastic surgery*. New York: Raven Press; 1987.
14. Ellenbogen R. Transcoronal eyebrow lift with concomitant upper blepharoplasty. *Plast Reconstr Surg* 1983;71:490–499.
15. Bostwick J, Eaves FF, Nahai F. *Endoscopic plastic surgery*. St. Louis: Quality Medical Publishing; 1995.

Subject Index